D1683903

Aligner Orthodontics
Diagnostics, Biomechanics, Planning and Treatment

Werner Schupp, Julia Haubrich

Aligner Orthodontics

Diagnostics, Biomechanics, Planning and Treatment

QUINTESSENCE PUBLISHING

London, Berlin, Chicago, Tokyo, Barcelona, Beijing, Bucharest, Istanbul, Milan, Moscow, New Delhi, Paris, Prague, Riyadh, São Paulo, Seoul, Singapore, Warsaw and Zagreb

Contents

	Foreword	VI
	Acknowledgments	VII
	Introduction	VIII
Chapter 1	Diagnostics	1
Chapter 2	Biomechanics of invisalign	25
Chapter 3	Treatment planning and treatment with aligners	31
Chapter 4	Treatment of different malocclusions with aligners	41

Topic 1	Deangulation of the maxillary incisors to remove an existing black triangle	42
Topic 2	Derotation of mandibular canines	46
Topic 3	Lingual tipped premolar, crowding and extrusion	49
Topic 4	Crowding	53
Topic 5	Buccal black corridors	57
Topic 6	Closing unwanted spacing	61
Topic 7	Spacing with periodontitis and bone loss	64
Topic 8	Bone and periodontium: General considerations	67
Topic 9	Missing maxillary lateral incisors	70
Topic 10	Crowding with insufficient space for full eruption of a retained tooth	74
Topic 11	Missing maxillary lateral incisor	80
Topic 12	Spaces with missing teeth	84
Topic 13	Agenesis of six teeth and migration of maxillary canines into spaces	88
Topic 14	Spaces after traumatic tooth loss with migration of neighboring teeth	93
Topic 15	Gummy smile in a young patient	97
Topic 16	Build up a "Speed Up"	102
Topic 17	Anterior open bite	105
Topic 18	Asymmetry of gingival height and crowding	109
Topic 19	When to use interproximal enamel reduction	114
Topic 20	Mandibular crowding: Extraction of a mandibular incisor	119
Topic 21	Bialveolar protrusion: Extraction of a mandibular incisor	122
Topic 22	Crowding in the lower arch with crossbite: Extraction of lower second premolars	125
Topic 23	CMD with unilateral class II relationship: Extraction of a single upper premolar	128
Topic 24	Unilateral class II relationship: Extraction of a unilateral premolar with sectional fixed mechanics followed by Invisalign treatment	134
Topic 25	Bialveolar protrusion: Extraction of four premolars	137
Topic 26	Class II treatment: General considerations	142
Topic 27	Class II with highly erupted upper canines	144
Topic 28	Class II/2 treatment	149

Topic 29	Class II pretreatment with Carrière distalizer in a teenager with all permanent teeth erupted	156
Topic 30	Class II pretreatment with Carrière distalizer in an adult	160
Topic 31	Craniomandibular disorder and class II relationship	164
Topic 32	Class II with open bite	171
Topic 33	Class III relationship and tongue dysfunction	177
Topic 34	Class III relationship treated without surgery	182
Topic 35	Intrusion of a maxillary molar with aligner therapy and miniscrews	186
Topic 36	Intrusion of a maxillary molar with aligner therapy	188
Topic 37	Tipped molars	190
Topic 38	Child with early loss of baby teeth	194
Topic 39	Creation of space for the eruption of a tooth in a young patient	201
Topic 40	Teenager with spaces and agenesis of two teeth	206
Topic 41	Teenager with agenesis of four teeth and an impacted tooth	213
Topic 42	Skeletal class II relationship in a teenager	224
Topic 43	Skeletal class II relationship in a teenager	228
Topic 44	Periodontitis with bone loss, extruded teeth, and spaces	232
Topic 45	CMD and bone loss in a patient with class II/2 relationship	235
Topic 46	Class II relationship treated with alignment before surgery	240
Topic 47	Class III relationship treated with alignment before surgery	244
Topic 48	Craniomandibular dysfunction: General considerations	249
Topic 49	Craniomandibular dysfunction: diagnosis and treatment planning	251
Topic 50	Craniomandibular disorder in a teenager	256
Topic 51	Craniomandibular disorder with pain	265
Topic 52	Craniomandibular disorder with pain treated with the Invisalign system followed by prosthodontics	270
Topic 53	Craniomandibular disorder with headache and cervical spine syndrome	277
Topic 54	Craniomandibular disorder with a crossbite and only partial centric contact on two molars	282
Topic 55	CMD and chronic pain, partial centric contact only on two molars	288
Topic 56	Craniomandibular disorder with partial centric contact on two incisors	295
Topic 57	Craniomandibular disorder with centric contact only on first premolars	302
Topic 58	Craniomandibular disorder with anterior disc displacement	308
Topic 59	Digital workflow in interdisciplinary dentistry	313
Topic 60	Posterior open bite at the end of Invisalign treatment	334
Topic 61	Selective tooth grinding in centric and/or excentric supraocclusions	336
Topic 62	Retention after the Invisalign technique	341
Topic 63	Scanning procedure with the iTero scanner	342

Chapter 5 Advantages of the invisalign system 351

Foreword
Prof R-R Miethke

In 1993, Toni Morrison received the Nobel Prize for literature. Of what relevance is this fact to this textbook? Well, Mrs Morrison once said: "If there's a book you really want to read but it hasn't been written yet, then you must write it." This was, in all likelihood, the motive behind Julia Haubrich and Werner Schupp's work on this textbook given that, in my opinion, it is the only one of its kind.

The authors are experienced orthodontists who work in the same private practice and who began using the Invisalign System shortly after its introduction into Europe. Very soon after this, they became devotees of this novel treatment modality, in which they have gained extensive experience since then.

This textbook opens with a chapter on diagnostics. It is for the reader to decide whether to examine patients to the extent and depth that is described here. One should at least be aware of the complex, interrelated physiology of the human being who exists at the end of every tooth, and be prepared to make individualized and appropriate referrals to other disciplines, which are specialized in muscle or joint problems.

Guest author John Morton has contributed a short chapter on the biomechanics of aligners. This is followed by a broad presentation of all kind of malocclusions, the accompanying symptoms, the rationale behind the selected treatment approaches, and the various outcomes achieved. Each patient is documented with high quality intra- and extraoral photos and radiographs. Every reader stands to benefit from this chapter irrespective of his or her level of experience with the Invisalign System. Impressive as the treatment results are, the authors, in their admirable self-criticism, still point out minor flaws.

The last chapter of the textbook deals with the advantages (and some disadvantages) of the Invisalign System. Its content may help patients and clinicians alike in deciding whether this system is the optimal choice for a particular situation.

This author does not wish to take any more time from the reader who has ahead of him or her a challenging, but worthwhile read. Study the text, read sections of it selectively, or skim through return to it over and over again in the best interest of your patients.

Acknowledgments

This book would not have been possible without the cooperation and understanding of our patients, many friends, colleagues, practice staff and that of our families.

The first idea for this book came from our friend and colleague Kenji Ojima. The Book Aligner Orthodontics was first published in Japan.

This book does not claim to consider the issues within aligner orthodontics as being purely scientific. It is rather supposed to give some assistance for the orthodontic practitioner with the aligner diagnosis, treatment planning, and treatment with aligners. One main focus of this book is the function of the craniomandibular system and the occlusion. The treatment of complex functional disorders, as well as of esthetic deficits, is often only possible in the interdisciplinary concept. This is why we have described in some patients not only the functional pretreatment with removable splints, but also in singular cases the necessary supply with prosthodontics after orthodontic therapy.

All shown treatments were performed with the Invisalign system. In this respect, the book can and should not make any comparisons to other aligner systems. This book ends with the description of the evolution of the Invisalign treatment with the G6 generation. Within the framework of research and development, the attachments are applied to the teeth even before the scanning/taking an impression, in some patients' examples. Since the G6 clinical innovations, it is possible for the clinician to plan the attachments himself in the ClinCheck software, modify, or change position as desired. This and many other developments, including the new aligner material SmartTrack, help in the treatment of our patients. The treatments are improving in detail, they are more accurately predictable, and the treatment time is reduced more and more.

We were particularly pleased to have found co-authors that we were able to convince to support us in this book. In the field of biomechanics in orthodontics, there are few who can so precisely and competently articulate this complex subject as John Morton. He deserves our very special thanks, as well as Mitra Derakshan, Srini Kaza and Bob Boyd, who were significantly involved with the development of the Invisalign technique and still have considerable influence on the evolution of this technology.

We were able to gain Wolfgang Boisserée, with whom we have written the book *Kraniomandibuläres und Muskuloskelettales System (2012)*, to participate with the chapter "Diagnosis," which deliberately focuses on the theme of "function." He has also contributed many documentaries for interdisciplinary dentistry showing the continued restorative treatment after orthodontic treatment.

Dr Kenji Ojima distributed an additional chapter concerning extractions, showing a premolar extraction case.

Our thanks go also to our teachers Ulrike Ehmer, Harold Gelb, Rainer-Reginald Miethke, Robert M. Ricketts, and Douglas Toll.

We would also like to thank Toni Graf-Baumann, Rainer Heller, Stefan Kopp, Gerhard Marx and Peter Zernial, with whom we have developed diagnostic and therapeutic procedures in an interdisciplinary approach, between orthodontics and manual and osteopathic medicine.

We also thank the dental laboratory Läkamp, in particular Manfred Läkamp and Max Mainzer for many innovative ideas and images, most notably with the technique Zirkonzahn (Inventor Enrico Steger).

In addition, we are grateful to Rainer Reginald Miethke, who has not only written a foreword, but also has contributed many suggestions for improvement.

Tommaso Castroflorio and Francesco Garino, we thank you for leaving the excellent "Torque study" article for disposal and sharing new thoughts and ideas concerning aligner treatment with us.

ACKNOWLEDGMENTS

With one exception, all the MRI scans of the TMJ are from the Media Park Clinic, Cologne. For this we thank Dr Andersson, Dr Steimel and colleagues.

We thank all patients and patients' parents, allowing us to treat them or their children. We would like to thank them deeply for the trust that they have given to us.

Most treatments were only possible in a close interdisciplinary team. Our thanks here go to our colleagues Carsten Appel, Margret Bäumer, Wolfgang Boisserée, Frank Bröseler, Elisabeth Janson, Ulrich Joos, Stefan Kopp, Sofia Krings Vogeler, Roland Mansch, Pascal Marquardt, Ulrich Meyer, Ingolf Säckler, Christina Tietmann, and Marit Wendels.

Our sincere thanks go to the entire team of our orthodontic office and laboratory, in particular to Maria Habrecht for her meticulous assistance with the photo documentation and our master technician Mario Klingberg, who have both contributed with their cooperation and support to make this book possible.

Introduction

Every scientific field including medicine, as well as orthodontics, is in continuous development and therefore subject to change. Some orthodontic inventions, as for an example the *Funktionsregler* named after Professor Fränkel, become an integral part of the orthodontic practice, while others cannot fulfill expectations or prove to be too complex and slip back into oblivion.

The movement of teeth using aligners was founded in 1926 by Remensnyder; Kesling popularized this method in 1945 and described it as the "Tooth positioning appliance." Later, Sheridan invented the "Essix Tooth Moving System." Using the Essix technology is quite similar to the conventional fixed appliances, as the therapy can be constantly modified because of the multiple variables that arise during treatment. With the Essix aligners, mild to moderate crowding can be solved.

Align Technology was founded in 1997, being the first company to use the former aligner techniques and combine them with CAD/CAM (computer-aided design/computer-aided manufacture) technology. Advances and innovations in this technology have further improved and enhanced the Invisalign system. The Invisalign system is unique in that the clinician is able to plan the final result and the path of the treatment virtually with the ClinCheck Software, even before the real treatment starts in the patient's mouth. In former days, Invisalign has been described as a successful tool for treating mild to moderate crowding, the closure of naturally occurring spaces, as well as tipping movements. After years of experience with the system, almost all tooth movements (see Chapter 3) can be performed with the Invisalign therapy. The Invisalign system has become established worldwide and counts as being one of the most innovative orthodontic techniques.

As per every orthodontic appliance, no matter if removable or fixed, the Invisalign system, too, needs a high level of education, training, and experience. This book may give to the beginner, as well as to the experienced user, tips and techniques on how to integrate the Invisalign System smoothly and successfully into the orthodontic office.

DIAGNOSTICS 1

1 DIAGNOSTICS

A complete orthodontic diagnosis includes:
- a complete history
- extra- and intraoral findings
- functional diagnostics
- model findings
- radiography findings.

It is important to consider the possibility of potential genetic causes of disorders during history taking. Further attention should be paid to previous disease, actual medications, trauma, habits, breathing patterns, and speech. If patients are experiencing pain, a pain questionnaire allows this to be assessed. This chapter describes the extra- and intraoral findings in an orthodontic context.

Myofunctional diagnosis will require some patients to be referred to a myofunctional therapist, in particular often to "Padovan" therapy for neurologic reorganization (Padovan, 1995). Special attention should be given to the diagnosis of craniomandibular system (CMS) and musculoskeletal system (MSS) disorders, which will be described in more detail in the following, together with diagnosis using modeling and radiography findings. Specialist orthodontic modeling and radiography analysis are also covered in the general literature.

The orthodontic diagnosis sheet part I

A basic record sheet is shown in Fig 1-1.

Goal.   Recording the case history and documenting the biologic and esthetic analysis. In addition, an orthopantomogram should be available at this point.

Action. After taking a general and specific case history, biologic parameters are recorded: dental status; periodontal findings; function; habits.

Fig 1-1 The orthodontic diagnosis sheet part I.

Biologic analysis

Biologic analysis examines the teeth, periodontium, and the position, projection, and characteristics of the lips and cheek ligaments.

Teeth. A record of missing and replaced teeth, untreated dead teeth, carious lesions, recessions, abrasions, all preserving and prosthetic measures, as well as chronic inflammation that will require endodontic measures.

Periodontal parameters. Use of a screening process (e.g. the Periodontal Screening Index) to determine the maintenance state, plaques and concrements, sulcus probing depth, and degrees of mobility.

For all biologic findings it is necessary to refer to the suitable specialty: dentist; periodontist; endodontist; or oral surgeon. These pathologies should be treated prior to starting orthodontic treatment.

Myofunctional analysis

Myofunctional diagnostics identifies potential speech or swallowing dysfunctions, considering whether there are any detrimental habits, if lip closure is competent, or if the patient is a mouth breather. It may be necessary to refer the patient to a myofunctional therapist.

Extra- and intraoral findings: photographic record

Goal. Extraoral and intraoral photographs document the current state. The extraoral photographs are fundamental for esthetic and functional analysis to document the external appearance of the teeth, gums, and the adjoining oral mucosa in regard to facial physiognomy. Furthermore, it is possible to make assessments about facial symmetry. The intraoral photographs document the position and form of the teeth and dental arches, as well as the adjacent soft tissues. The photographs are an important orientation guideline for treatment planning.

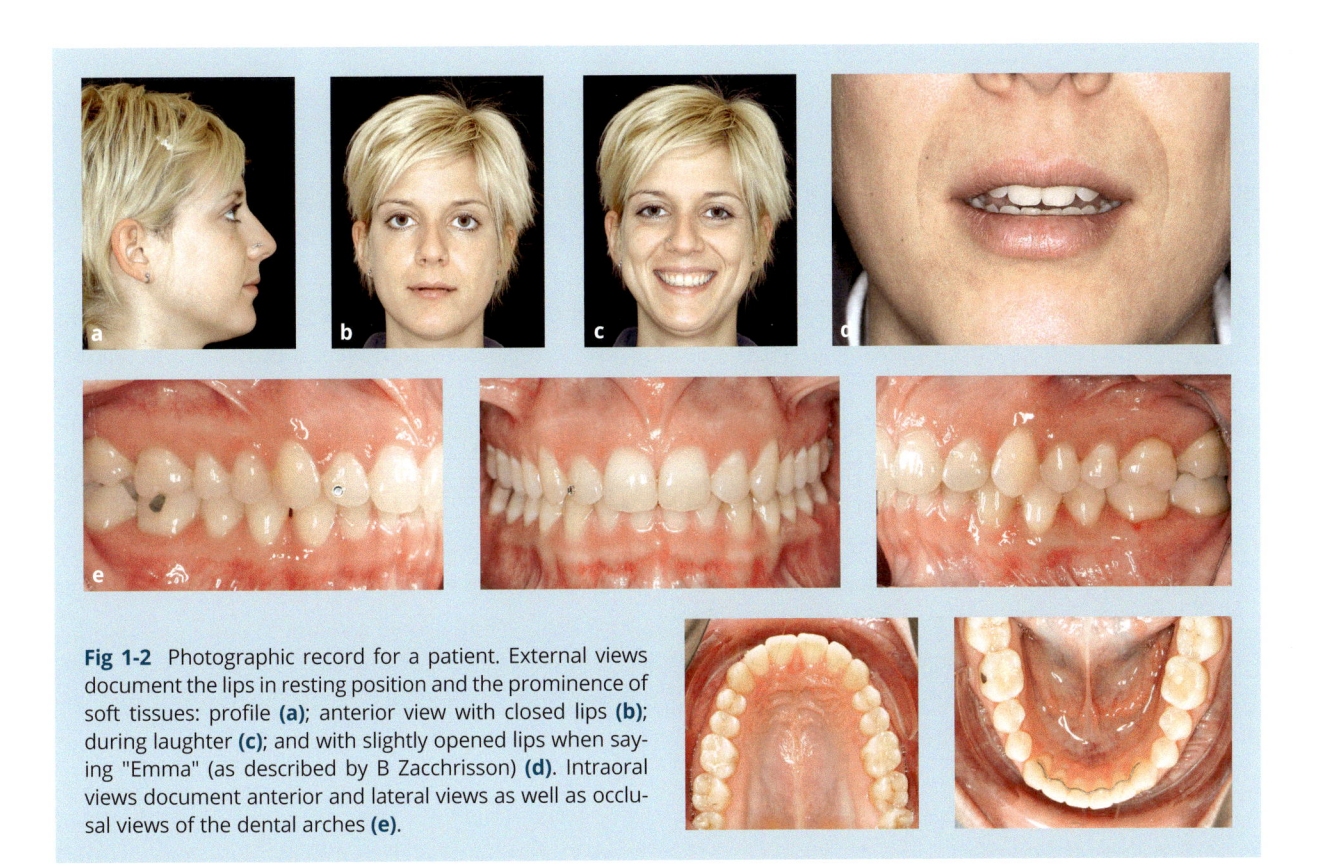

Fig 1-2 Photographic record for a patient. External views document the lips in resting position and the prominence of soft tissues: profile **(a)**; anterior view with closed lips **(b)**; during laughter **(c)**; and with slightly opened lips when saying "Emma" (as described by B Zacchrisson) **(d)**. Intraoral views document anterior and lateral views as well as occlusal views of the dental arches **(e)**.

1 DIAGNOSTICS

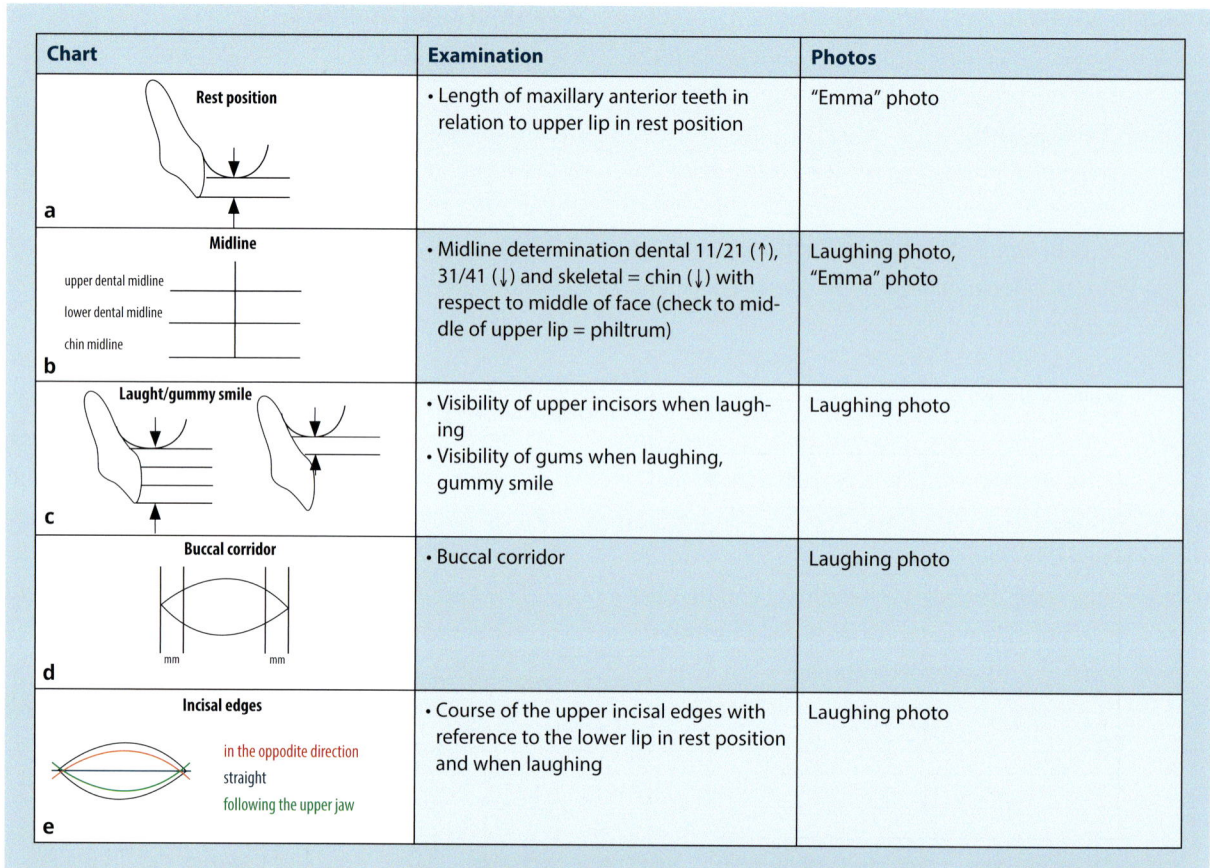

Chart	Examination	Photos
a **Rest position**	• Length of maxillary anterior teeth in relation to upper lip in rest position	"Emma" photo
b **Midline** (upper dental midline, lower dental midline, chin midline)	• Midline determination dental 11/21 (↑), 31/41 (↓) and skeletal = chin (↓) with respect to middle of face (check to middle of upper lip = philtrum)	Laughing photo, "Emma" photo
c **Laught/gummy smile**	• Visibility of upper incisors when laughing • Visibility of gums when laughing, gummy smile	Laughing photo
d **Buccal corridor**	• Buccal corridor	Laughing photo
e **Incisal edges** (in the oppodite direction, straight, following the upper jaw)	• Course of the upper incisal edges with reference to the lower lip in rest position and when laughing	Laughing photo

Fig 1-3 The examination sheet showing the graphics (column 1), the examination parameters (column 2), and the patient's photographs (column 3).

Action. Photographs are taken of the patient in external views to show the lips in resting position and the prominence of the soft tissues (Fig 1-2a to d) and for intraoral views (Fig 1-2e).

Esthetic analysis

Goal. Documentation of the current esthetic state. The results of the examination are entered on the examination form together with the graphics, taking in consideration the photographs and the intra- and extraoral appearance (Fig 1-3). The esthetic analysis forms the basis in planning esthetic aspects of therapy.

Action. The graphics of the examination sheet (column 1) are compared with the examination parameters (column 2), and the patient's photographs (column 3) (Fig 1-3).

The esthetic analysis begins with assessment of the position of the maxillary central incisors in relation to the upper lip (Fig 1-3a), which should ideally show about 2 mm visible tooth in rest position. The relation of the visible tooth surface to the upper lip can be influenced with orthodontic measures.

This is followed by examination of the dental upper midline in relation to the middle of the upper lip (philtrum; Fig 1-3b). A shift of more than 2 mm is detrimental to appearance. The course of the incisor teeth axis should also be evaluated.

The assessment of the gingival margin (Fig 1-3c) is an essential component of the esthetic evaluation. The vertical part of the visible maxillary anterior teeth or the part of the visible gingiva (gummy smile) is evaluated when laughing. The esthetic level is not more than 3 mm of visible gingiva when laughing.

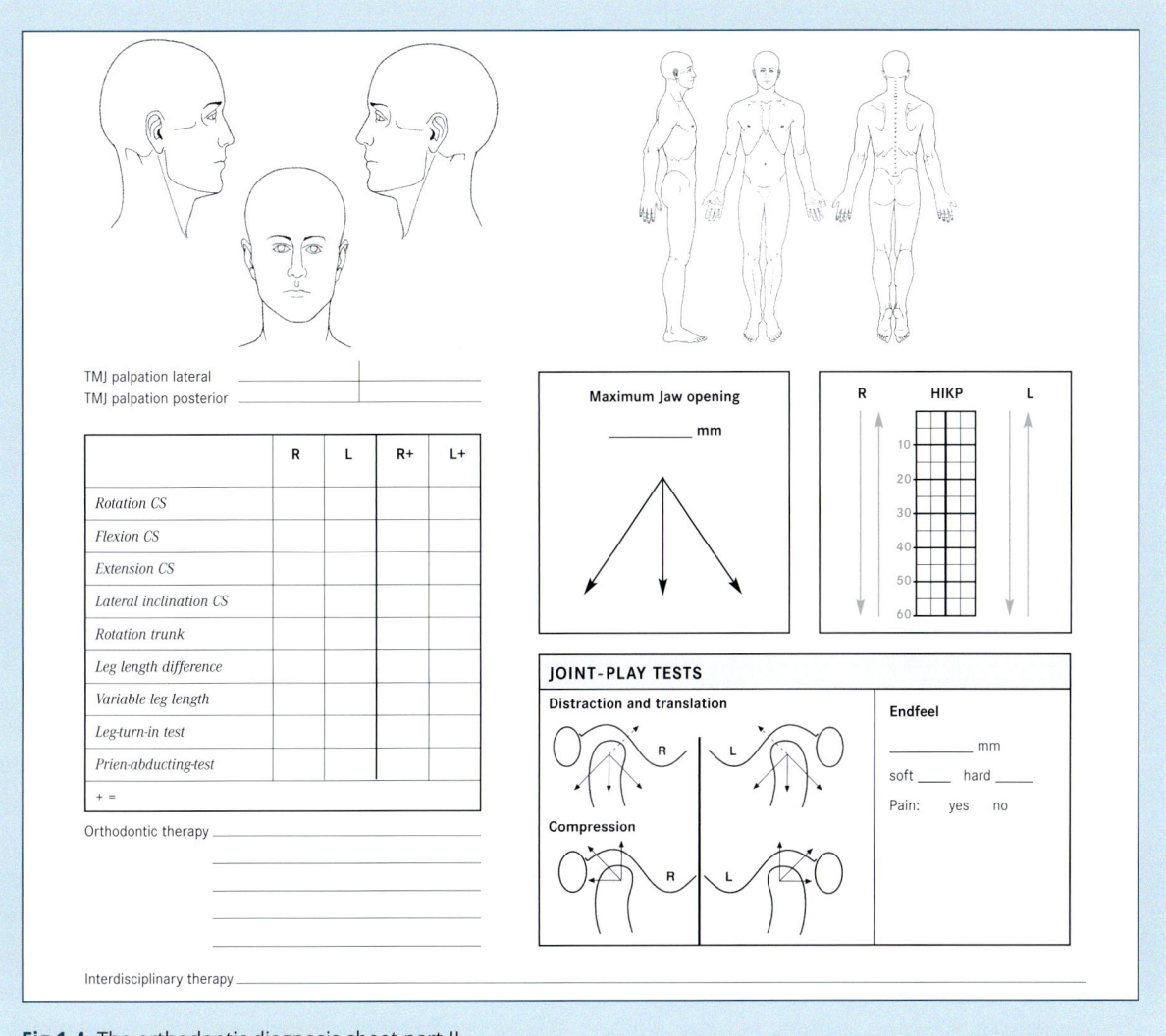

Fig 1-4 The orthodontic diagnosis sheet part II.

An ideal tooth–lip relationship can frequently only be achieved with orthodontic intrusions and extrusions, or periodontal or orthognathic surgical methods.

The mandibular anterior teeth are integrated into the evaluation only after planning of the maxillary teeth has been completed.

The buccal corridor should be completely filled by the dental arches (Fig 1-3d).

Of special significance is the incisal contour of the maxillary teeth relation to the lower lip (Fig 1-3e). Ideally, the course of the maxillary teeth follows the curvature of the lower lip. The straight or opposed course of curvature appears esthetically disadvantageous.

The orthodontic diagnosis sheet part II

The functional examination takes always place at the beginning of the diagnostics.

Goal. *This examination concerns the identification of occlusion disorders that can lead to indicators and symptoms of a craniomandibular dysfunction (CMD).*

Action. *The following sequence is recommended for the functional examination and the results are filled into the chart shown in Fig 1-4.*

1. Document information from the case history

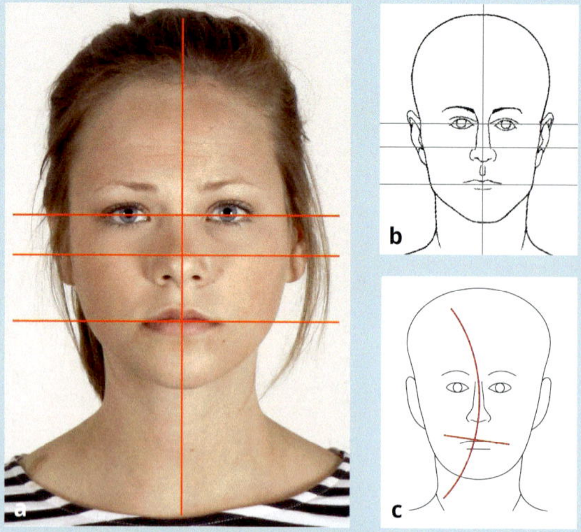

1 DIAGNOSTICS

Fig 1-5 Facial symmetry. **(a,b)** Photograph and drawing of the face to show parallelism. **(c)** Facial scoliosis.

2. Examination of the CMS
   - evaluation of facial symmetry (additionally using the photographic records)
   - palpation of the most important muscles of the CMS: masseter; pterygoideus medialis; and temporalis anterior
   - examination of the TMJ: palpation lateral and posterior; measure path of motion; endfeel test;- joint play test
3. Centric occlusion (occlusion of opposing teeth when the mandible is in centric relation)
   - determination of the centric relation
   - determination of the therapeutic relation
4. Analysis of centric occlusion with an instrumental function examination
5. Supplementary imaging: cone beam computed tomography (CBCT) and magnetic resonance tomography (MRT), based on the findings.

These steps are discussed further below.

1. Case history

Data are drawn into the head and body chart based on the case history:
- facial asymmetries and distinctive features for the body stance
- pain (intensity documented as: X, discomfort, slight pain; XX, significant pain; XXX, strong pain, possibly with radiation) as reported by the patient
- muscle palpation findings.

These issues are then further covered during the examination.

2. Functional examination of the temporomandibular joint

Facial symmetry

Goal. *Facial symmetry is evaluated to determine potential deviations in the positioning of the mandible, which can be caused by the occlusion. In reduced vertical dimensions, even small faults have a serious influence. The mandible shows a shift to the side with the loss of height, leading to TMJ compression on the reduced posterior supported side. Such an occlusal malfunction should be compensated with occlusal therapy.*

Action. *The examiner is positioned symmetrically in front of the patient and examines with the dominant eye.*

Please note that close attention should be paid to the head form and face (Fig 1-5a,b). Attention is paid to the parallelism of eye level, auditory canal level, lip closure line, and occlusion level. The mandible should be centered in the face. The center of chin and the maxilla midline should always be evaluated in relationship to the philtrum, not the tip of the nose, since the nose is frequently asymmetrical. Facial scoliosis based on findings should be drawn into the examination form (Fig 1-5c). The examination sheet shows a left convex face with an inclination of the occlusal plane of a face shortened to the right. The mandible is shifted to the right. The cause can be a loss or absence of vertical dimension on the right side, with potential TMJ compression of the right side.

Musculature

Goal. *Muscle palpation provides information about muscular hyperactivity. This can be caused by occlusal malfunction, which leads to chronic compensatory muscular activity. Typical muscular symptoms are*

DIAGNOSTICS 1

Fig 1-6 Muscle palpation: **(a)** m. masseter; **(b)** m. pterygoideus medialis.

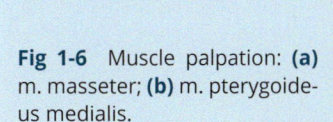

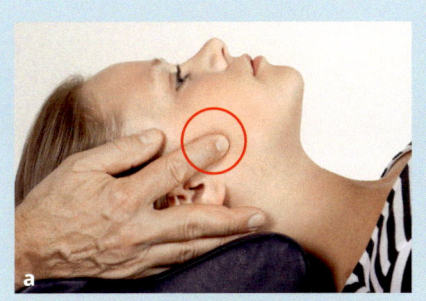

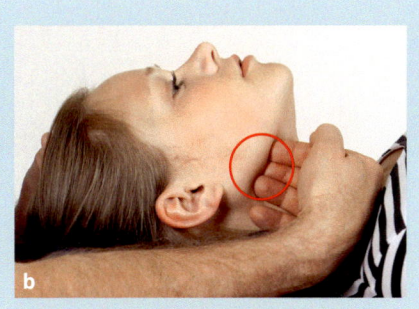

Fig 1-7 Assessment of pain. Trigger points **(a)** and their radiated pain areas **(b)**. This example shows the trigger points of the m. temporalis (x). The radiation zone with pain pattern is shown in red and the radiation zone with less intensive pain pattern is shown in orange.

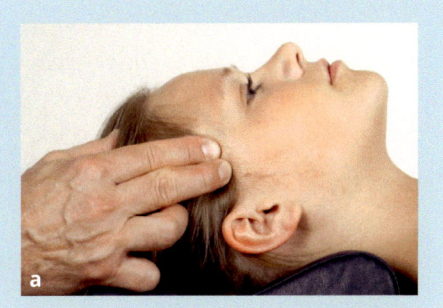

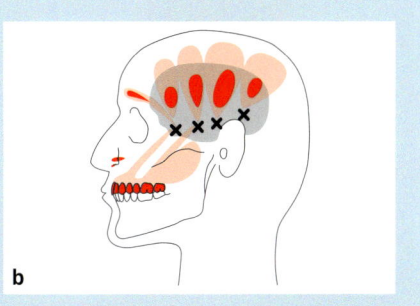

tension, pain, hypertrophies, and trigger points. Palpation provides information on whether muscular hyperactivity is present.

Action. Before palpation, the technique is explained to the patient, who is asked to provide information on the intensity of pain in the individual palpation areas.

Palpation is performed transverse to the fiber direction. The individual muscles are located symmetrically on both sides in sequence and palpated smoothly (Fig 1-6). Palpation needs to be performed with continuous increasing pressure. The pain builds up a little at a time to a pain maximum that should be held constant for about 5 seconds (Fig 1-7).

Muscle size/hypertrophy, palpation pain, and trigger points are evaluated by comparing the sides, since these are indicators of activity (Fig 1-7). The intensity of pain is documented for each muscle and side (X, discomfort/slight pain; XX, significant pain; XXX, strong pain, possibly with radiation). Trigger points and their radiated pain areas are noted based on patient feedback. Trigger points are small, very painful nodules of degenerated and long-standing hyperactive muscle tissue. They lead to myofascial pain. On palpation with the fingertips, they can be detected in compressed, hypertrophied muscle areas as tightly limited zones that are very painful and radiating.

Temporomandibular joint assessment

Goal. Assessment of TMJ function and pathologies.
Action. Lateral and intra-auricular TMJ palpation.

In lateral palpation, the lateral condyle pole immediately anterior of the tragus on both sides is located with the forefinger (Fig 1-8a). From the closed position, the patient successively

- opens and closes the mouth
- protrudes and retrudes the mandible
- moves the jaw to right and left.

Lateral palpation (Fig 1-8a,b) provides information about:

- pain and pain localization, particularly of the articular capsule
- joint noises (clicking, crepitation)
- condyle mobility (simultaneous or time-delayed start of movement, unilateral or bilateral limitations).

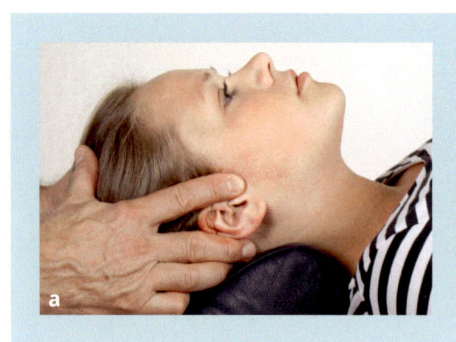

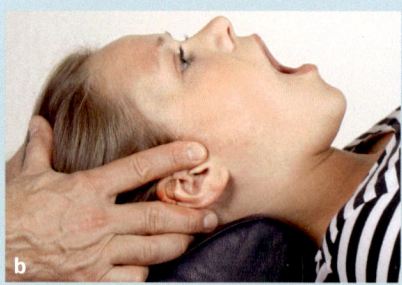

Fig 1-8 The lateral condyle pole immediately anterior of the tragus is located with the forefinger. The examiner assesses the TMJ while the patient moves the jaw.

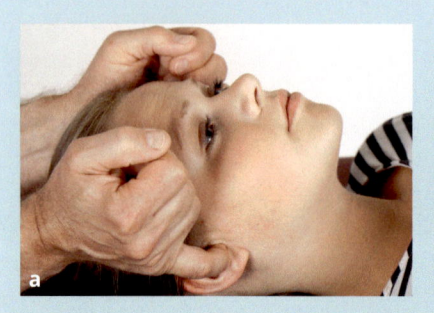

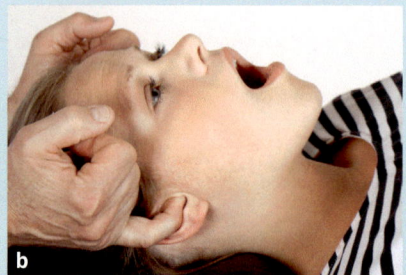

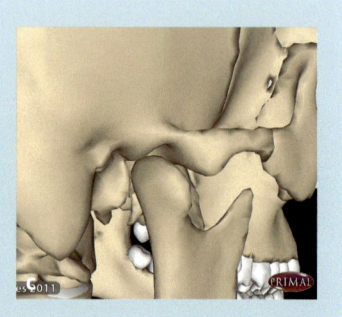

Fig 1-9 Intra-auricular palpation. **(a)** The fingertips of the little fingers are placed in the porus acusticus externus pointing in the direction of the cranial posterior condyle pole. **(b)** The patient performs the movements described for lateral palpation. **(c)** Skeletal relationship.

Intra-auricular palpation is performed bilaterally in the porus acusticus externus with the fingertips of the little fingers. The little fingers point in the direction of the cranial posterior condyle pole. The patient performs the movements described above for lateral palpation. Palpation is carried out with slight local pressure, while pain, movement restrictions, clicking, crepitation, and joint shifts are noted.

Intra-auricular palpation (Fig 1-9a,b) provides information about:
- pain and pain localization, particularly in the bilaminar zone
- inflammation
- joint noises (clicking, crepitation)
- condyle mobility (simultaneous or time-delayed start of movement, unilateral or bilateral limitations)
- anterior/posterior position of the condyle in habitual intercuspation (where the mandible position creates the maximum multipoint contact between mandibular and maxillary teeth).

Mandible mobility

Goal. *After palpation of the TMJs, the mobility of the mandible is examined. This provides additional information about the TMJs and muscle function. The extent of the movements, the path of motion as well as the presence of TMJ noises are examined (Fig 1-10). The endfeel test can provide supplementary information about the origin of pain and restrictions of joint movement. If the origin is more a muscular problem, the endfeel is painful, soft, and more than 4 mm. If the origin is more arthrogenic, the endfeel is hard, blocked, and less than 1 mm.*

Action. *The maximum active opening of the mouth, any shifts in the movement curve on opening and closing, any clicking or rubbing noises are assessed, and an endfeel test is carried out.*

The maximum active opening of the mouth should be at least three fingerbreadths of the patient. The

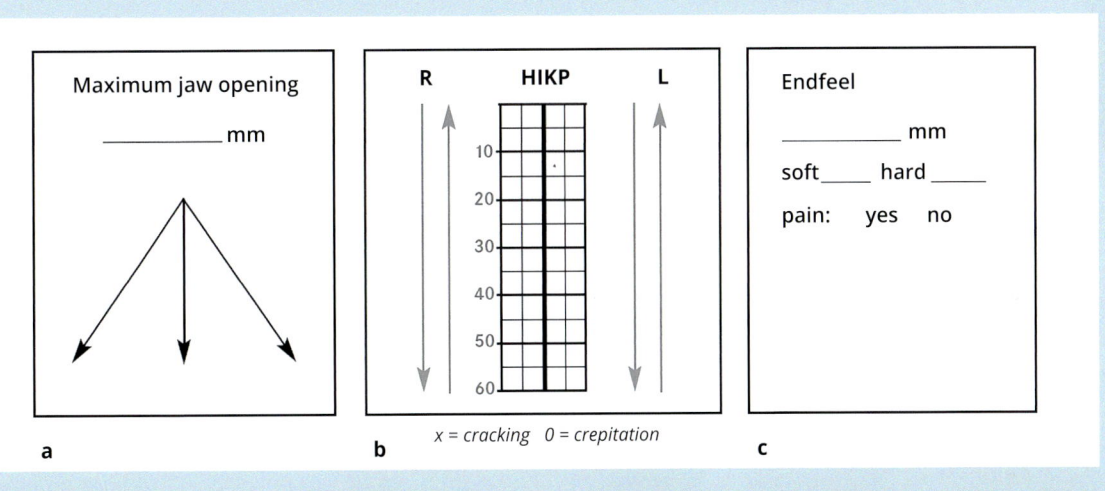

Fig 1-10 Mobility of the mandible. **(a,b)** Maximum active opening of the mouth, which should be at least three fingerbreadths of the patient. The course of the laterotrusion to the right and left, as well as the protrusion is noted. Shifts in the movement curve on opening and closing are noted, along with clicking and rubbing noises and the location of their occurrence. **(c)** The endfeel test is the passive continuation of the active maximum mouth opening by the examiner. HIKP, habitual maximal intercuspation.

course of the laterotrusion to the right and left as well as the protrusion are noted (Fig 1-10a). Shifts in the movement curve on opening and closing can be drawn in; clicking and rubbing noises can likewise be noted at the location of their occurrence (Fig 1-10b).

The endfeel test is the passive continuation of the active maximum mouth opening by the examiner (Fig 1-10c). In the healthy joint, the passive endfeel is about 2 mm and ligamental but not painful. This examination can provide supplementary information about the origin of pain and restrictions of the joint movement. If the origin is more a muscular problem, the endfeel is painful, soft, and more than 4 mm. If the origin is more arthrogenic, the endfeel is hard, blocked, and less than 1 mm.

Joint play in the temporomandibular joints

Goal.   The joint play examination is a supplementary examination in patients with CMD. The term joint play is related to the movements of the synovial joint, which are independent of arbitrary motor behavior and which can also not be triggered by it. They are the basis for the painless and free movement of the joint. These movements are determined by the form of the joint surface. A loss of joint play can be equated with joint dysfunction. Normal arbitrary movements are then restricted and frequently associated with pain. Causes for a joint play restriction can be overloading of the joint surface as a result of a continual shift of the condyle in the TMJ.

Action.   Movement of the synovial joint is examined in distraction and in compression.

The examiner sits laterally and slightly behind the patient and enfolds the mandible with the contralateral hand, while the forefinger on the same side monitors the position of the lateral condyle pole (Fig 1-11a). Joint play is examined in distraction. In traction, the translation leads to a sliding motion of the joint. The quality of sliding motion is more important than the quantity of the movement extent. The feeling should be smooth and elastic and in no case blocked. Barriers to movement can be simultaneously treated by traction and translation. This leads to a loosening of the joint surfaces as well as a tightened articular capsule

1 DIAGNOSTICS

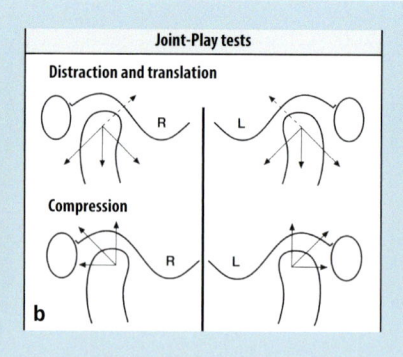

Fig 1-11 Examination of joint play of the TMJs. **(a)** The examiner is seated laterally and slightly behind the patient and enfolds the mandible with the contralateral hand, while the forefinger on the same side monitors the position of the lateral condyle pole. **(b)** The examination sheet.

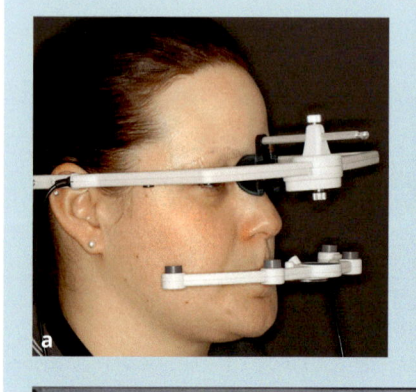

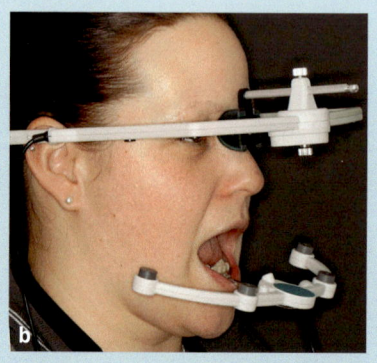

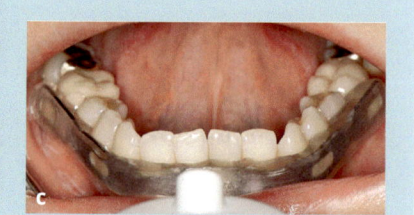

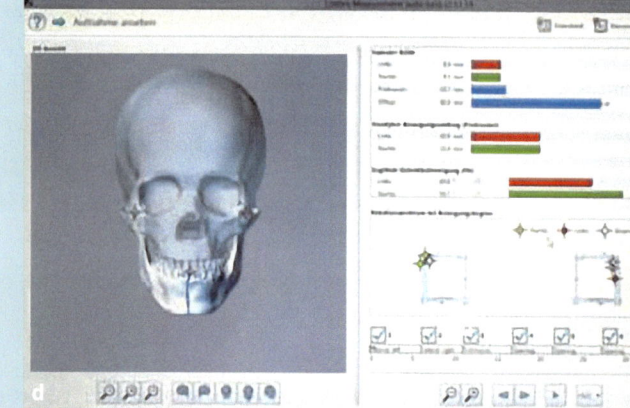

Fig 1-12 The JMA System (Zebris). **(a,b)**. The digital registration system inserted during closure and opening of the mouth. **(c)** Close up of the system fixed on the mandibular arch. **(d)** Zebris software with the collected data.

and its reinforcement ligaments, and to stretching of the shrunken parts of the flexor retinaculum of the hypomobile joint. The starting point of traction treatment is not the physiologic neutral position but rather the endpoint of joint mobility. The next step includes the examination of the joint play in compression in order to localize painful structures that can be attributed to condylar overloading. The location of the painful structures can provide hints about occlusal disorders that are causes for a condylar shift. This is the reason why the condyle assessment needs to be conducted in compression in all directions of movement, anteriorly, posteriorly, laterally, and medially. The findings are noted in the examination sheet (Fig 1-11b).

Functional jaw movement analysis can be performed digitally, for example with digital registration using the JMA System (Zebris) or SAM System. The

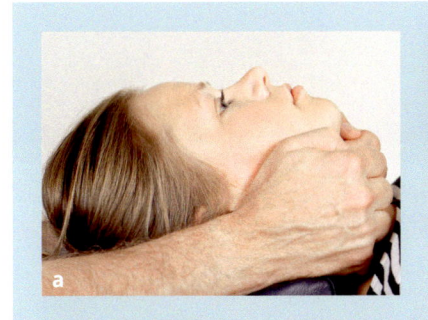

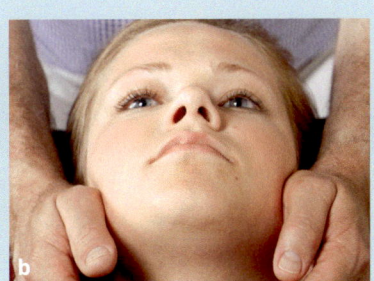

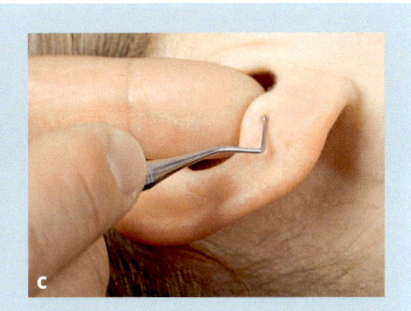

Fig 1-13 Adjustment of the position of the TMJs. **(a,b)** Traction using an osteopathic technique to move the condyle. **(c)** Ear acupuncture showing the needle position used for the temporomandibular joint according to Prof H Gumbiller.

JMA system uses the travel time of ultrasound impulses to assess joint play (Fig 1-12). Simple, rapid, and high-precision measurements are possible with extremely light sensors. A sensor pen, which is included in the system, allows the input of the profile as well as points on the occlusal area. This newly developed system determines the optimum kinematic axis from protrusion and opening movements. Misinterpretations of the functional evaluation of the condyle paths will be minimized and measurement can be monitored in real time. The parameters of functional analysis, in addition to the settings of the fully adjustable articulators, are issued in an automatically produced report. Today it is possible to use this report and, therefore, the obtained data with other software programs, offering the opportunity to extend to various applications, ranging from the recording of myographic data to analysis of functional disturbances of the cervical spine.

3a. Centric occlusion: determination of the centric relation

Every functional (functional diagnostics) and orthodontic diagnosis should occur in centric relation. The orthopedic situation should be assessed prior to orthodontic diagnosis. As Harold Gelb (1994) accurately commented:

> "Think orthopedic first – then teeth!"

Consequently, it is essential first to determine the centric position. The following discusses the preparatory measures needed and the final determination of the "centric bite relation."

Preparatory measures

Goal. To determine the exact jaw relationship and achieve the most physiologic relation, it is necessary first to eliminate as many proprioceptive disorders of the CMS and MSS as possible.

Action. Adjustment of the CMS can be made using
- osteopathic traction of the TMJ
- acupuncture for the CMS
- osteopathic cranial base release for normalizing cervical spine function
- reduction of intercuspation in a malocclusion pattern using an aqualizer.

The following methods can be applied to adjust the CMS:
- traction of the TMJs (Fig 1-13a,b), where an osteopathic technique is used to move the condyle into a physiologic position (see film at www.youtube.com/user/PraxisDrSchupp)
- acupuncture for TMJ dysfunction uses a long-term needle for a total of 10 days in an area of the outer ear (Fig 1-13c) before the determination of centric occlusion
- cranial base release is an osteopathic technique for atlas decompression and is effective for the normal-

1 DIAGNOSTICS

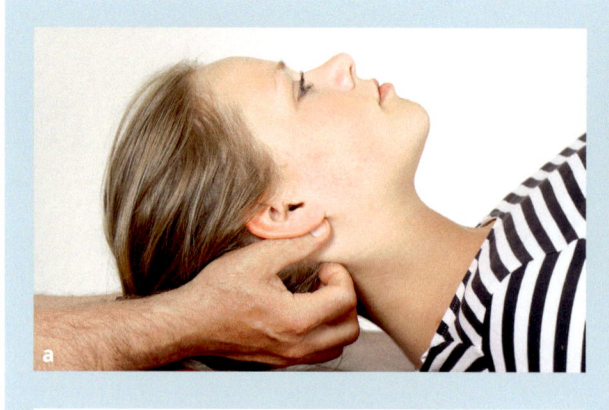

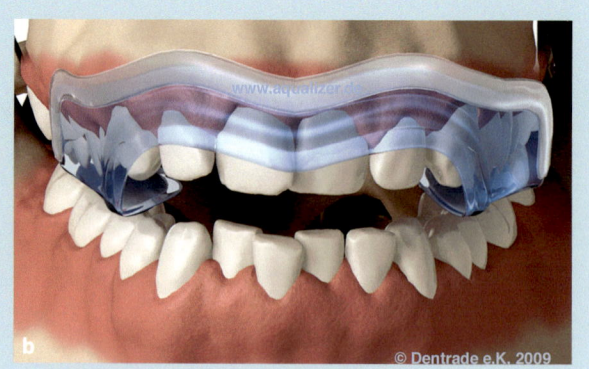

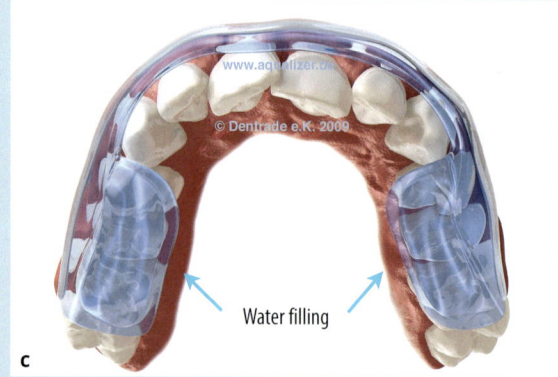

Fig 1-14 Adjustment of the position of the TMJs. **(a)** Osteopathic cranial base release for atlas decompression. **(b,c)** The Aqualizer (Dentrade, Cologne).

ization of cervical spine function and an outstanding supplement for TMJ traction (Fig 1-14a)
- use of an aqualizer, which is a water pad that prevents intercuspation in the existing malocclusion pattern; the pad is worn for several hours, removed, and then centric occlusion is determined before the patient occludes the teeth again.

If a patient has had manual treatment prior to the dental appointment, the patient should wear an aqualizer in order to avoid occlusal contact until centric occlusion can be determined.

Examination of the musculoskeletal system
Goal. To detect with reasonable certainty whether the occlusion has elicited a compensatory reaction in the MSS.
Action. The use of manual tests and changing the proprioception of the TMJs to assess any reactions in the MSS.

The CMS is linked to the MSS. Malfunctions in the CMS can affect the entire MSS and be the initiating cause of an MSS dysfunction. Thus occlusal problems can have effects on the entire MSS, and vice versa.

The most important manual diagnostic tests to demonstrate correlations between the CMS and MSS are:
- rotation of the cervical spine
- flexion of the cervical spine
- extension of the cervical spine
- lateral inclination of the cervical spine
- rotation of the trunk
- leg length difference
- leg-turn-in test
- Prien abduction test.

Figure 1-15 shows the Prien abduction test, introduced in 2000 by Marx. This assesses hip abduction as well as the quality of the joint play during active movement by an evaluation that always compares

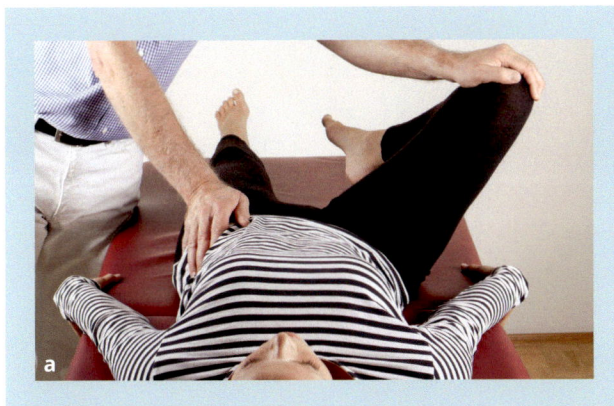

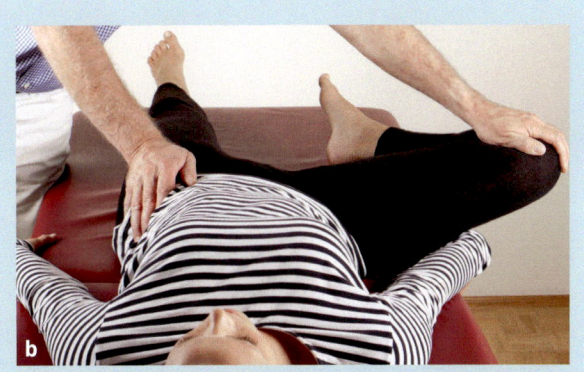

Fig 1-15 The Prien abduction test. The patient's pelvis is fixed on one side by pressing on the spina iliaca anterior superior. The contralateral knee is bent to 90 degrees and then allowed to sink passively into abduction at the hip joint. **(a)** The test with fixed endfeel at maximum occlusion. **(b)** The physiologic endfeel with an occlusal splint in a patient with descending problems.

the two sides. The hip is held in position on one side while the contralateral knee is bent at 90 degrees and then allowed to sink passively into abduction.

Determination of the jaw relationship

Goal. Registration of the (physiologic) centric relation.

Action. The centric relation is measured using a wax plate between the teeth of a relaxed seated patient without any manipulation of the mandible.

The patient sits for the registration process with head posture upright and never extended. The patient determines his or her neuromuscular-guided centric position after preparatory measures (Fig 1-16). The patient should never occlude the teeth between the impressions. To avoid any occlusion, cotton rolls or an aqualizer can be used.

A 3 mm thick Beauty-Pink wax extrahard plate is warmed in a water bath at 52°C, cut out trapezoidally, and adapted to the maxillary teeth. The still soft sheet is cut back circularly up to the dental impressions and then set on the maxillary teeth. The patient bites down on the wax until the mandibular incisors also perforate the wax wafer. The bite registration is cooled in iced water and all impressions of the mandibular teeth are cut back with a sharp knife (e.g. X-Acto No. 5, blade 22) on the underside of the registration, until only traces of the impressions are still recognizable.

Upon trimming the front of the wax, a plateau is established, on which the mandibular incisors can contact at a right angle without being displaced anteriorly or posteriorly, right or left. The wax wafer, which is again cooled, is reinserted and the patient requested to bite onto it. Now the contacts are presented with black occlusion foil on the bottom side of the wax wafer. This is further reduced until only a uniform contact plateau in region 33 to 43 still remains (Fig 1-16c).

Finally, the impressions of the mandibular teeth are outlined with aluminum wax. Aluminum wax sticks, heated with a gas flame, are ideal for this purpose. At first, the warmed and soft wax is thinly applied on the anterior area and the patient is subsequently requested to bite down again after it is inserted. After application of aluminum wax in the posterior teeth area, the patient bites down again to create impressions of all the mandibular teeth (Fig 1-16d).

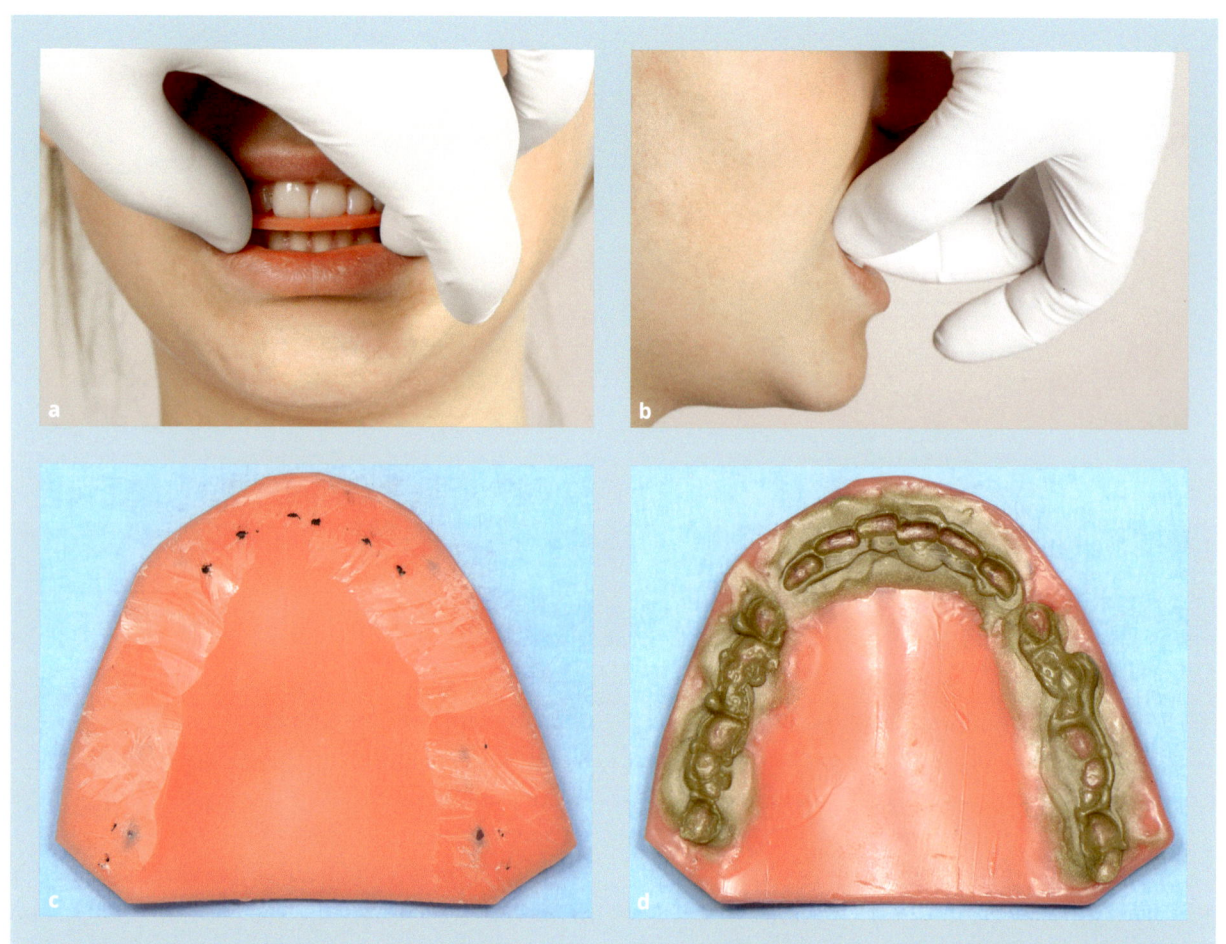

Fig 1-16 Determining the jaw relationship in centric relation. **(a)** The patient should be seated with the head upright and not extended. **(b)** The mandible is not manipulated by the therapist. **(c)** Contacts can be seen with black occlusion foil on the bottom side of the wax wafer. **(d)** Impressions of the mandibular teeth in aluminum wax in the anterior and posterior regions.

3b. Centric occlusion: determination of the therapeutic relation

In patients with pathologic condyle positions, it is necessary to place the condyles in a therapeutic condyle position. Once this has been achieved, the therapeutic construction bite can be taken to show the therapeutic position of the mandible. The therapeutic construction bite is then used to transfer the optimal relationship of the mandibular arch to the maxillary arch into the articulator and the mounted plaster casts. The occlusal splint is fabricated in this therapeutic relation on the mounted plaster casts. The described technique can also be used for the making of functional appliances, such as e.g. the Fraenkel Appliance.

The condyle lies in the mandibular fossa with a relationship distally to the petrotympanic fissure (Fig 1-17). During the examination of the TMJ in the porus acusticus externus, the upper distal part of the condyle is palpated together with the joint capsule. During palpation of a joint, changes of joint width or of the capsule can be assessed and potential malpositions of the joint can be determined. This would include functional response interference (Frisch, 2009).

The three-dimensional graphic of the TMJ in Figure 1-18 shows the physiologic joint position and a posterior condyle position, a diagnostic finding which can often be seen by CBCT.

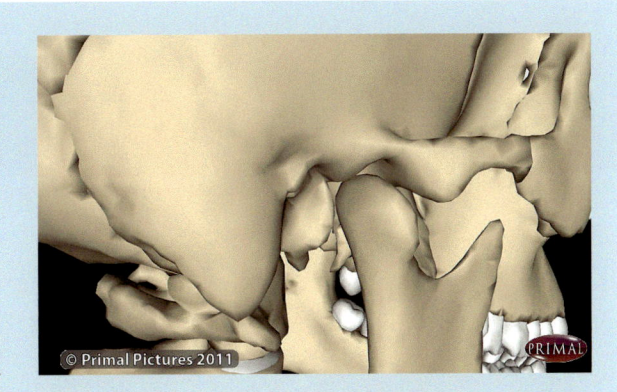

Fig 1-17 Position of the condyle in the mandibular fossa.

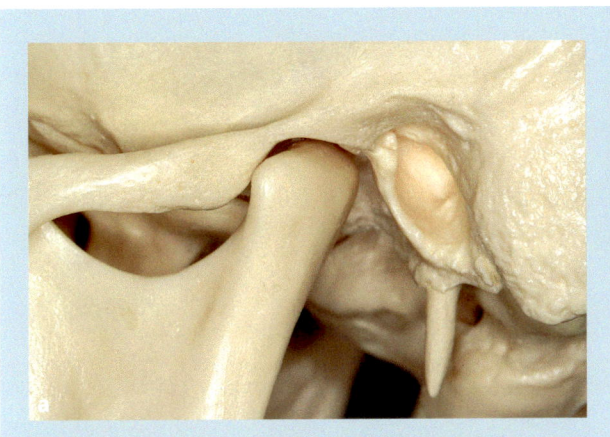

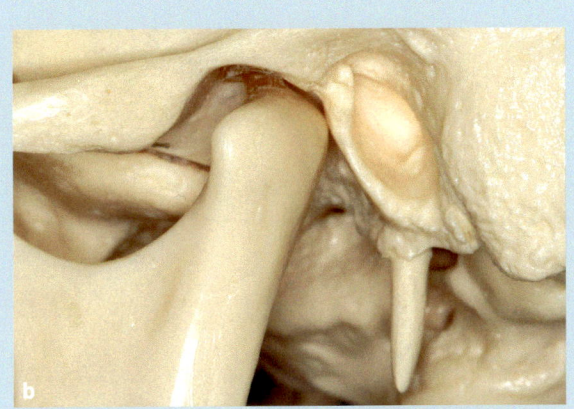

Fig 1-18 TMJ in a physiologic position **(a)** and with a posterior condyle position **(b)**.

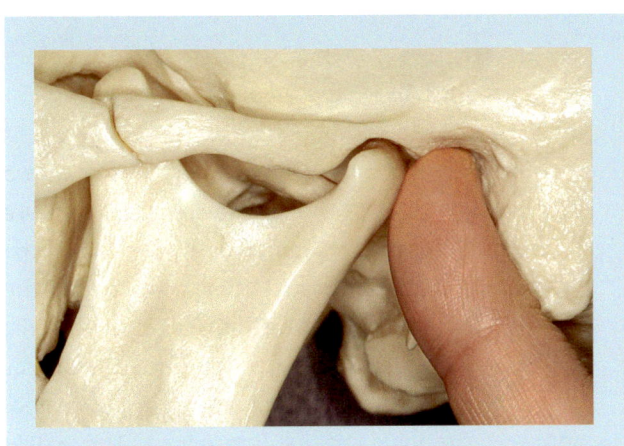

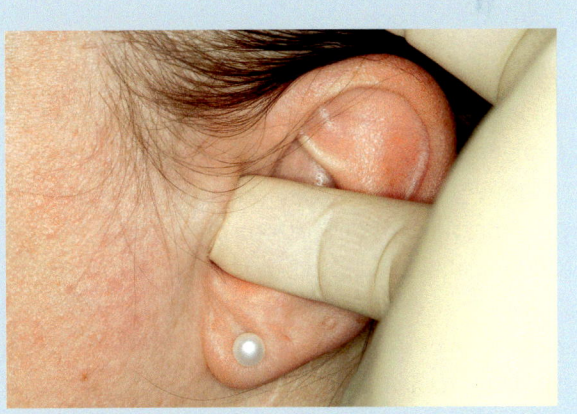

Fig 1-19 Palpation to examine the TMJ is performed bilaterally with the little finger.

Palpation to examine the TMJ is performed bilaterally with the little finger (Fig 1-19). The fingertip is positioned on the posterior part of the joint capsule. During palpation, the patient is asked to open the mouth, to close the mouth, and to protrude the mandible: protrusive movements should be performed while maintaining tooth contact.

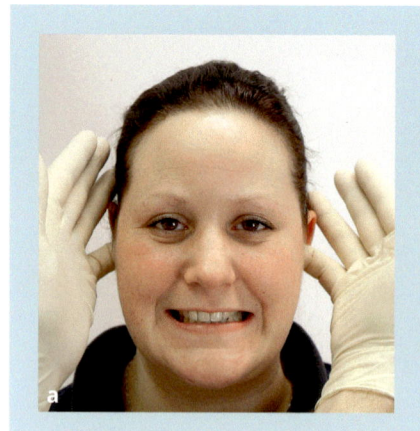

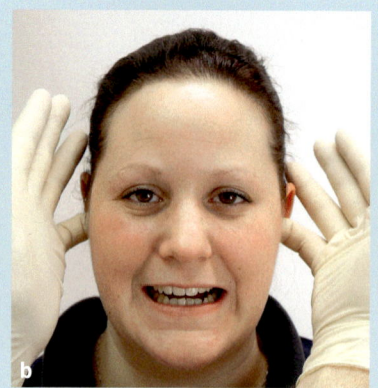

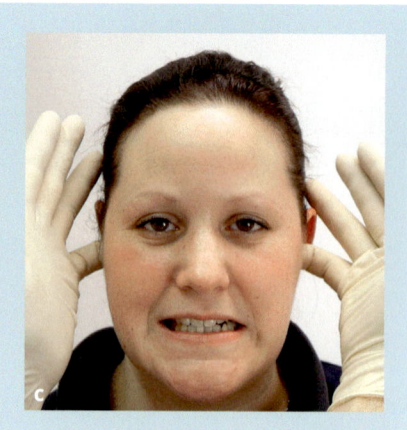

Fig 1-20 Palpation for the therapeutic construction bite. **(a)** Normal maximal intercuspation. **(b)** The mouth is opened a couple of millimeters. **(c)** The mouth is closed again, and from this point the patient moves the mandible forward.

Assessment of the position of the condyles

Palpation for the therapeutic construction bite takes place bilaterally on the upright sitting patient, while the patient is taking his or her normal intercuspation (maximal multipoint contact between mandibular and maxillary teeth; Fig 1-20a). From this position, the patient opens the mouth a couple of millimeters (Fig 1-20b), closes the mouth again, and from this point moves the mandible forward (Fig 1-20c). The protrusive movements need to be performed while keeping the teeth always in contact, without opening the mouth completely again. The movement to the anterior should be performed to a maximum of 2 mm. Palpation during this functional movement gives an idea of the position or malposition of the condyles.

Formation of the therapeutic construction bite

The therapeutic construction bite is created in a series of steps. First a 3-mm thick Beauty-Pink extrahard wax plate is formed on the plaster cast of the maxillary arch. This wax plate covers the molars, premolars, and canines, leaving free only the incisors. The wax plate is formed towards the palate to avoid interference with the tongue (Fig 1-21a).

The wax plate is warmed and softened in a waterbath at 52°C before being positioned on the patient's maxillary teeth. The patient is asked to bite slightly into the wax, in a more retral than anterior position.

There is no manipulation by the therapist. The therapist's finger tips palpate bilaterally the position of the condyles. If there is retral/cranial condyle position during compression, the patient is advised to protrude the mandible slightly to the anterior until palpation demonstrates a physiologic and neutral position of the condyles. Once this physiologic position has been reached, the patient is asked to gently bite onto the soft wax. During the biting too, the position of the condyles, particularly equality of both sides, is controlled by the therapist based on palpation.

The wax plate is then cooled in iced water before being set into the patient's mouth for testing. To obtain neurologic reorganization, the patient is advised to swallow several times and take a couple of steps. After this, the manual medical testing takes place (Fig 1-21c). If there is descending dysfunction, the endfeel should be more physiologic than without the therapeutic bite (Boisserée and Schupp, 2012).

The accuracy of the wax plate is more than sufficient to mount the plaster casts in an average movement articulator, which is used to produce the removable or the fixed occlusal splints (Fig 1-21d,e). For the making of functional orthopedic appliances, such as the Bionator or Fraenkel, the plaster casts can be mounted with the therapeutic construction bite in a split fixator without additional mounting procedures.

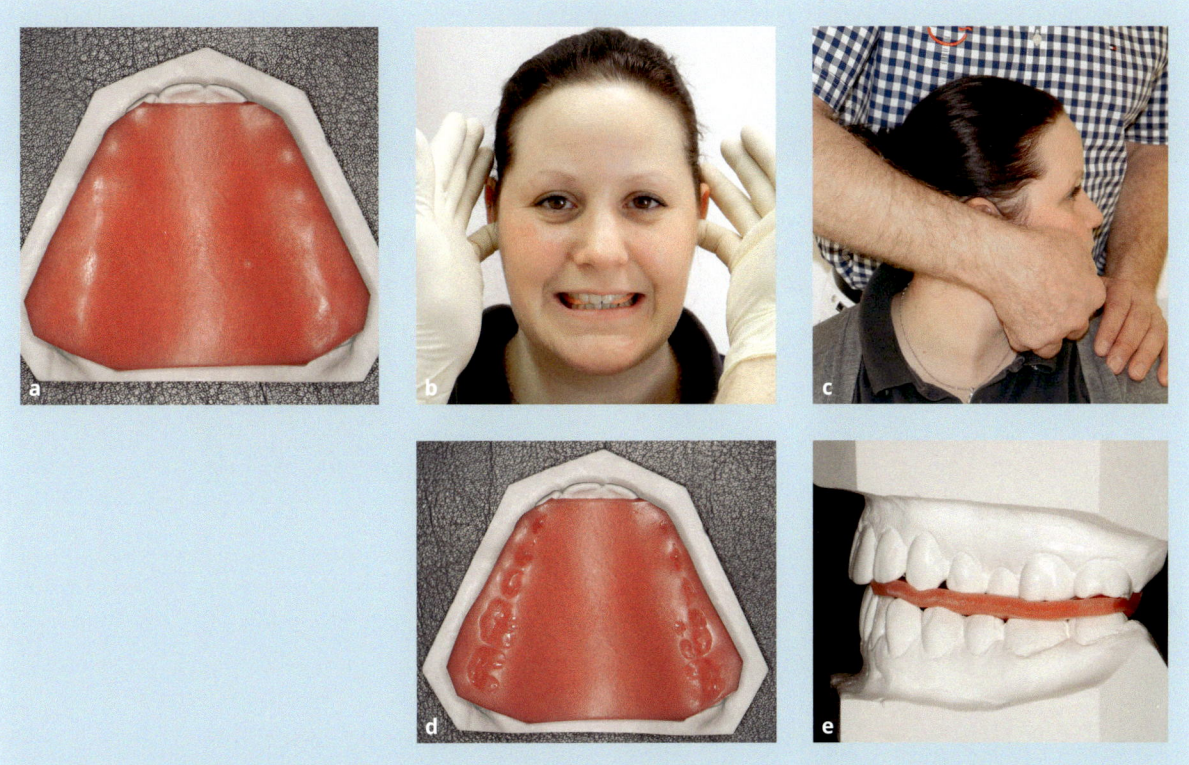

Fig 1-21 Creation of the therapeutic construction bite. **(a)** The hard wax plate is formed on the plaster cast of the maxilla to cover the molars, premolars, and canines, leaving the incisors free. **(b)** The patient bites into the softened wax to create an impression, with the position of the condyles assessed by the therapist, who instructs the patient to adjust the jaw to maintain a physiologic and neutral position of the condyles. **(c)** Testing of joint play in rotation of the upper spine to the left with the therapeutic bite in situ. **(d, e)** The wax plate is used to mount the plaster casts in an average movement articulator in order to produce the removable or fixed occlusal splints.

Mounting the plaster casts
Mounting of the casts allows diagnosis with the bite in centric or therapeutic relation. The following describes mounting in a SAM articulator.

4. Model diagnostics: arbitrary facebow transfer

Goal. To transfer exactly the relationship between the maxillary teeth and the patient's head across to the maxillary cast so it is mounted on the articulator in the correct anatomic position. The mounted casts are the basis for simulating the static and dynamic occlusion in the articulator.

Action. A facebow transfer is used to establish the exact relationship between the maxillary teeth and the horizontal reference plane, so that the maxillary cast is mounted correctly on the articulator.

The arbitrary facebow is symmetrically applied to the patient's face. The ear plugs should sit in the same way in the two auditory canals (Fig 1-22a). For the assembly of the maxillary cast, the transfer fork should be supported in the articulator with a telescopic transfer fork support (Fig 1-22b) in order for the cast to be mounted in the correct position. There must be no downward bending of the fork under the

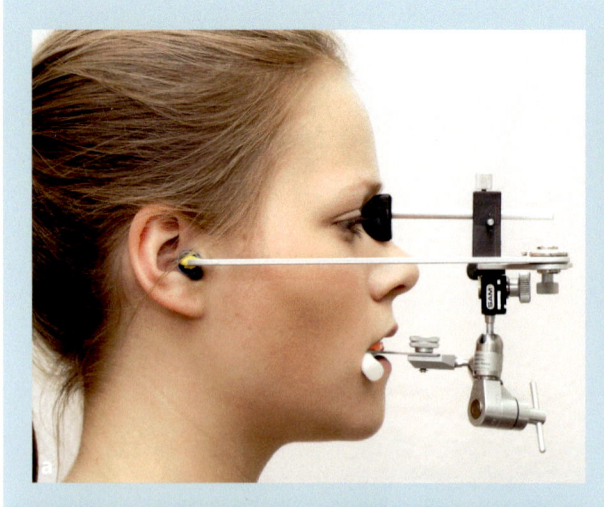

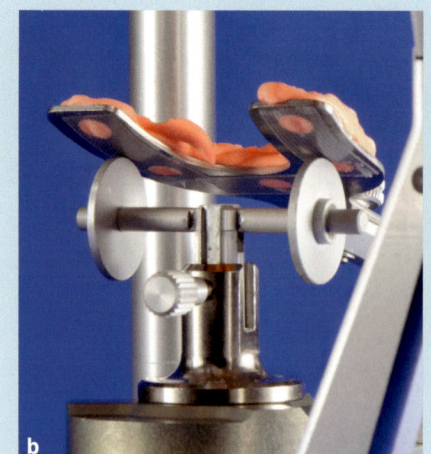

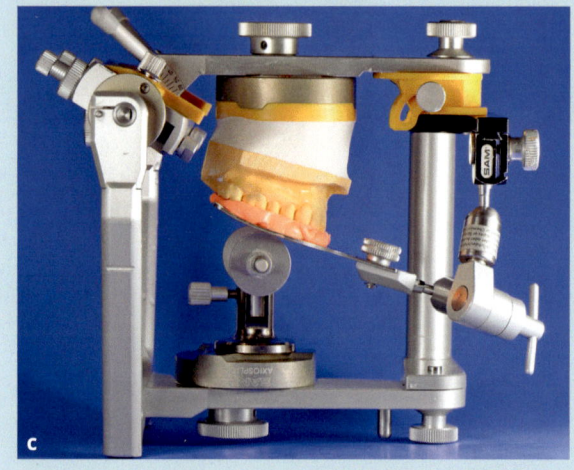

Fig 1-22 Use of the arbitrary facebow to adjust the maxillary cast mounted in the articulator. **(a)** The ear plugs should sit on both sides in the auditory canals. **(b)** The transfer fork should be supported in the articulator with a telescopic transfer fork support. **(c)** It is important to assure the transfer without any downward bending of the fork under the weight of the cast.

weight of the cast, which would prevent exact positioning of the cast (Fig 1-22c).

Mounting the casts with centric bite
Goal.   Cast diagnostics depend on precise fixation of the maxillary and mandibular casts with the tested centric bite in the articulator.
Action. The aluminum wax impressions of the mandibular arch are used to check the centric bite registration for a swing-free position on the plaster cast. The casts need to be fixed in the articulator with the centric bite before assembly of the casts. Once this is achieved, the maxillary and mandibular casts are securely fixed together.

The aluminum wax impressions of the mandibular arch are slightly reduced to avoid excessive material (Fig 1-23a). The centric bite registration is checked for a swing-free position on the plaster cast (Fig 1-23b). The casts are securely oriented based on the centric bite (Fig 1-23c) and held together using wire pins on each side (Fig 1-23d). The embedding of the casts using the centric record prevents errors in cast assignment during the articulator assembly.

Mandible cast assembly
Goal.   To ensure the correctness of the mandibular cast assembly, which is a prerequisite for cast analysis, particularly in prothetics.

DIAGNOSTICS 1

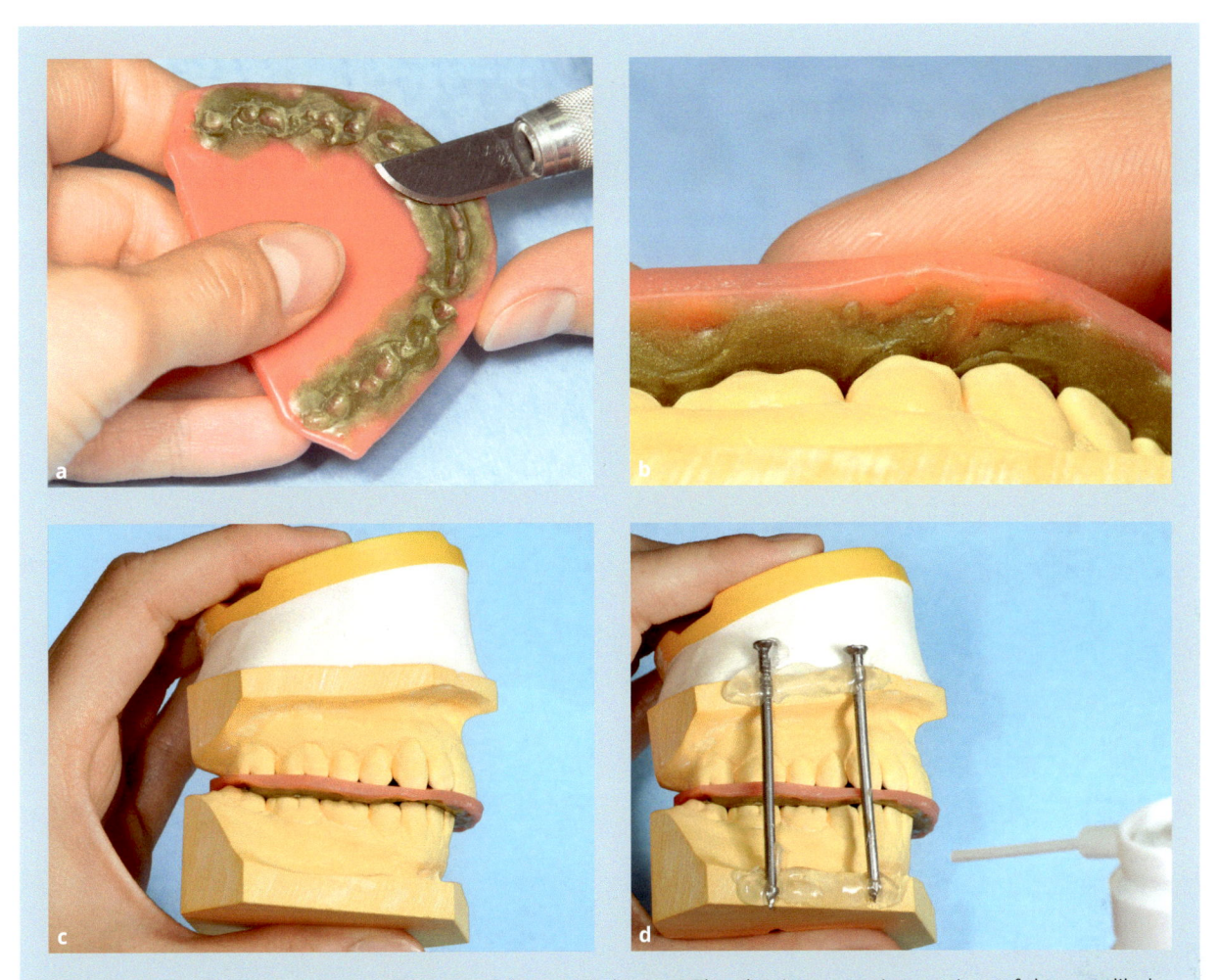

Fig 1-23 Mounting the casts with alignment of the centric bite. **(a)** The aluminum wax impressions of the mandibular arch are slightly reduced to avoid excessive material. **(b)** The centric bite registration is checked for a swing-free position on the plaster cast. **(c)**. The casts are securely orientated based on the centric bite. **(d)** Casts are held together using two wire pins on each side fixed using a glue gun. The cooling procedure can be accelerated with cold spray.

Action. Mandibular cast assembly in the articulator is ensured by a detailed split-cast inspection.

The mounted casts are placed in the upper part of the articulator and the assembly completed with plaster. For the split-cast inspection, the magnet is removed from the metal plate and the split-cast is checked to see if it closes precisely (Fig 1-24). If it does not, the cast can be reassembled until it is correct.

Functional occlusal analysis

Goal. To assess static and dynamic occlusion disorders by examining static occlusion in centric jaw relationship.

Action. Centric contacts and dynamic occlusion are checked:

- centric contacts are identified with Shimstock foil and marked for documentation, after the incisal pin has been opened and the upper part of the articulator lowered to the first contact

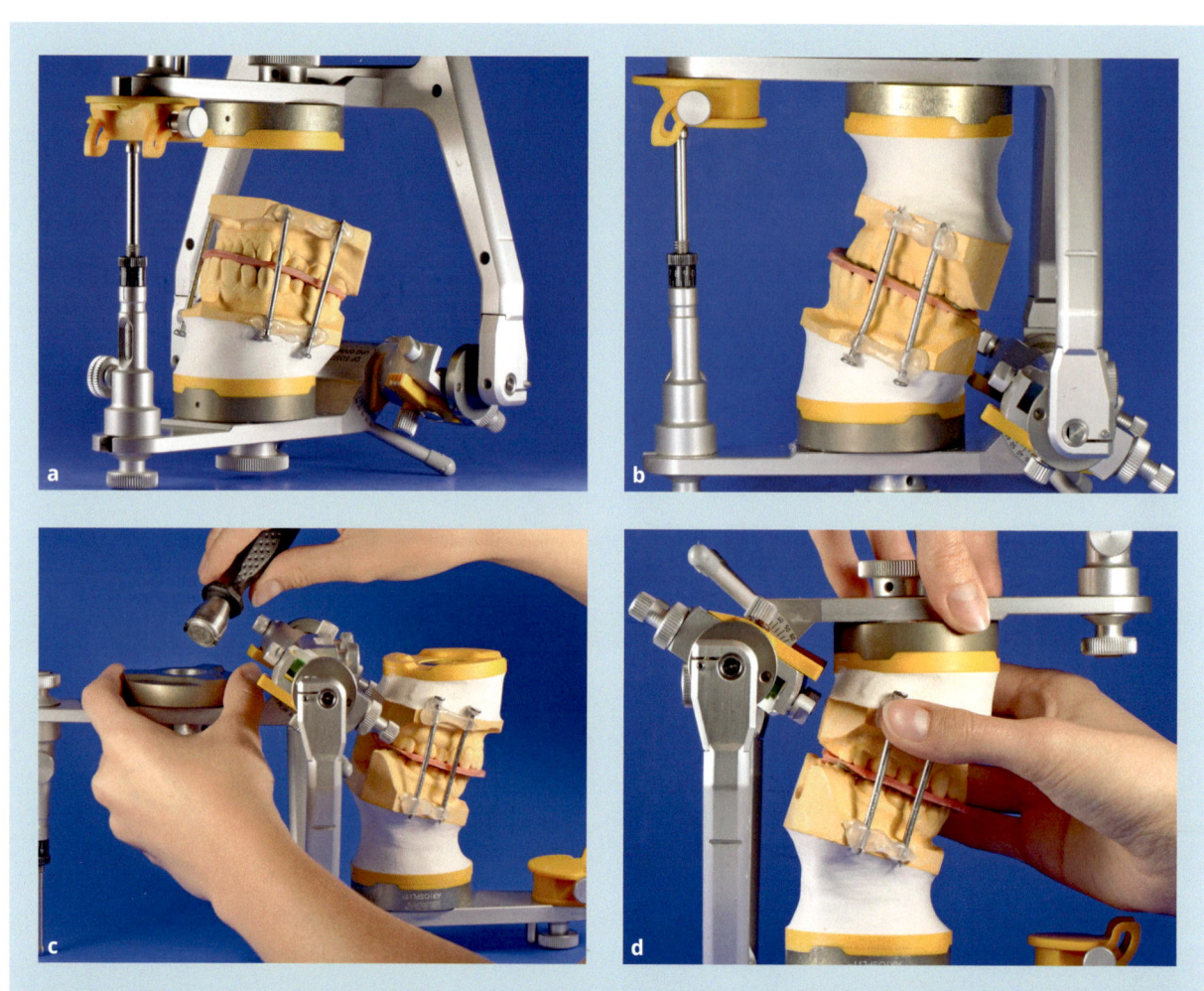

Fig 1-24 Mandible cast assembly. **(a,b)** The mounted casts are placed in the upper part of the articulator and the assembly completed with plaster. **(c,d)** The magnet is removed from the metal plate **(c)** and the split-cast is checked to see if it closes precisely **(d)**.

- *dynamic occlusion is assessed by checking the protrusion and laterotrusion to find the type of occlusal guidance.*

The centric cast assembly is also the starting position for the manufacturing of a therapeutic splint.

Static occlusion in centric jaw relationship is indicated by the position of the first contacts (centric precontacts; Fig 1-25a). This indicates the direction and amount of the mandibular shift from centric relation to its habitual centric occlusion.

Figure 1-26 shows analysis of static and dynamic occlusion in a patient with CMD. After centric cast assembly, static occlusion shows deviation from physiologic occlusion with no uniform and simultaneous contacts on all posterior teeth. Centric occlusion shows reduced initial contact exclusively on the last molars (black markings in Fig 1-28a). In dynamic occlusion, guidance differs from a physiologic canine or a unilateral guidance. The blue markings in Figure 1-28b show a bilateral balanced occlusion.

These findings of variation in static and dynamic occlusion can be the trigger for bruxism and this might be the reason for the pronounced abrasions of the second molars shown in the casts in Figure 1-26.

DIAGNOSTICS 1

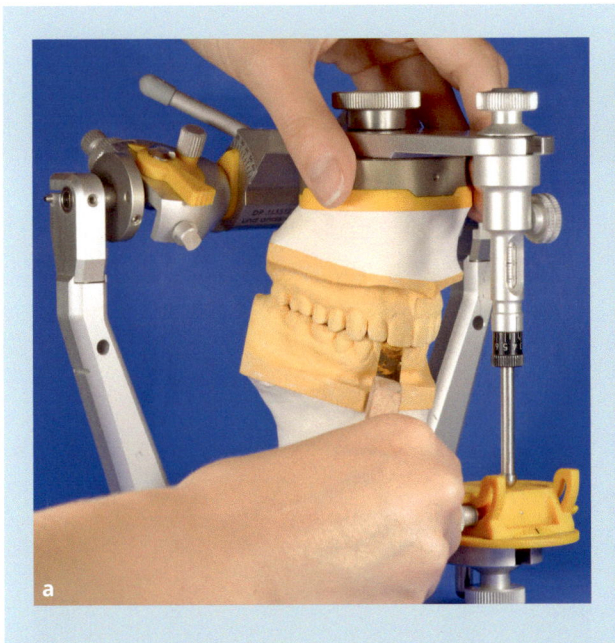

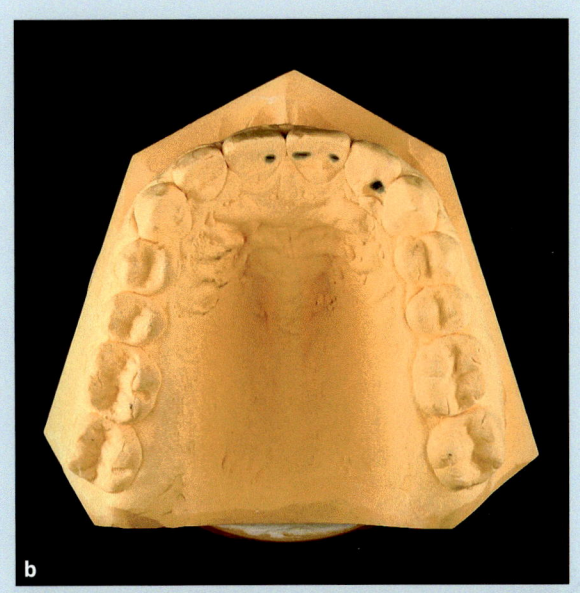

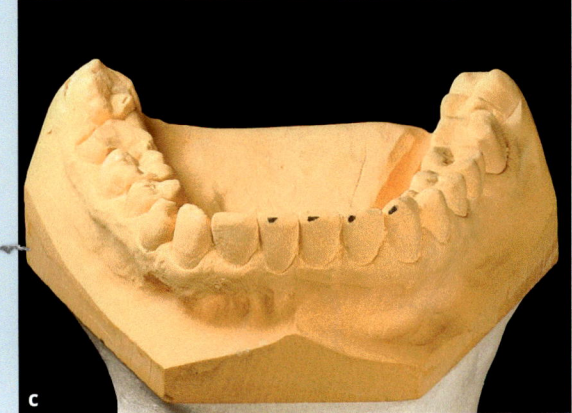

Fig 1-25 Functional occlusal analysis. **(a)** Examination of the position of the first contacts (centric precontacts) indicates the direction and amount of the mandibular shift from centric relation to habitual centric occlusion. **(b, c)** This example shows the centric contacts exclusively in the front, which leads to a high probability that in maximum occlusion the mandible will shift into a posterior and cranial direction, leading to compression of the bilaminar zone by the dorsal condyle position in the fossa.

5. Supplementary imaging

Cone beam computed tomography (CBCT)
Goal. In addition to manual and instrumental findings, CBCT can be an important diagnostic supplement for assessing bone structures and position of the condyle.
Action. CBCT can be used for the following indications:
- determination of condyle position in all dimensions (error is <0.15 mm)
- changes in the condylar shape
- arthritis, arthrosis
- erosions
- cysts
- trauma
- tumor (rare).

Figure 1-27 shows a normally positioned condyle as seen with CBCT. The cortical lining of the fossa is without any discontinuity. The condyle shows physiologic shape.

Magnetic resonance tomography (MRT)
Goal. MRT is the gold standard for the imaging of soft tissues, in particular for the discus articularis.
Action. Indications for use of MRT of the TMJs include:

21

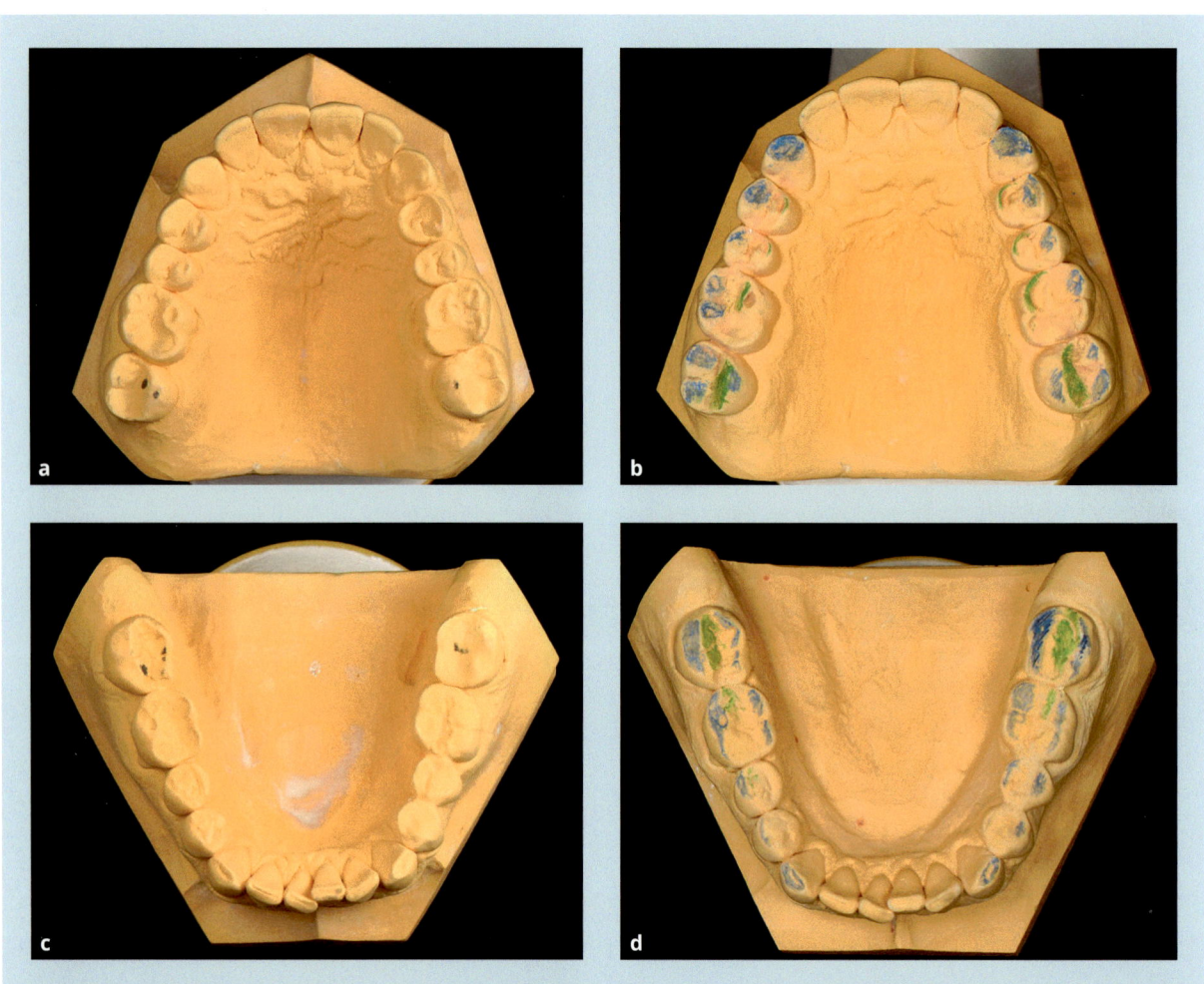

Fig 1-26 Analysis of occlusion after centric cast assembly. **(a,c)** Static occlusion with no uniform and simultaneous contacts on all posterior teeth, indicating deviation from physiologic occlusion. There is reduced initial contact exclusively on the last molars (black markings). **(b,d)** In dynamic occlusion, there is bilateral balanced occlusion (blue markings) but guidance differs from a physiologic canine or a unilateral guidance.

- position and shape of the condyle and the disc
- bilaminar zone inflammation
- arthritis
- cysts
- trauma
- tumor (rare).

Figure 1-28 shows MRT of a TMJ in normal physiologic occlusion and in joints with shifts in the discus articularis and condyle position.

References

Boisserée W, Schupp W. Kraniomandibuläres und muskuloskelettales System. Berlin: Quintessenz, 2012.

Frisch H. Programmierte Untersuchung des Bewegungsapparates. Berlin: Springer, 2009.

Gelb H (ed.). New Concepts in Craniomandibular and Chronic Pain Management. St. Louis, MO: Mosby-Wolfe, 1994.

Marx G. Über die Zusammenarbeit mit der Kieferorthopädie und Zahnheilkunde in der manuellen Medizin. Man Med 2000;38:342–345.

Padovan BA. Neurofunctional reorganization in myo-osteo-dentofacial disorders: complementary roles of orthodontics, speech and myofunctional therapy. Int J Orofacial Myol 1995;21:33–40.

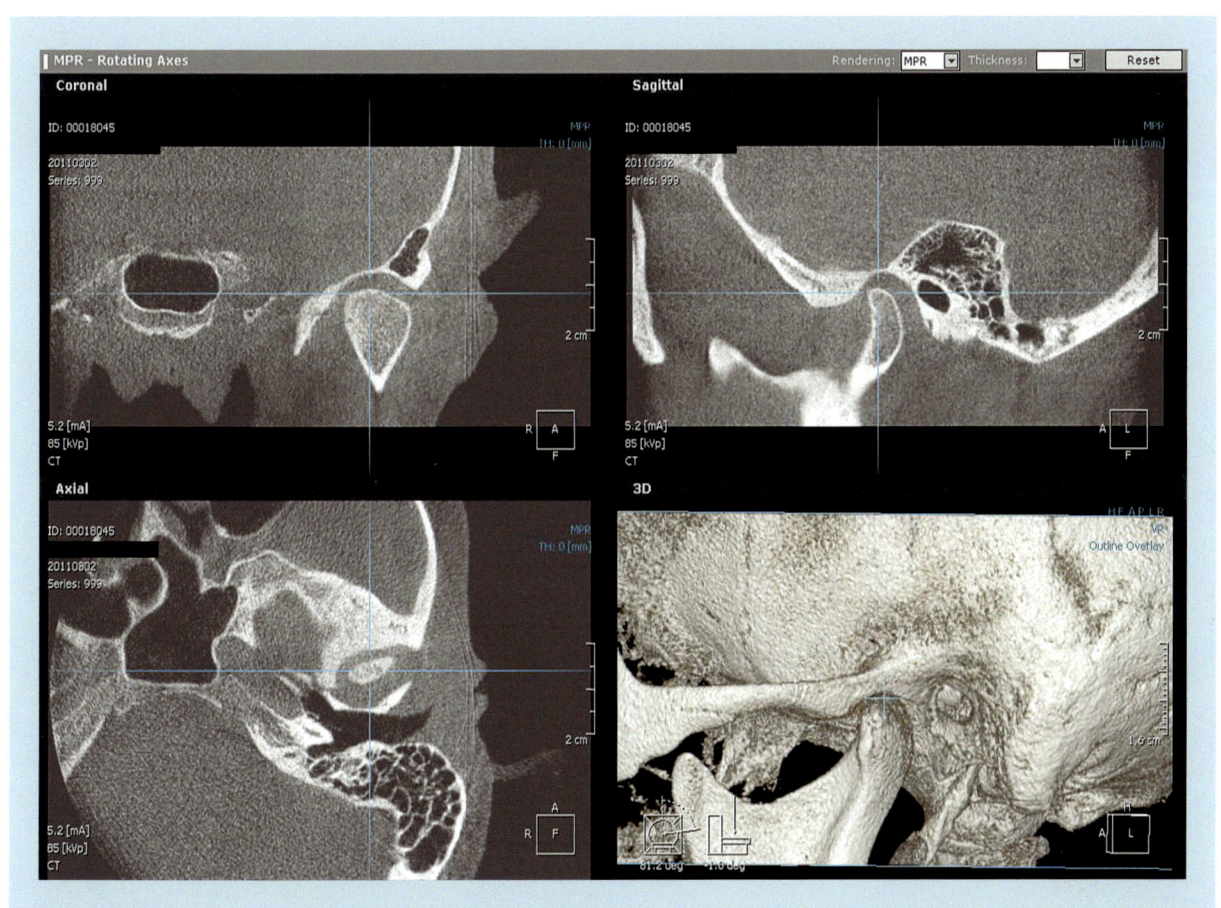

Fig 1-27 CBCT with a normally positioned condyle in all dimensions. (CBCT performed with Picasso Trio, Orange Dental.)

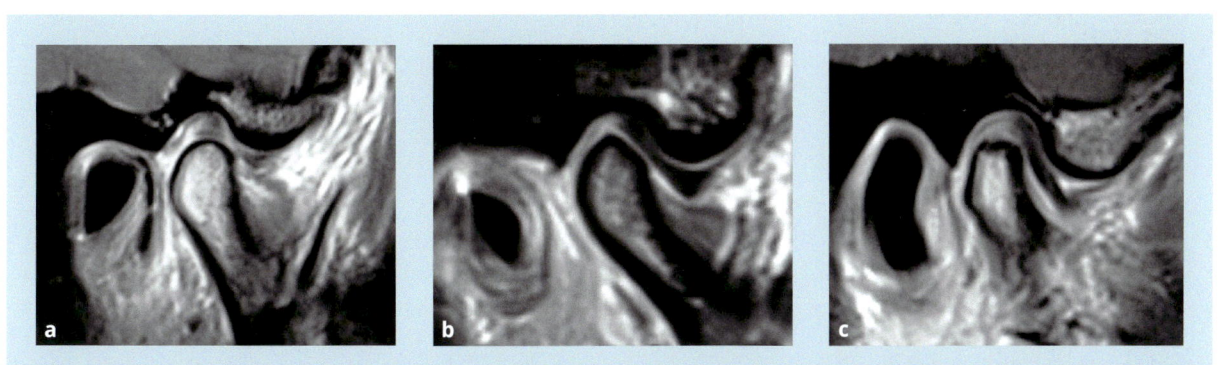

Fig 1-28 Magnetic resonance tomography. **(a)** A physiologic TMJ in habitual occlusion. The condyle is in a well-centered position, without cranial or retral shift. The discus articularis is in the correct position and and has physiologic shape with the pronounced double-concave structure. The condyle shows no pathologic changes. **(b)** The disc is partially shifted anteriorly; the posterior part is already flattened and clearly thinned out compared with normal **(a)**; the double-concave structure is lost. The condyle clearly appears medially/cranially flattened. **(c)** A condyle position in habitual occlusion with retral and cranial shift. The disc is shifted to anterior. The thinned out pars posterior of the disc barely lies in the anterior joint space. The double concave structure of the disc is lost. The condyle is flattened cranially.

BIOMECHANICS OF INVISALIGN 2

John Morton

The content of this chapter is approved by Align Technology and is provided independent of the content of all other chapters. The content of other chapters of this book has not been endorsed by Align Technology.

Biomechanics of Invisalign

Orthodontics is both an art and a science. The quest for beauty and balance in appearance is art. Putting a plier to a wire at each appointment to attain that perfect treatment outcome is analogous to putting a brush to canvas and seeing a painting come to life. Both are dependent on the knowledge and vision of the expert. The science of orthodontics is the understanding of the biologic basis of tooth movement and the functioning of the orthodontic appliance itself. Mathematics, computer science, material science, and biomechanics lie at the heart of optimal appliance design.

Recent improvements of the Invisalign clear aligner appliance are based on principles from each of these scientific disciplines. To improve the functioning of an orthodontic appliance, one must first understand how it works. How does an Invisalign aligner control tooth movement? This question can be answered from two very different perspectives: a displacement-driven system, or a force-driven system. In a displacement-driven system, the aligner is formed with the geometry of the tooth crown in the next staged location of the treatment plan, and it is considered that the tooth will move until it lines up with its shape in the aligner. This displacement-driven concept, of forming the aligner with the next location of the crown, is effective when tipping a tooth is required but it is less effective in controlling the movement of the root. In a force-driven system, the aligner is formed in a shape that is intended to impart specific forces to the tooth crown that will result in the desired movement of the tooth.

The shape of the aligner capable of producing these forces is not necessarily the shape of the tooth. The system of force required to move the tooth and the shape of the aligner are determined by the principles of biomechanics. It is the biomechanical principles of a force-driven system that are used in the Invisalign system to provide improved control of movement for the entire tooth, both crown and root.

In a force-driven system, the fundamental concept of biomechanics in orthodontics is used: to achieve a desired tooth movement, first the force system to be applied to the tooth must be determined and then the appliance designed. It is well accepted in orthodontics that if the force system produced by the appliance is correct for the movement, then the probability of accomplishing the movement is greater. Force systems required for various tooth movements have been studied since the 1960s and remain the topic of investigations worldwide. The orthodontic literature is replete with articles defining the force systems necessary to accomplish different types of tooth movement. For example, should the tooth require tipping, a single force applied to the crown will accomplish the movement. Should controlled tipping, translation, or root movement be required, the aligner appliance must deliver the correct forces and moments to the tooth. A moment is the tendency of a force to produce a rotational movement of the tooth. Rotation as used here includes angulation and inclination, which are also rotational movements. The proportion of the moment to the force is termed the moment-to-force ratio (M/F) (Fig 2-1). This ratio describes the type of tooth movement and values of this ratio to accomplish different types of tooth movement.

The introduction of a force-driven concept to the Invisalign aligner treatment has provided improved control of the M/F ratio, resulting in improved control

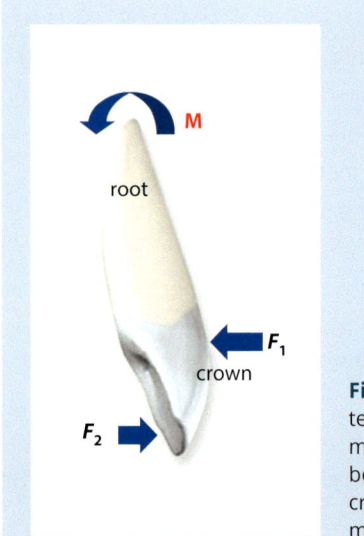

Fig 2-1 Force systems for tooth movements. A force (F) can be applied to the crown to created a moment (M).

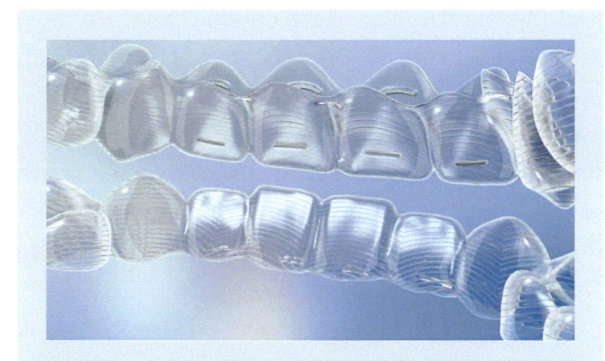

Fig 2-2 The Power Ridge feature is a specific aligner shape that produces a force system to control lingual movement of the root with respect to the crown. This shows a buccal–lingual ridge pair on the maxillary incisors.

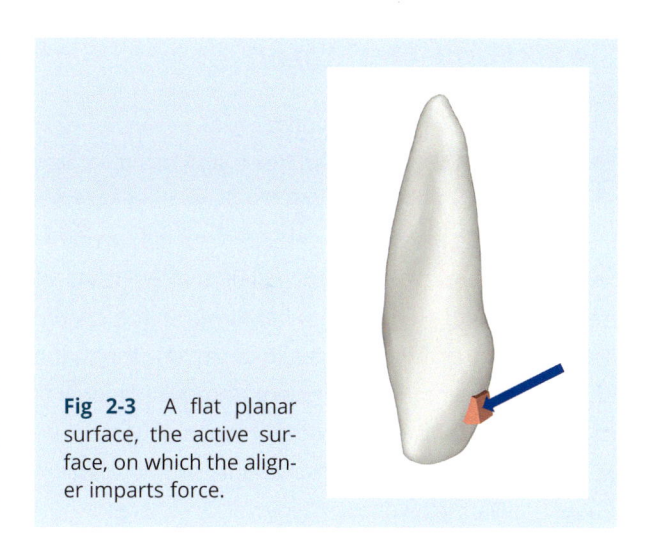

Fig 2-3 A flat planar surface, the active surface, on which the aligner imparts force.

of the root movement with respect to the crown. The movement required for each individual tooth from the beginning to the end of treatment is entered into the ClinCheck software. The software then determines the movement of a tooth and the type of movement the tooth is to undergo during treatment. The force system needed to accomplish this movement is calculated and the aligner shape is determined. The principle is movement, force system, and then appliance design. The aligner can easily exert force on a surface of the tooth to accomplish intrusion or tipping. Movements such as lingual root torque and angulation can be more difficult to achieve because of the complex force system (a group of forces and moments) that must be delivered to the tooth. To produce the correct force system for these movements, the shape of the aligner cannot be the same as the shape of the tooth. It must be modified. Features that are a change in the shape of the aligner are the power ridge and the pressure point.

The power ridge is a specific change in the shape of the aligner that has been engineered to produce the force system necessary to control the lingual movement of the root with respect to the crown. Differences in tooth morphology require that there be individual designs for the maxillary central incisors, maxillary lateral incisors, and mandibular incisors. The power ridge feature is designed to apply a lingual force to the tooth and to control the distortion of the aligner near the lingual incisal edge, which produces the moment required to control the movement of the root (Fig 2-2).

Treatments requiring lingual root torque with retraction result in removal of the contact on the lingual incisal edge that is required for control of the root; hence, a lingual power ridge has been designed to restore the contacts in these treatments.

Extrusion is a movement where the tooth does not have a surface on which the aligner can exert the required force. An artificial surface must therefore be fabricated on the tooth, so that the aligner can exert a force in the extrusive direction. This artificial surface is called an "attachment." All recent attachment designs have a flat planar surface, the "active surface," on which the aligner imparts force (Fig 2-3). The active surface of the attachment is the only surface of importance, because it is the surface engaged by the aligner. The rest of the attachment material exists only to hold the active surface in place. The aligner is designed to alleviate contact with the other surfaces of the attachment; in this way, force can be applied at a specific location on the tooth and in a specific direction. Control of the direction and magnitude of force is essential in providing accurate force systems and controlling tooth movement.

SmartForce Optimized Attachments

The family of Invisalign SmartForce Optimized Attachments was introduced in 2009. These attachments are engineered to produce a force system that is favorable for the desired movement. Research conducted at Align Technology has shown that the shape of the tooth must be considered when determining the shape of the attachment. The use of computer simulation has enabled a customized attachment to be provided that is specific for each tooth movement outlined in the patient's treatment plan, if needed. The software automatically places the attachment needed for the movement with no input required from the practitioner. This family of SmartForce attachments includes the Optimized Extrusion attachment, Multi-tooth Anterior Extrusion attachment, Optimized Rotation attachment, Multi-plane attachment, and Root Control attachment. Forces of very low magnitude are required to accomplish extrusion. When deflected vertically, an aligner can produce very high levels of force because of its material composition and shape. Figure 2-4 shows the Optimized Extrusion attachment, which is designed to distribute this energy in a manner that delivers the appropriate levels of force to accomplish extrusion.

When extrusion of all four incisors is required, the Multi-tooth Anterior Extrusion attachment is needed (Fig 2-5) to ensure that nearly equivalent force is delivered to each tooth. This force system is considered to provide more successful extrusion of all incisors as a unit and is being used effectively in the treatment of open bite. Practitioners indicate that extrusion of teeth with Invisalign aligners is now much more predictable than prior to the development of these innovative attachments.

Rotation of a tooth around its cross-section, long considered difficult to achieve with aligners, has been improved using a fundamental biomechanic approach. Rotation of canines and premolars may now be accomplished more predictably using the Optimized Rotation attachments (Fig 2-6). The software automatically positions the active surface of the attachment on the buccal surface, as far from the long axis of the tooth as possible and designs the aligner to apply force to this surface. The result is a substantial moment of the force to rotate the tooth in the desired direction. A practitioner would not bond a button at a location on the tooth that would create any interference during the derotation; the software is configured to mimic this decision process and places an attachment only at a location that does not produce interference during treatment.

Tooth movements prescribed throughout treatment are not always pure movements, such as extrusion along the long axis of the tooth. For example, the movement of a maxillary lateral incisor during treat-

Fig 2-4 The Extrusion attachment, delivering an aligner force with components that are extrusive and lingual.

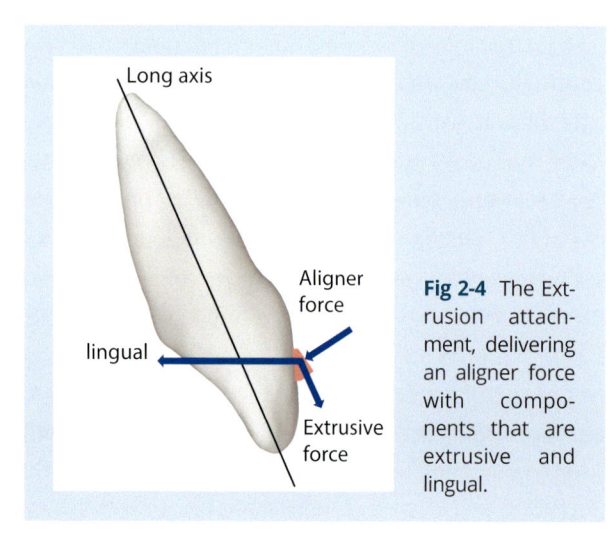

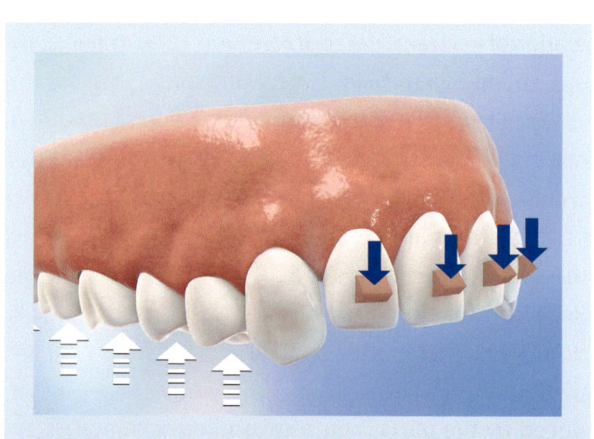

Fig 2-5 The Multi-tooth Anterior Extrusion attachment, designed to extrude all four incisors.

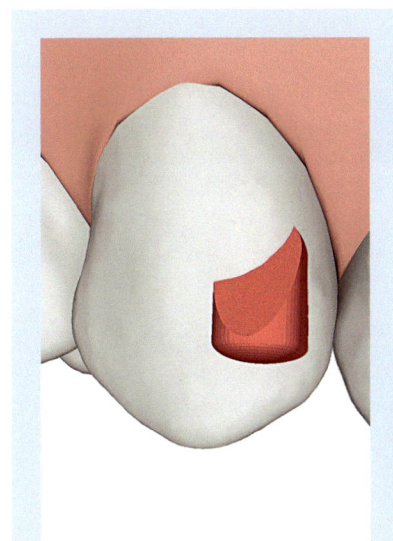

Fig 2-6 Rotation of canines and premolars using the Optimized Rotation attachment.

Fig 2-7 Creation of a force system with several movements. **(a)** The Multi-plane attachment on the labial surface of the tooth at a point determined by the software. **(b)** A pressure point fabricated in the aligner to produce a second force on the lingual face.

ment may be partly extrusive, partly labiolingual tipping, and combined with rotation. A major advancement in aligner treatment is in determining the force system that is optimal to move the tooth along this compound pathway comprising many movements, and then determining the combination of features required to produce the force system necessary for this movement. Use of an attachment on the labial surface of the tooth (Fig 2-7a) and a pressure point fabricated in the aligner to produce a force on the lingual face of the aligner (Fig 2-7b) provide a force system that is favorable to complex three-dimensional movement. The Multi-plane attachment is part of a software-enabled generation of a system that addresses the three-dimensional movement of a maxillary lateral incisor.

Excellent treatment outcomes require excellent control of root angulation and alignment (Fig 2-8). A change in angulation requires a force system comprising a mesial or distal force and a second-order moment. This force system can be achieved using the Root Control attachments. The aligner is designed to produce a force on the gingival attachment in the direction of movement of the root. A force is produced by the aligner on a second attachment placed occlusally, to provide the counter-moment necessary to control the movement of the root. Should the tooth be too small to bond two attachments, one attachment with a pressure point is placed to produce the force system. A pressure point is a modification to the shape of the aligner that concentrates force at a specific location on the tooth. The ClinCheck software determines the tooth movements needed in a set-up approved by the practitioner and places any features intended to produce the force system to support the desired movement. There is no design action required on the part of the practitioner. Should the practitioner wish to use a feature other than one placed by the software, an interface allows

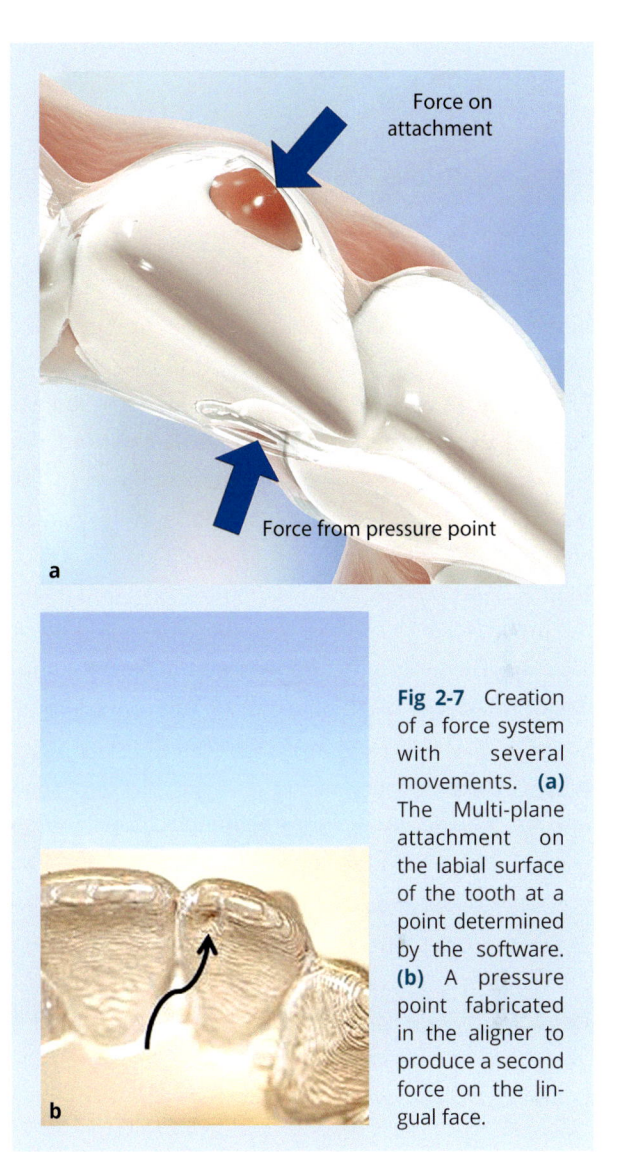

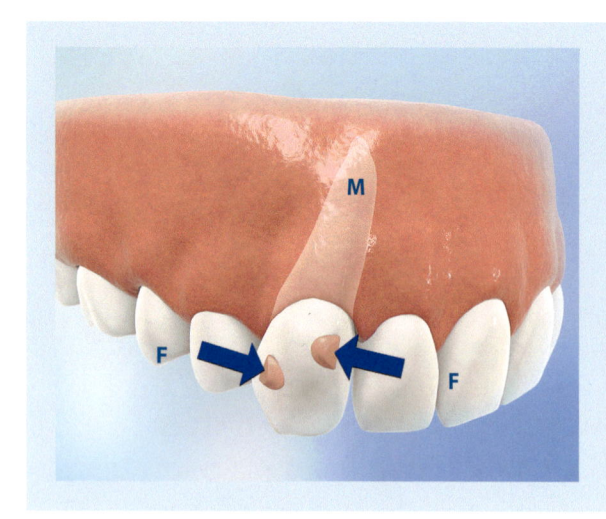

Fig 2-8 Control of root angulation and alignment. A change in angulation requires a mesial or distal force (F) and a second-order moment (M). The aligner is designed to produce a force on the gingival attachment in the direction of movement of the root. A second attachment placed occlusally provides the counter-moment necessary to control root movement.

the practitioner to remove the attachment and place another. Thus, the practitioner remains in total control of the design of the appliance. The fundamental scientific principles of biomechanics advanced computer simulation being used to provide features such as SmartForce Optimized Attachments, power ridge features and pressure point features to better control tooth movement and improve treatment outcomes with the Invisalign system. Science in combination with the vision and knowledge of the expert serve to deliver the best possible orthodontic treatment to the patient.

TREATMENT PLANNING AND TREATMENT WITH ALIGNERS 3

Orofacial orthopedic treatment always start with the case history, the patient records, and then the diagnosis. Treatment planning for use of Invisalign system differs from other techniques such as fixed appliances. The Invisalign system can be used to treat almost all problems and it can be combined with other techniques. Strategic planning with the Invisalign system is crucial and one of the main factors that contributes to its success. This chapter describes strategic planning of orthodontic treatments with the Invisalign system.

Diagnosis of function, esthetics, biology, and structure is necessary for every orthodontic treatment, but the sequence followed can vary. Although initially we commenced with the biologic and structural analysis, Kokich et al (2006) suggested an algorithm starting with an esthetic analysis. We start with the functional analysis (1), followed by esthetic analysis (2), biologic analysis (3), and then structural analysis (4) (Fig 3-1). If a musculoskeletal or craniomandibular disorder (CMD) is diagnosed that requires treatment, we start with functional treatment of the CMS. Planning of the esthetics is a backward process. Use of a wax-up followed by a mock-up, as in traditional prosthetics, will be increasingly displaced by digital systems. When using the Invisalign system in orthodontic treatment of complex situations, we analyze the end result in the ClinCheck software together with the dentist and the laboratory technician (pathway *a* in Fig 3-1). Before the orthodontic and, if needed, restorative treatment starts, the periodontal, endodontal, and tooth status is assessed and the treatment goal is redetermined after any periodontal, endodontal, or restorative dentistry (pathway *b* in Fig 3-1). Finally, structural analysis is used to plan orthopedics/orthodontics, implantology, and/or prosthetic and restorative dentistry.

In the treatment of patients using fixed appliances, the finishing phase was started and designed during the last few months of treatment. When patients are treated with the Invisalign system, treatment planning includes the finishing phase right from the start using the ClinCheck software. Whenever you start an ortho-

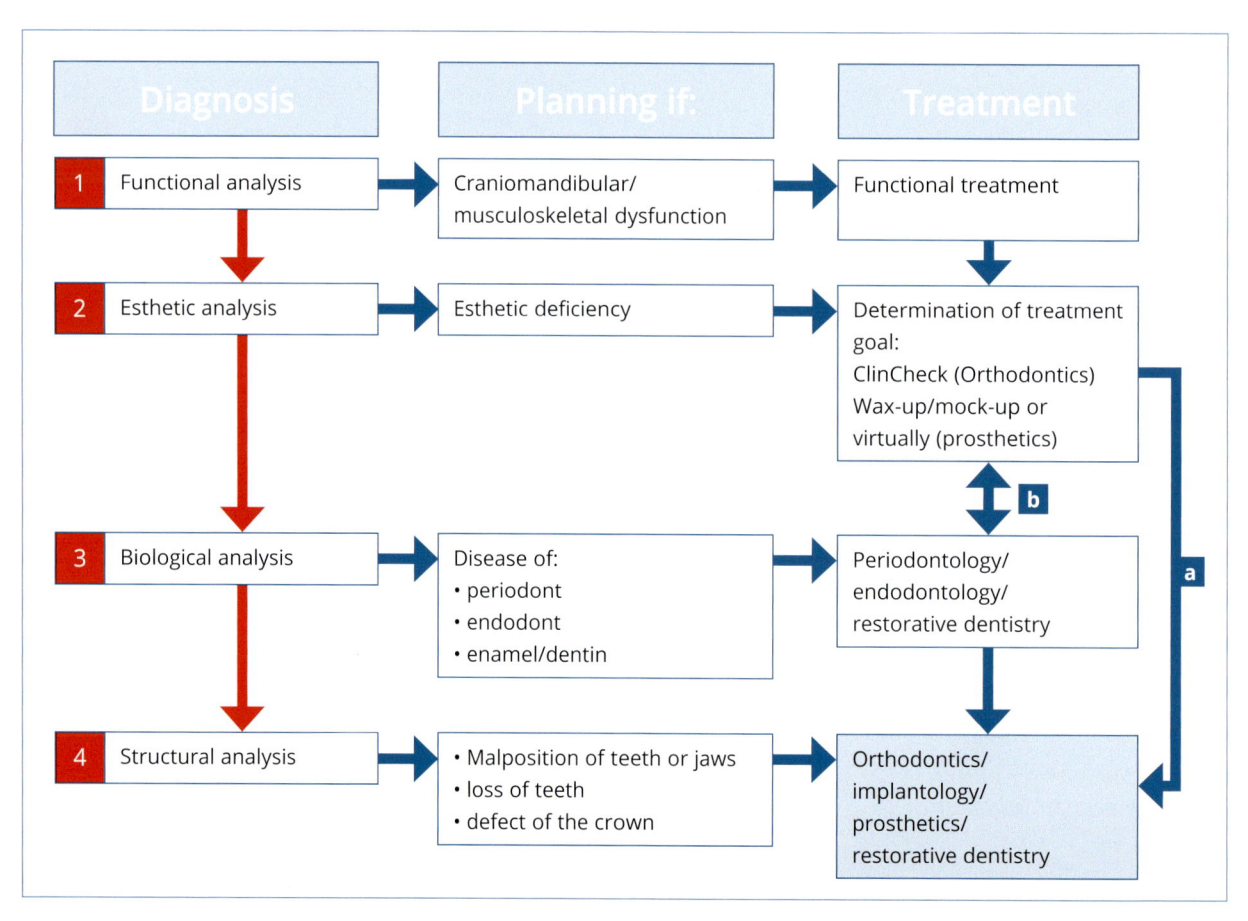

Fig 3-1 Planning algorithm for diagnosis and treatment. **(a)** Periodontics, endodontics, or restorative dentistry not needed; **(b)** determination of treatment goal after the decision that periodontics, endodontics, or restorative dentistry would be needed.

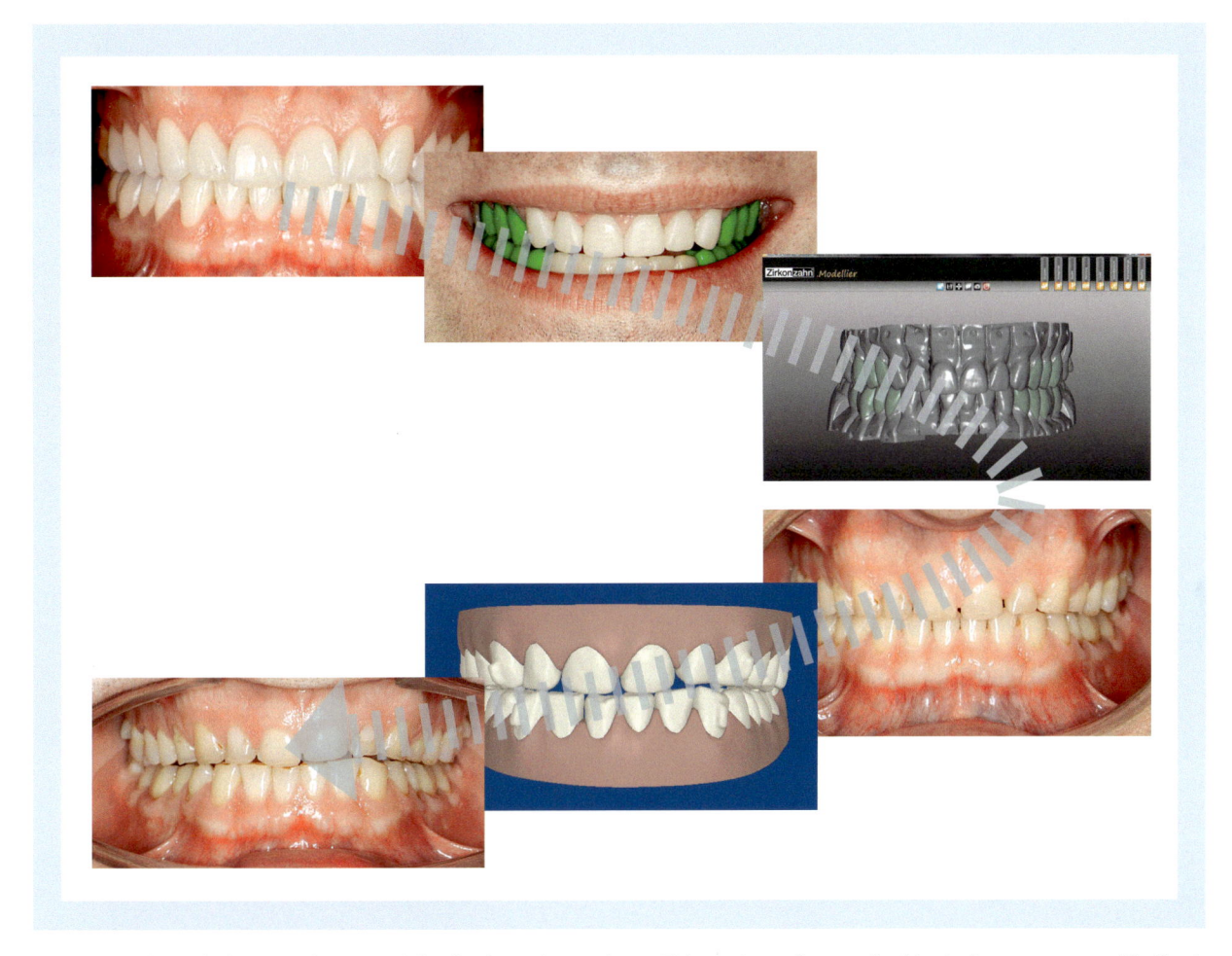

Fig 3-2 Backward planning (from top left): final result; mock up; Zirkonzahn software; final Invisalign treatment; ClinCheck software; start.

dontic treatment, start with the end in mind. Whenever a complex treatment including prosthodontics is planned, it should be commenced with the intended results clearly envisaged.

With the advent of virtual systems for planning, backward planning is the gold standard in dentistry (Fig 3-2), with the goal of achieving excellent results core to the treatment right from the beginning. The ClinCheck finishing checklist is divided into three parts:
1. occlusion: static and dynamic
2. bone and periodontium
3. esthetics.

Occlusion

Occlusion has been described by many authors in the past, with some fundamental differences. In the following, as well as in all the treatments described later in the book, tooth anatomy and occlusion will be described within the meaning of Polz (2012). Figure 3-3a shows the static occlusal points in ideal occlusion and with perfect tooth anatomy. In this contact relationship, the chewing forces lead to a sliding into the opposite direction. If the contact relationship is not ideal, the chewing forces lead to a precontact with loading of the tooth and, therefore, loosening and moving of the tooth. Even if it is not very evident during swallowing and chewing, parafunctions may lead to damage in the whole CMS.

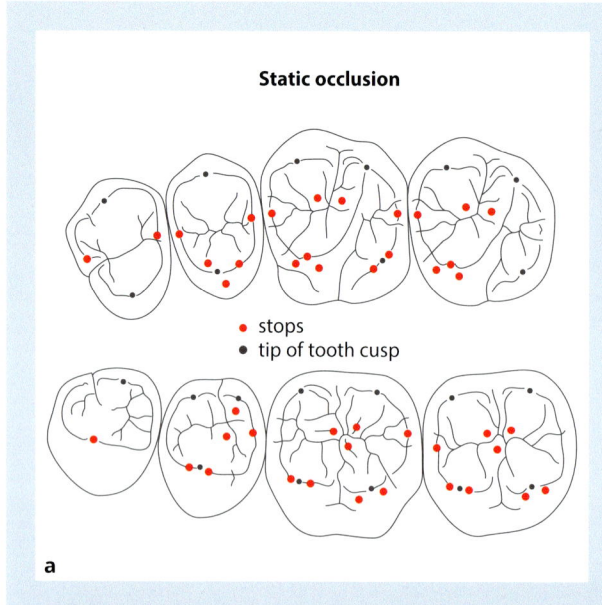

Fig 3-3 Occlusion: **(a)** static occlusal points in ideal occlusion and with a perfect tooth anatomy; red indicates the stops and black the tips of the cusps as they might occur in a class I relationship; **(b)** the three dimensions of dynamic occlusion.

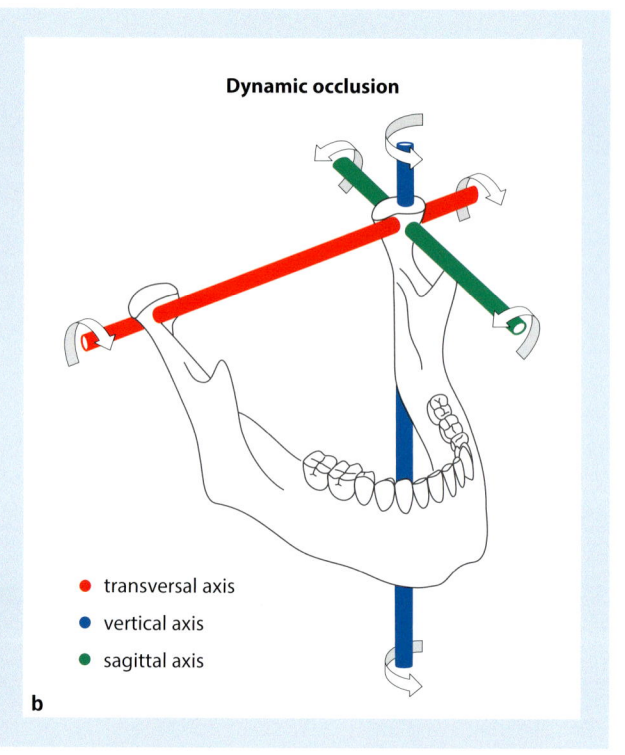

As tooth anatomy cannot be changed orthodontically, so orthodontics alone cannot generate perfect occlusal patterns in teeth with anatomical defects. However, new techniques such as digital scanning, set-up software, and registration (recording) of individual movement patterns, and their transfer into a virtual articulator, can help us to get closer in achieving this goal. Orthodontic treatment should end with:
- full contact of premolars and molars
- overbite in relation to excentric movement (anterior guidance)
- canines with minimum contact, incisors without contact, "Shimstock open" (= 8 μm)
- overjet open (as shown with Shimstock foil; no incisor contact in maximal intercuspation).

From the static occlusion the dynamic occlusion develops in three dimensions (Fig 3-3b):
- transversal
- vertical
- sagittal.

During dynamic occlusion, the mandible is moving around all three axes. Particular emphasis in orthodontic treatment is given to laterotrusion, mediotrusion, and protrusion (Fig 3-4). If precontacts or hyperbalance contacts lead to disorders, the physiologic movement of the condyles is also disturbed, and structural changes in the TMJ can develop.

The incisors are feelers and have, therefore, managerial function in guiding mandibular movement. The canines also contribute to mandibular movement and unloading of the posterior teeth, which leaves their contact position in excursion and, thus, leads to release of the TMJs. The premolars too, particularly the first premolars, contribute to leading mandibular movement. The premolars and molars in their orthographic position capture the occlusal force of the molars and are responsible for masticating of the food.

Orthodontic treatment should end with achieving:
- canine guidance, possibly canine and premolar guidance
- no balance or hyperbalance contacts in mediotrusion
- incisor guidance in protrusion.

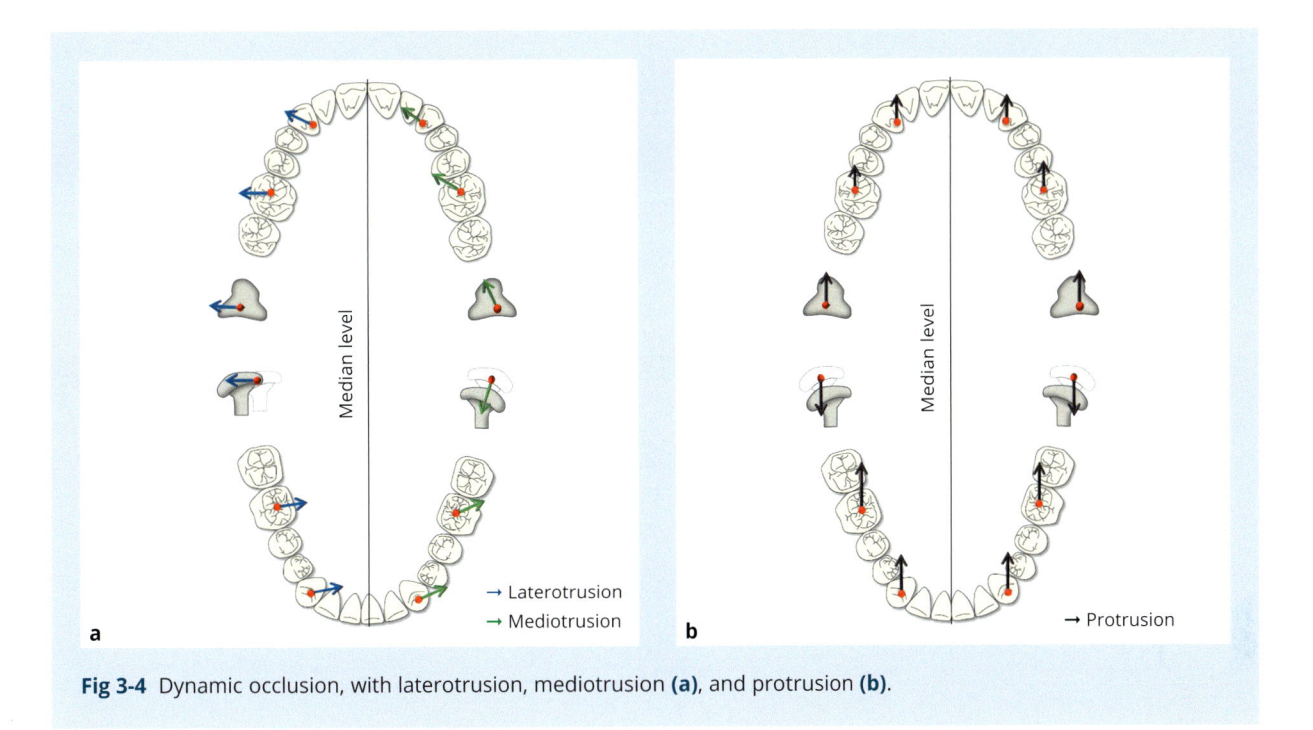

Fig 3-4 Dynamic occlusion, with laterotrusion, mediotrusion **(a)**, and protrusion **(b)**.

Bone and periodontium

Several factors affect treatment:
- Intermittent and low forces (<0.3 N/cm²) initiate an inflammation process in the periodontal ligament that leads to tooth movement via resorption in bone. This causes minimal root resorption compared with continuous forces. Consequently, staging should be slowed (number of aligners increased) if bone loss exists (Fig 3-5).
- If lower forces are used (below the capillary blood pressure, 0.20 to 0.26 N/cm²), blood supply is maintained to the area and there is less cell damage.
- More interproximal bone will provide greater resistance to periodontal bone loss. Root angulation should be planned in the ClinCheck software with consideration of the radiographic findings. Optimized attachments will help to perform angulations.
- In adults with former periodontal disease and interproximal bone loss, the incisal edges do not determine the vertical position of the teeth, and sometimes bone level will need to be aligned.

These finishing decisions should be made at the very beginning.

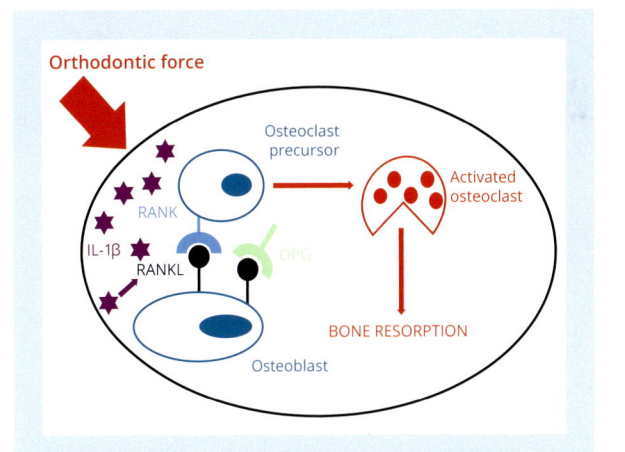

Fig 3-5 Receptor activator of NF-κβ ligand (RANKL) and its receptor RANK have a role in osteoclastogenesis in periodontal disease. Periodontal ligament fibroblasts produce primarily osteoprotegerin (OPG), a decoy receptor that prevents RANKL binding and thus inhibits osteoclastogenesis (increasing bone resorption). The type of force used should be adjusted if bone loss has occurred: intermittent or low forces stimulate RANKL production more than continuous forces do; they also cause less cell damage than continuous/larger force. Staging can be slowed if bone loss exists. Graphic: modified according to Yasuda

a **Visible upper incisors in rest position of upper lip**
- 2–3 mm visible upper incisors while speaking is perfect
- Be careful to avoid too much intrusion and therefore unesthetic results with need for extrusion in the refinement
- If you start with more than 3 mm visible incisors and gummy smile, plan overcorrection for the intrusion

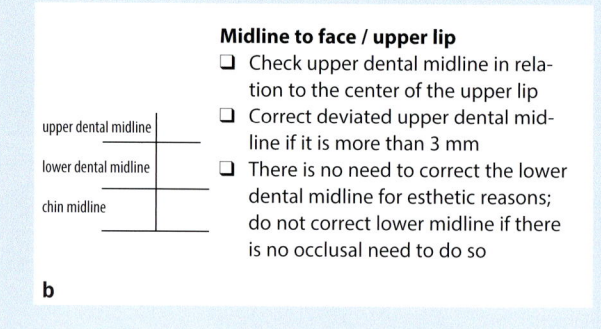

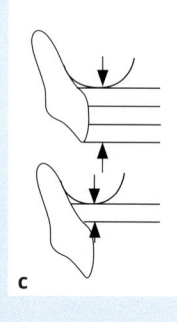

b **Midline to face / upper lip**
- Check upper dental midline in relation to the center of the upper lip
- Correct deviated upper dental midline if it is more than 3 mm
- There is no need to correct the lower dental midline for esthetic reasons; do not correct lower midline if there is no occlusal need to do so

c **Visible teeth / gingiva during smile**
- To correct a gummy smile without orthognathic surgery, plan overcorrection for intrusion according the amount of desired intrusion
- If periodontal surgery is planned after the Invisalign treatment, plan and discuss the ClinCheck together with the periodontist before accepting it

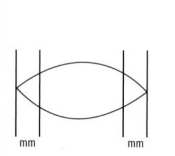

d **Buccal corridor**
- The size of the buccal corridor depends on the width of the smile and the width of the dental arches
- We can change the archform, not the smile width
- Plan overcorrection for expansion in the first online treatment plan

e **Curve of upper teeth to curve of lower lip**
- The curve of the upper dentition should follow the curve of the lower lip in the vertical dimension
- Examine the patient and the extraoral pictures to describe the movement that is needed in the vertical to harmonize the curve of the upper dentition
- If interdisciplinary dentistry is required, discuss the ClinCheck with the dentist and the lab – technician to optimize the situation for later restoratives and an esthetic result

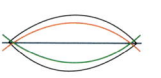

opposing
straight
following the lower lip line

f **Gingival levels**
- Relationship of the gingival margins of upper incisors and canines is important for dentofacial esthetics.
- Gingival margins of the central incisors should be exactly on the same level and positioned more apically than the laterals but at the same level as the canines.
- End with gingival margins on the correct level, not with aligned incisal edges. If a crown is shorter after orthodontic alignment, the dentist can build it up with composite or veneers. BUT: discuss this with the patient and dentist using the ClinCheck software beforehand, keeping in mind also the risk of overcorrection

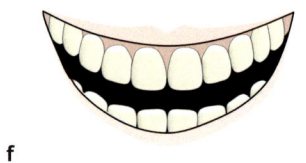

g **Papilla form**
- Visible black triangles reduce esthetics dramatically
- If you have to treat crowding of incisors and canines, do not end with black triangles: consider finishing and keep roots together from the beginning on; do not forget IPR if needed
- Close existing black triangles as much as possible, especially if restoration for these teeth will not be needed. Keep roots together – optimized attachments will help you to finish in an optimal condition

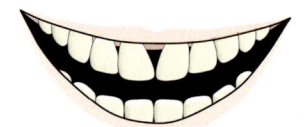

Fig 3-6 The ClinCheck finishing checklist: esthetics.

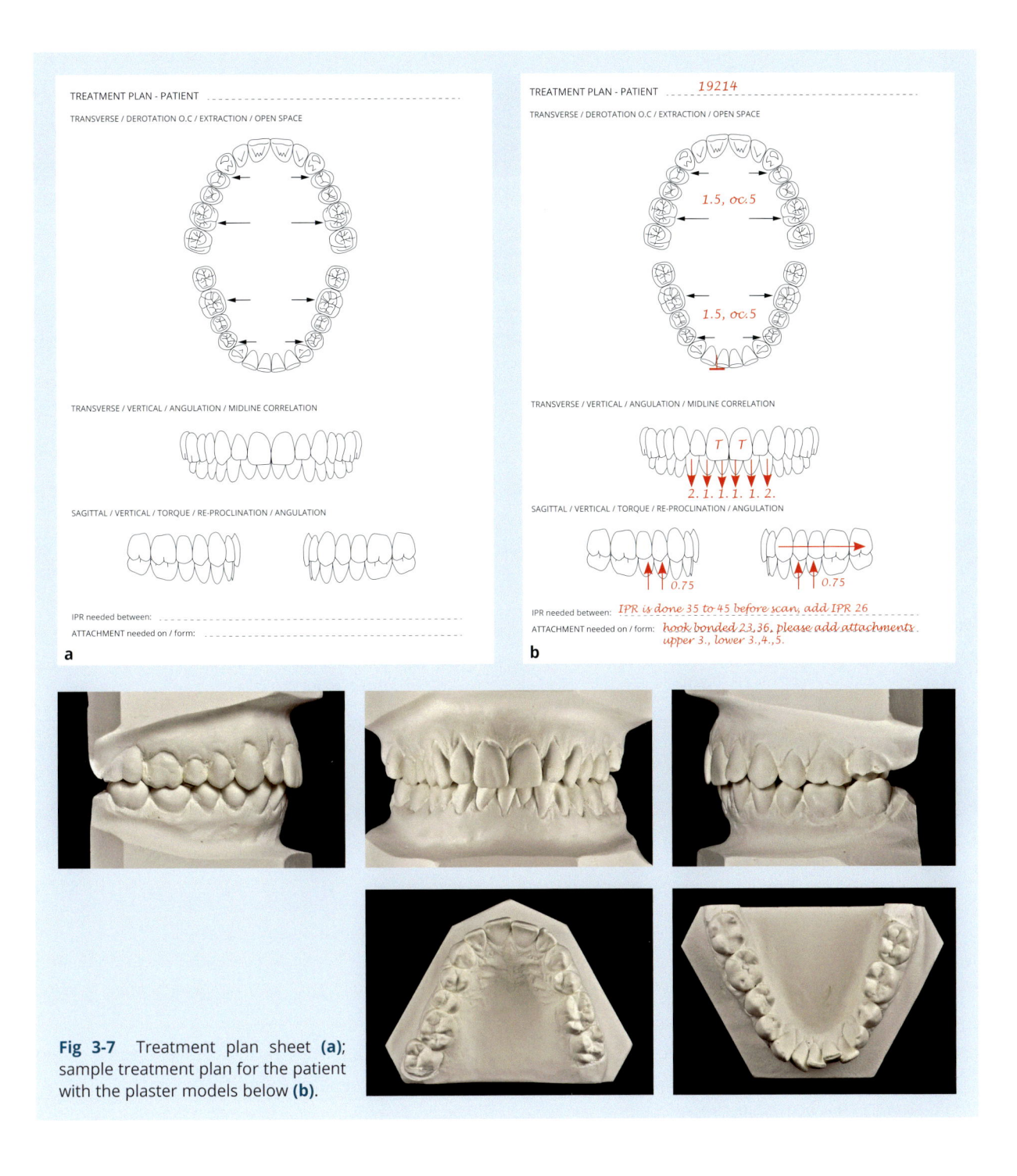

TREATMENT PLANNING AND TREATMENT WITH ALIGNERS 3

Fig 3-7 Treatment plan sheet **(a)**; sample treatment plan for the patient with the plaster models below **(b)**.

Esthetics

It is recommended that treatment is planned right from the start with the final esthetic finish in mind (Fig 3-6). The planned tooth movements are entered into the office treatment plan when the whole orthodontic treatment is decided. The planned movements can be sketched in detail in all dimensions, including any overcorrections wanted for individual tooth movements (Fig 3-7). Any desired interproximal enamel reduction

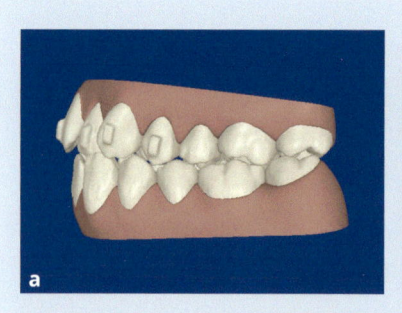

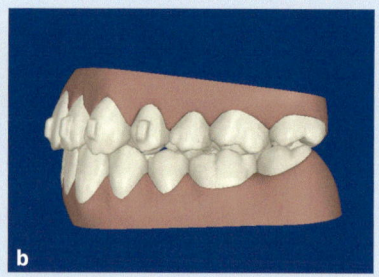

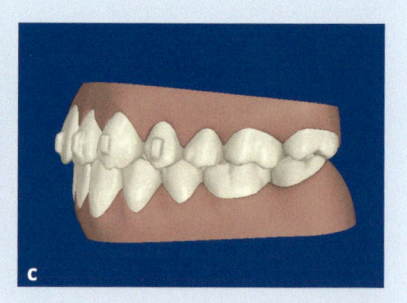

Fig 3-8 ClinCheck software for treatment planning and adjustment. **(a)** Initial situation with crowding in both arches and transversally constricted arch forms. **(b)** First version with aligned arches but insufficient occlusal contact of premolars and molars on the left posterior side. **(c)** Second and final version with corrected posterior left occlusion and hard collision of all premolars and molars.

(IPR), potential conventional attachments and possible auxiliaries, such as buttons, can be decided and identified right at the start of treatment.

An example treatment plan

To level a curve of Spee, there are various possible pathways:
- intrusion of incisors
- intrusion of incisors and canines
- extrusion of premolars
- extrusion of molars
- combination of all these options.

As there are many possibilities, the orthodontist has to decide which one is best for the patient. If the online treatment plan simply says "please level curve of Spee," this is not useful or informative.

The plan for this patient (Fig 3-7) was as follows:
1. Intrusion of the mandibular incisors
2. Intrusion of the mandibular canines
3. During both intrusive movements, a simultaneously extrusion of the mandibular premolars by 0.75 mm.

Torque is needed for teeth 11 and 21, expansion of the maxillary and mandibular arches 1.5 mm with overcorrection 0.5 mm, and distalization of the upper left. Tooth 42 is proclined and cannot be moved further labially without creating gingival recessions. At the very beginning, everything in the "treatment plan" is documented and then transferred into the Invisalign online treatment plan:

It is very important to review the ClinCheck result carefully.
- Is the mounting of the maxillary and mandibular arches correct?
- Is the occlusion at the end correct in detail?
- Is the contact of molars and premolars sufficient?
- Do black triangles exist at the end or within the movement?
- Is there enough overjet?
- Is there enough anterior space?
- Are the movements as requested or do they need to be separated (e.g. first uprighting, then derotation)?
- Is the staging correct or too fast? Are some of the planned movements too fast?
- Does the amount of requested IPR in the ClinCheck seem satisfactory? Or is IPR also needed on other interproximal contact points?
- Are the attachments appropriate for the movement and are they at least 2 mm away from the gingival margin to guarantee appropriate function of the attachments?

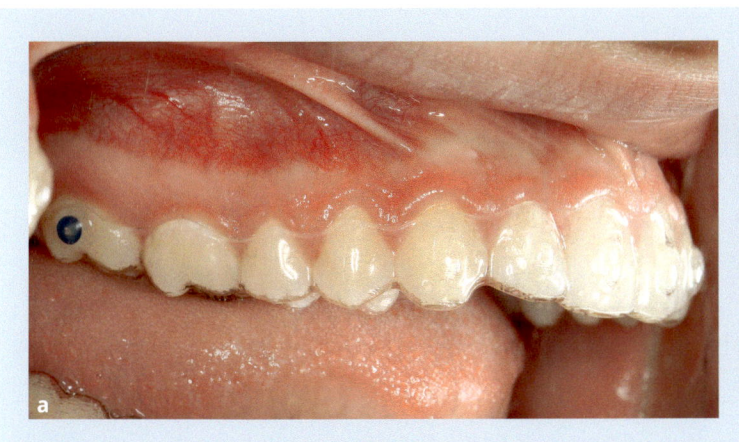

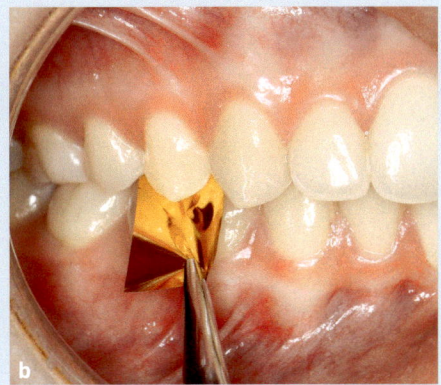

Fig 3-9 Checking of the aligner fitting **(a)** and control of the occlusal contacts with Shimstock foil **(b)**.

Figure 3-8 shows the ClinCheck software in the initial situation and for two versions of the treatment planned.

Course of therapy

A number of points need to be checked during the course of treatment (Fig 3-9):
- Is the patient comfortable with the aligners and the treatment?
- Is the patient wearing the aligners sufficiently?
- Do the aligners fit well?
- Are all attachments covered correctly by the aligner?
- Is the occlusion in the mouth exactly as planned in the ClinCheck?
- Is oral hygiene satisfactory?
- Have recessions developed?
- Are there signs of CMD, muscle pain, or trigger points?

Once treatment has started, the next step in the ClinCheck software should be compared with the situation in the mouth:
- Is there enough space approximally to perform the planned movement or is additional space needed?
- Based on the IPR chart, does IPR still need to be performed?
- Will additional bonding of attachments be needed during the course of treatment (as shown in the treatment panel of the ClinCheck software)?

A decision is then made for the time of the next patient visit.

At the end of the first phase, the following points will need to be considered:
- Is a refinement for finishing required?
- Will overcorrections be necessary?
- Are there spaces or black triangles that still need to be corrected?
- Is the level of the gingiva correct or are there unacceptable vertical height differences?
- In habitual intercuspation, do all posterior teeth have heavy occlusal contact and can the premolars and molars hold Shimstock foil?
- In habitual intercuspation, are the anterior teeth slightly out of contact (Shimstock foil can be pulled through)?
- Is mounting in the articulator needed to check static and dynamic occlusion?
- Is tooth shaping or grinding of interrupting contacts necessary?
- If restorative dentistry is planned, should the patient see the dentist before the Invisalign treatment is finished?
- If refinement is not required, which retention is preferred?

References

Kokich VG, Spear FM, Mathews DP. Interdisziplinäre Behandlungsplanung: Am Anfang steht die Ästhetik. InfOrthodKieferorthop 2006;38:211–220.

Polz M. Anatomy of teeth. In: Boisserée W, Schupp W. Kraniomandibuläres und muskuloskelettales System. Berlin: Quintessenz, 2012.

Yasuda H. Bone and bone related biochemical examinations. Bone and collagen related metabolites. Receptor activator of NF-kappaB ligand (RANKL)]. Clin Calcium 2006;16:964-970.

TREATMENT OF DIFFERENT MALOCCLUSIONS WITH ALIGNERS 4

This chapter will provide examples of different malocclusions and their treatment with the Invisalign system step by step. The topics will show different malocclusions, but with a focus on one main aspect of the malocclusion when determining treatment for this particular problem. No further details will be given for treatment of other issues in the patient.

4 TREATMENT OF DIFFERENT MALOCCLUSIONS WITH ALIGNERS

Topic 1
Deangulation of the maxillary incisors to remove an existing black triangle

- removal of black triangle
- deangulation of maxillary incisors

The patient had had a fixed appliance in another office before presenting for treatment. He had a palatal maxillary fixed retainer and was not satisfied with the black triangle mesial to teeth 11 and 21 (Fig 4-1).

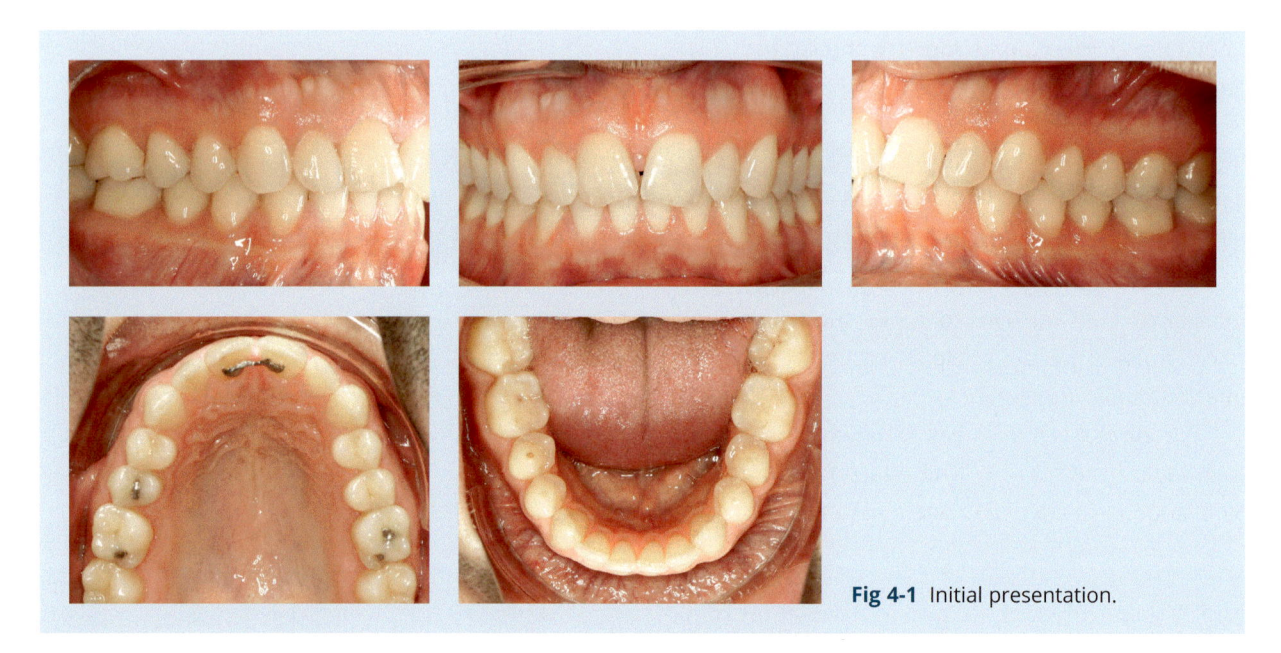

Fig 4-1 Initial presentation.

Diagnosis:
- previous orthodontic treatment with a fixed appliance
- Class I relationship
- diastema in the maxilla
- slight crowding in the mandibular arch
- deep bite.

Therapy:
- alignment of maxilla and mandible
- deangulation of teeth 11 and 21 with closure of diastema
- intrusion of lower incisors and canines.

Treatment

The main objectives were to deal with the extreme distal angulation of the roots of teeth 11 and 21, which had led to the severe black triangle, and to move from the use of a palatal retainer, which was maintaining the black triangle.

One of the first steps is deangulation. To deangulate the central incisors, attachments (Fig 4-2) are necessary on both teeth and interproximal enamel reduction (IPR) is needed on the mesial aspect to move the contact points more to the gingiva. If both incisors are in a crowded position that is going to be solved, the online treatment plan will need to indicate that the roots of the incisors need to be deangulated with the start of movement of the incisor crowns. With this additional deangulation of the roots, a black triangle cannot evolve. Additionally, IPR mesial of both incisors to move the contact point more apically will also help to prevent the development of a black triangle.

The palatal retainer was removed and Invisalign therapy started (Fig 4-3). The attachments used were conventional rectangular ones, as treatment started before the G4 generation of attachments was available. To avoid a black triangle, the roots must be kept together over the whole treatment time. IPR can be added as needed.

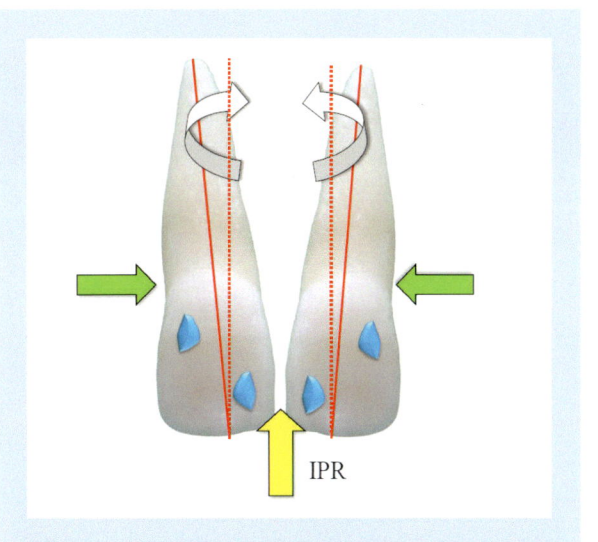

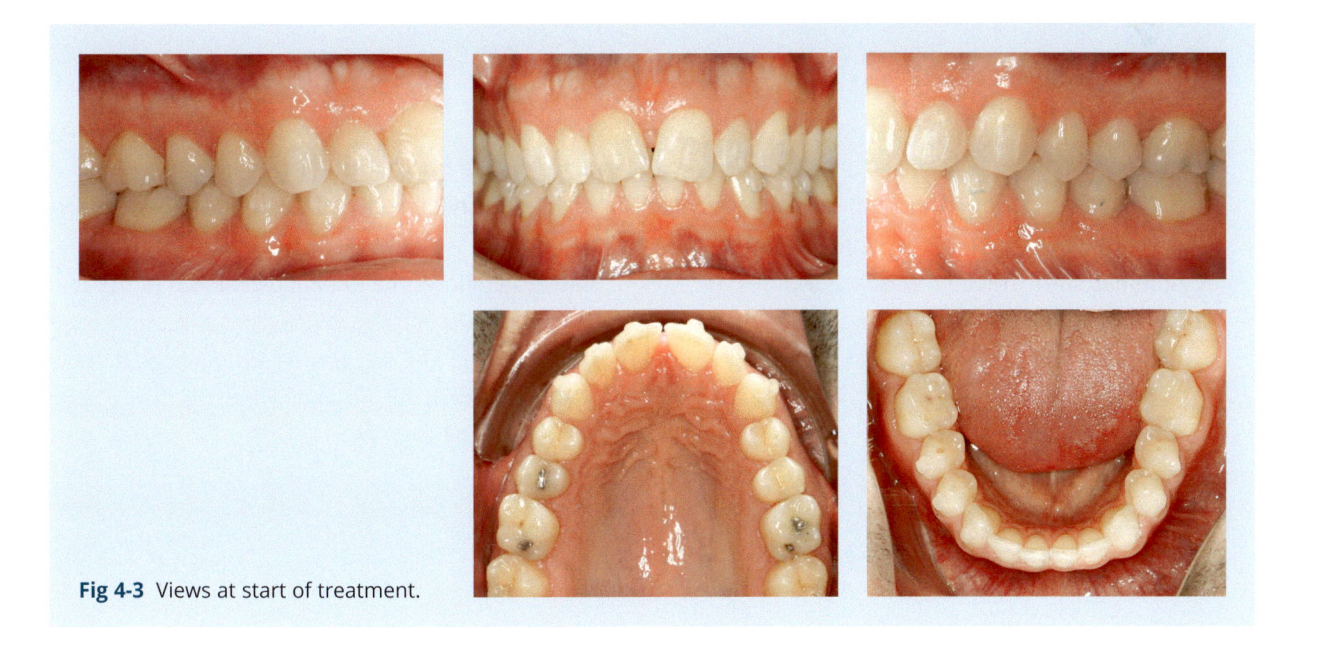

Fig 4-2 Attachments of the G4 generation can be used to deangulate the central incisors attachments (alternatively conventional vertical rectangular attachments can be used).

Fig 4-3 Views at start of treatment.

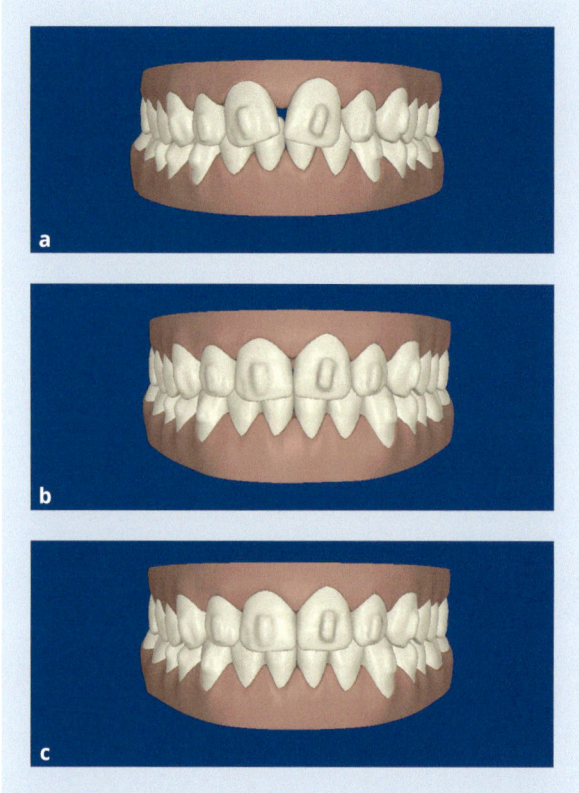

Fig 4-4 Planned treatment in the ClinCheck software. **(a)** Initial anterior findings. **(b)** Planned final findings at the end of phase 1 and remaining with insufficient deangulation of teeth 11 and 21 and remaining black triangle mesial 11 and 21. **(c)** Final situation after refinement aligners and additional angulation with a further six aligners for deangulation of teeth 11 and 21 with IPR 0.2 mm mesial on teeth 11 and 21.

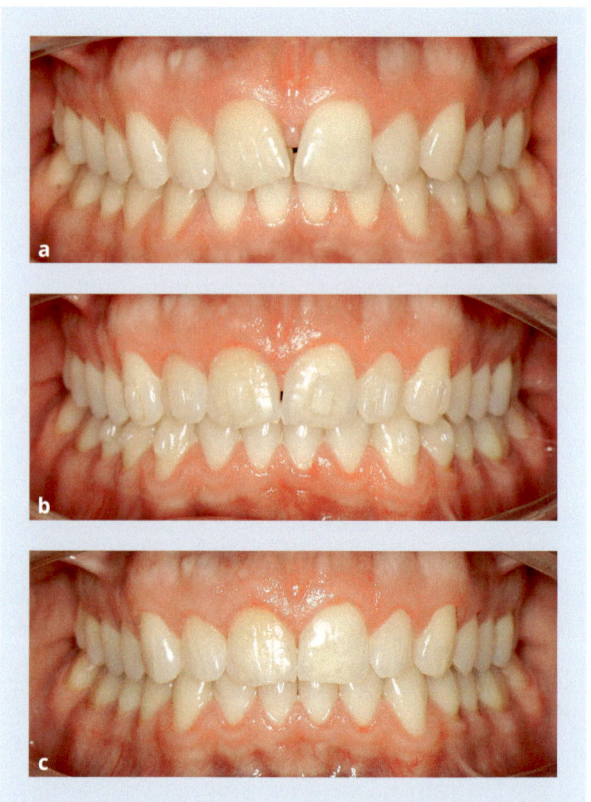

Fig 4-5 Intraoral findings at start of treatment **(a)**; at end of the first phase **(b)**; and final result **(c)**.

Angulation of the roots is not an easy movement and so care must be taken that the staging is not too quick and, therefore, the force was reduced.

Figure 4-4 shows the planned treatment in the ClinCheck software. The first treatment phase included 25 aligners.

Figure 4-5 shows the intraoral findings during treatment. It can be seen that treatment of crown angulation is highly predictable with the Invisalign system.

Figure 4-6 shows the patient's dentition at the end of treatment. The black triangle and diastema have been closed and the roots of teeth 11 and 21 have been deangulated. All other corrections have been accomplished completely.

Fig 4-6 Intraoral views at the end of treatment.

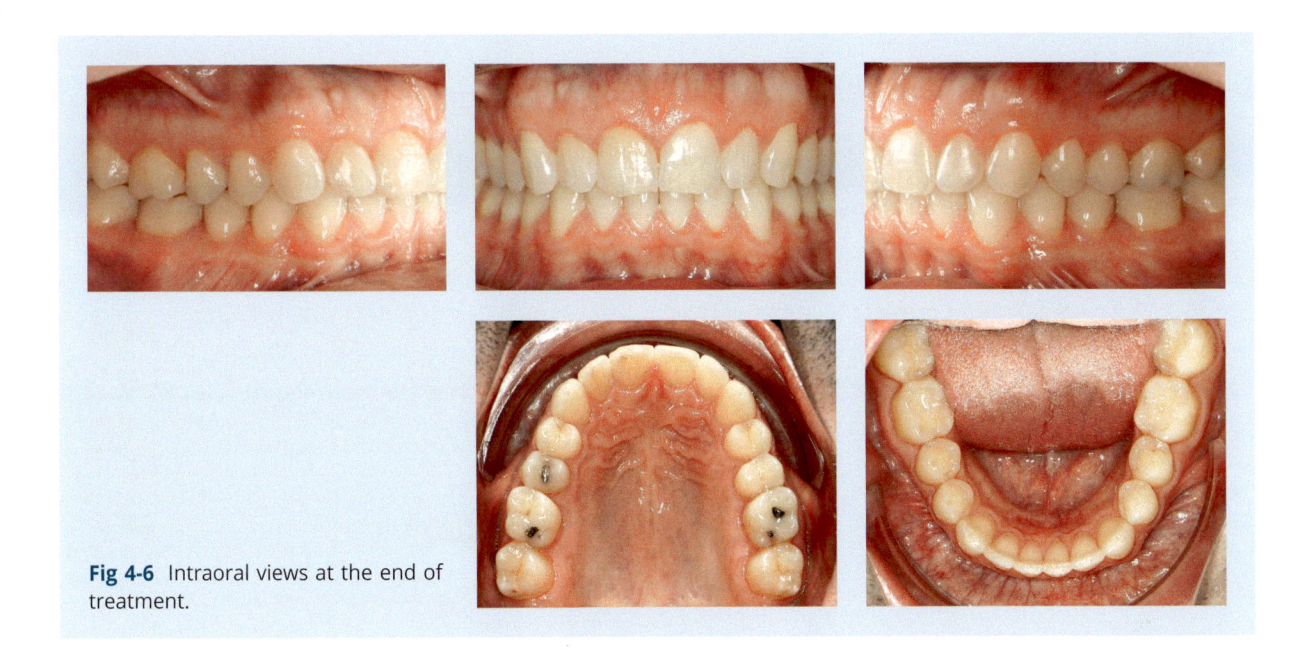

Topic 2
Derotation of mandibular canines

- rotation of canines
- derotation with Invisalign treatment only

This patient had several problems but the focus here is on the mandibular canines with severe rotation. At the age of 8, the patient started orthodontic treatment with a Quad Helix to solve her existing crossbite; this was followed by functional therapy with a Frankel appliance treating the class II relationship. After the Frankel therapy, a full class I relationship was obtained (Fig 4-7). Invisalign treatment was started when she was 13 years of age.

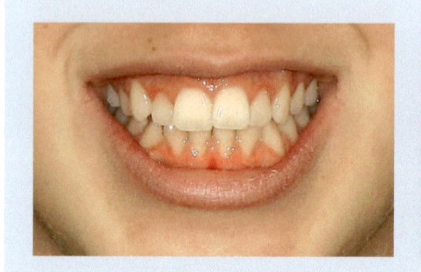

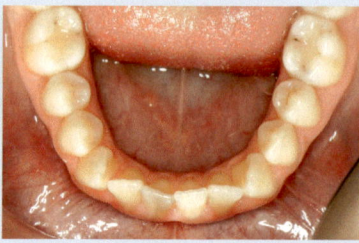

Fig 4-7 Initial presentation.

Diagnosis:
- class I relationship after orthodontic functional pre-treatment
- crowding and rotation in the mandibular arch, particularly of teeth 33 and 43.

Therapy:
- alignment of maxilla and mandible
- derotation of mandibular canines.

Treatment

The main objective was to to create space at the mandibular canines to allow for their derotation. The expansion was more a crown uprighting to labial than a bodily movement with root movement to buccal. The total amount of IPR included 0.4 mm up to 0.5 mm from each canine to molar, followed by distalization of the premolars. Overcorrection of both mandibular canines was requested, with additional rotation of the mesial aspect to lingual 0.4 mm (Fig 4-8). The intraoral views show teeth positions before starting Invisalign treatment (Fig 4-8). Invisalign treatment used conventional rectangular attachments on teeth 33 and 43 for major anchorage during the planned derotation (treatment took place before the launch of the G4 generation of attachments).

Figure 4-9 shows the ClinCheck result with IPR and the visualizations of the treatment path.

A comparison of initial and final views shows the perfectly derotated teeth 33 and 43 (Fig 4-10). Canines, premolars, and molars had been uprighted with expansion to achieve more space for the canines in addition to that from IPR. The derotation was planned with overcorrection of the canines with rotation of the mesial aspect to lingual. The expansion together with the derotation and uprighting of the mandibular

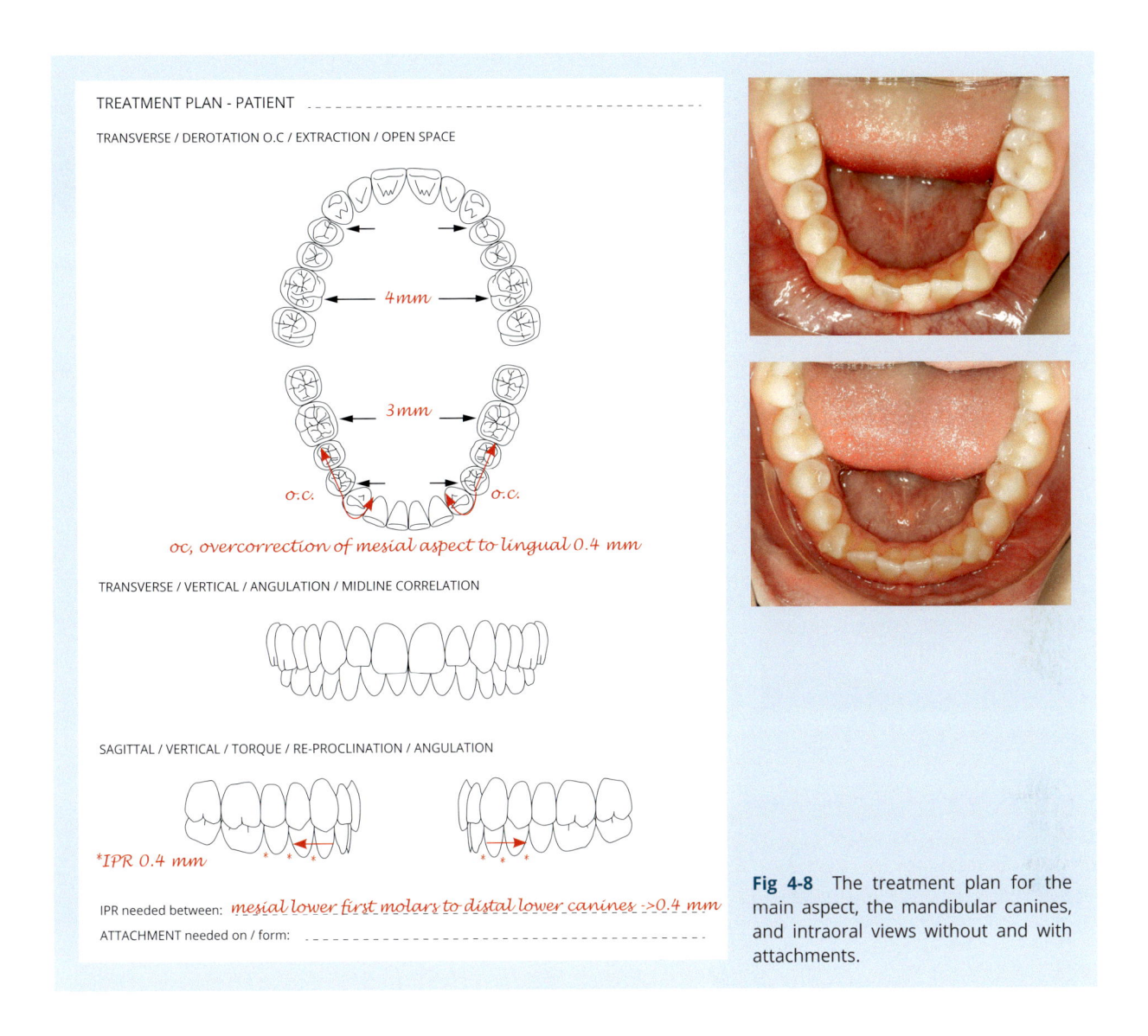

Fig 4-8 The treatment plan for the main aspect, the mandibular canines, and intraoral views without and with attachments.

canines has had a positive effect on the dentofacial esthetics. Retention was performed with a removable splint in the maxilla and a fixed retainer in the mandibular arch from canine to canine.

4 TREATMENT OF DIFFERENT MALOCCLUSIONS WITH ALIGNERS

Fig 4-9 ClinCheck software results. **(a)** The IPR checklist with 0.2 mm up to 0.5 mm on mandibular incisors, canines, and premolars to create space for alignment of canines. **(b)** The initial situation with rotated mandibular canines and crowding of mandibular anterior teeth. **(c)** Final situation with aligned mandibular arch due to expansion and IPR with derotated mandibular canines after use of 23 aligners. **(d)** Use of an additional three aligners for overcorrection and further derotation 0.4 mm of mandibular canines with mesial aspect to lingual.

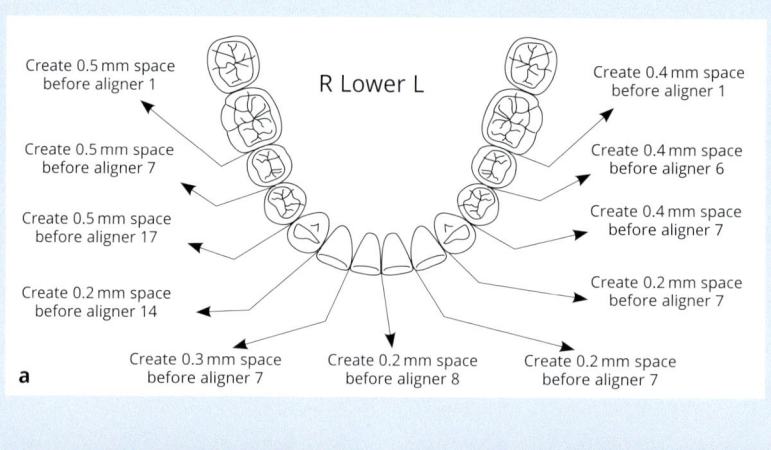

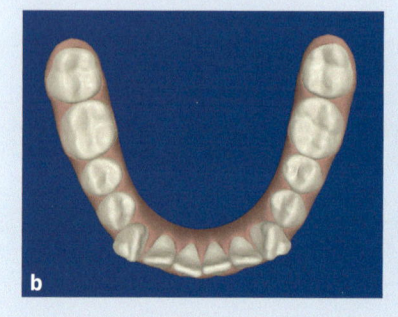

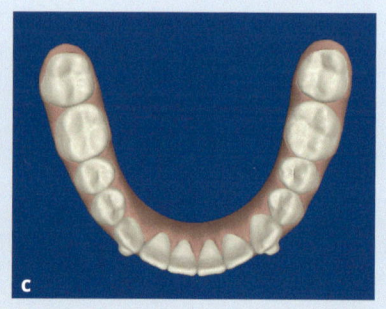

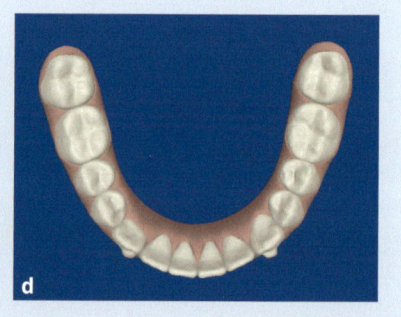

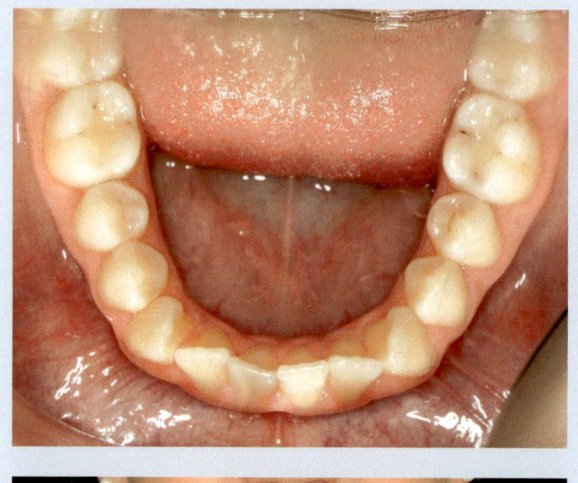

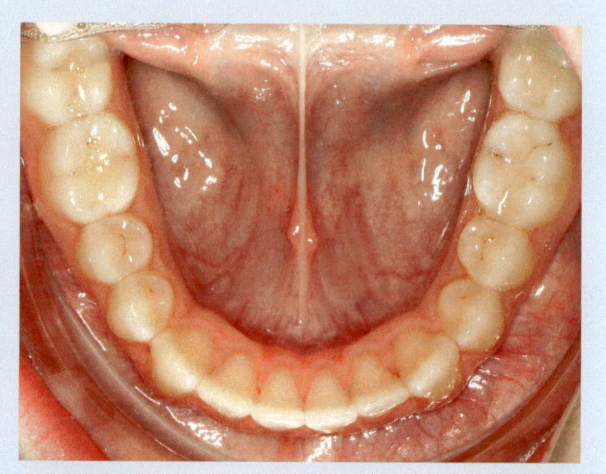

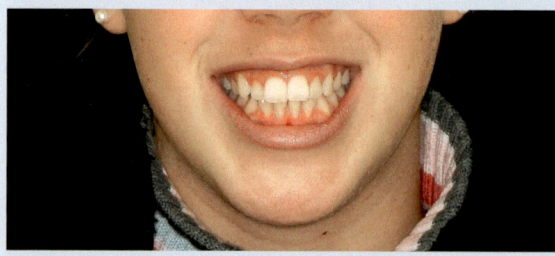

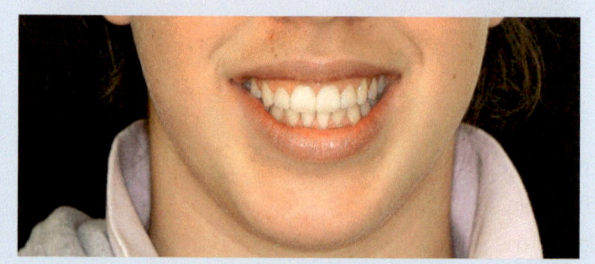

Fig 4-10 The initial **(left)** and final **(right)** intraoral and extraoral views.

Topic 3
Lingual tipped premolar, crowding and extrusion

Treatment:
- uprighting of a lingual tipped premolar
- intrusion and derotation of mandibular canines and incisors
- aligning mandibular arch

The patient showed a dental deep bite with extruded teeth 11 and 21. The dentist asked for alignment of the maxillary anteriors with maintained spaces mesial and distal of teeth 12 and 22 for later restoratives on the small laterals with veneers at later time. The patient did not show any craniomandibular (CMD) disorders.

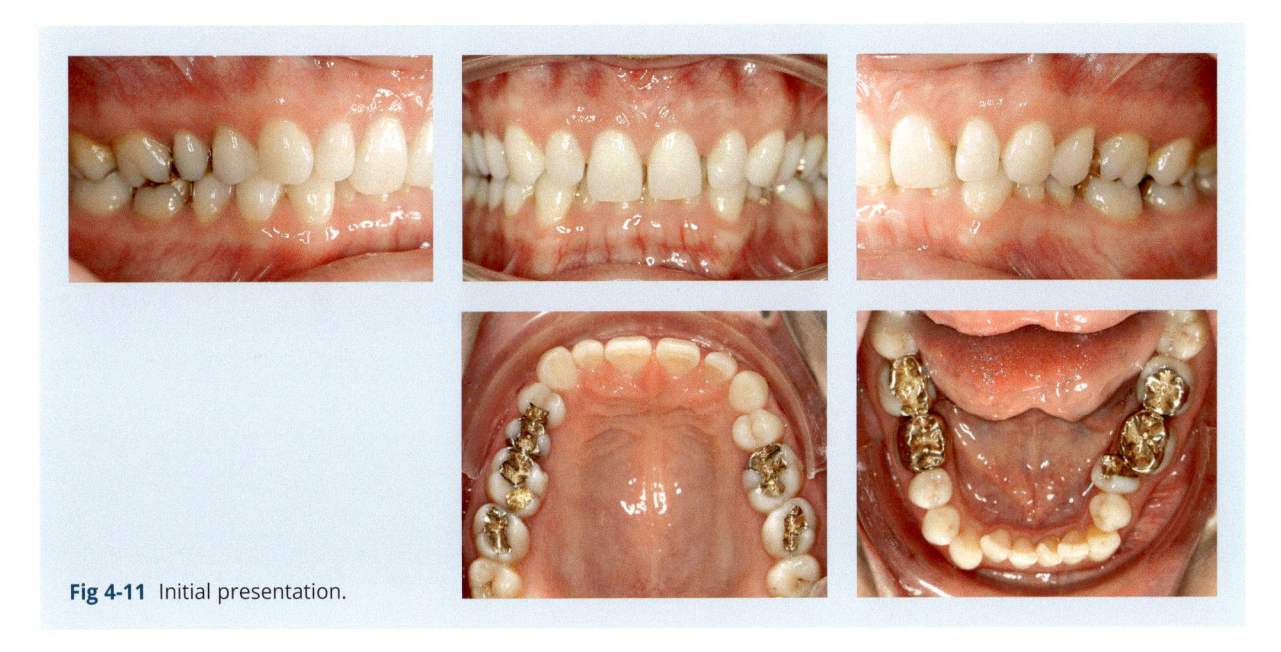

Fig 4-11 Initial presentation.

Diagnosis:
- class I relationship
- spaces in the maxillary arch
- crowding and rotations in the mandibular arch with lingually tipped tooth 35
- deep bite.

Therapy:
- alignment of both arches with maintained space mesial and distal of teeth 12 and 22 and leveling of gingival height for optimal positioning for later restoratives (veneers)
- uprighting of tooth 35
- correction of deep bite.

Treatment

The main objectives were to upright tooth 35 and correction of the severe rotation in mandibular anterior teeth.

The severity of the tipping of tooth 35 made the placement of the aligner problematic. This topic focuses on treatment in the mandibular arch, with uprighting of tooth 35 making the placement of the aligner problematic (Fig 4-12). The mandibular arch was expanded 3 mm and the mandibular incisors were proclined. Teeth 33 and 43 were derotated with an

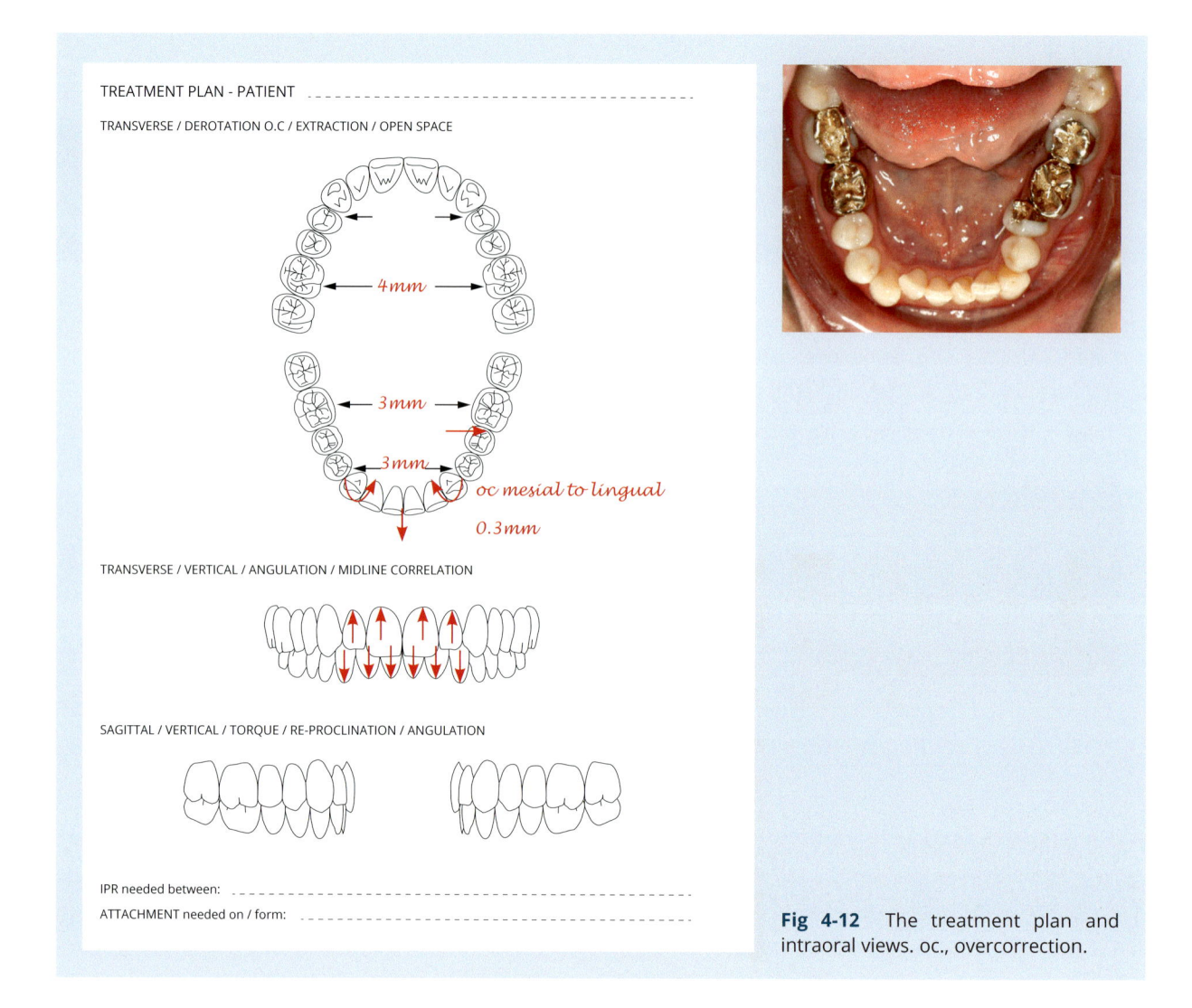

Fig 4-12 The treatment plan and intraoral views. oc., overcorrection.

overcorrection of the mesial aspect to lingual 0.3 mm. Ending with the mesial part of the mandibular canine in a more lingual position than the distal part of the lateral incisor helps to lead to better retention results.

With the endresult in mind, the finishing phases and the overcorrection were factored in at the beginning of the Invisalign planning. In corrections of crowding, care should be taken to avoid protruding the incisors and canines first and then retracting them, as might be suggested by the ClinCheck software under a protocol to obtain better access to perform IPR (Fig 4-13). This rocking forward and then backward movement should be avoided, particularly in patients with bone loss and recessions. IPR of 0.4 mm mesial of teeth 36, 35, and 34 was planned to create space for uprighting and alignment of the posterior mandibular left side. The first treatment phase included 35 aligners in the mandibular arch and 23 in the maxillary arch, follwed by a refinement phase with additional 8 upper and 11 lower aligners.

The final result showed uprighting of tooth 35 and well-aligned arch forms (Fig 4-14). The arches were aligned with expansion and IPR. Anterior recessions have not developed during treatment as care was taken to avoid excessive protrusive movements of the incisors.

Orthopantomography at the end of treatment showed no root resorption and physiologic interproximal bone (Fig 4-15).

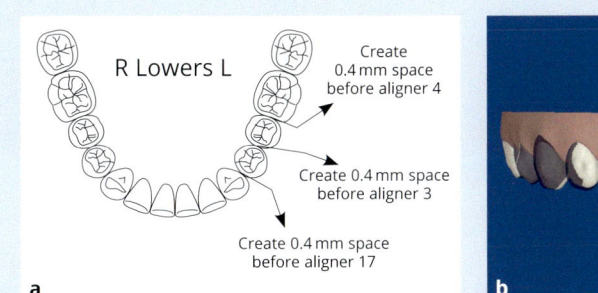

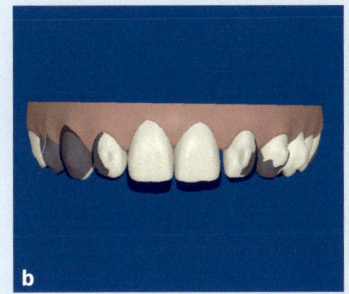

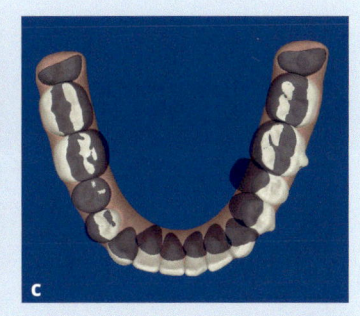

Fig 4-13 ClinCheck software results. **(a)** IPR chart. **(b)** Frontal superimposition with the planned intrusive movement of maxillary central incisors to obtain optimal gingival heights for the later restoratives. **(c)** Superimposition of the mandibular arch with uprighting of teeth 34 and 35 and proclination and alignment of mandibular anterior teeth, as well as transversal expansion of mandibular first and second molars (original tooth position in blue, planned final tooth position in white).

Fig 4-14 The final intraoral views.

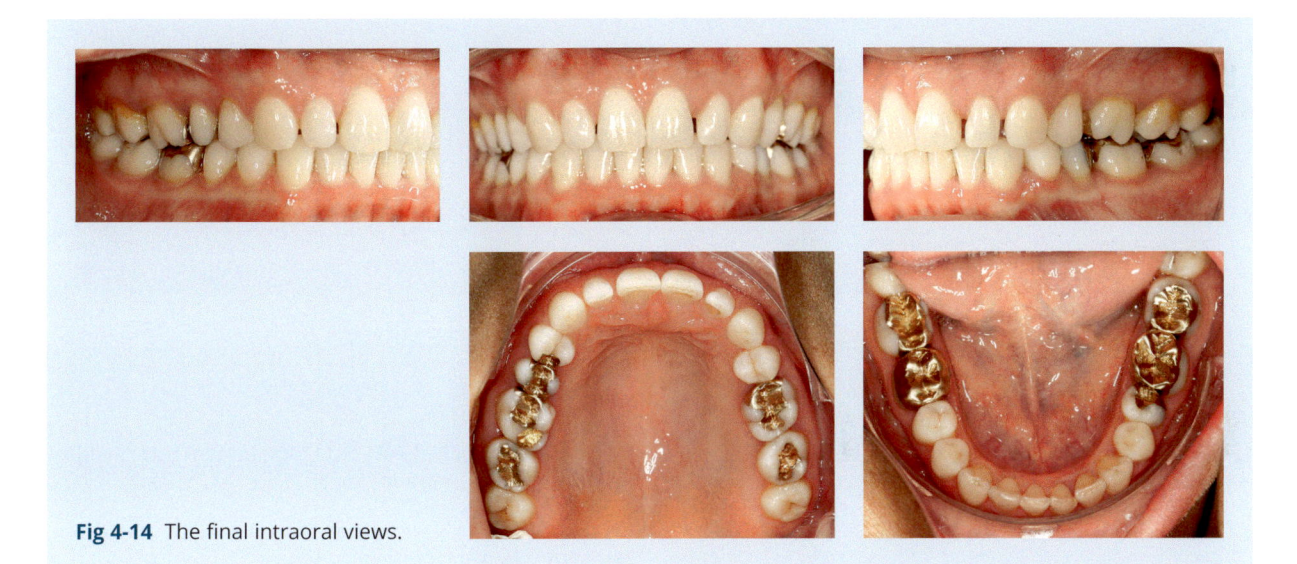

Fig 4-15 Orthopantomography, showing no root resorption and physiologic interproximal bone.

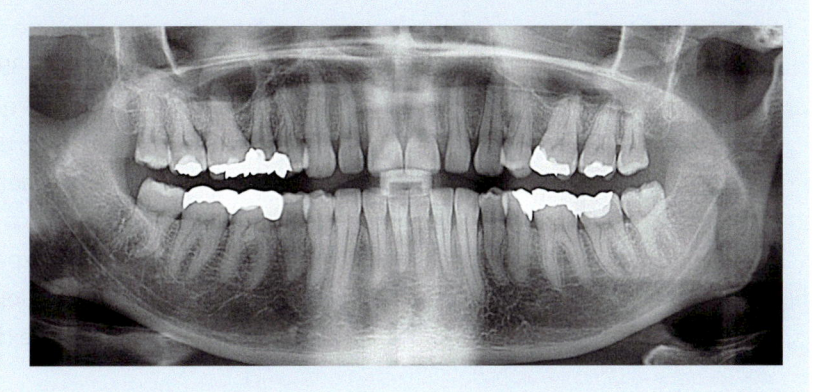

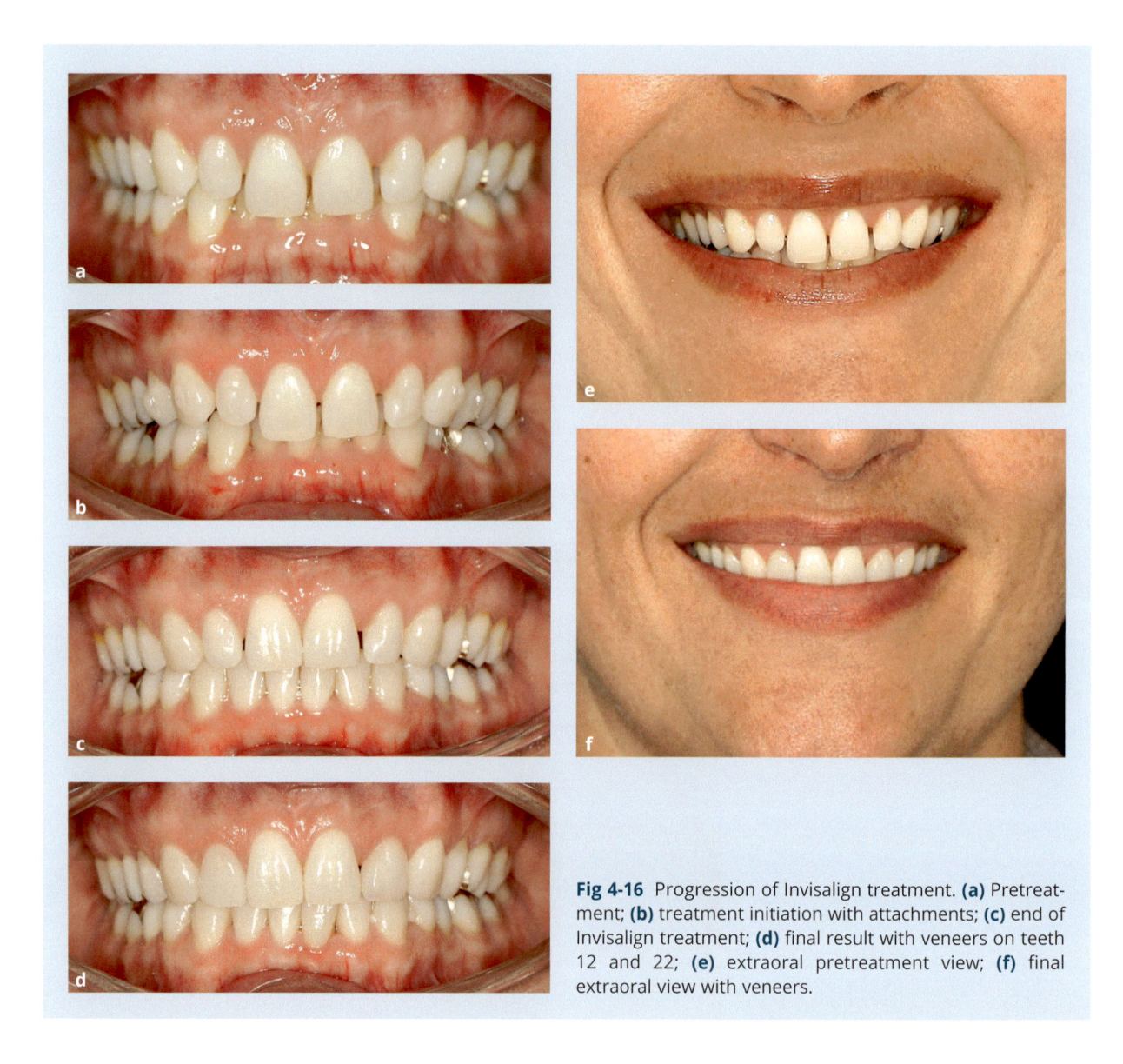

4 TREATMENT OF DIFFERENT MALOCCLUSIONS WITH ALIGNERS

Fig 4-16 Progression of Invisalign treatment. **(a)** Pretreatment; **(b)** treatment initiation with attachments; **(c)** end of Invisalign treatment; **(d)** final result with veneers on teeth 12 and 22; **(e)** extraoral pretreatment view; **(f)** final extraoral view with veneers.

Figure 4-16 shows the progression of treatment using Invisalign. The complete treatment included:
- uprighting of tooth 35
- derotation of incisors, but also of canines with mild overcorrection and premolars
- IPR on mandibular left premolars as well as on each interproximal contact from distal 33 to distal 43 in the refinement phase.
- dental deep bite correction with intrusion of teeth 11 and 21, as well as of the mandibular anterior teeth (intrusion of incisors first, then canines)
- leveling gingival heights in the maxillary anterior region to 1.5 mm deeper than the central incisors to achieve harmonious gingival position
- optimizing the positions of teeth 12 and 22 for later restoratives (veneers; planned using the ClinCheck software in interdisciplinary consultation with the dentist and dental technician at the start of treatment).

The patient was transferred to an oral surgeon for control of mucoceles.

Topic 4
Crowding

> **Treatment:**
> - expansion and solving of crowding
> - reduction of unesthetic buccal corridors

In patients with narrow arches, space can be created with expansion to solve the crowding and reduce unesthetic buccal corridors. It is important to understand that retention should be lifelong. Although expansion in the molar area is stable, that in the mandibular canines requires retention. Like Björn Zacchrisson, we prefer a mandibular 3–3 multistrand wire for fixed retention, sometimes even a 4–4 lingual retainer.

Expansion is possible in a periodontally healthy patient without recessions and buccal bone loss. To evaluate bone, cone beam computed tomography (CBCT) can be advised to show the bone in all dimensions. If expansion is needed to solve crowding because IPR is exhausted and extraction impossible (e.g. a patient who has already had premolar extraction), treatment is discussed with a periodontal surgeon to decide if a gingival graft might be necessary before or after orthodontic treatment. Staging should be slower to minimize the force from aligner to the next aligner: the best force is an intermittent force less than $0.3\ N/cm^2$. The new Smart Force material delivers a better force ratio.

This patient has had orthodontic treatment as a teenager with extraction of first premolars and he showed no signs of CMD. At the beginning of this orthodontic treatment the patient showed a root filling on tooth 16 and healthy gingiva without recessions (Figs 4-17 and 4-18).

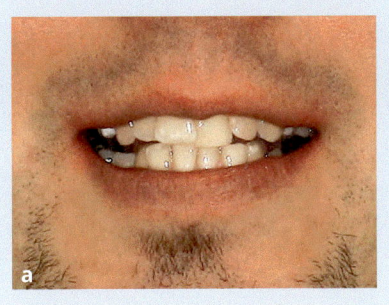

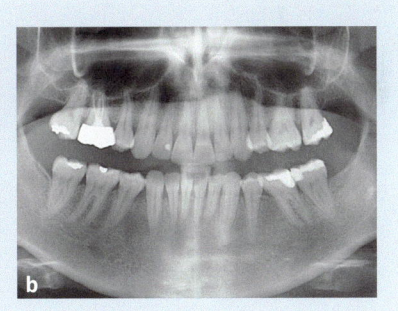

Fig 4-17 Initial presentation. **(a)** Frontal view; **(b)** orthopantomogram.

Diagnosis:
- class II
- crowding and rotations in the maxilla and mandible
- deep bite.

Therapy:
- solving of crowding and aligning of arches
- expansion.

Fig 4-18 Initial intraoral views.

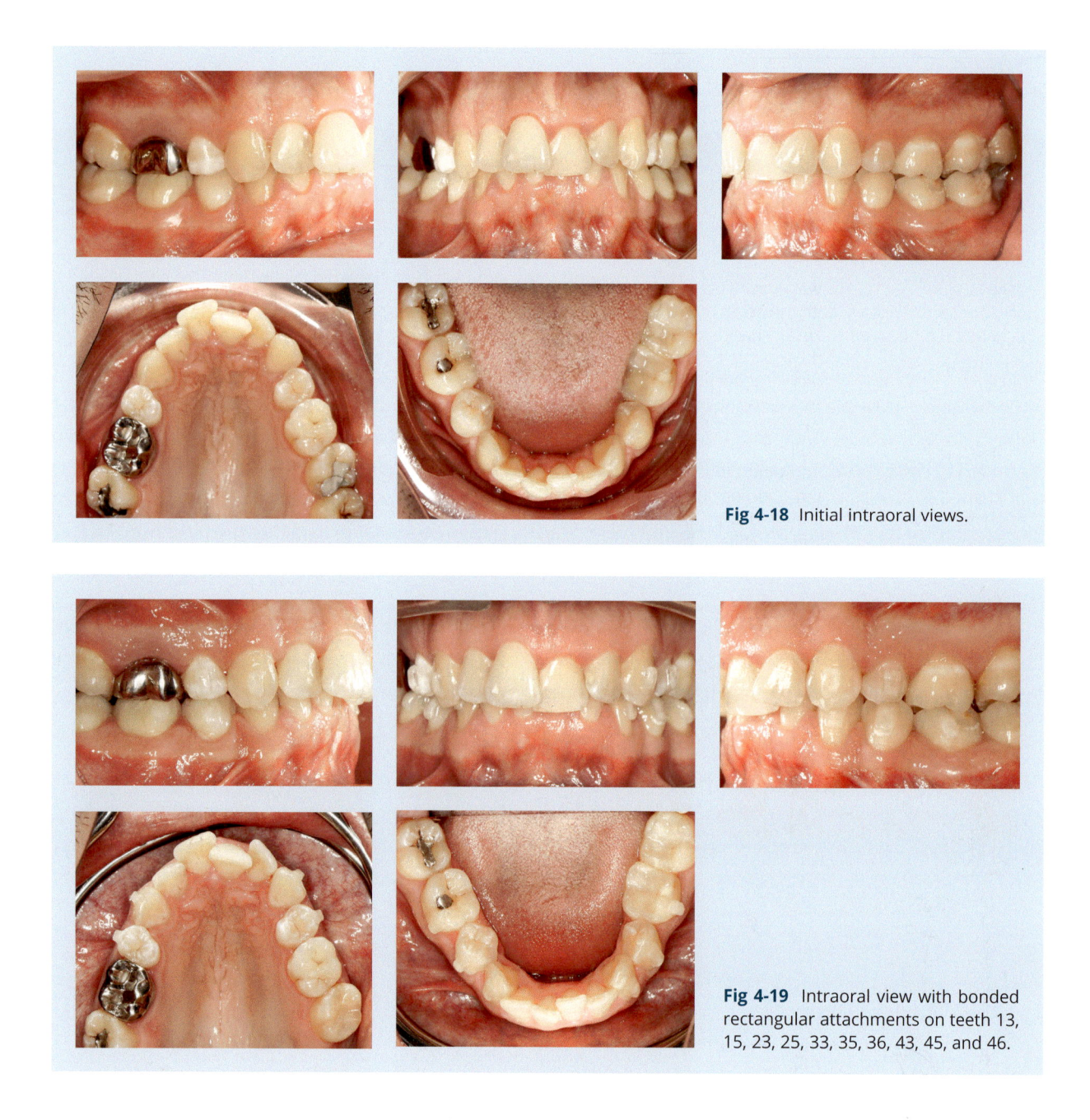

Fig 4-19 Intraoral view with bonded rectangular attachments on teeth 13, 15, 23, 25, 33, 35, 36, 43, 45, and 46.

Treatment

Because of the fragile root situation with the root filling of tooth 16, it was decided not to distalize the maxillary dentition and consequently to maintain the class II dental relationship. Healthy gingiva without recessions is the precondition for expansion in the maxillary and mandibular arches. The gingiva height showed different levels on teeth 11 and 21 and was planned to be corrected with the alignment of the maxillary anterior teeth.

Bonded rectangular attachments were placed on 10 teeth (Fig 4-19).

Fig 4-20 ClinCheck software results. **(a)** The IPR chart shows the need for 0.5 mm IPR between teeth 11 and 21 to avoid a black triangle after the alignment of the maxillary anterior teeth. **(b)** Superimposition shows the initial and final anterior view. **(c)** Superimposition of maxillary arch showing the planned amount of transversal expansion and proclination for the alignment of the maxillary arch (blue, initial tooth position; white, final tooth position).

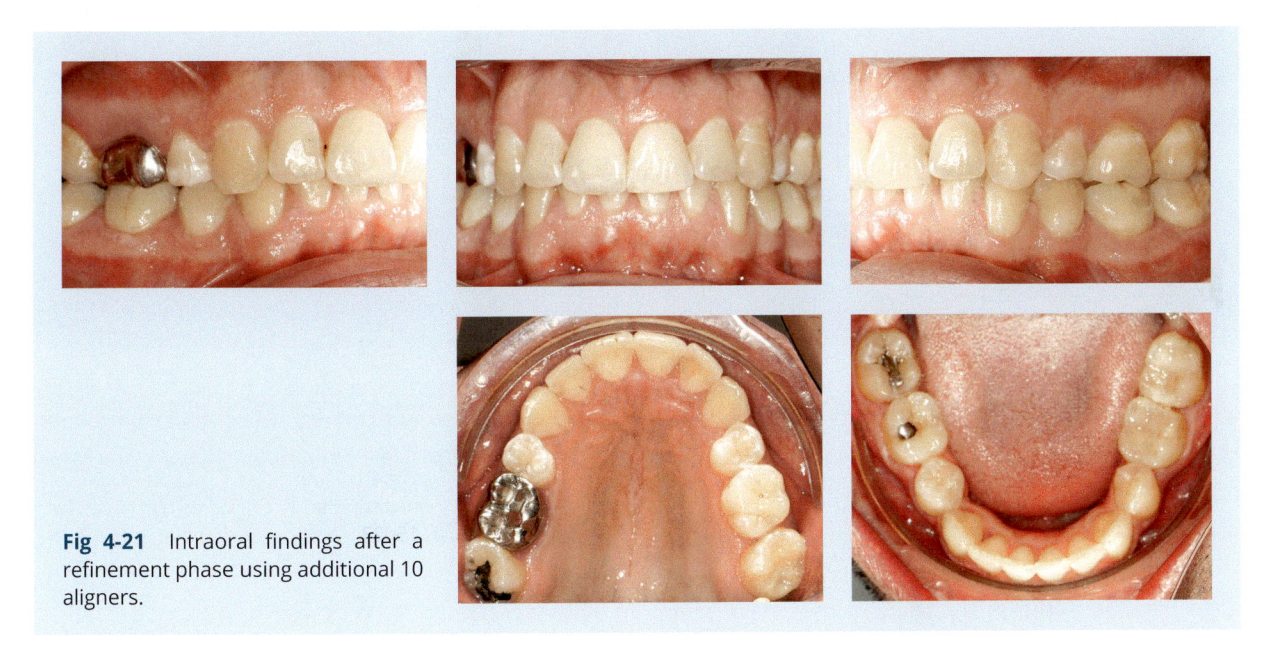

Fig 4-21 Intraoral findings after a refinement phase using additional 10 aligners.

Figure 4-20 shows the ClinCheck software results. It is advisable to overcorrect the deangulation of the maxillary central incisors with IPR to avoid opening a black triangle mesial 11 and 21; this can be done using three additional overcorrection aligners to mesialize teeth 11 and 21 using a power chain effect, which in the virtual planner can be seen to overcorrect anterior teeth mesialization. The treatment plan included 28 aligners in the maxillary arch and 20 aligners in the mandibular arch.

Figure 4-21 shows the intraoral findings after an additional refinement phase of 10 aligners at the end of treatment. Because of the expansion achieved, it was possible to solve the crowding with minimal IPR. The expansion in the formerly constricted maxillary arch led to better esthetics. At the end of orthodontic

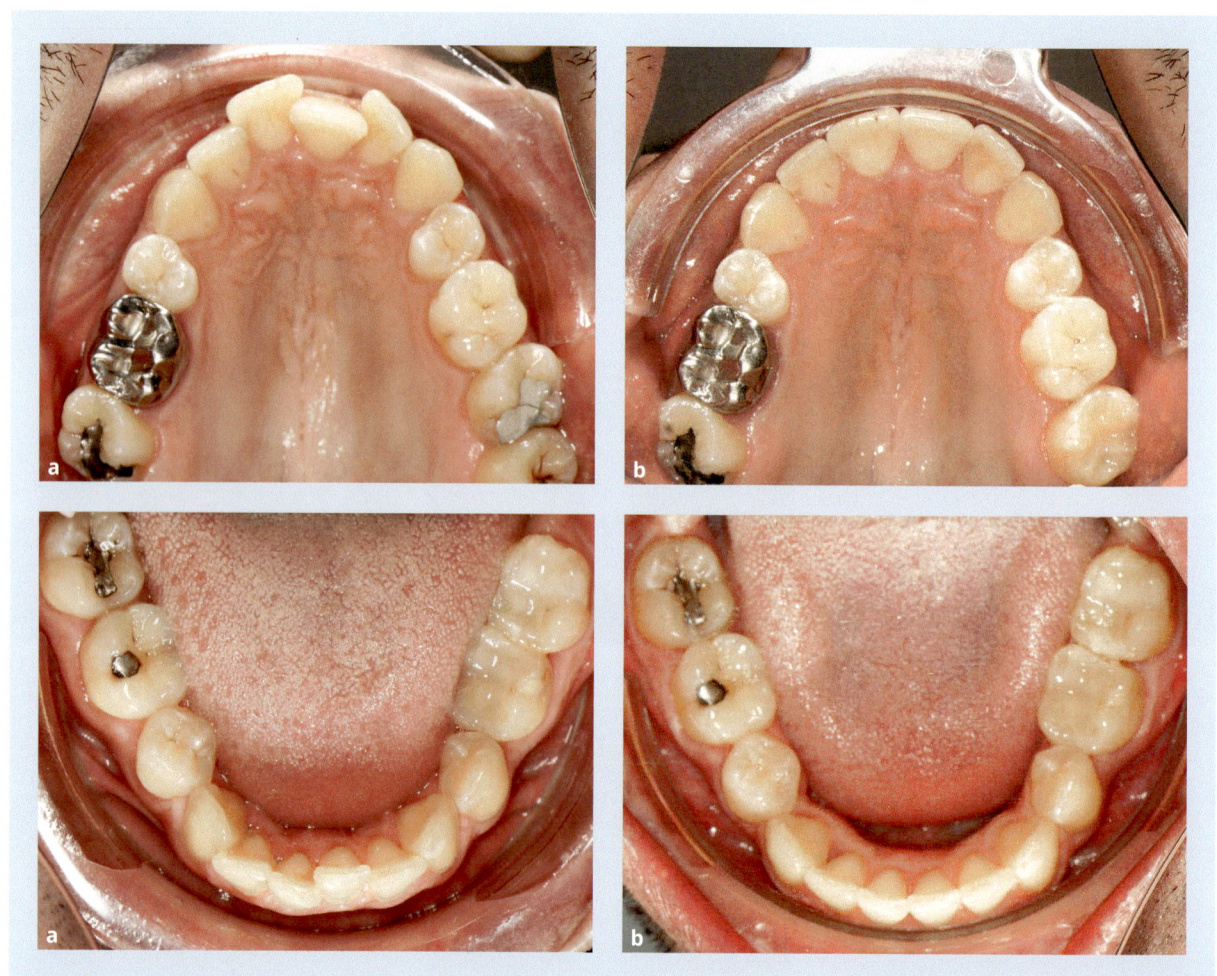

Fig 4-22 Comparison of situation before **(a)** and after **(b)** Invisalign treatment.

treatment, the patient showed healthy gingiva without recessions. The gingiva of teeth 11 and 21 is about the same height, which is important for the dentofacial esthetics.

Comparison of the situation before and after Invisalign treatment shows that both arches have been expanded and IPR had achieved harmonically aligned arches with an overcorrection of the mandibular canines (Fig 4-22). The mandibular incisors still show abrasions from the traumatizing incisor contacts before treatment. The premolars have not been completely derotated, in order to maintain the existing stable occlusion in the premolar and molar area.

Topic 5
Buccal black corridors

> **Treatment:**
> - removal of buccal black corridors
> - expansion

The buccal corridor is the space between the posterior teeth and the corner of the mouth during smiling. Buccal black corridors during smiling disturbs the dental esthetics. Displaying the first molar is ranked as the best esthetic result (Sabri, 2005). However, there are ethnic differences in preferences and a study of esthetic scoring with Korean and Japanese dental students indicated that both the Koreans and the Japanese tended to prefer broader smiles to medium or narrow smiles (Ioi and Nakata, 2009).

This patient presented with narrow maxillary and mandibular arches and crowding in the mandibular anterior teeth. When she smiled, black buccal corridors were apparent (Figs 4-23 and 4-24).

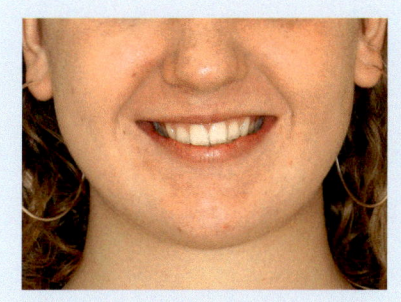

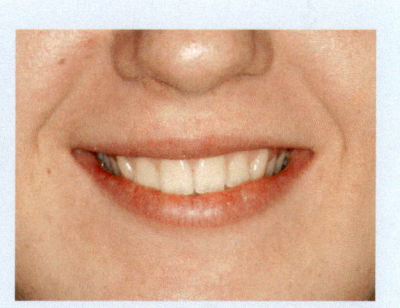

Fig 4-23 Initial presentation.

Diagnosis:
- class I
- crowding and tooth rotation in the maxillary and mandibular arches
- buccal black corridors, the maxillary teeth from canine to canine are visible but the premolars and first molars almost do not show.

Therapy:
- expansion in both arches and correction of buccal black corridors
- solving of rotations and crowding in the maxillary and mandibular arches.

4 TREATMENT OF DIFFERENT MALOCCLUSIONS WITH ALIGNERS

Fig 4-24 Intraoral views showing the narrow maxillary and mandibular arches and crowding in the mandibular anterior teeth.

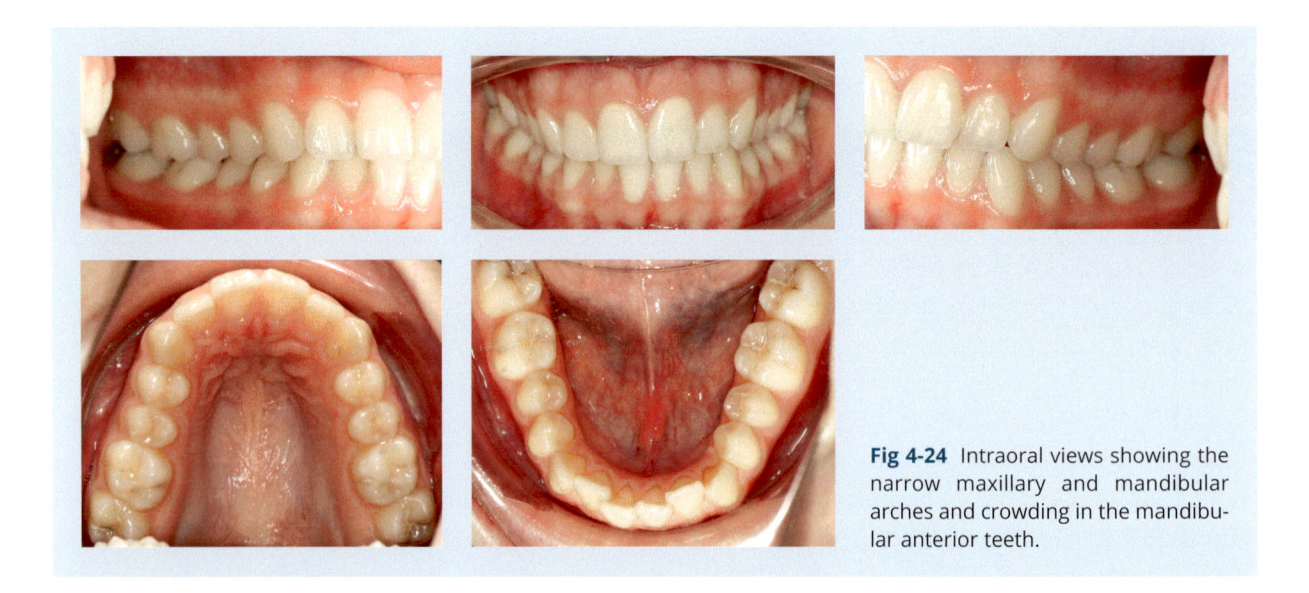

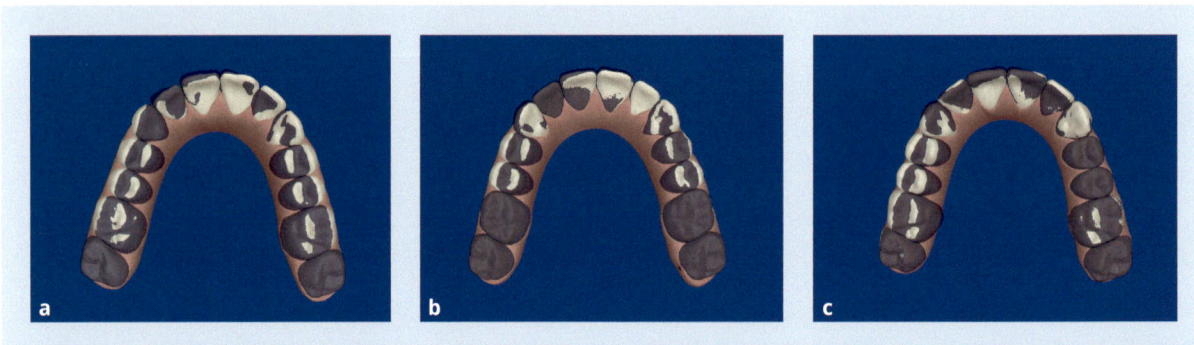

Fig 4-25 ClinCheck software results. **(a)** Superimposition of the first treatment phase in the maxillary arch. Treatment goal was the expansion of all premolars and molars for better esthetics and to reduce the buccal black corridors. **(b)** Superimposition after the first phase of treatment (11 aligners in the maxillary arch) and at the first refinement. As the expansion was not sufficient in phase 1, the refinement adddded another 10 aligners to create additional expansion in the premolar region. **(c)** Superimposition after the second refinement, showing still need for expansion to obtain optimal results.

Treatment

The main objective was to obtain a full smile and show complete teeth surfaces of teeth 16 to 26.

It was planned to upright the mandibular canines, premolars, and first molar crowns with tipping of the crowns to buccal. Expansion in the maxilla is depending on the amount of expansion in the mandibular arch. It is advantageous to plan overcorrection of the expansion from the beginning of treatment and to incorporate this into the treatment plan (Fig 4-25), using the software-enabled assessment of the effectiveness of treatment at each stage. The first phase used 11 aligners in the maxillary arch but as this did not give sufficient expansion, the plan was refined to create more expansion in the premolar region using another 10 aligners (Fig 4-25b). Even after this first refinement, transverse expansion was not sufficient and a further refinement was needed to achieve the desired planned result.

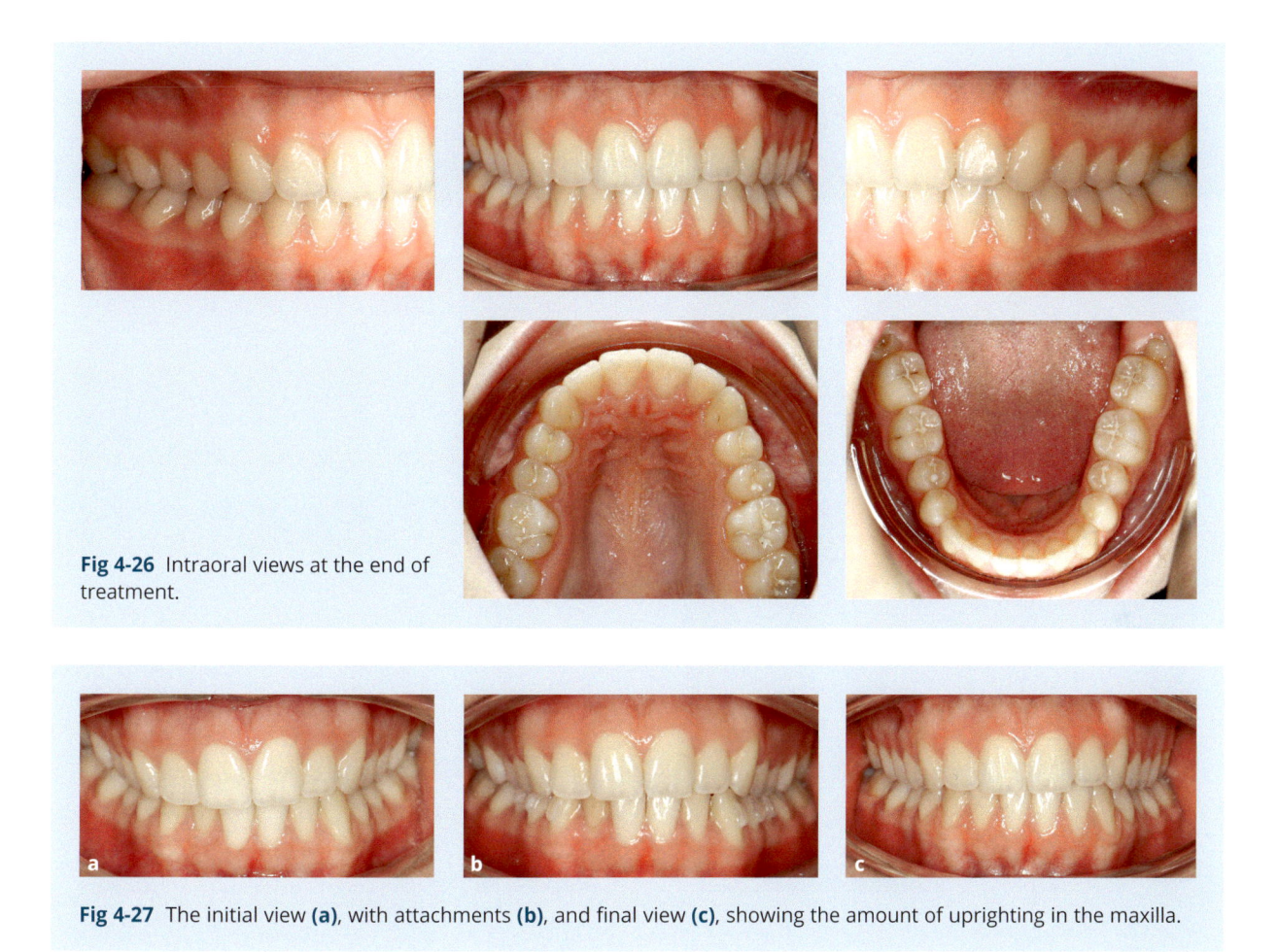

TREATMENT OF DIFFERENT MALOCCLUSIONS WITH ALIGNERS 4

Fig 4-26 Intraoral views at the end of treatment.

Fig 4-27 The initial view **(a)**, with attachments **(b)**, and final view **(c)**, showing the amount of uprighting in the maxilla.

The need for further refinements of the treatment pathway in this patient shows how important sufficient expansion right from the beginning is. At the end of the first phase, the need for a first or even second refinement should be avoided, as in this patient. Figure 4-26 shows the final intraoral views after treatment.

Now, we plan more transverse correction from the beginning because experience has shown that we usually do not achieve the total amount of expansion planned in the ClinCheck software. The course of treatment is shown in Figure 4-27.

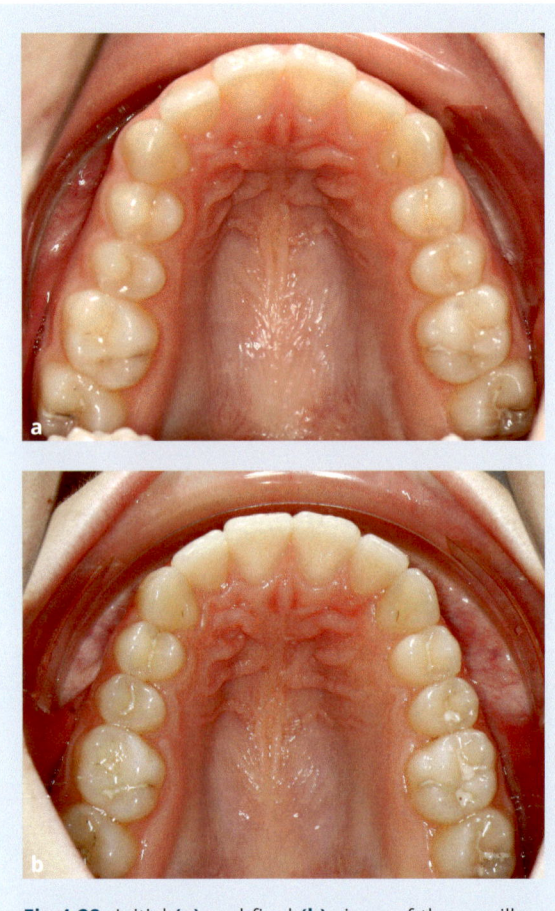

Fig 4-28 Initial **(a)** and final **(b)** views of the maxillary arch, showing expansion in the region of maxillary premolars and molars.

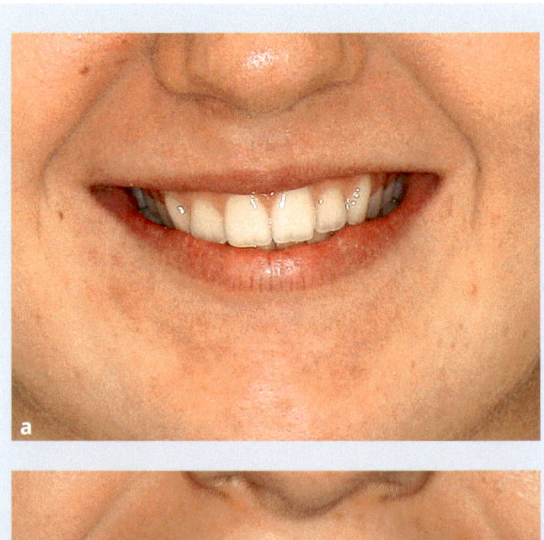

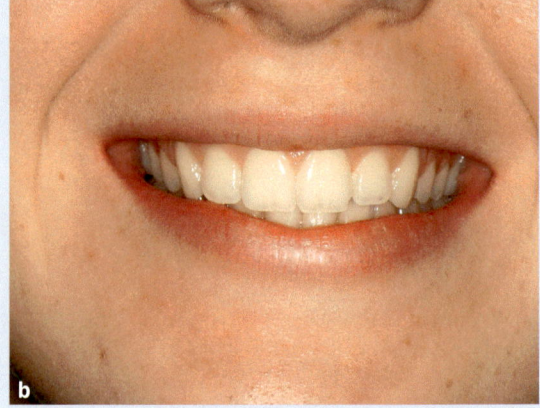

Fig 4-29 Initial **(a)** and final **(b)** views of the patient's smile, showing reduction in the buccal corridor and increased view of the buccal surfaces of the maxillary premolars and molars.

Figure 4-28 shows the changes in the maxillary arch, with considerable expansion in the premolar and molar region. The maxillary incisors have been aligned harmonically; overcorrection was planned for the derotation of the lateral incisors. Figure 4-29 shows the effect on the patient's smile, with a reduction in the buccal corridor and increased view of the buccal surfaces of the maxillary premolars and molars.

Topic 6
Closing unwanted spacing

Treatment:
- closing of spaces
- bodily movement of teeth

Space closure is one of the easiest movements to perform with the Invisalign system, as an aligner can cover the complete tooth crown because of the gaps existing between the teeth.

This patient had a large diastema between the maxillary central incisors in addition to other spacing (Fig 4-30).

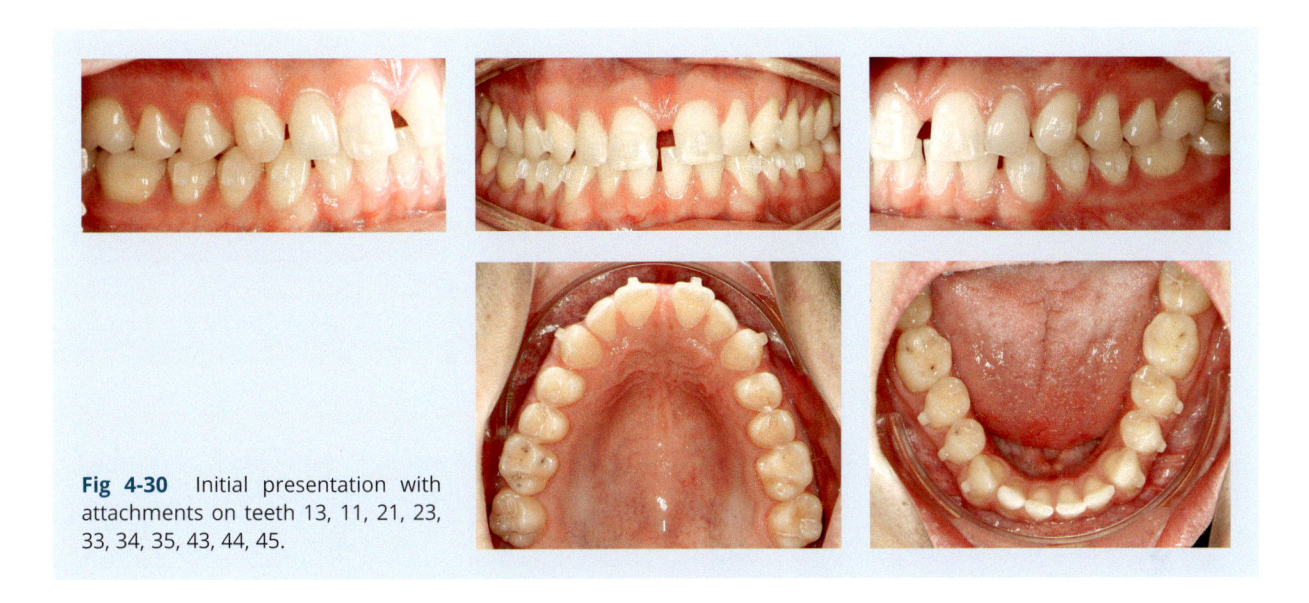

Fig 4-30 Initial presentation with attachments on teeth 13, 11, 21, 23, 33, 34, 35, 43, 44, 45.

Diagnosis:
- class I
- spaces in the maxillary and mandibular arches
- deep bite.

Therapy:
- alignment of maxillary and mandibular arches
- closure of spaces.

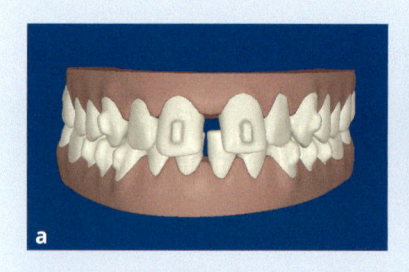

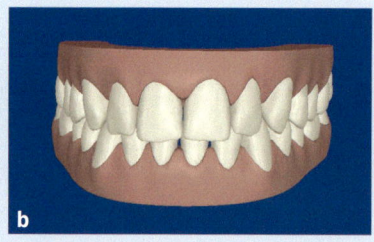

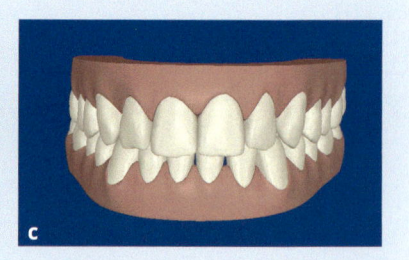

4 TREATMENT OF DIFFERENT MALOCCLUSIONS WITH ALIGNERS

Fig 4-31 ClinCheck software results. **(a)** Initial findings in anterior view with diastema mesial 11 and 21. **(b)** At the end of first phase of treatment, some diastema mesial 11 and 21 remained. Refinement of treatment added four more aligners in the maxillary and mandibular arches to close the diastema completely. **(c)** Final findings with complete closure of diastema mesial 11 and 21.

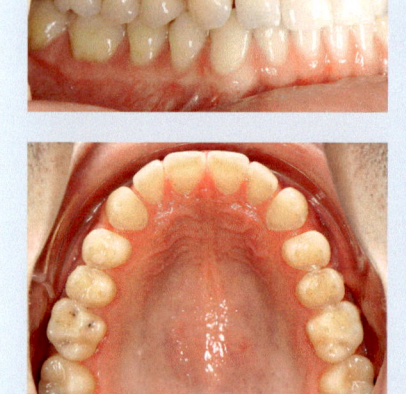

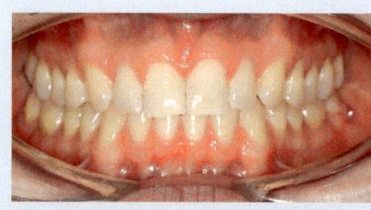

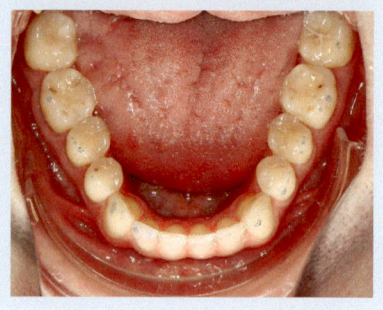

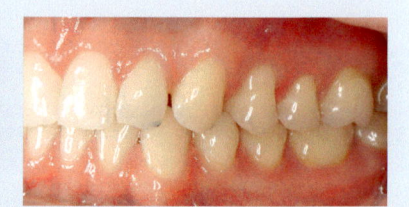

Fig 4-32 Intraoral views showing perfect space closure of teeth 11 and 21. Static occlusal contact points are marked in blue. All canines, premolars, and molars demonstrate full occlusal contact.

Treatment

The main objective was the closure of spaces to improve esthetics.

Invisalign treatment used rectangular attachments (nowadays G 4 optimized attachments can be used), which help to transfer optimal forces onto the tooth and to obtain even more predictable tooth movements. Figure 4-31 shows the ClinCheck software results. The maxillary and mandibular arches were treated with 15 aligners in the first phase. As some diastema mesial 11 and 21 remained, four more aligners were added to refine the treatment. To avoid having spaces remaining at the end of treatment, it is advisable to use overcorrection for space closure right from the beginning.

Final views (Figs 4-32 to 4-34) show perfect space closure of teeth 11 and 21. Due to Bolton discrepancy, spaces were maintained on canines which can be closed with restoratives later on. The refinement to the treatment plan asked for space closure with power chain effect, which overcorrects the anterior teeth mesialization virtually with overlapping approximal surfaces.

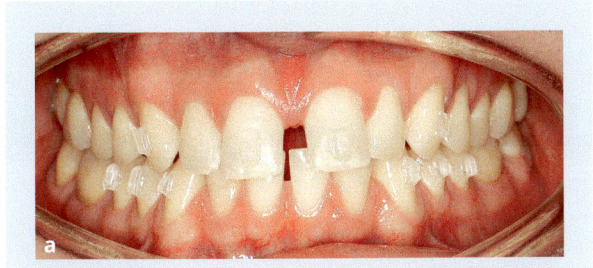

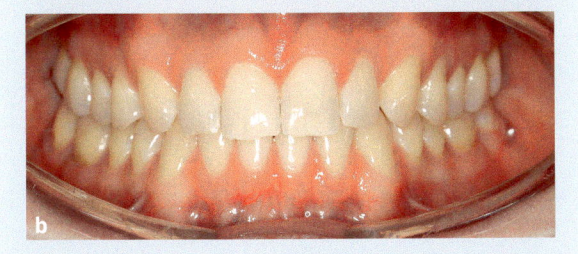

TREATMENT OF DIFFERENT MALOCCLUSIONS WITH ALIGNERS 4

Fig 4-33 Initial (a) and final (b) anterior views. Both arches have been aligned and space closure was performed with bodily tooth movement.

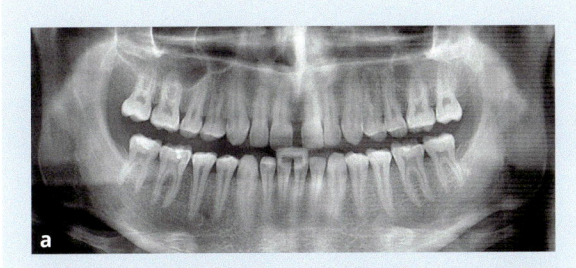

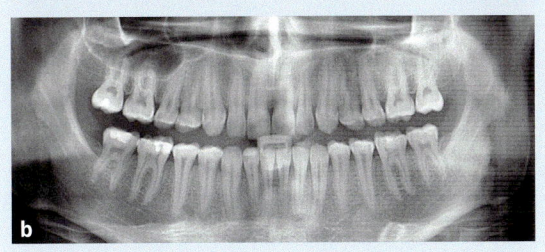

Fig 4-34 Initial (a) and final (b) orthopantomograms showing the bodily movement involved in space closure.

4 TREATMENT OF DIFFERENT MALOCCLUSIONS WITH ALIGNERS

Topic 7
Spacing with periodontitis and bone loss

Treatment:
- bodily movement with slow staging
- myofunctional therapy
- periodontal pretreatment

The optimum of orthodontic force lies between 0.2 and 0.3 N/cm². Particularly in patients with periodontal disease and bone loss, the orthodontic force should be small and well controlled. The Invisalign system offers the possibility of reducing forces for every tooth movement, or for a single tooth showing reduced periodontal bone. Forces can be reduced by increasing the number of aligners and asking for slower staging, which reduces the force from one aligner to another. In every case, periodontal treatment needs to be successfully accomplished before orthodontic treatment can begin. During the orthodontic treatment, the patient should remain closely monitored periodontally.

This patient presented needing space closure but had severe bone loss in both arches (Fig 4-35). Initial radiography and CBCT showed the degree of bone loss (Fig 4-36).

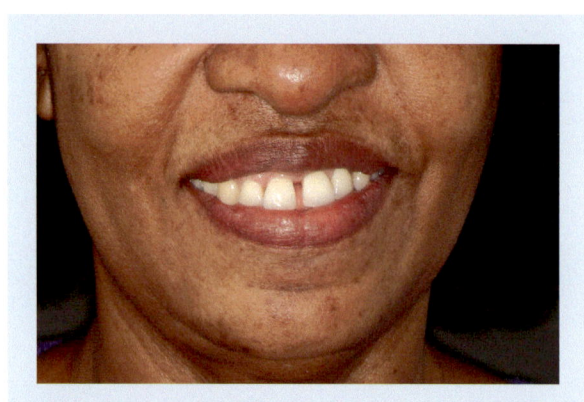

Fig 4-35 Initial presentation.

Diagnosis:
- severe bone loss in the maxilla and mandible
- spaces in the maxillary and mandibular arches
- dental open bite.

Interdisciplinary therapy:
- periodontal treatment and myofunctional therapy
- Invisalign treatment accompanied by periodontal recall.

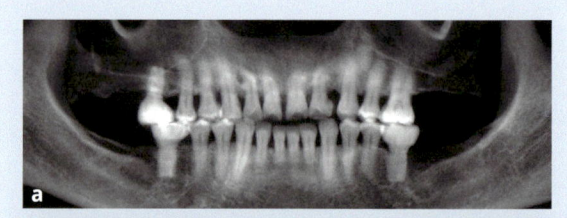

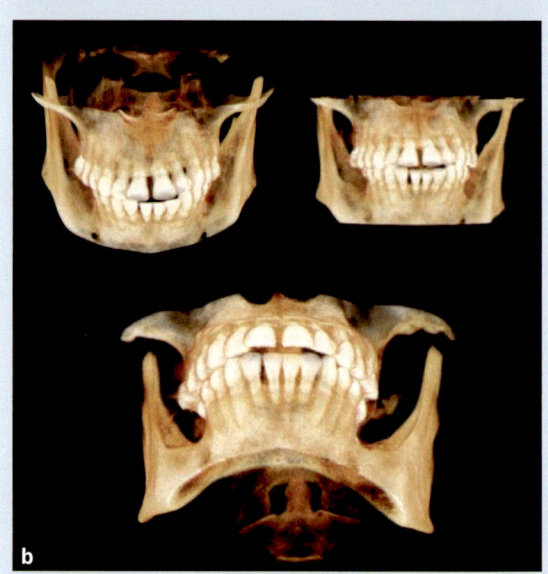

Fig 4-36 Severe bone loss. **(a)** Orthopantomogram; **(b)** CBCT (Picasso, Orange Dental), transferred into the Invivo Software (Anatomage).

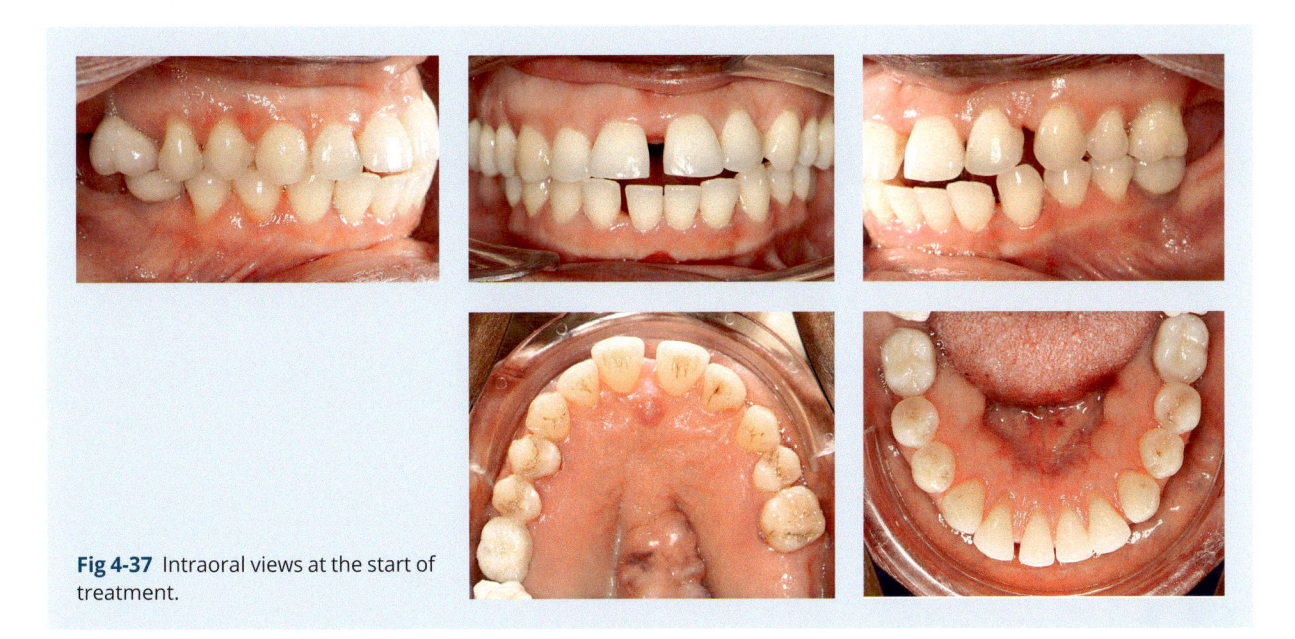

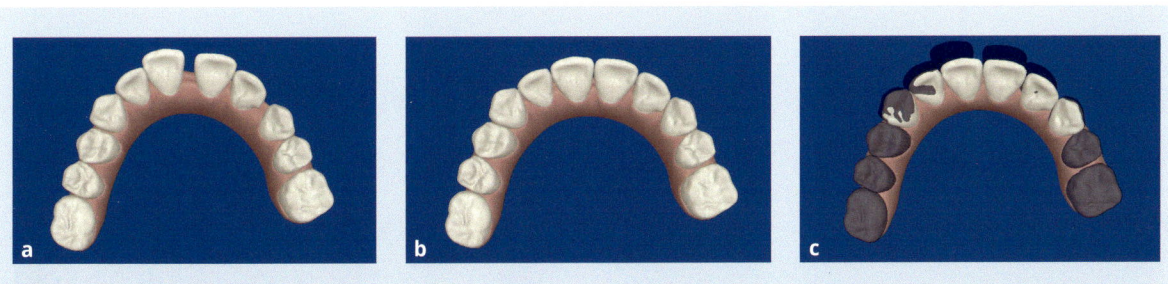

TREATMENT OF DIFFERENT MALOCCLUSIONS WITH ALIGNERS 4

Fig 4-37 Intraoral views at the start of treatment.

Fig 4-38 ClinCheck software results. **(a)** Initial findings for the maxillary arch. Because of the patient's periodontal situation, a large number of aligners (30) were used for very slow staging. **(b)** The situation at the end of treatment after retraction of the maxillary anterior teeth and closure of all spaces. **(c)** Superimposition showing the amount of planned retraction and space closure (blue, initial tooth position; white, final tooth position).

Treatment plan

The main objectives were the initial treatment of periodontitis, myofunctional therapy to adjust tongue dysfunction, and space closure with minimized orthodontic forces.

The patient was pretreated by a periodontal specialist to ensure that Invisalign treatment started in a healthy periodontal situation (Fig 4-37). The patient was also advised to undergo myofunctional therapy to deal with her tongue dysfunction.

Treatment was designed with 30 aligners, which is twice the number normally used. In the online treatment plan, this was called "staging ×2." During Invisalign treatment, the patient has to remove the aligners for eating and tooth cleaning. This leads to an interruption of the applied aligner force, making the treatment an intermittent force system. Figure 4-38 shows the ClinCheck software results.

Fig 4-39 Views at the end of treatment.

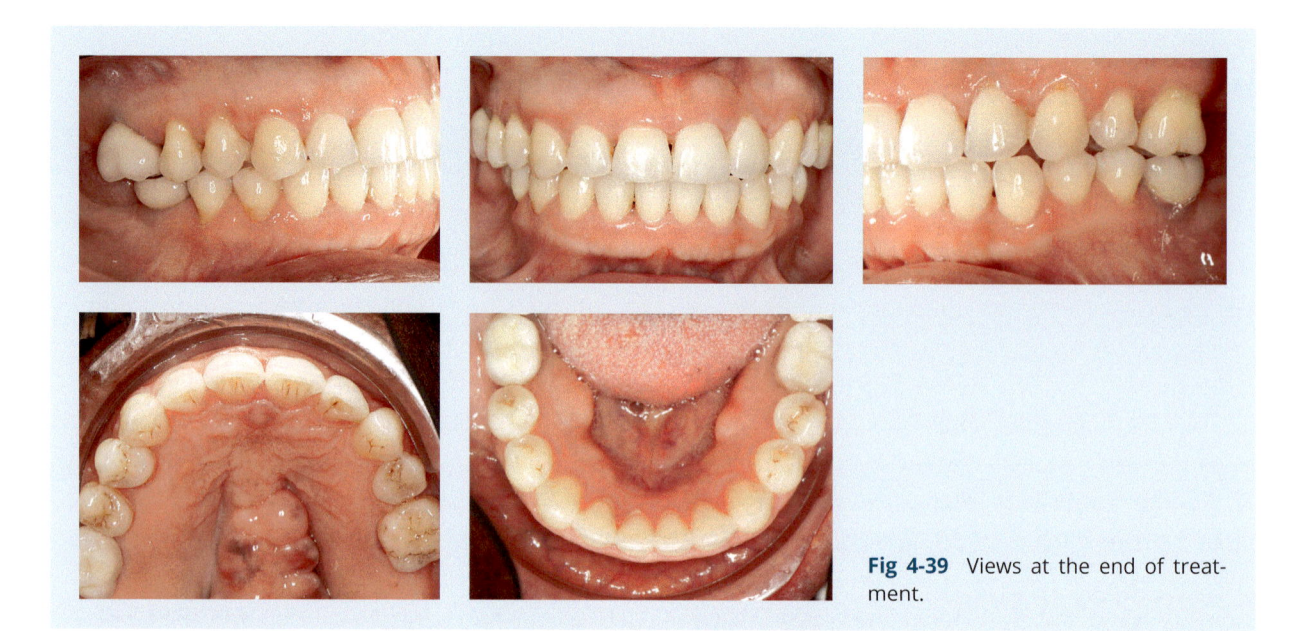

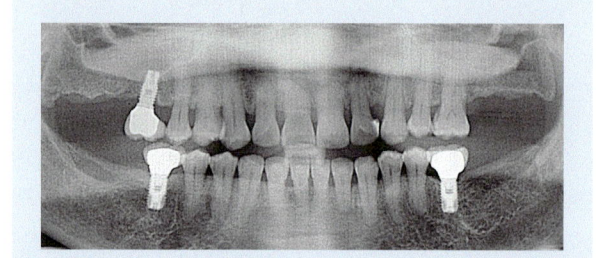

Fig 4-40 Final digital orthopantomogram showing stable bone.

At the end of treatment, the patient had space closure and a stable healthy periodontal situation (Fig 4-39). The periodontal recall was easy to organize, as with Invisalign treatments there is no need to remove and religate archwires or ligatures before or after professional oral hygiene (as needed with fixed appliance treatment).

The final digital orthopantomogram shows the stable bone situation (Fig 4-40).

Comparison of the extraoral views before and after treatment shows the maxillary curve of the dentition following exactly the curve of the lower lip. The gummy smile had been reduced and there is an esthetic maxillary arch with parallel orientation of the maxillary incisors (Fig 4-41).

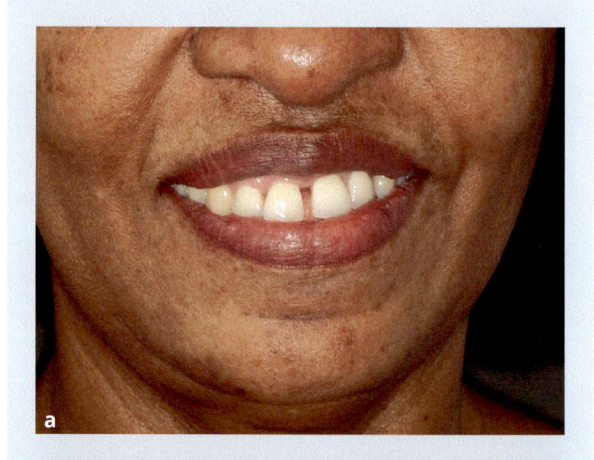

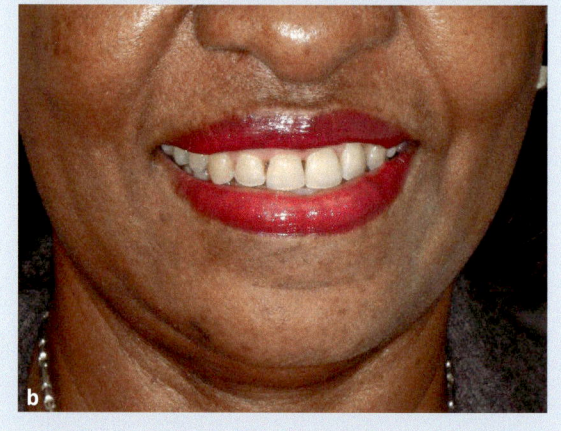

Fig 4-41 The initial **(a)** and final **(b)** extraoral views.

Topic 8
Bone and periodontium: General considerations

Treatment:
- transversal bone remodeling
- bone and papilla remodeling

The biochemic response to an orthodontic force is an extremely complicated and yet largely unexplored process (Yasuda, 2006). The periodontal ligament, consisting of Sharpey fibers and cells of the alveolar bone, converts mechanical force into molecular activity and thus into orthodontic tooth movement (Masella and Meister, 2006). If, over an extended period of more than 18 days, an orthodontic force of 0.15–0.2 N/cm^2 is applied, an inflammatory process is initiated in the periodontal ligament, leading to tooth movement via resorption in the bone. Sterile inflammation, therefore, forms the basis of every orthodontic tooth movement. Optimum orthodontic force is between 0.2 and 0.3 N/cm^2 root surface. The force should always be less than the capillary blood pressure, which is 0.20–0.26 N/cm^2. Under this pressure, blood vessels remain open, cells continue to be adequately supplied with blood, and bone modeling can occur. If the force becomes too large, tooth movement will stop as physiologic resorption cannot take place. In this case, only hyalinization occurs. Hyalinization comprises disappearance of connective tissue cells and osteoclasts, which can lead to severe tooth loosening and root resorption. The continuous forces arising from fixed appliances have more side effects than seen with the intermittent forces occurring in removable appliance therapy (Knak, 2004). Nakao et al (2007) investigated molecular mechanisms in human periodontal ligament after continuous or intermittent force application. Intermittent forces led to less cell destruction than continuous orthodontic forces, as indicated by lactate dehydrogenase release. Intermittent forces can initiate production of receptor activator of NF-kb ligand (RANKL) and its receptor RANK, which have a role in osteoclastogenesis in periodontal disease, in the periodontal ligament more effectively than continuous forces.

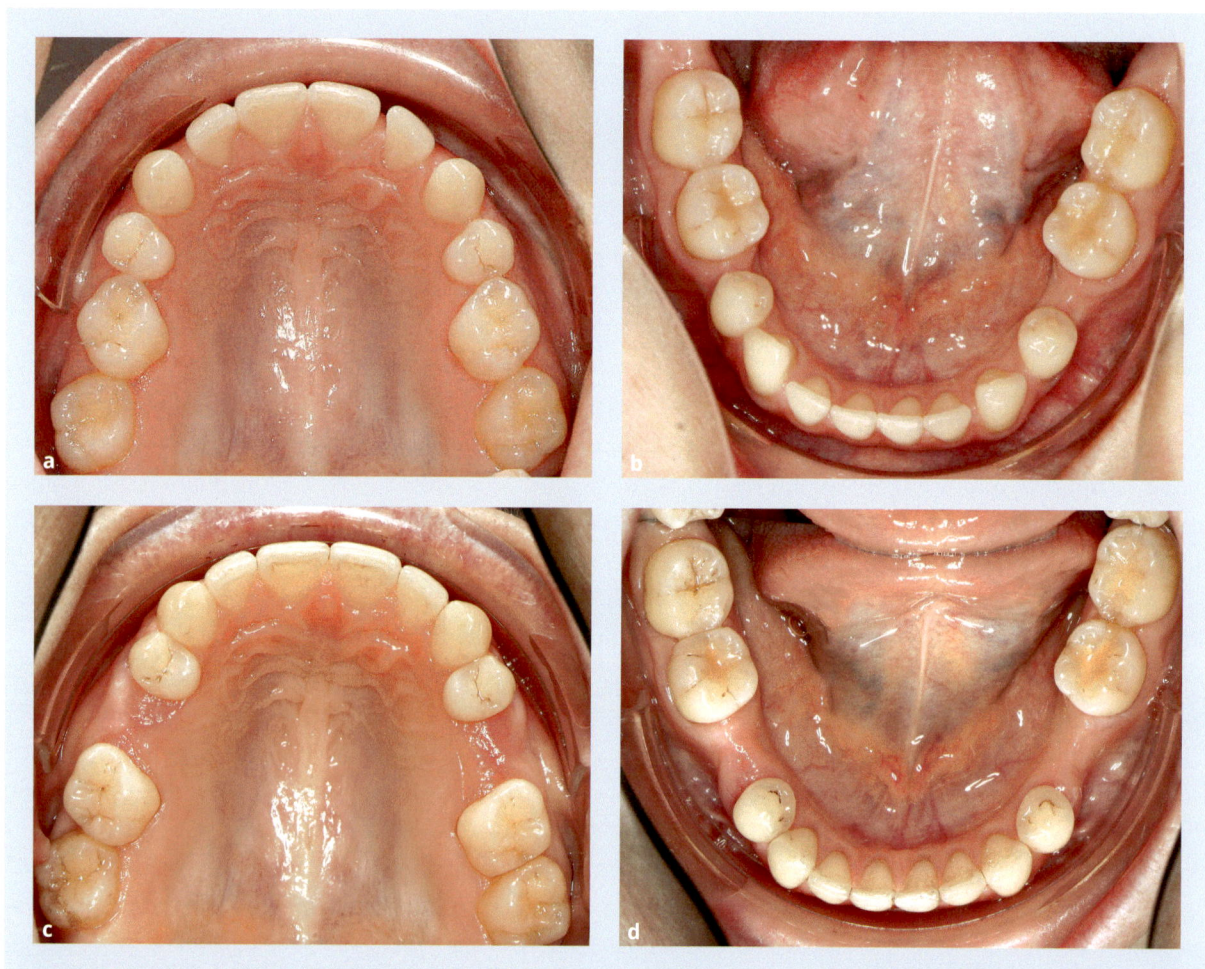

Fig 4-42 A patient with spaces after loss of teeth 15, 25, 35, and 45 and migration of neighbored teeth into the spaces. **(a,b)** Before treatment. **(c,d)** Orthodontic Invisalign treatment opened spaces for the insertion of implants in regions 15, 25, 35, and 45.

Transversal bone remodeling

With a movement of a tooth, new bone develops (Zachrisson, 2009).

Figures 4-42 and 4-43 show a patient after loss of teeth 15, 25, 35, and 45 and migration of the neighbored teeth into the spaces.

Bone and papilla remodeling

Interdisciplinary therapy is required in patients with reduced periodontal support. Figure 4-44 shows a patient with a severely reduced periodontal situation and extruded tooth 22. The periodontist sent the patient for orthodontic treatment to manage the space 21/22 and to intrude and retract maxillary incisors to obtain greater support of bone and gingiva.

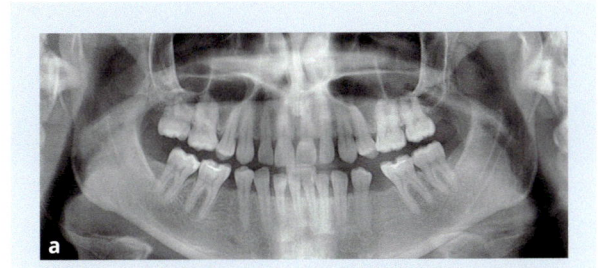

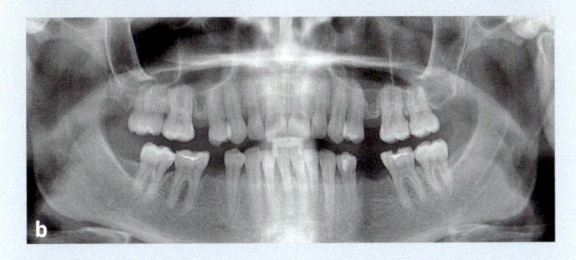

Fig 4-43 Orthopantomography. **(a)** Initial view showing tipping of the premolars and molars into the space left by loss of the second premolars. **(b)** After uprighting and mesialization of the neighboring teeth, there is sufficient alveolar bone for insertion of implants.

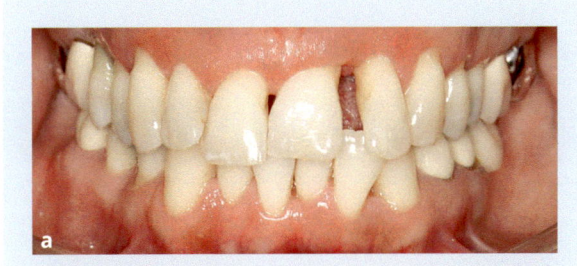

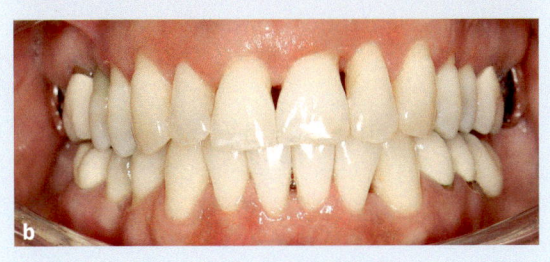

Fig 4-44 Severely reduced periodontal state and extruded tooth 22. **(a)** Before orthodontic treatment to manage the space 21/22 and to intrude and retract maxillary incisors. **(b)** After Invisalign treatment, there is improved esthetic appearance and increased bone support and papilla in region 21/22.

Topic 9
Missing maxillary lateral incisors

Treatment:
- space closure
- combination of Frankel and Invisalign treatment
- later restoratives on maxillary incisors and canines

In growing patients with skeletal class II relationship, a functional appliance is normally used; for most we use the Frankel appliance. However, in a large percentage, orthodontic finishing is required, which traditionally was with a fixed appliance. The problem is that teenagers usually do not like fixed appliances and very often their oral hygiene is not good enough for fixed appliances, thus risking white spot lesions and decalcifications. Invisalign offers the possibility to finish orthodontic treatment with a minimal invasive treatment option, allowing optimal oral hygiene. For this reason we now prefer to treat these patients with Invisalign Teen instead of fixed multibracket appliances.

This patient had class II occlusion and a dental deep overbite, with biting of the mandibular incisors into the upper palatinal gingiva, because of the extent of the overbite (Fig 4-45).

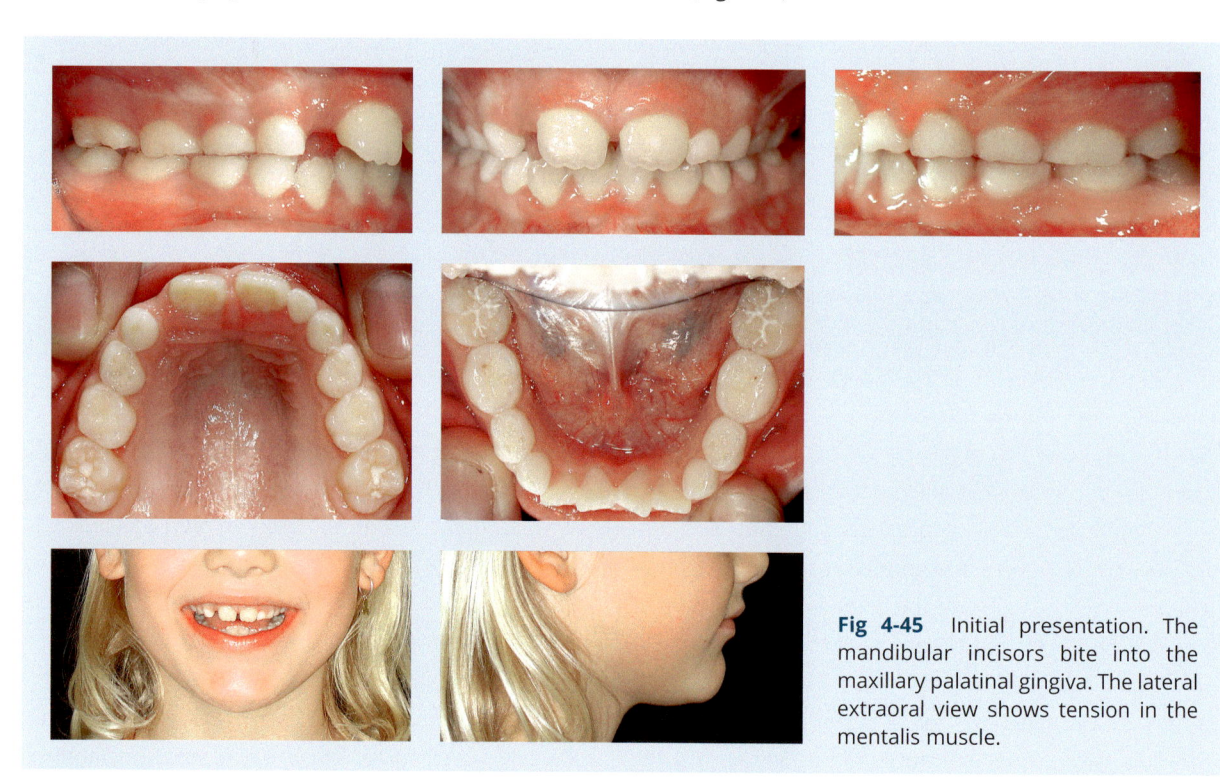

Fig 4-45 Initial presentation. The mandibular incisors bite into the maxillary palatinal gingiva. The lateral extraoral view shows tension in the mentalis muscle.

Diagnosis:
- class II
- deep bite
- missing teeth 12 and 22.

Therapy:
- Frankel appliance
- Invisalign system
- reshaping of teeth 13 and 23 with composite resin.

Fig 4-46 At the end of the functional treatment phase, showing the mesial position of canines.

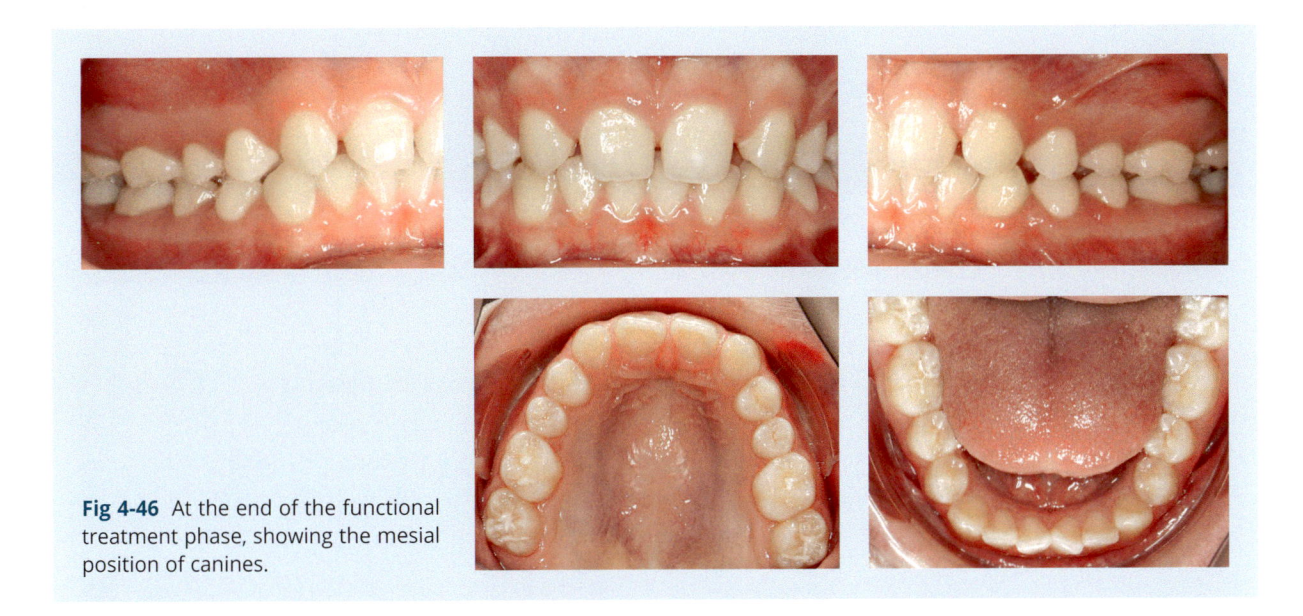

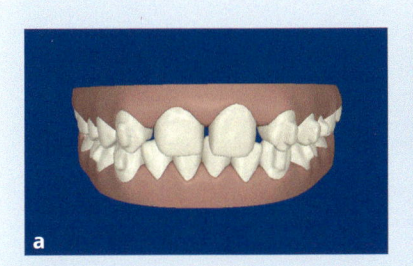

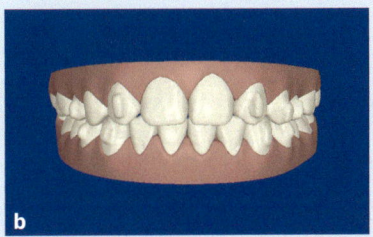

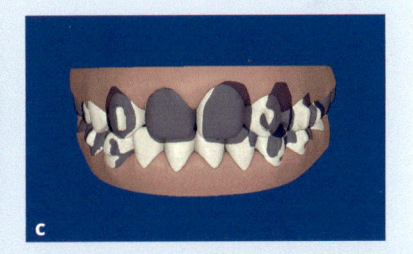

Fig 4-47 ClinCheck software results. **(a)** Initial situation with missing maxillary lateral incisors and diastema and spaces in the maxillary anterior region. **(b)** Final planned ClinCheck situation with space closure and optimal position of teeth 13 and 23 for later restoratives. **(c)** Superimposition showing the amount of retraction and mesialization of maxillary anterior teeth (blue, initial tooth position; white, final tooth position).

Treatment

At the end of the functional treatment phase using the Frankel appliance, the overbite was improved and the maxillary canines were in a good, but not perfect, position (Fig 4-46). Jointly with the dentist, it was decided to mesialize the maxillary canines into the position of the missing maxillary lateral incisors and to reshape them after orthodontics for a better esthetic result. There was mild crowding in the mandibular arch.

The treatment plan asked for rectangular attachments on all the maxillary teeth requiring mesialization. Treatment in the mandibular arch started with rectangular attachments on 33, 34, 43, and 44 for derotation (Fig 4-47). The treatment used 21 aligners in the maxillary arch and 12 in the mandibular arch.

Figure 4-48 shows the intraoral findings after alignment of both arches and closure of spaces in the maxillary arch. The canines are in an optimal position for the reshaping and restorative phase.

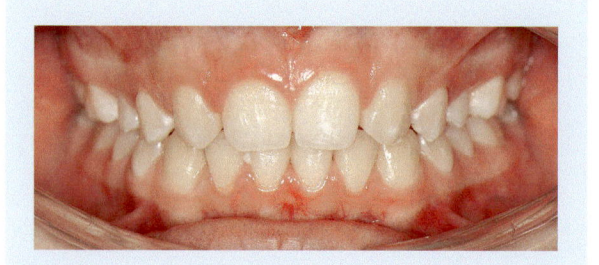

Fig 4-48 Intraoral findings after alignment of both arches and closure of spaces in the maxillary arch. The canines are in an optimal position for reshaping and restoratives to substitute the missing teeth 12 and 22.

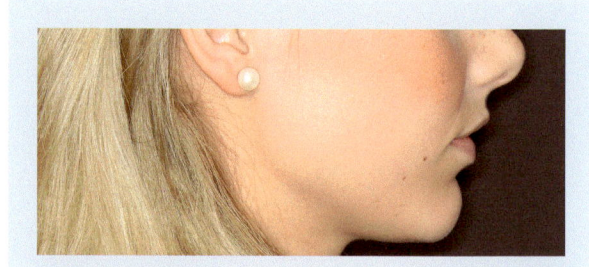

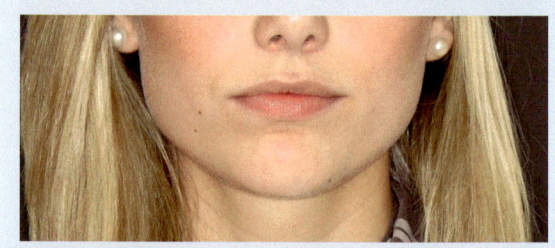

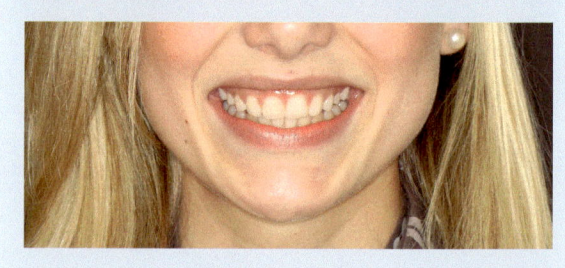

Fig 4-49 External views after reshaping of teeth 13 and 23, showing the improved dental esthetics. (Reshaping of teeth 14, 13, 11, 21, 23, and 24 was performed by Dr Boisserée (Cologne, Germany) with Enamel Plus (Vanini).)

Figures 4-49 and 4-50 show the external views after reshaping of teeth 13 and 23, with improved dental esthetics. The teeth were reshaped and built up based on functional and esthetic tooth anatomy in orientation to the curve of the lower lip. The tooth size relies on the norm of the regular relation of central to lateral incisors according the divine proportions. The intraoral views show closure of all spaces and the mandibular arch in perfect harmony. The class II relationship was maintained and represents a stable one tooth to two teeth occlusion.

Figure 4-51 shows views during the course of treatment.

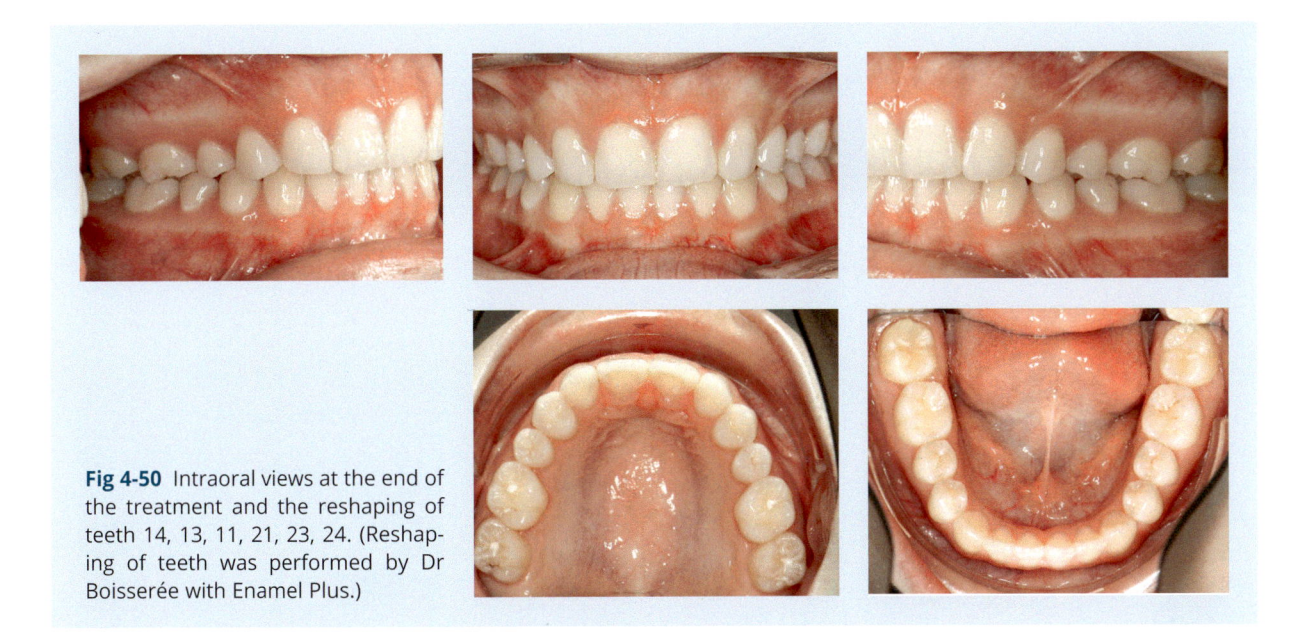

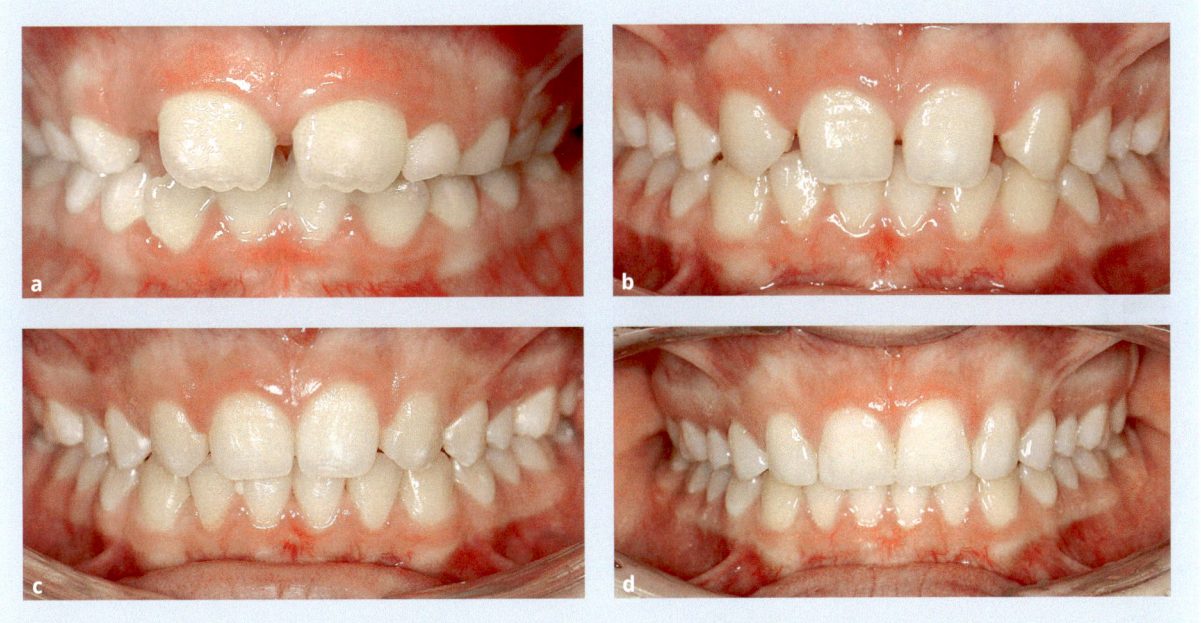

Fig 4-50 Intraoral views at the end of the treatment and the reshaping of teeth 14, 13, 11, 21, 23, 24. (Reshaping of teeth was performed by Dr Boisserée with Enamel Plus.)

Fig 4-51 Views during the course of treatment. **(a)** Before treatment; **(b)** after Frankel treatment; **(c)** after Invisalign therapy; **(d)** after reshaping of upper teeth.

Topic 10
Crowding with insufficient space for full eruption of a retained tooth

Treatment:
- opening space for retained but not fully erupted tooth

This woman has crowding that has resulted in insufficient space for tooth 13 to complete eruption (Figs 4-52 and 4-53).

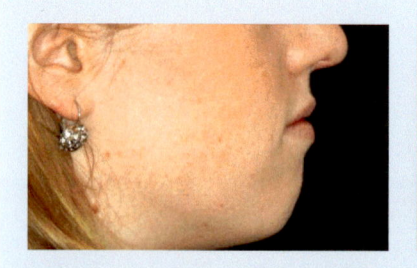

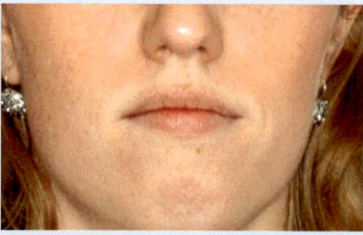

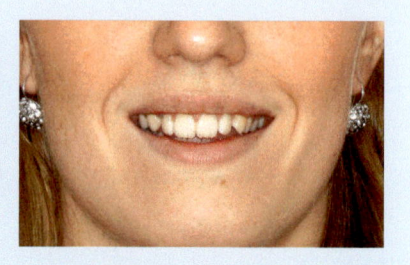

Fig 4-52 Initial presentation. The patient does not show a right maxillary canine while smiling.

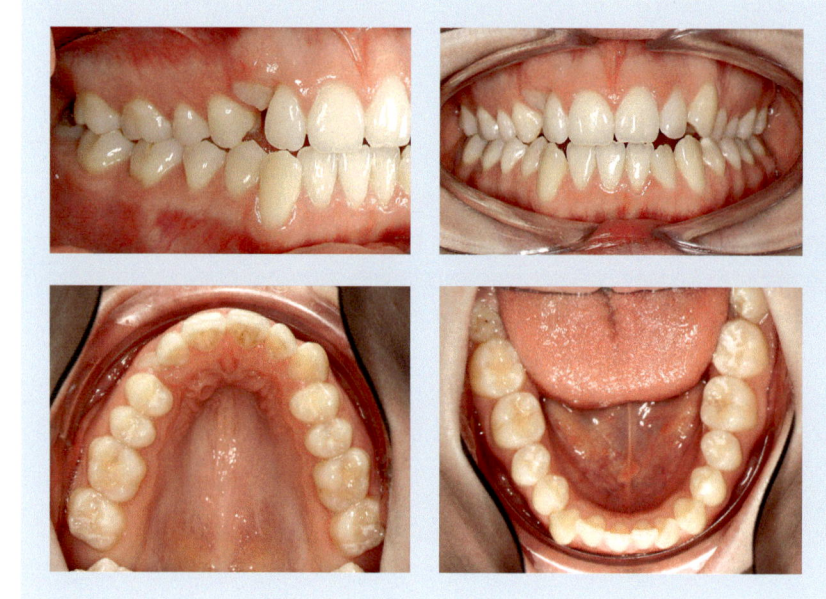

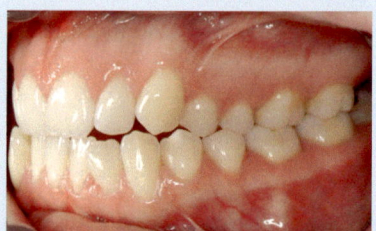

Fig 4-53 The initial intraoral views show insufficient space for retained tooth 13, crowding in the maxillary and mandibular arches, and anterior open bite.

Diagnosis:
- crowding
- insufficient space for tooth 13 to complete eruption
- crossbite situation tooth 12 to 43, 24, 25 to 35
- midline deviation
- anterior open bite.

Therapy:
- to create spaces between the maxillary incisors
- to harmonious profile and create an esthetic full smile.

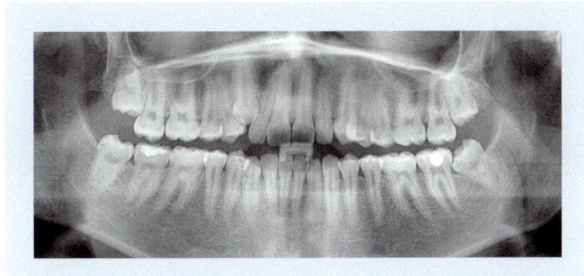

Fig 4-54 Orthopantomogram showing the retained tooth 13.

Treatment

The main objectives were to create space for tooth 13 to complete eruption and to maintain a harmonious facial pattern.

Orthopantomography shows the retained tooth 13. Teeth 18, 28, 38, and 48 were advised for extraction. Lateral cephalometric radiography was used to provide data for determining the facial pattern (Fig 4-55).

Use of IPR initially created some space between the maxillary incisors before Invisalign treatment was commenced (Fig 4-56).

If IPR occurs before impression/digital scanning, the patient needs to wear retention aligners to retain the spaces before the first treatment aligners are set in place.

Attachments were bonded on teeth 14, 15, 24, 25, 33, 34, 35, 43, 44, and 45. The first phase of treatment planned distalization of the maxillary right premolars and protrusion of the maxillary incisors to open sufficient space for the extrusion of tooth 13. Tooth 13 was not covered with the aligner but substituted with a pontic in this first aligner phase.

After 15 months of aligner treatment, distalization in the maxillary right had created a class I relationship with sufficient space distal of tooth 13 for extrusion and derotation (Figs 4-57 and 4-58). New scans were taken to start the refinement phase of treatment.

At stage 19 of the refinement, tooth 13 was not following the planned extrusion predicted by the ClinCheck software. To obtain an additional extrusive force on tooth 13, a hook was added palatal and

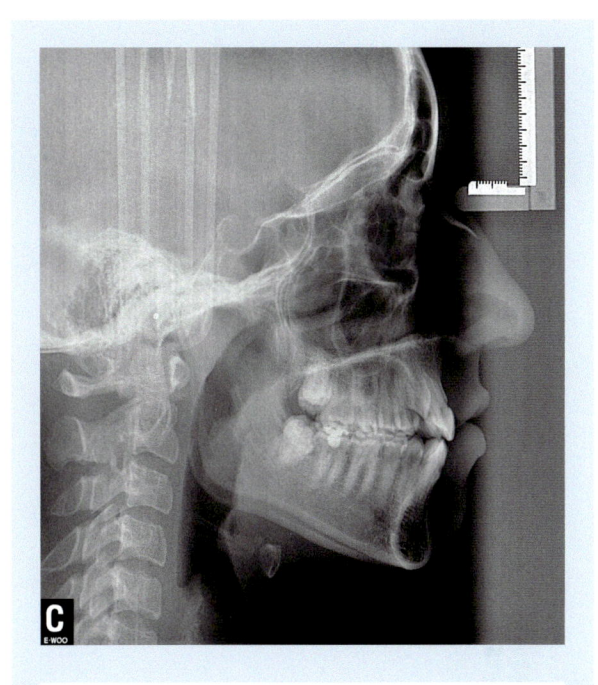

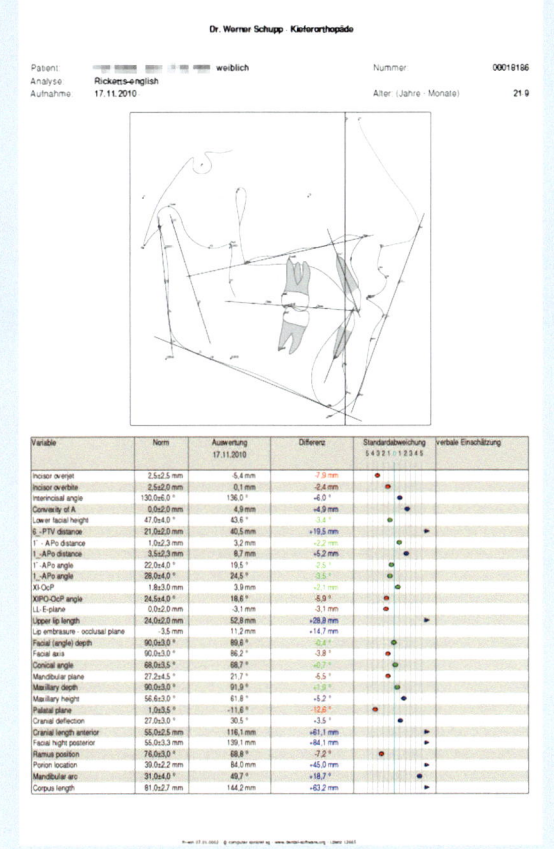

Fig 4-55 Lateral cephalometric radiography with landmarks for Ricketts analysis to determine the facial pattern.

4 TREATMENT OF DIFFERENT MALOCCLUSIONS WITH ALIGNERS

Fig 4-56 Intraoral views after IPR and before Invisalign treatment showing the spaces created between maxillary incisors.

Fig 4-57 Intraoral views after 15 months of aligner treatment.

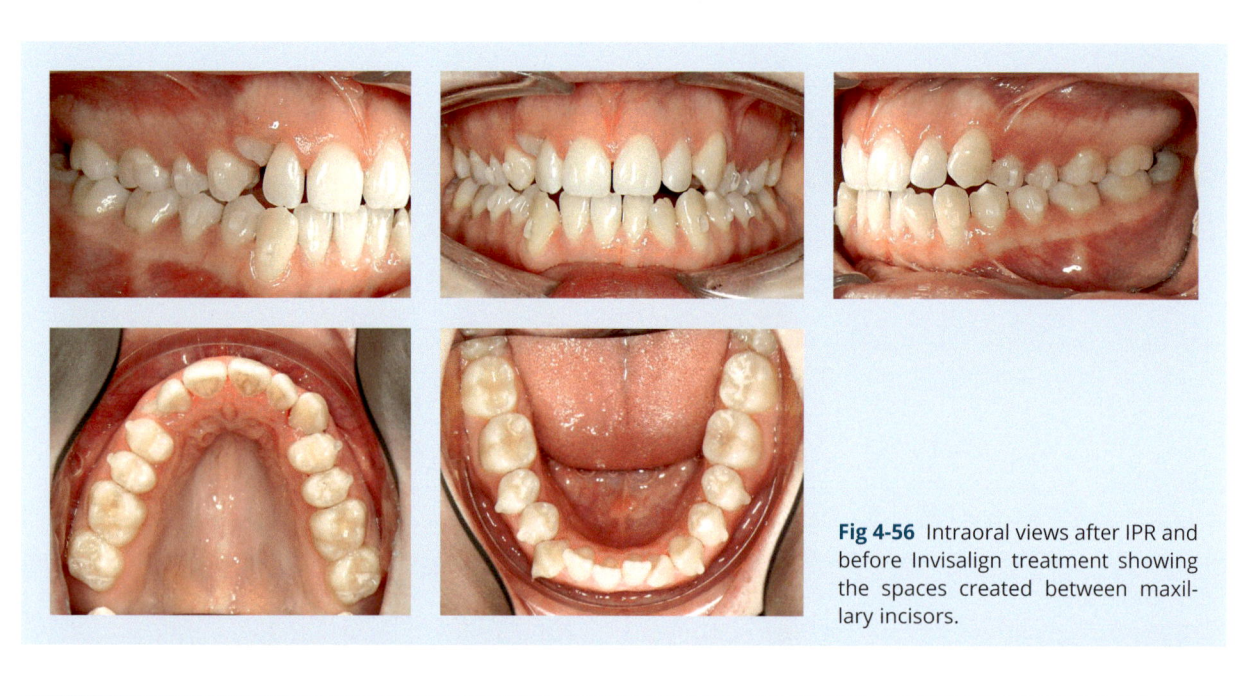

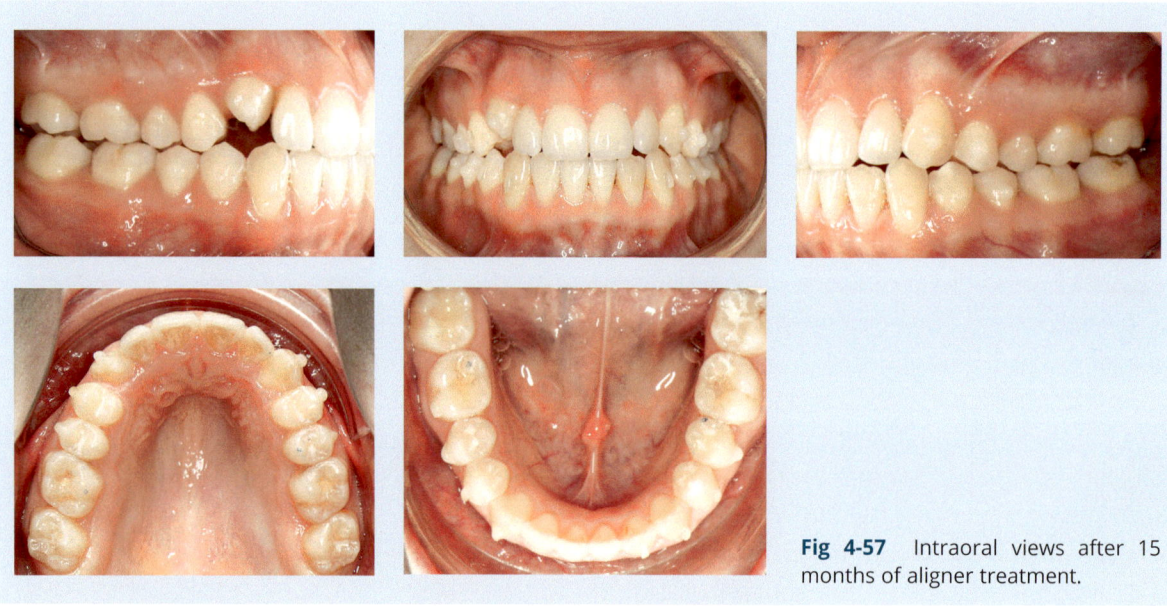

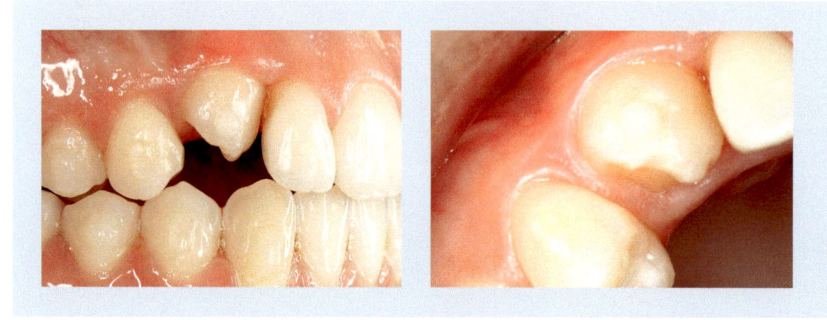

Fig 4-58 Intraoral view of tooth 13 with the attachments in detail.

76

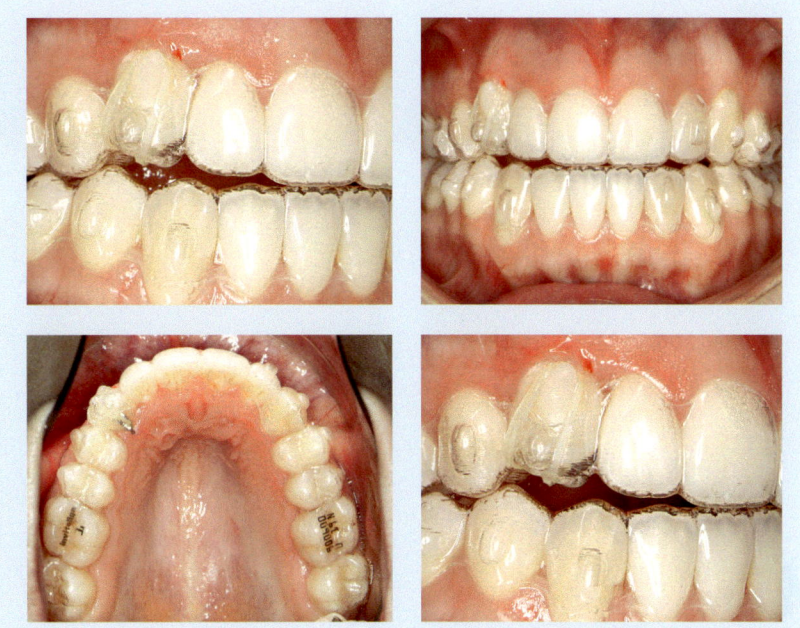

Fig 4-59 Intraoral findings at stage 19 of the refinement, showing that tooth 13 had failed to follow the the planned extrusion. Hooks have been bonded on the buccal and palatal surface of tooth 13 to obtain increased extrusive force with additional elastic wear.

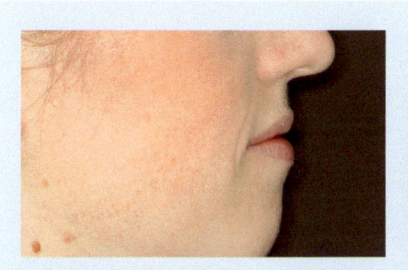

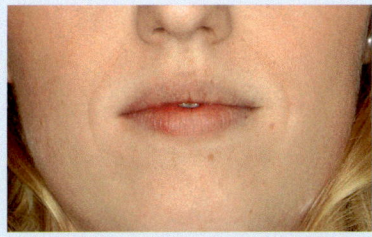

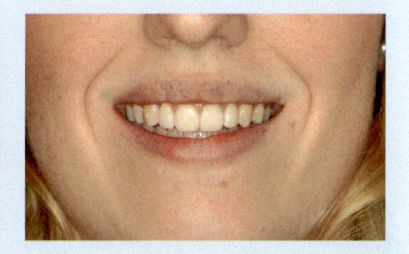

Fig 4-60 Extraoral findings at the end of treatment, showing harmonious profile and esthetic full smile.

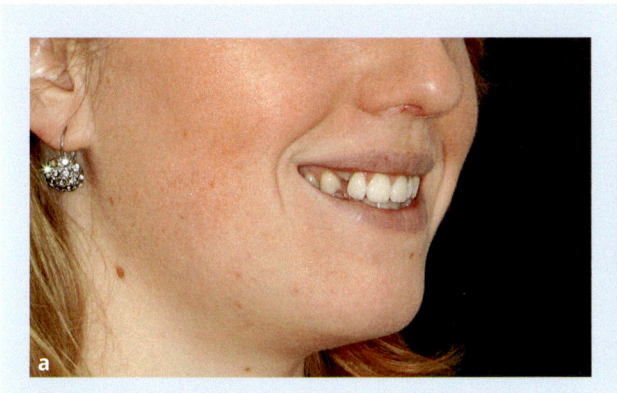

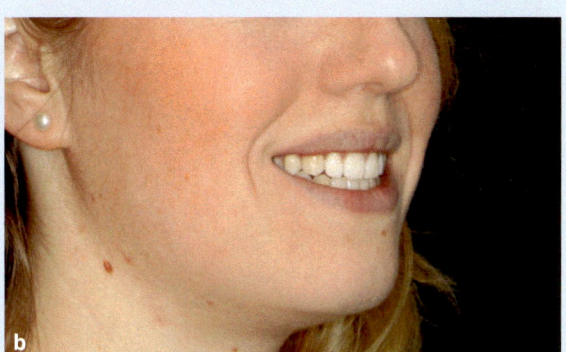

Fig 4-61 Comparison of the extraoral view before **(a)** and after **(b)** treatment.

Fig 4-62 Intraoral final situation.

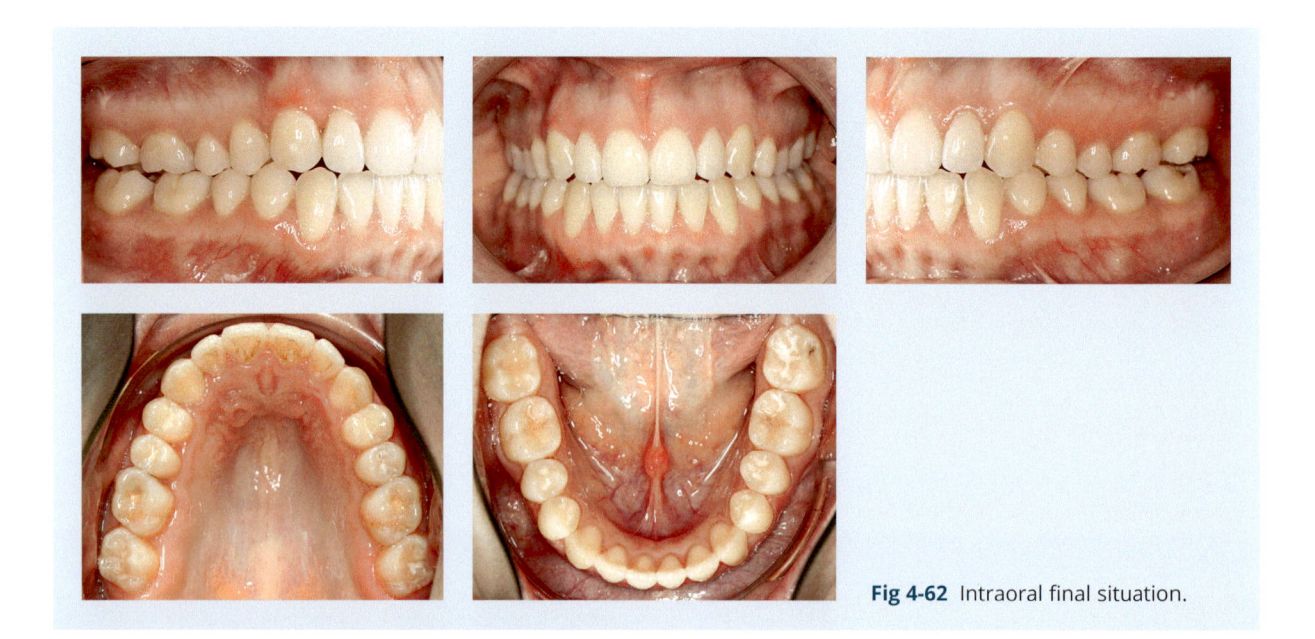

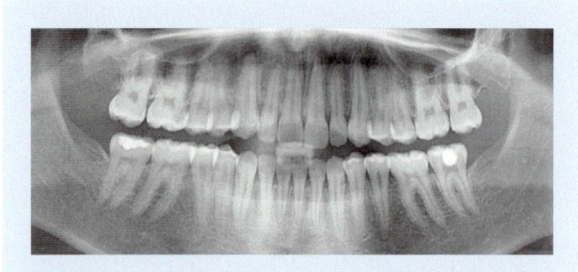

Fig 4-63 Final orthopantomogram with correct position of tooth 13; all wisdom teeth had been extracted.

buccal on the tooth and the patient was advised to wear elastics from palatinal to buccal over the aligner (Fig 4-59).

At the end of treatment, a harmonious profile and esthetic full smile had been achieved (Figs 4-60 to 4-63). This had required the use of 30 aligners in the first treatment phase, an additional 33 aligners in the maxillary arch, and 15 aligners in the mandibular arch in a second phase.

Figure 4-64 shows views before and after treatment.

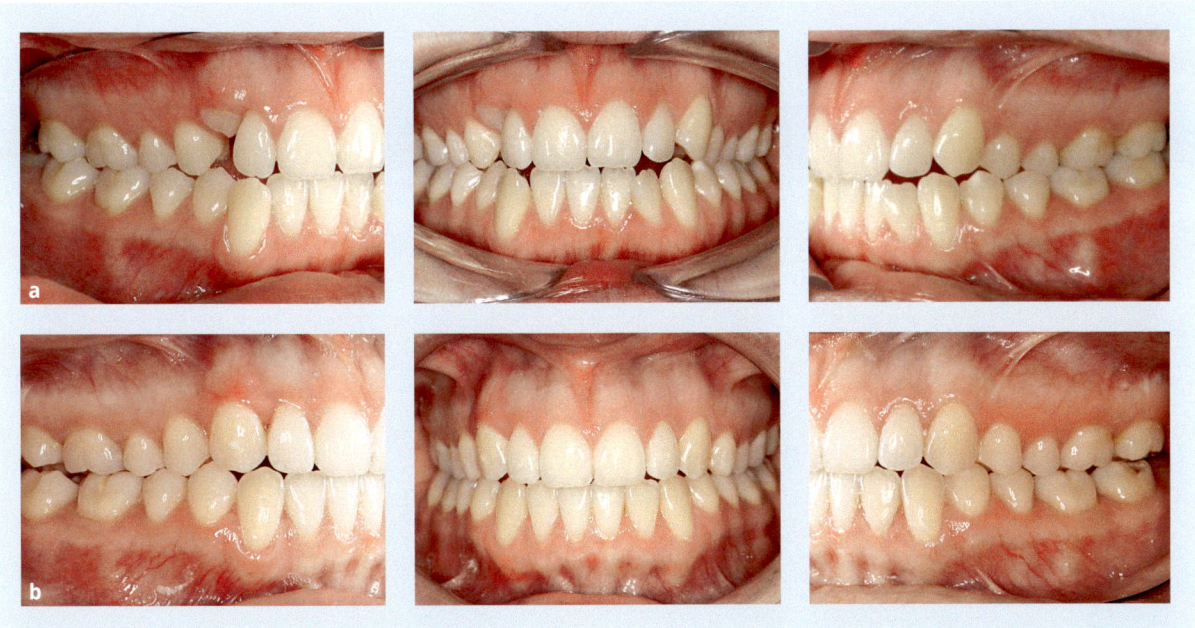

Fig 4-64 Views before **(a)** and after **(b)** treatment.

Topic 11
Missing maxillary lateral incisor

Treatment:
- space opening for an implant to replace tooth 12

This topic describes the use of an interdisciplinary approach to improve esthetics using Invisalign therapy initially to open sufficient space in area 12 for subsequent implant insertion and finally new restoratives.

This 32-year-old woman had agenesis of tooth 12 and an adhesive fixed partial denture on teeth 13 to 11 (Figs 4-65 and 4-66).

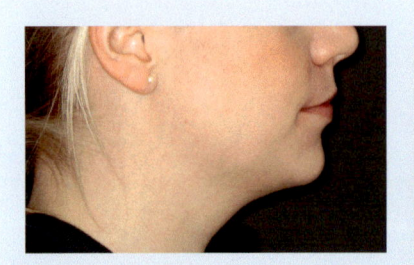

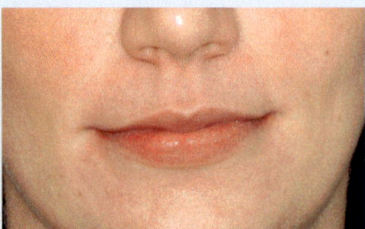

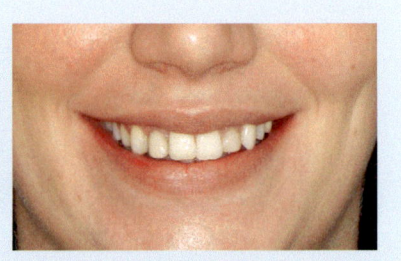

Fig 4-65 Extraoral views at the beginning of the Invisalign therapy, showing harmonious profile and smile line.

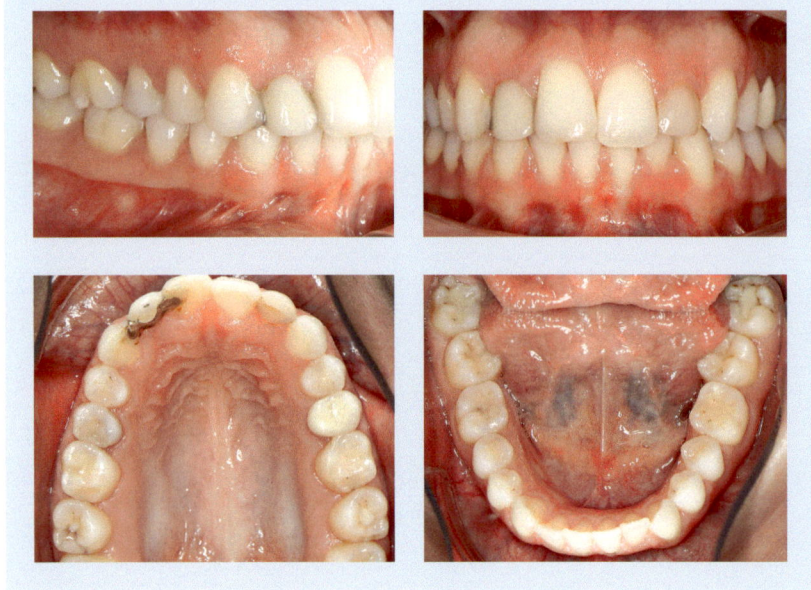

Fig 4-66 Intraoral views showing the adhesive fixed partial denture on teeth 11 to 13 after an orthodontic fixed appliance treatment as a child and agenesis of tooth 12.

Diagnosis:
- class I relationship on the right side and class II on the left
- slight anterior crowding
- insufficient adhesive fixed partial denture on teeth 13 and 11 to substitute missing tooth 12.

Therapy:
- opening of space for planned implant area 12
- alignment of both arches.

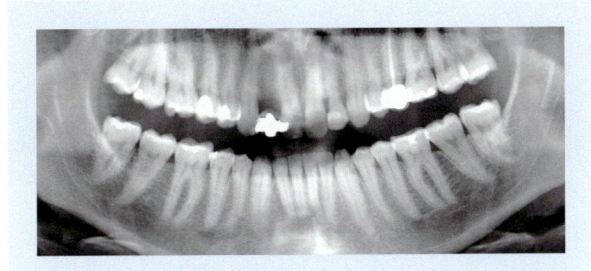

Fig 4-67 The initial orthopantomogram showing the lack of space for implant insertion at position 12 because of tipped roots of teeth 13 and 11.

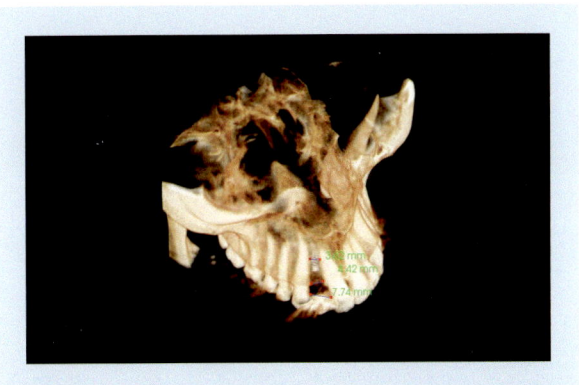

Fig 4-68 CBCT (Anatomage) showing insufficient space for implant insertion in area 12 in detail, with an apical space of 3.62 mm, mesial space of 4.42, and gingival space of 7.74 mm.

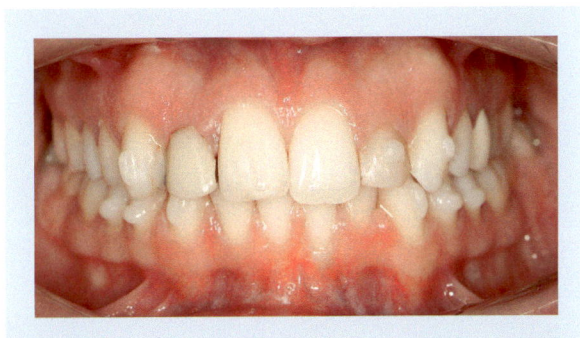

Fig 4-69 Intraoral situation at the start of Invisalign treatment, showing attachments on maxillary canines and tooth 22, as well as on all mandibular canines and premolars.

Treatment

The main objective was to create space to allow an implant to be positioned to carry a replacement for tooth 12.

Orthodontic therapy was to be followed by insertion of an implant and restoratives. The initial orthopantomography and digital volume tomography showed insufficient space for implant insertion at position 12 because of tipping of the roots of teeth 13 and 11 (Figs 4-67 and 4-68).

At the start of Invisalign treatment, attachments were placed on maxillary canines and tooth 22, as well as on all mandibular canines and premolars. The fixed partial denture was separated mesial of tooth 12 and remained fixed only on tooth 13 for esthetic reasons. Tooth 13 was moved together with the attached pontic tooth 12 (Fig 4-69).

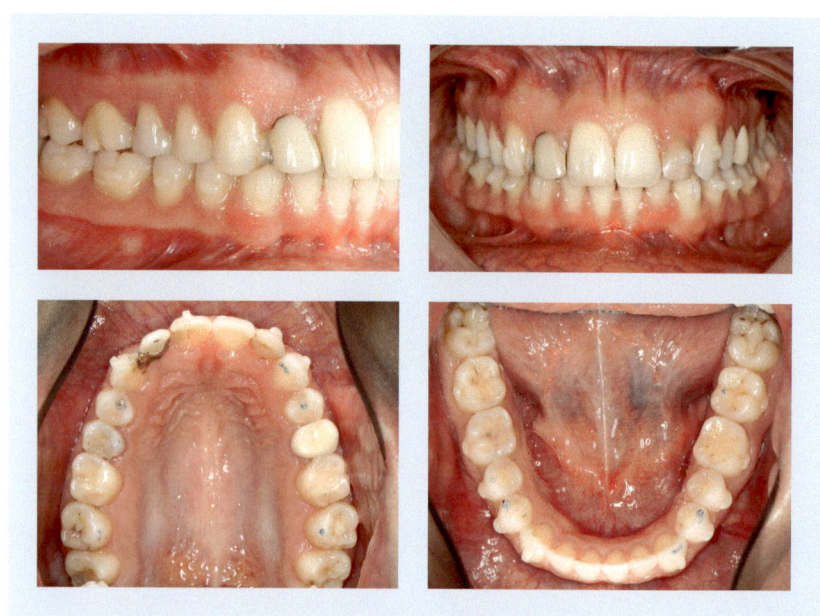

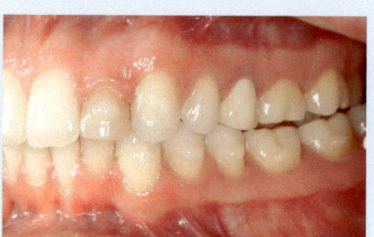

4 TREATMENT OF DIFFERENT MALOCCLUSIONS WITH ALIGNERS

Fig 4-70 Intraoral view at the end of the first phase of treatment. There has been transversal expansion, leading to slight opening of the bite on the left posterior side.

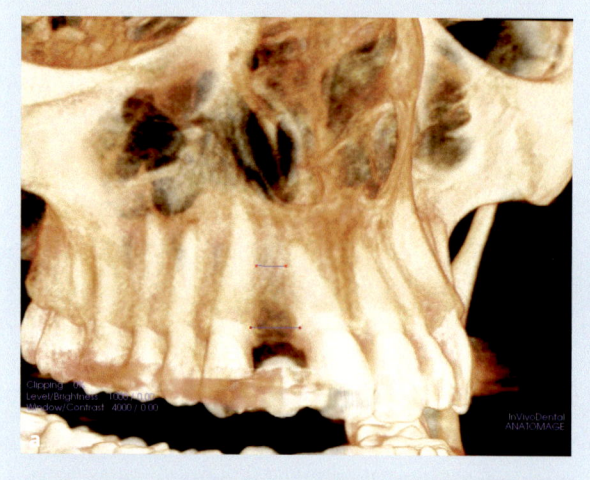

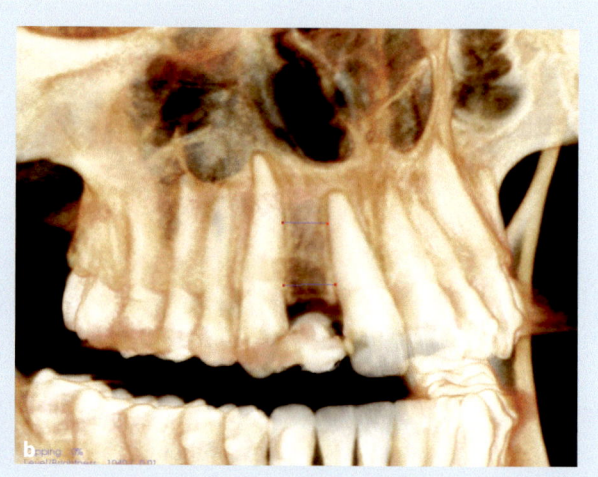

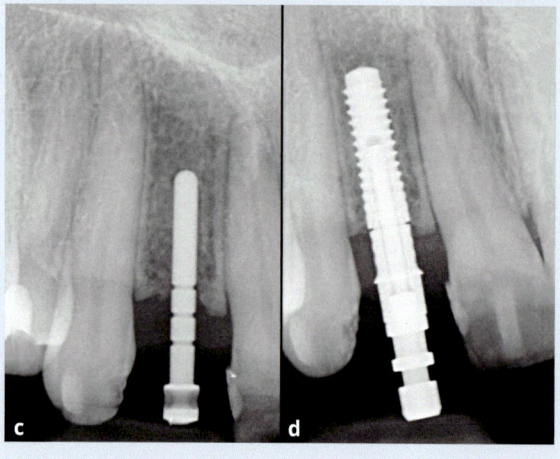

Fig 4-71 CBCT (Picasso, Orange Dental), transferred into the Invivo Software (Anatomage). **(a)** Before treatment. **(b)** After the first phase, almost sufficient bone and, therefore, space for the planned implant in area 12 has been achieved. **(c)** The refinement phase provided additional root deangulation of teeth 13 and 11. **(c)** The implant site with the inserted direction indicator after the refinement phase. **(d)** The implant in situ. (Implant insertion by Dr M Bäumer, Cologne.)

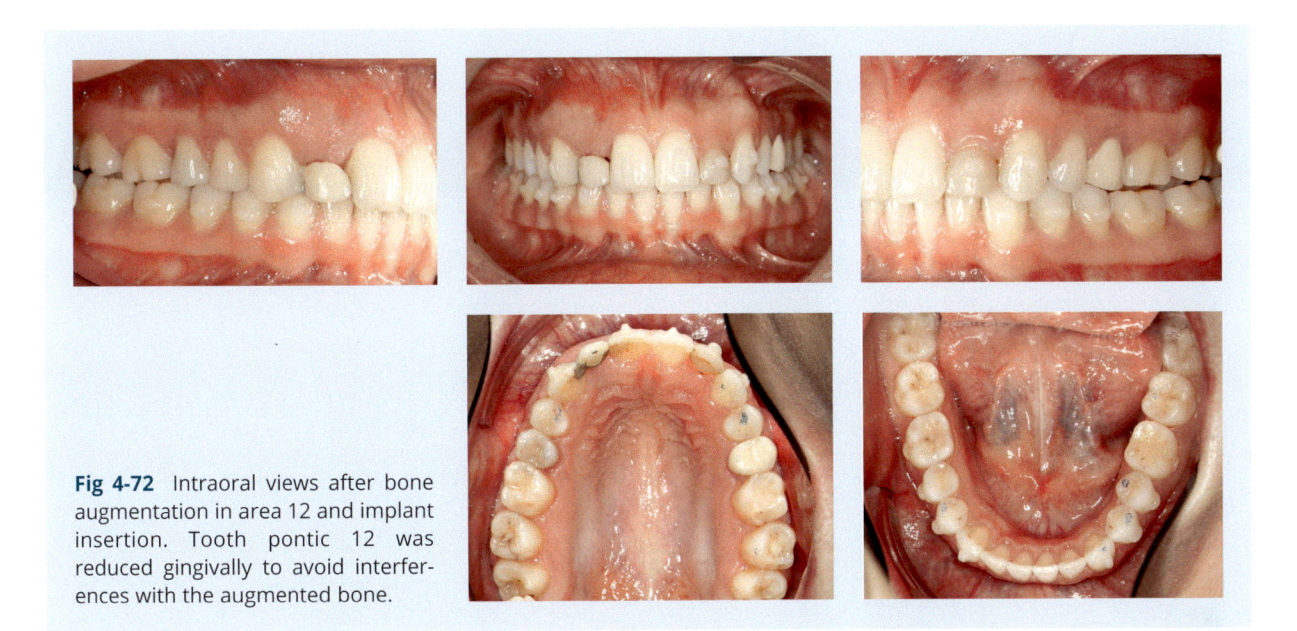

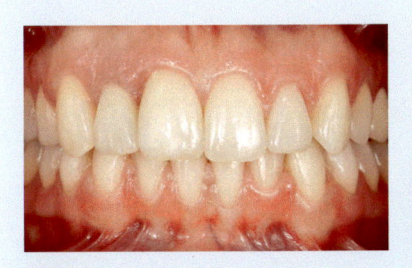

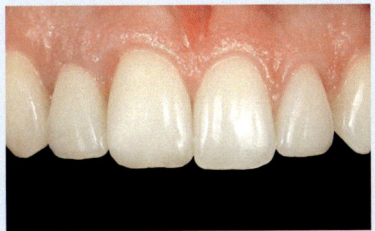

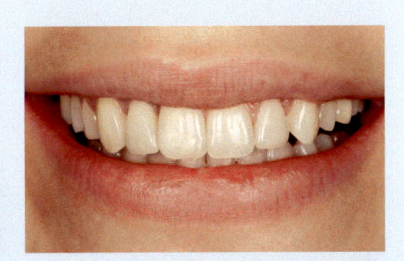

Fig 4-72 Intraoral views after bone augmentation in area 12 and implant insertion. Tooth pontic 12 was reduced gingivally to avoid interferences with the augmented bone.

Fig 4-73 Intra- and extraoral views at the end of treatment with inserted implant crown on tooth 12 and composite restorations on tooth 22.

The first phase of treatment used 23 aligners. Due to the transversal expansion, slight opening of the bite occurred on the left posterior side (Fig 4-70); extrusion of the posteriors is necessary and was planned with the refinement. At the end of this phase, there was not quite sufficient space for the implant to be inserted and so the refinement also provided root deangulation of teeth 13 and 11.

CBCT showed an opening of sufficient space for implant insertion during the two phases of Invisalign treatment (Fig 4-71).

Figure 4-72 shows the final view at the end of orthodontic Invisalign treatment and Figure 4-73 the extra- and intraoral views after insertion of the implant and crown, as well as the new restoratives (Dr Wolfgang Boisserée, Cologne).

4 TREATMENT OF DIFFERENT MALOCCLUSIONS WITH ALIGNERS

Topic 12
Spaces with missing teeth

Treatment:
- open space and creating new bone for an implant at position 42

This topic describes the use of an interdisciplinary approach involving an oral surgeon and dentist to create an opening for an implant and to ensure new bone in the implant area.

The patient had two missing teeth, 42 and 47, and resulting spaces (Figs 4-74 and 4-75). Tooth 43 had migrated, the crown of tooth 25 was tipped to buccal and that of tooth 35 to lingual, creating buccal non-occlusion. The alveolar bone between 43 and 44 was narrow, a so-called "hourglass defect."

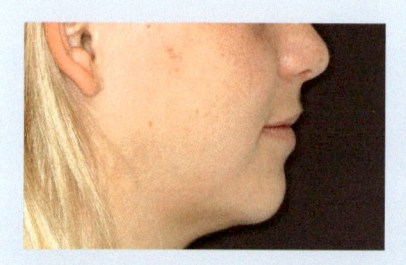

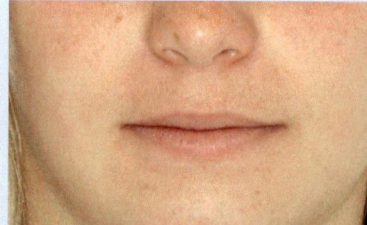

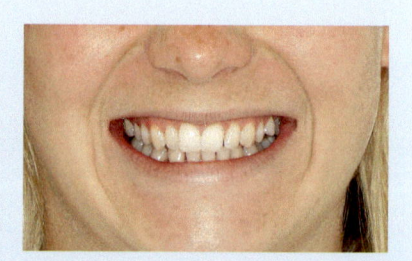

Fig 4-74 Extraoral views at the start of treatment.

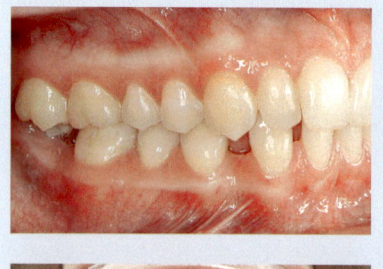

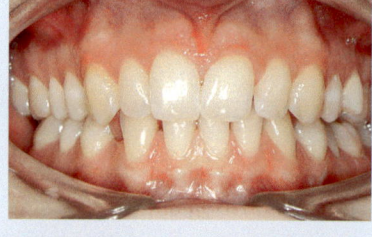

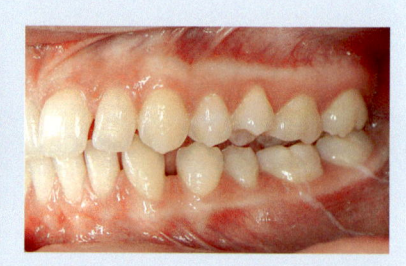

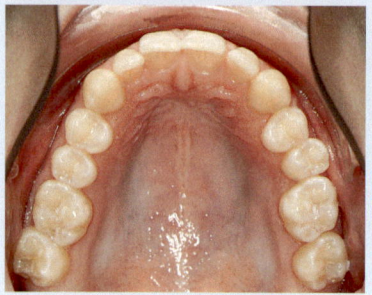

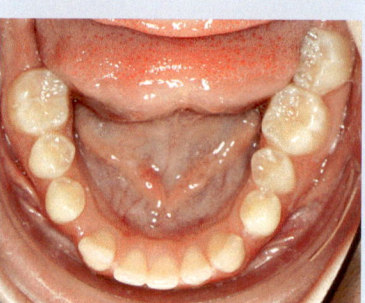

Fig 4-75 Intraoral views showing the spaces in the mandibular arch, missing teeth 42 and 47, and migrated tooth 43. The crown of tooth 25 is tipped to buccal and the crown of tooth 35 tipped to lingual, showing buccal non-occlusion.

Diagnosis:
- missing tooth 42
- hourglass defect in planned implant area
- buccal non-occlusion tooth 25 to 35.

Therapy:
- open space for later implant in area 42 by distalization of tooth 43 and bone remodeling
- correct buccal non-occlusion of teeth 25 to 35
- implant and prosthetics.

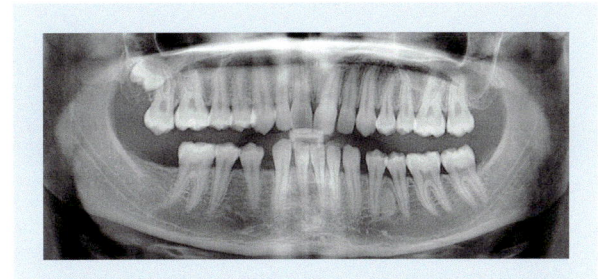

Fig 4-76 Orthopantomogram showing spaces in the mandibular arch. Wisdom tooth 18 is visible and region 34/35 shows sclerotic bone.

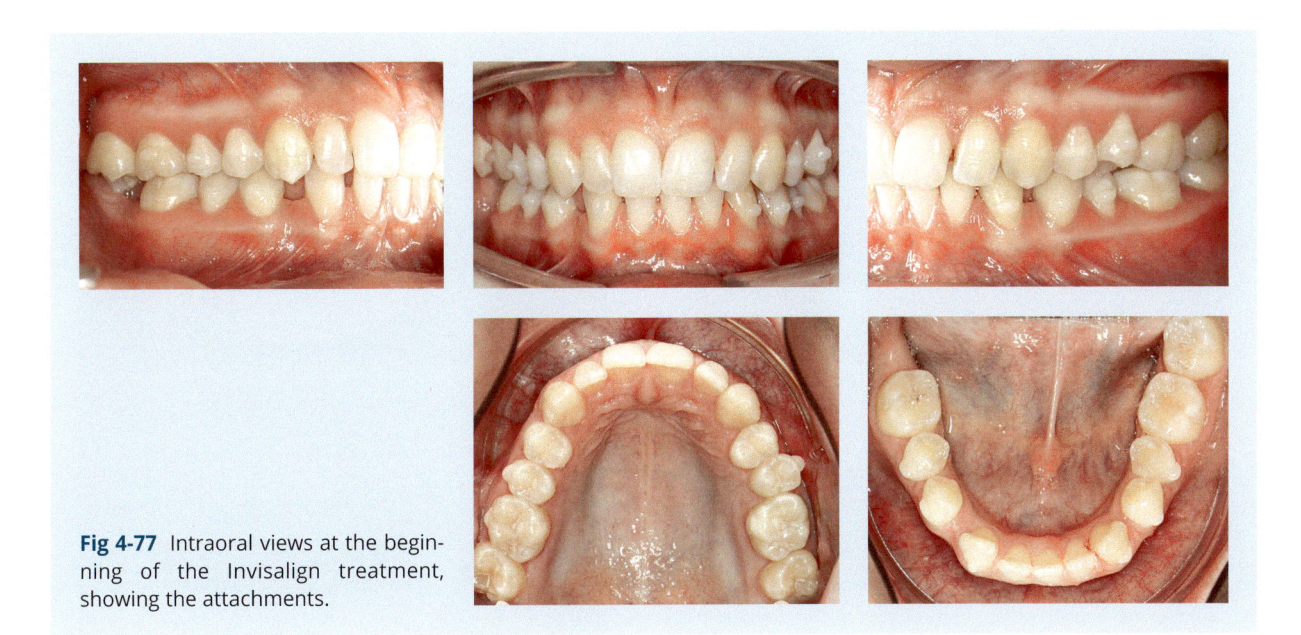

Fig 4-77 Intraoral views at the beginning of the Invisalign treatment, showing the attachments.

Treatment

The main objectives were to create an opening and sufficient new bone for an implant at position 42 and to correct buccal non-occlusion.

The alveolar bone between 43 and 44 is too narrow transversally and sagittally to place an implant. Simply opening a space between tooth 43 and tooth 44 will not provide sufficient bone for implant insertion. If teeth are moved into bone with an hourglass defect, bone remodeling can be initiated and sufficient bone in the horizontal direction can be achieved.

Orthopantomography showed spaces in the mandibular arch and sclerotic bone in region 34/35 (Fig 4-76).

Figure 4-77 shows the attachments in place at the start of Invisalign treatment.

The ClinCheck software shows the projected treatment path with IPR and distalization of teeth (Fig 4-78). Planned tooth movements for distalization of mandibular right posterior teeth included IPR 0.6 mm mesial on tooth 46; distalization of teeth 43, 44, and 45 with complete space closure; distalization of teeth 33, 32, and 31; and mesialization of tooth 41 to open space for the planned implant at position 42. For esthetic reasons, a pontic was planned between teeth 41 and 43. Teeth 37 and 46 were maintained in their position to increase anchorage.

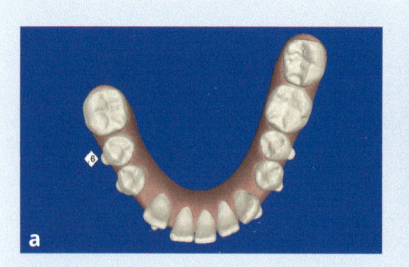

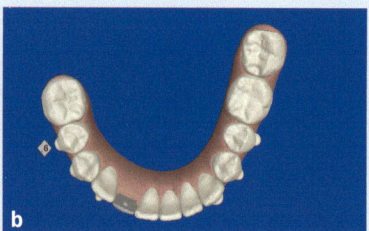

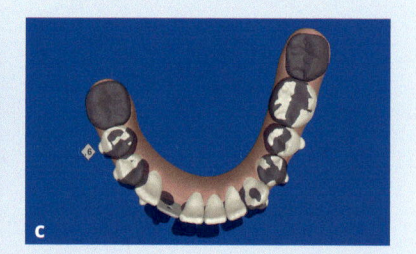

Fig 4-78 ClinCheck software results. **(a)** IPR was planned 0.6 mm mesial of tooth 46. **(b)** The planned final result at the end of treatment with space opening for later implant at position 42. **(c)** Superimposition shows the amount of planned tooth movements (blue, initial tooth position; white, final tooth position).

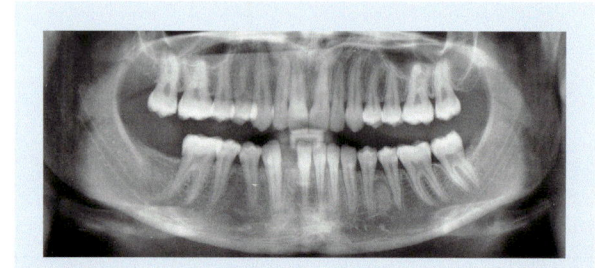

Fig 4-79 Orthopantomogram showing space created with the orthodontic treatment.

At the end of orthodontic treatment, orthopantomography showed space opening for implant insertion in area 42 (Fig 4-79). Invivo software shows the bone situation in area 42 (Fig 4-80).

Figure 4-81 shows the placement of the implant in area 42.

At the end of treatment, a restorative had been added to the implant in area 42. Implant placement in area 47 was planned and recommended for major occlusal stability. To avoid an extrusive movement of tooth 17 and maintain the orthodontic result, the patient was advised to wear removable retainers at night in both arches. Distalization into class I relationship would have presupposed opening of spaces lateral of maxillary incisors, but this was declined by the patient.

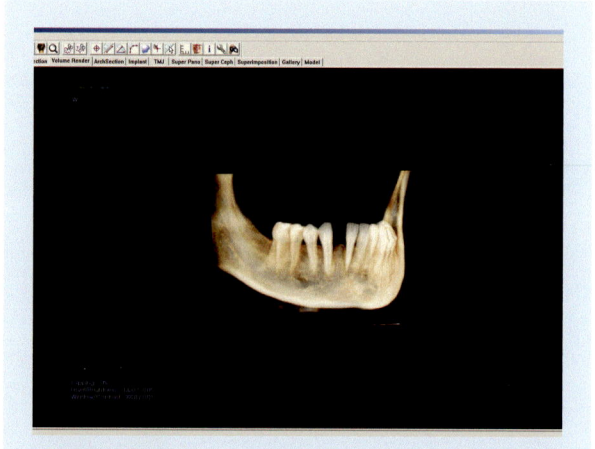

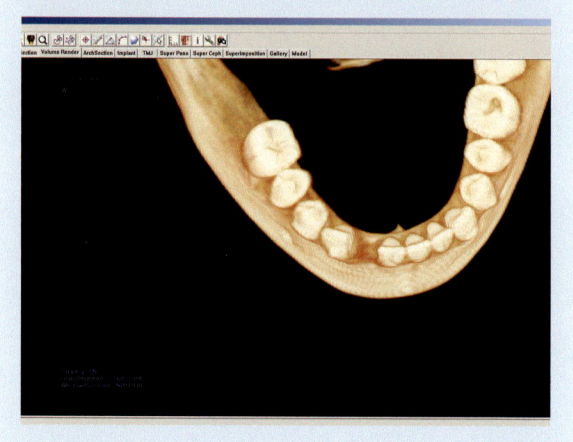

Fig 4-80 Invivo software showing bone in area 42 after the orthodontic treatment (Invivo Software, Anatomage).

TREATMENT OF DIFFERENT MALOCCLUSIONS WITH ALIGNERS 4

Fig 4-81 Intraoral view **(a)** and orthopantomogram **(b)** after implant placement. (Implant insertion by Dr P Marquardt, Cologne.)

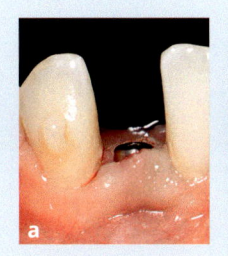

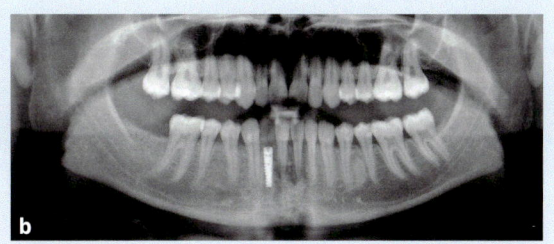

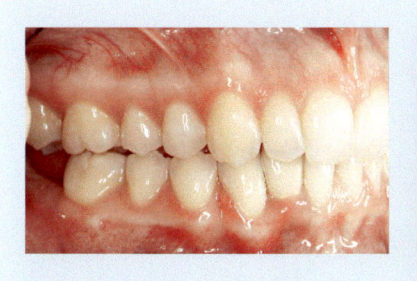

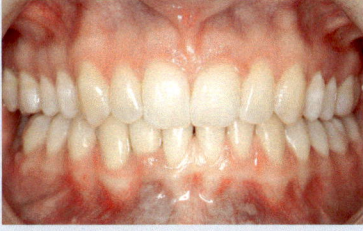

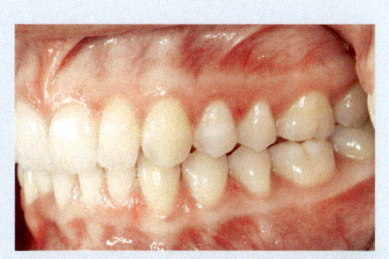

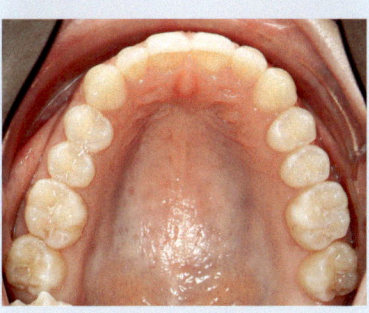

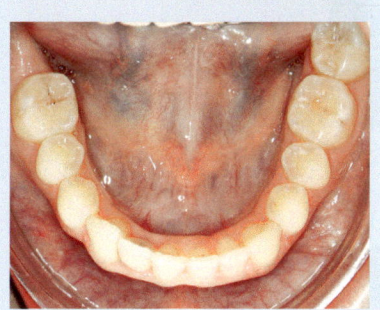

Fig 4-82 Intraoral views at the end of treatment with a restorative on an implant in area 42 by Dr P Marquardt, Cologne.

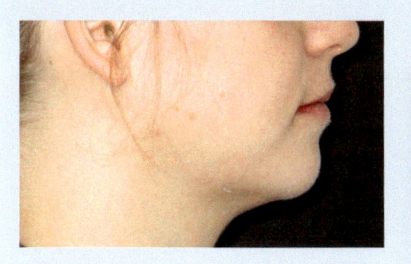

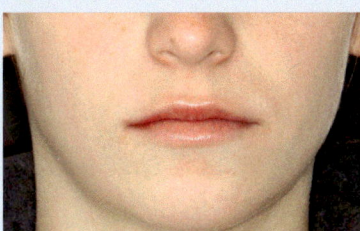

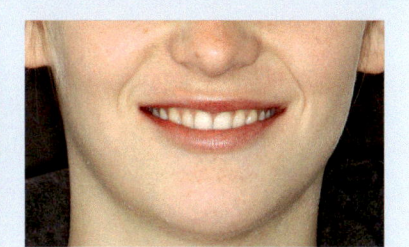

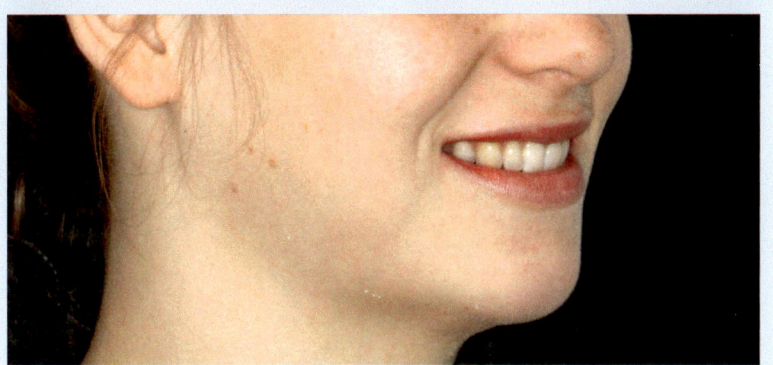

Fig 4-83 Extraoral views at the end of treatment with harmonious lip relation and profile.

87

Topic 13
Agenesis of six teeth and migration of maxillary canines into spaces

Treatment:
- open space for implants

In adults, interdisciplinary dentistry is often essential and this topic involves both an oral surgeon and a dentist. Backward planning can be easily performed with the ClinCheck software, thus allowing treatment to be discussed by all the specialists who will need to be involved with a particular patient. With desktop sharing software, it is nowadays easy to discuss the ClinCheck outcome regardless of the location of each of the specialists.

This patient had agenesis of teeth 12, 22, 15, 25, 35, and 45. The intraoral initial views showed both maxillary canines in a class II relationship. There were gaps between the maxillary canines and the first premolars and between the central incisors and canines. Teeth 11/21 showed a diastema (Fig 4-84).

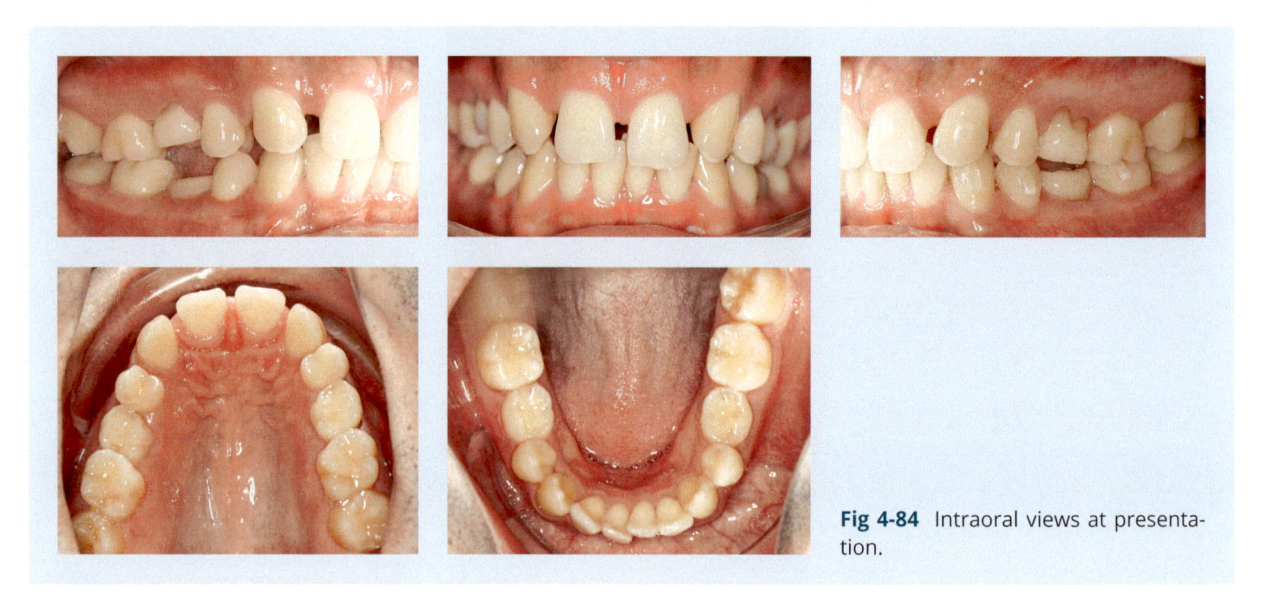

Fig 4-84 Intraoral views at presentation.

Diagnosis:
- missing teeth 12, 22,15, 25, 35, and 45
- persistent teeth 55, 65,75, and 85.

Therapy:
- alignment of maxilla and mandible
- opening of spaces 12 and 22 for implants
- implants and restoratives.

Fig 4-85 Attachment positions at the start of treatment.

Treatment

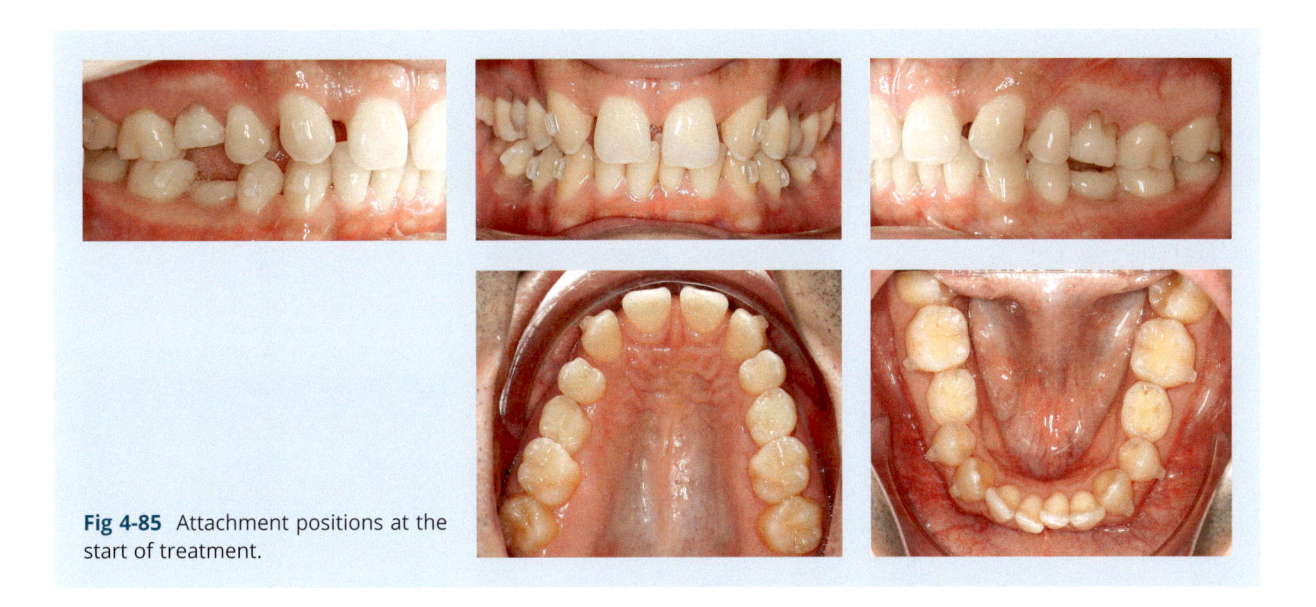

The main objective was to balance issues of crowding, missing teeth, and spaces by combining space opening for implants with use of restoratives.

At presentation, the gaps were too big to build up the canines and central incisors with restoratives to close all spaces. The potential positions for implants was discussed with the oral surgeon to find the best solution: should implants be inserted to replace the missing lateral incisors or should the canines be mesialized to open up space for implants in the canine region. In the latter approach, additional veneers on the canines would be necessary to build them up according to the shape of lateral incisors. It was decided to reduce the size of primary teeth 55 and 65 and gain this space for the distalization of teeth 14 and 24 first, then 13 and 23; this would create space for implants in regions 12 and 22. In the mandibular arch, crowding would be solved with IPR.

As the spaces mesial and distal of the central incisors allowed optimal aligner capture of the crowns, attachments were not made on teeth 11, 21 but exclusively on teeth 13, 23 for the distalization and tipping of the canine roots. (Fig 4-85). In the mandibular arch, intrusion of the incisors was to occur first, followed by the canines for a predictable leveling of the curve of Spee. To obtain maximum anchorage for the intrusive force, rectangular attachments were bonded on the mandibular canines, first premolars, and first molars. During the anterior intrusion, simultaneous extrusion of 0.4 mm of the first premolars and molars was performed.

ClinCheck software shows the proposed orthodontic treatment (Fig 4-86). IPR would be needed mesial to some teeth to create space for the later implants. The maxillary arch would have 25 aligners.

After the first phase of treatment, ClinCheck was used to assess what further treatment was needed (Fig 4-87). The patient was transferred to the dentist to reduce mesial aspects of primary teeth 55 and 65 to gain even more space for the distalization of first premolars and canines to open increased space for later implants. A further phase with an additional 18 aligners in the maxillary arch would open more space for implants in areas 12 and 22.

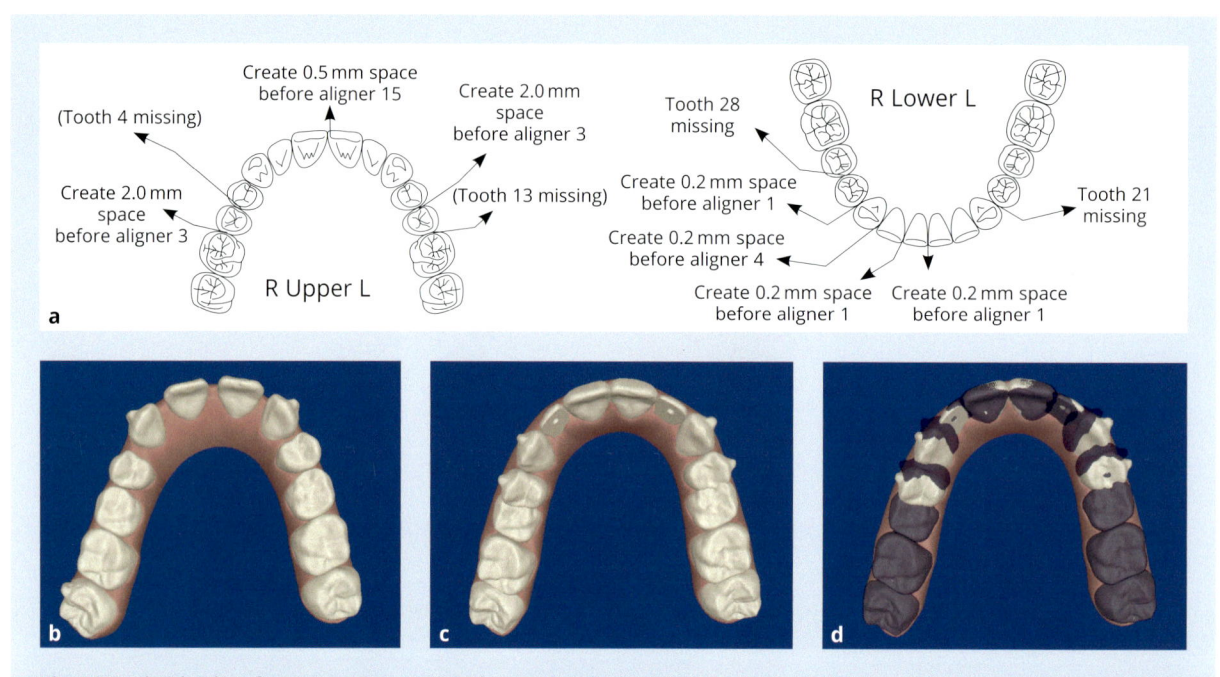

4 TREATMENT OF DIFFERENT MALOCCLUSIONS WITH ALIGNERS

Fig 4-86 ClinCheck software results. **(a)** IPR chart with IPR mesial of teeth 11 and 21 as well as 2.0 mm IPR mesial on maxillary primary teeth 55 and 65 to obtain space for later implants in regions 12 and 22. **(b)** Initial view with insufficient spaces for later implant supply and diastema mesial of 11/21. **(c)** Planned situation after the first phase of treatment with closure of diastema 11/21 and opening of spaces for implants. Teeth 14, 55, 24, and 65 are in an overlapping positions because of excessive IPR (2 mm). Spaces in areas 12 and 22 are closed with virtual pontics. **(d)** Superimposition for planned movements in the maxillary arch (blue, initial tooth position; white, final tooth position).

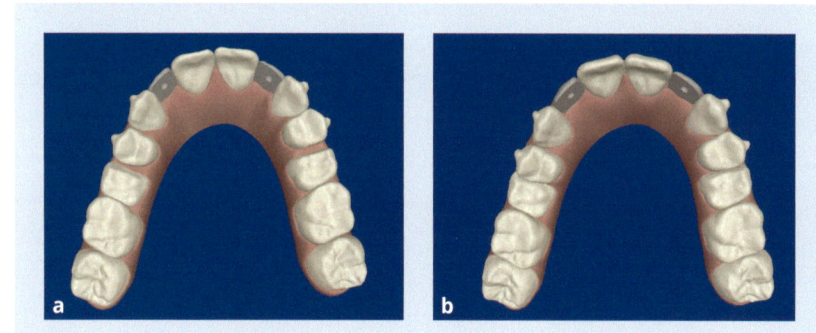

Fig 4-87 ClinCheck software results at the end of the first phase. **(a)** Teeth position with virtual pontics on teeth 12 and 22, indicating that more IPR was needed to reduce the mesial aspects of primary teeth 55 and 65. **(b)** Planned treatment outcome in the next stage to open more space for implants in areas 12 and 22.

After IPR and distalization of the maxillary first premolars and canines, there was sufficient space for the planned implants 12 and 22 (Figs 4-88 to 4-90). There was still a physiologic overbite and overjet.

Figure 4-89 shows before and after Invisalign treatment. The maxillary canines are in a physiologic position for dynamic occlusion at the end of treatment. Teeth 11 and 21 showed slight gingival recessions, which seemed to improve after the next prosthodontic stage (see Figs 4-91 and 4-92, overleaf).

Implant placement then took place in regions 12 and 22 (Fig 4-89).

Figures 4-91 and 4-92 show the effects of treatment.

Fig 4-88 Final intraoral views showing sufficient spaces for the planned implants in regions 12 and 22.

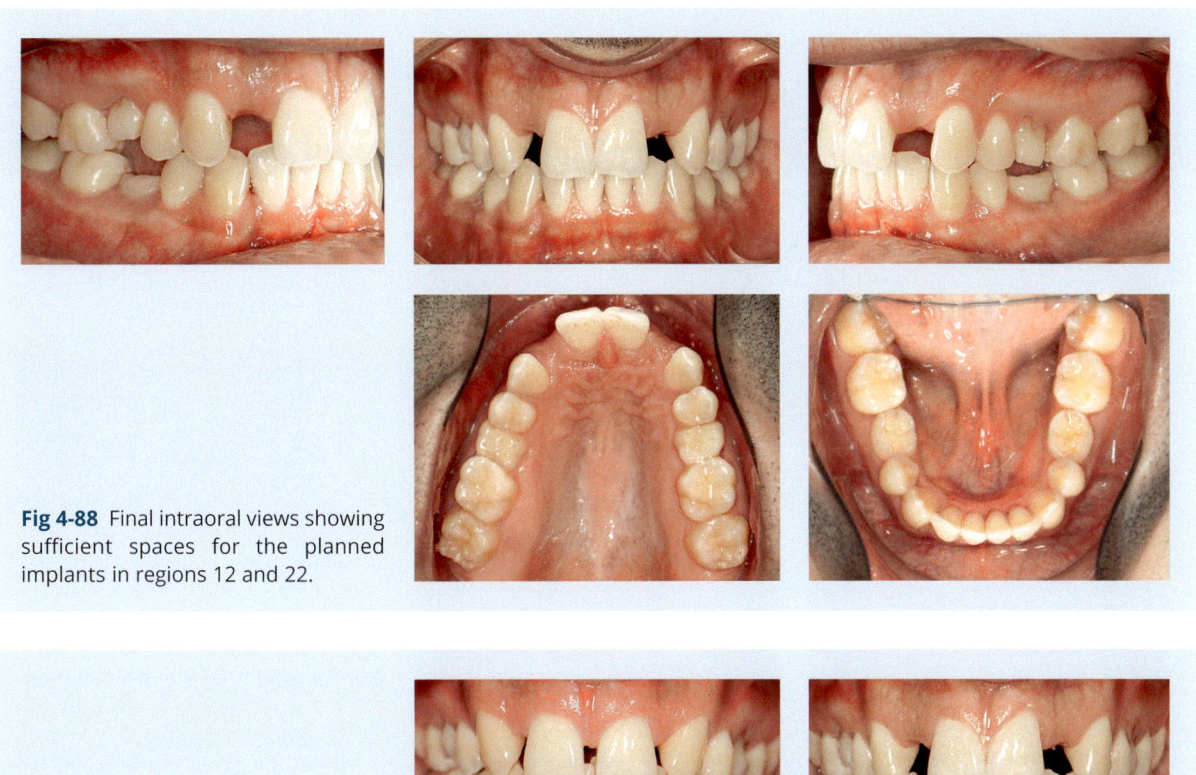

Fig 4-89 Before **(left)** and after **(right)** Invisalign treatment. The maxillary canines are in dynamic occlusion at the end of the treatment. Teeth 11 and 21 showed slight gingival recessions.

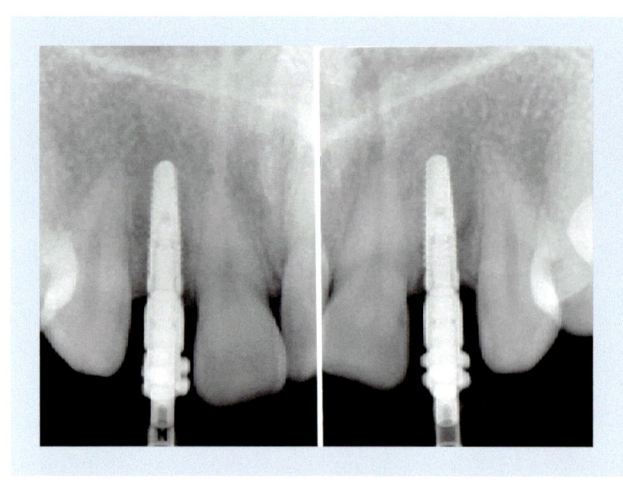

Fig 4-90 Radiography showing optimal placement of implants in regions 12 and 22. (Implant placement by Dr S Vogeler-Krings, Cologne.)

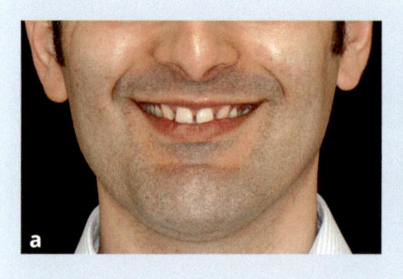

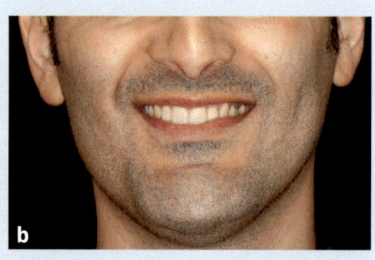

Fig 4-91 The space mesial and distal of the central incisors before treatment **(a)** and the improved smile esthetic at the end of combined Invisalign, implantology, and prosthodontics **(b)**.

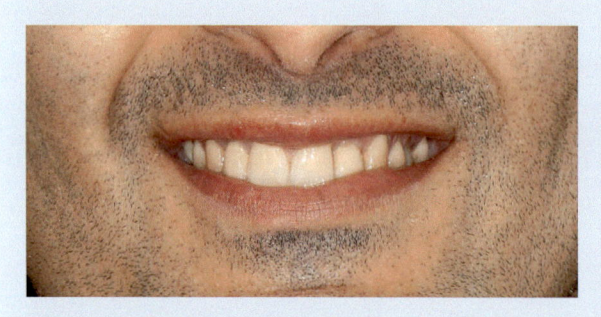

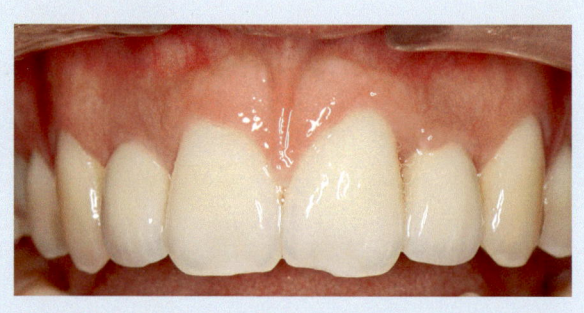

Fig 4-92 The gingiva of the maxillary canines and incisors is healthy at the end of treatment. Gingiva on implant site 22 is still undergoing remodeling healing. The enamel defect on tooth 21 was not adjusted. (Implants and prosthodontics by Dr S Vogeler-Krings, Cologne.)

TREATMENT OF DIFFERENT MALOCCLUSIONS WITH ALIGNERS 4

Topic 14
Spaces after traumatic tooth loss with migration of neighboring teeth

Treatment:
- open space for a fixed partial denture

Often a decision needs to be made by the clinician and patient together as to whether spaces should be closed completely or if space needs to be opened up. If there is a need to open space, how should the gap be restored: with a fixed partial denture or with an implant? This topic deals with space opening for later restoratives after traumatic loss and attrition of anterior teeth.

The length and the shape of the clinical crown cannot be modified with orthodontics and so interdisciplinary dentistry is recommended and should be planned before orthodontic treatment starts. One of the major benefits of Invisalign treatment is the ability to discuss and visualize the end-result of orthodontic treatment using the ClinCheck software.

This patient lost parts of the maxillary and mandibular incisor enamel as well as tooth 22 in an accident (Fig 4-93). He also had severe injuries to his upper lip and below his left eye.

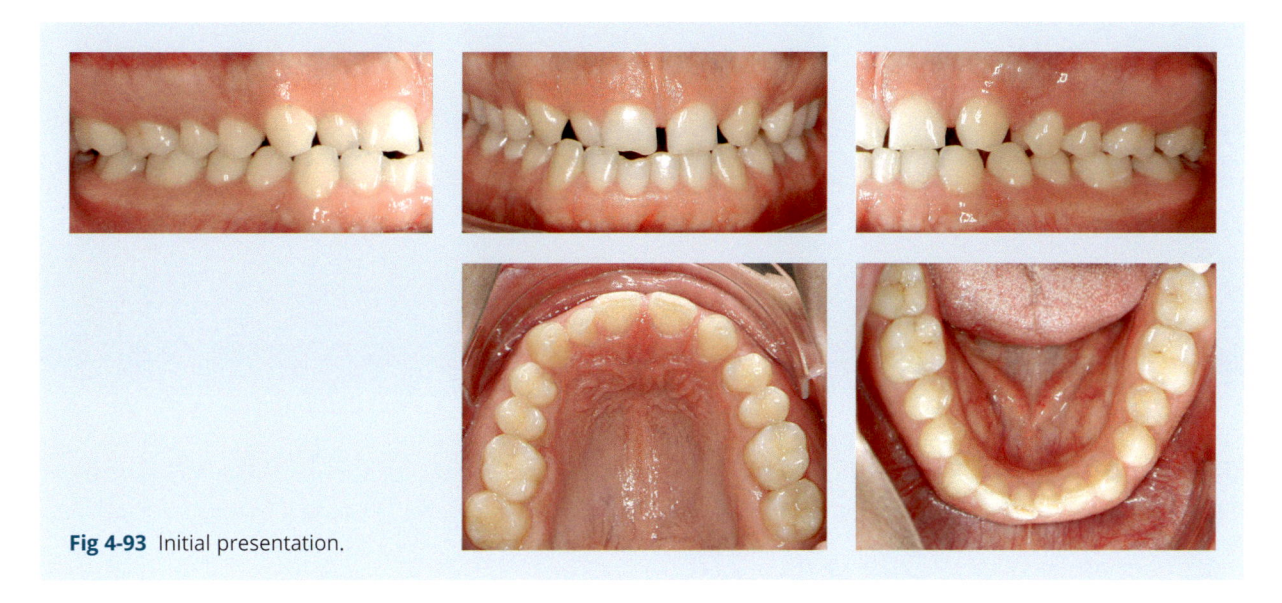

Fig 4-93 Initial presentation.

Diagnosis:
- traumatic loss of tooth 22 with mesial migration of tooth 23
- attrition from dental trauma
- severe cicatricial pull from upper lip scar.

Therapy:
- opening of space 22
- correction of anterior crossbite
- correction of overjet to obtain optimal situation for later restoratives
- crowns, fixed partial denture, and veneers to finish.

Fig 4-94 Start of Invisalign treatment with rectangular attachments.

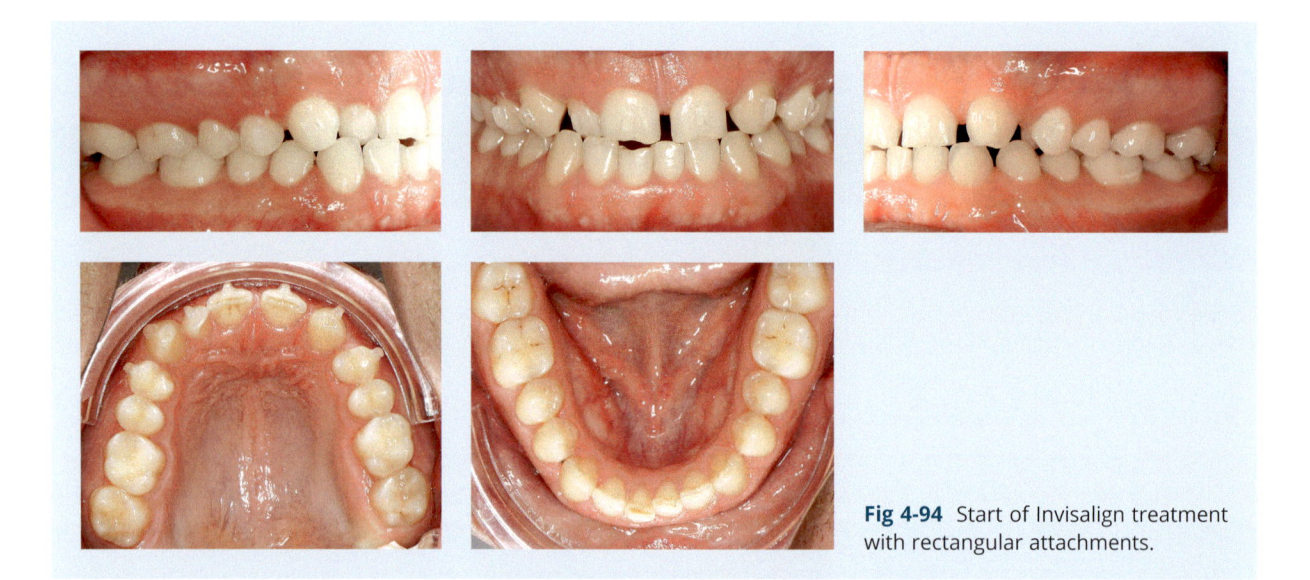

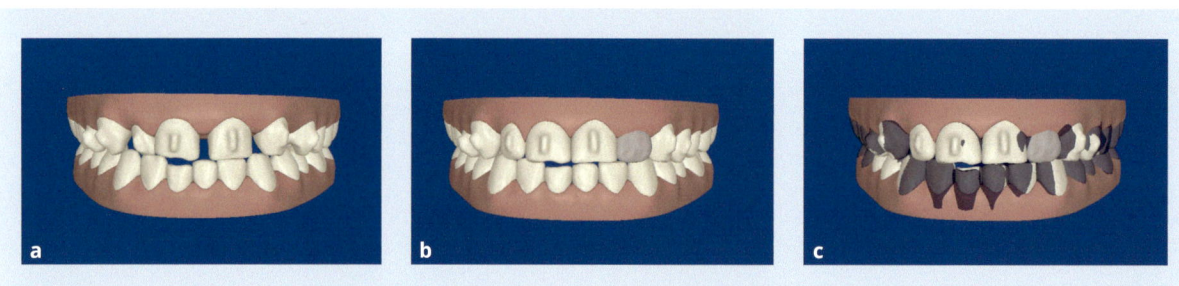

Fig 4-95 ClinCheck software results. **(a)** Initial findings with spaces in the maxillary arch. **(b)** Final findings with opening of space for later restorative tooth 22 with inserted virtual pontic, alignment of maxillary and mandibular anterior teeth, and increased overjet for later restoratives. **(c)** Superimposition showing the planned teeth movement (blue, initial tooth position; white, final tooth position).

Treatment

Because of the fractured enamel and the short crowns of the maxillary canines and incisors, it was decided to open the space for a fixed partial denture from 21 to 23 and to place veneers on teeth 13, 12, and 11 and the mandibular incisors.

Invisalign treatment used rectangular attachments (before G4 attachments were available) (Fig 4-94). During aligner therapy and afterwards for retention, pontics were inserted in the aligners until the insert of restoratives.

Figure 4-95 shows the ClinCheck software results. The first phase used 20 aligners in the maxillary arch and 15 aligners in the mandibular arch.

Figure 4-96 shows before and after Invisalign treatment with opening of space in region 22 for later restoratives.

Before initiating any orthodontic treatment where an interdisciplinary approach is needed, a treatment plan is worked out between all the specialists concerned. It was decided to open the space to substitute missing tooth 22, correct the crossbite at tooth 12, and create increased overjet and a slight open bite to obtain sufficient space in the vertical dimension for the planned fixed partial denture and veneers (Fig 4-97).

Treatment was completed with veneers and a fixed partial denture. To reduce the unfavorable aspect of

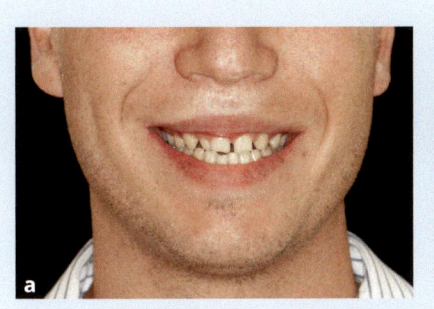

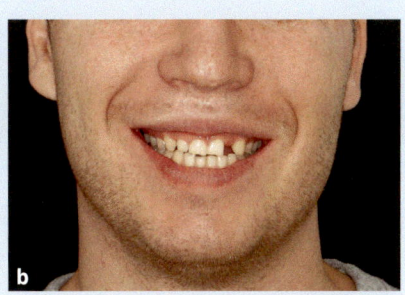

TREATMENT OF DIFFERENT MALOCCLUSIONS WITH ALIGNERS 4

Fig 4-96 Before Invisalign treatment **(a)** and after **(b)** showing opening of space in region 22.

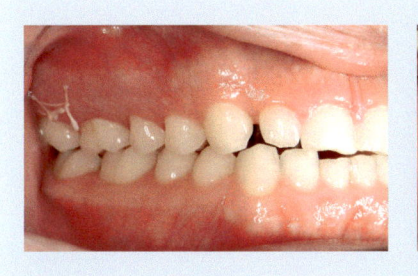

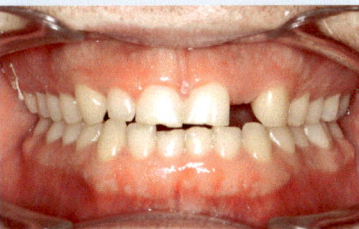

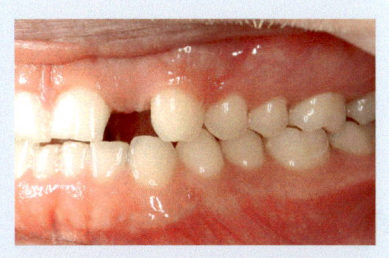

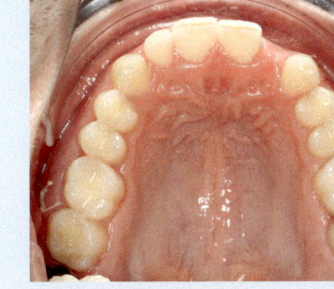

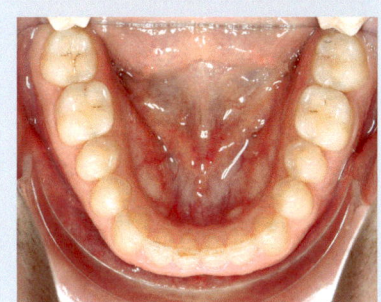

Fig 4-97 Views at the end of Invisalign treatment with space for substitution of tooth 22 and sufficient space in the vertical dimension for the planned fixed partial denture and veneers.

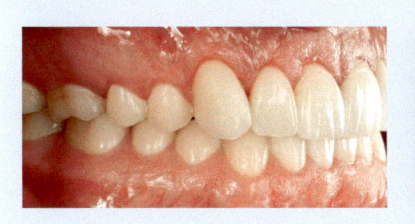

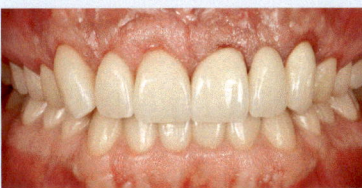

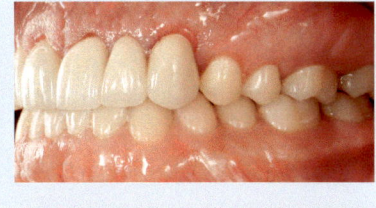

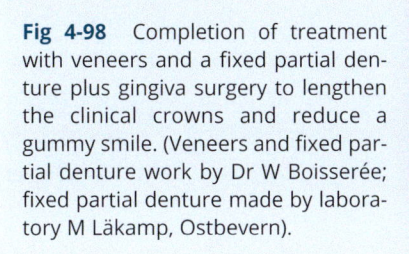

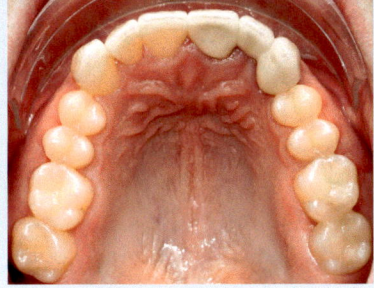

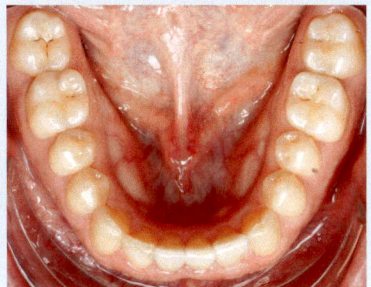

Fig 4-98 Completion of treatment with veneers and a fixed partial denture plus gingiva surgery to lengthen the clinical crowns and reduce a gummy smile. (Veneers and fixed partial denture work by Dr W Boisserée; fixed partial denture made by laboratory M Läkamp, Ostbevern).

95

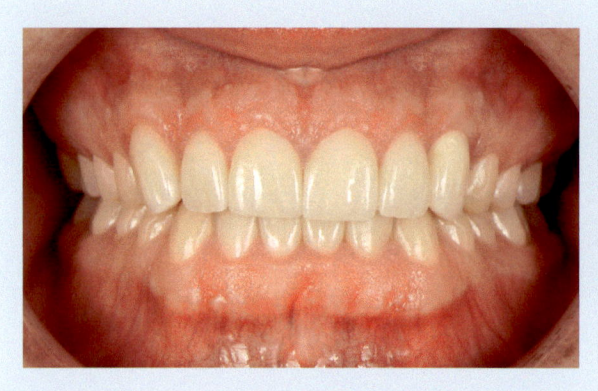

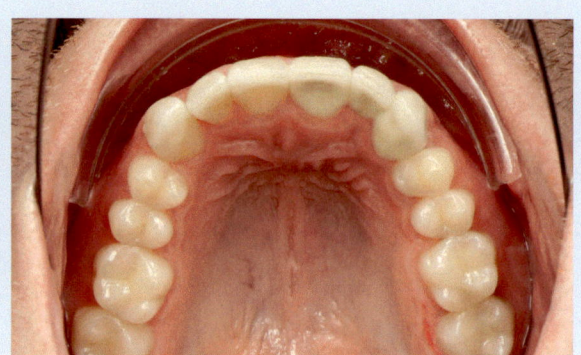

Fig 4-99 Intraoral view after gingival healing.

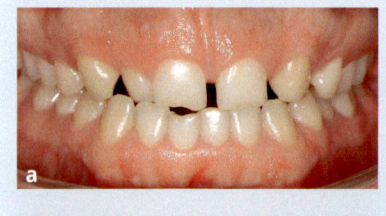

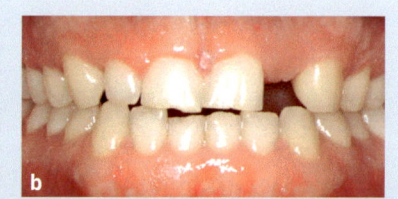

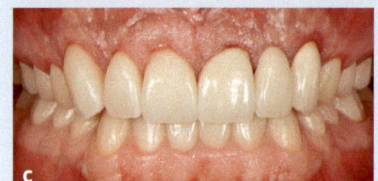

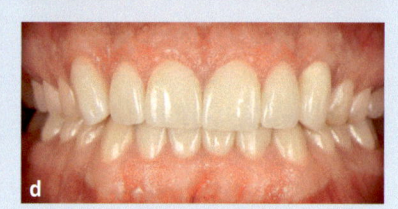

Fig 4-100 Intraoral views of treatment progress. **(a)** Initial situation; **(b)** at the end of Invisalign treatment; **(c)** after esthetic and prosthodontic therapy including surgical crown lengthening **(d)** the final result after an additional 2 months of gingival healing.

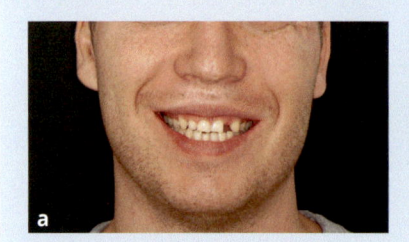

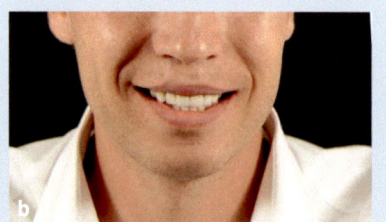

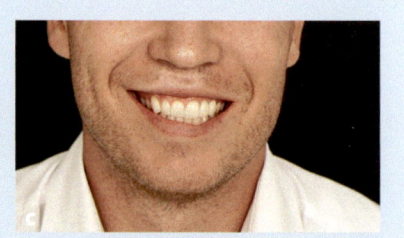

Fig 4-101 Extraoral views of treatment progress. **(a)** After orthodontic treatment with missing tooth 22, gummy smile, and very short clinical crowns due to abrasion and attrition. **(b,c)** The smile after the periodontal and restorative esthetic dentistry.

the gummy smile, gingiva surgery lengthened the clinical crowns using an apically repositioned flap with osteoplasty. Veneers were inserted on teeth 13 to 11, a ceramic fixed partial denture on zircon base (Prettauer) on teeth 21 to 23, and Non Prep veneers on teeth 31 to 42 (Fig 4-98).

Figure 4-99 shows the intraoral view after several months of gingival healing.

Figures 4-100 and 4-101 show treatment progression.

Topic 15
Gummy smile in a young patient

Treatment:
- intrusion of teeth

There are several orthodontic options to open the bite in an anterior deep bite:
- intrusion of maxillary incisors, sometimes canines
- intrusion of mandibular incisors, sometimes canines
- extrusion of mandibular posterior teeth
- a combination of all these.

A curve of Spee can be leveled by:
- intrusion of mandibular incisors and most often canines
- extrusion of mandibular premolars and molars
- a combination of intrusion and extrusion.

Intrusion is highly predictable with the Invisalign system. In deep bites or leveling of excessive curves of Spee, the decision needs to be made as to which movement combination is necessary and then this should be written precisely in the online treatment plan for the ClinCheck software.

This patient had a dental deep bite with extruded maxillary anterior teeth (Fig 4-102). The maxillary clinical crowns of the incisors are short and she had a significant gummy smile.

Diagnosis:
- class I relationship
- spaces in the maxillary and mandibular arches
- extruded maxillary anterior teeth
- gummy smile.

Therapy:
- Invisalign treatment with intrusion of upper incisors.

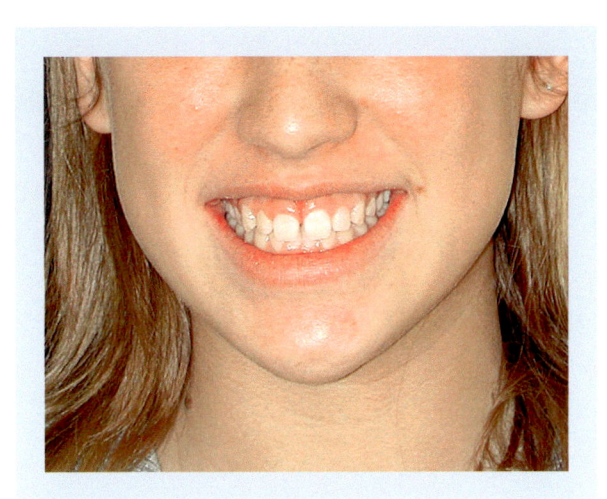

Fig 4-102 Initial presentation.

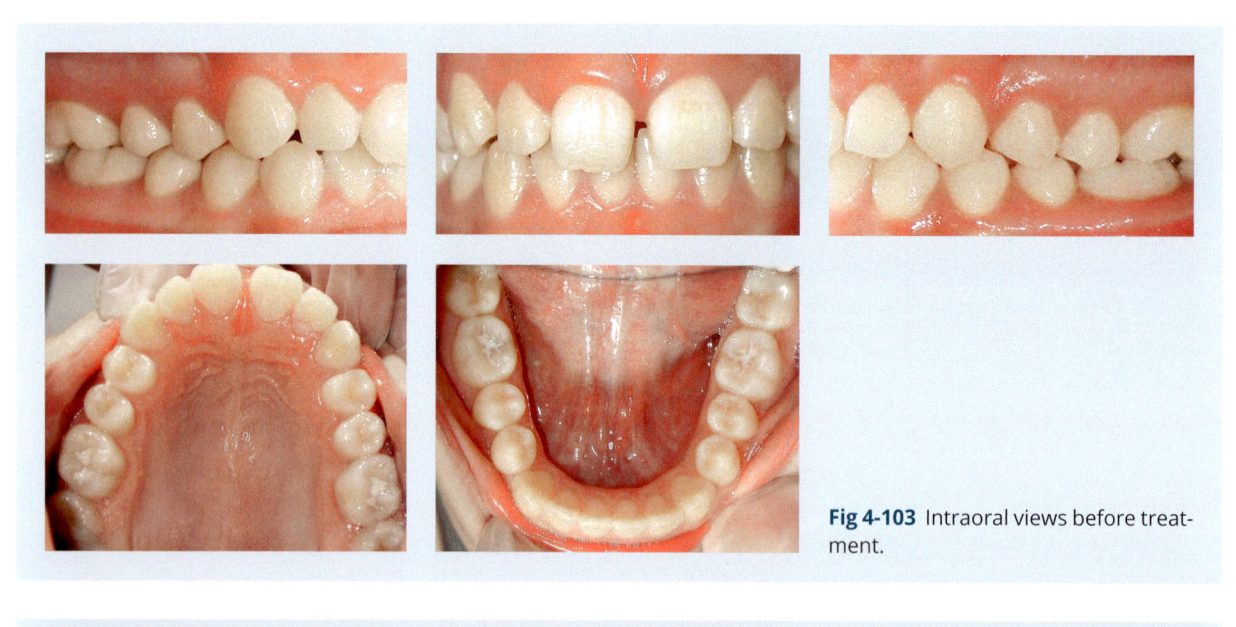

Fig 4-103 Intraoral views before treatment.

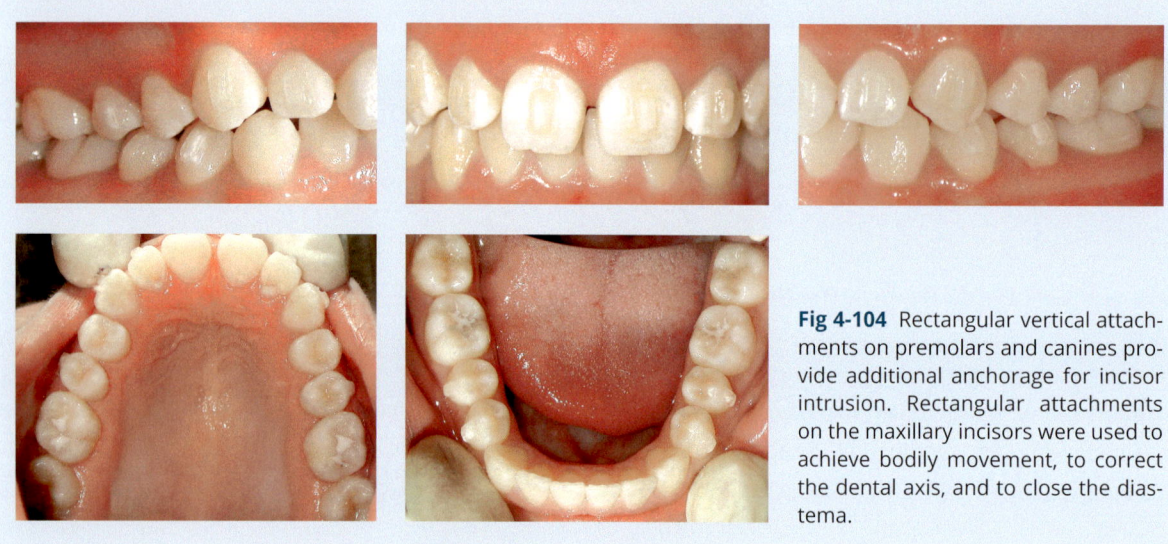

Fig 4-104 Rectangular vertical attachments on premolars and canines provide additional anchorage for incisor intrusion. Rectangular attachments on the maxillary incisors were used to achieve bodily movement, to correct the dental axis, and to close the diastema.

Treatment

A gummy smile can be treated orthodontically, surgically, with periodontal plastic surgery, or with combinations of these. For this patient, it was decided to intrude the maxillary incisors, given also consideration to the possibility of periodontal plastic surgery after the Invisalign therapy.

Intrusion of maxillary incisors is possible and should not exceed the amount of 2–3 mm visible incisors in rest position of the lips (Fig 4-103). Intrusion of maxillary incisors must be carried out cautiously as the esthetic result at the end is far from satisfactory if the maxillary incisors do not show during speaking.

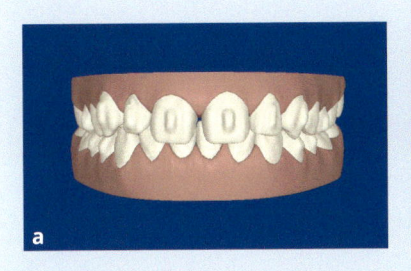

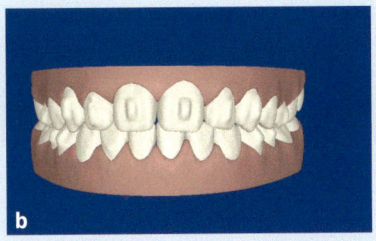

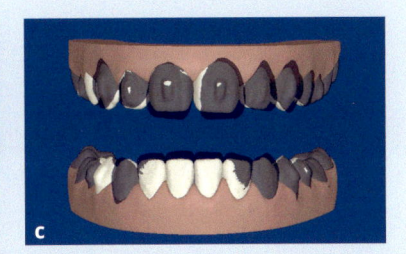

Fig 4-105 ClinCheck software results. **(a)** Initial situation. **(b)** Planned final situation. **(c)** Superimposition shows the initial and final position of teeth in both arches (blue, initial tooth position; white, final tooth position).

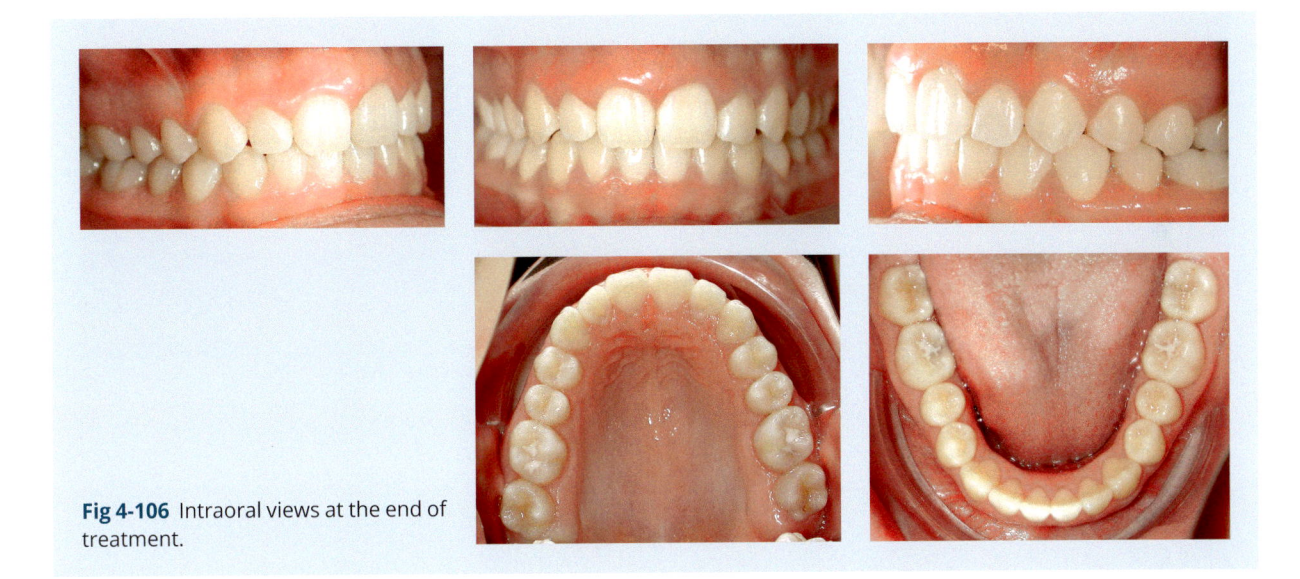

Fig 4-106 Intraoral views at the end of treatment.

The intraoral pictures (Fig 4-104) show the start of Invisalign treatment. Rectangular vertical attachments on premolars and canines help to provide additional anchorage to ensure predictability of incisor intrusion. Rectangular attachments on the maxillary incisors were used to achieve bodily movement, to correct the dental axis, and to close the diastema. Eight aligners were planned for the maxillary arch and 14 for the mandibular arch (Fig 4-105).

The planning for this young patient required simultaneous intrusion of mandibular incisors and canines, as well as a slight extrusion of the mandibular premolars. In adults, simultaneous intrusion of canines and incisors can be quite difficult and so this is often done sequentially (see separate treatment plan at the end of this topic).

Figure 4-106 shows the harmonically leveled curve of Spee at the end of treatment. All premolars and molars show occlusal contacts in habitual intercuspation. In the incisor region, teeth barely show anterior contact in habitual intercuspation, allowing the Shimstock foil (8 μm) to be pulled through the dental arches, which we consider to be an optimal anterior relationship. Laterotrusion is guided by canines, protrusion by incisors.

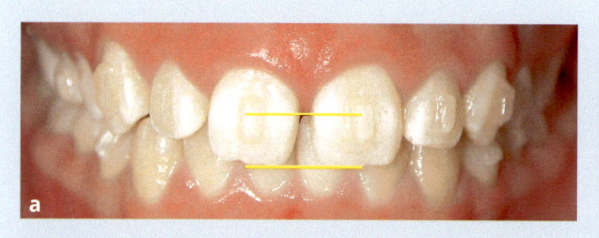

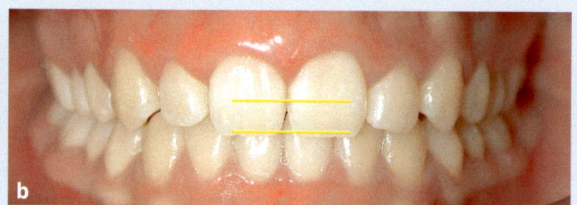

4 TREATMENT OF DIFFERENT MALOCCLUSIONS WITH ALIGNERS

Fig 4-107 Initial **(a)** and final **(b)** views showing distinct intrusion of maxillary and mandibular incisors, angulation of teeth 11 and 21, and closure of diastema.

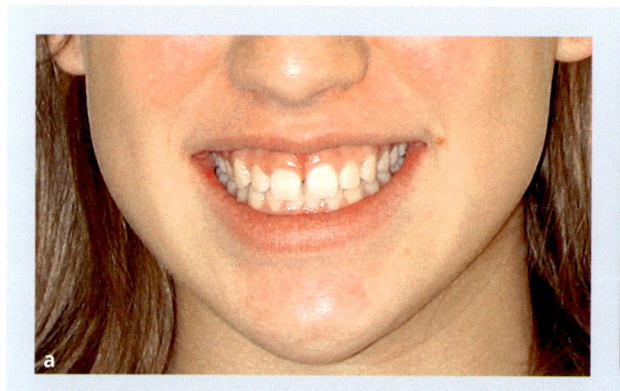

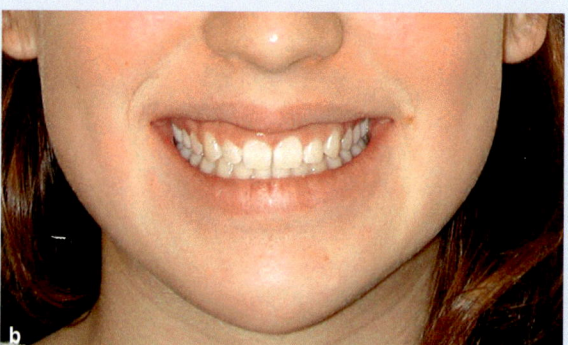

Fig 4-108 Extraoral initial **(a)** and final **(b)** views show the improved esthetic smile line, although the gummy smile is present.

Figures 4-107 and 4-108 shows distinct intrusion of maxillary and mandibular incisors with the Invisalign treatment. The angulation of teeth 11 and 21 was corrected and the diastema closed; this was achieved by asking in the online treatment plan for an overcorrection of the mesial teeth movement, thus ensuring complete space closure. She had an improved esthetic smile line although the gummy smile is still present because of the short crowns of the maxillary incisors. To obtain an optimum esthetic smile, periodontal plastic surgery might be an additional treatment in this patient.

Retention was performed with the last aligner, which was worn initially after the active treatment for an additional 3 months for 3–4 hours a day. At night, the patient was advised to wear an occlusal retention splint (see Topic 62).

Treatment plan for intrusion of teeth in an adult

To level the curve of Spee in adults, teeth can be intruded in the mandibular arch. Because simultaneous intrusion of canines and incisors can be quite difficult in adults, the incisors are intruded first; the canines are then intruded, with simultaneous extrusion of mandibular premolars 0.3 to 0.5 mm, depending on requirements. This sequence guarantees major anchorage during the intrusive movements.

The described path is carried out using the Ricketts technique (utility arch for intrusion, Rickets 1976), which can be transferred into the Invisalign system.

Attachments are placed on the mandibular canines and premolars for major anchorage and also on the first molar if it needs extrusion. The optimized extrusion attachments are ideal (Fig 4-109 and 4-110).

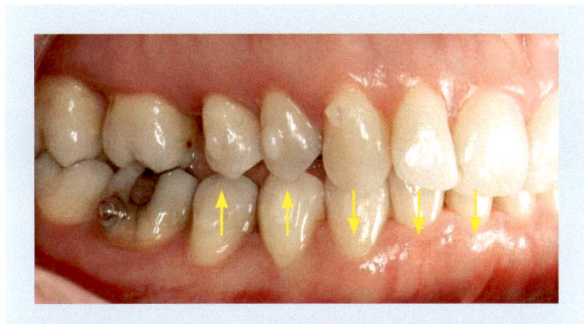

TREATMENT OF DIFFERENT MALOCCLUSIONS WITH ALIGNERS 4

Fig 4-109 Movement required for mandibular teeth.

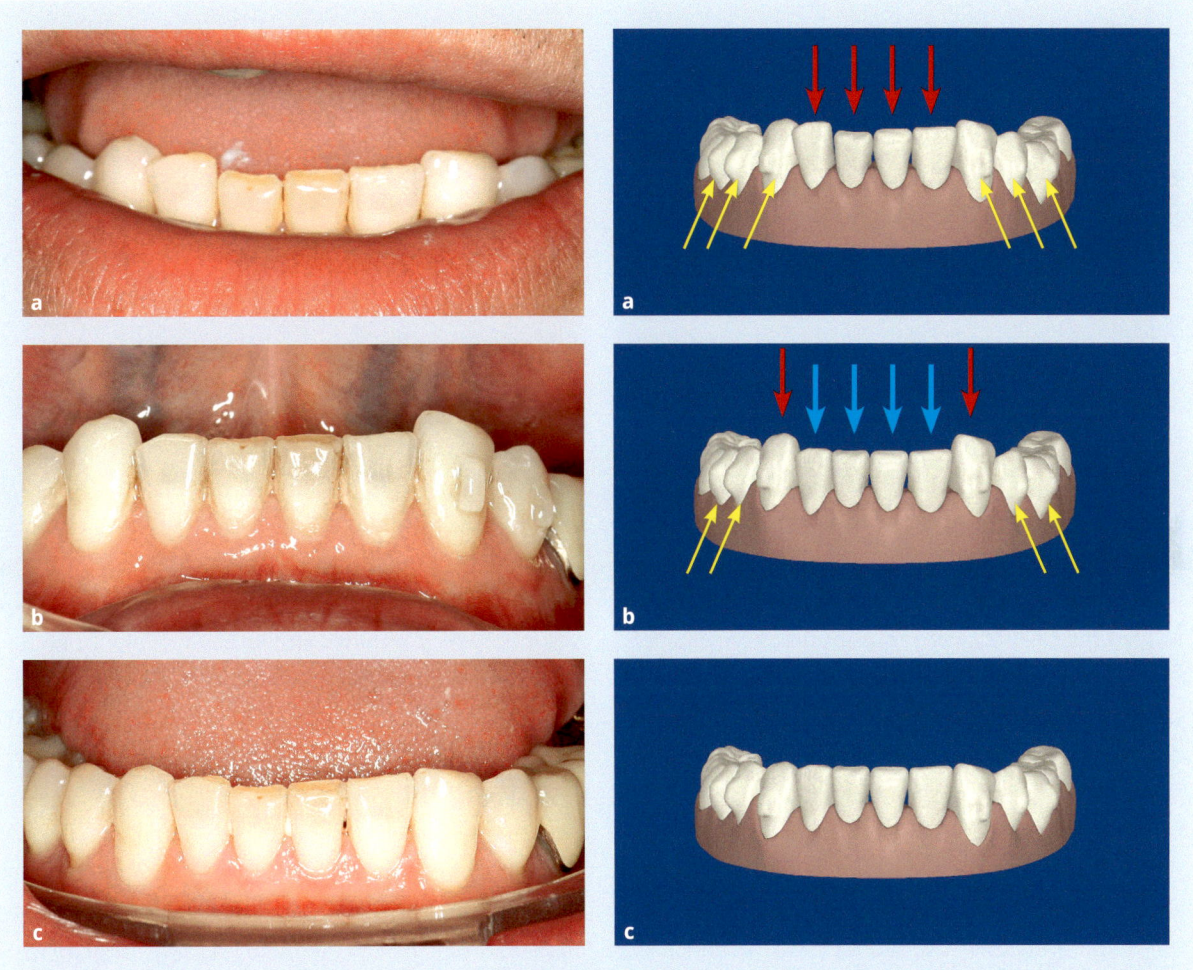

Fig 4-110 Treatment pathway with intraoral views **(left)** and the ClinCheck simulation **(right)**. **(a)** Initial view with extruded mandibular incisors and canines. With the first aligners, intrusion was planned only on incisors (red arrows), vertical rectangular attachments were bonded prior to the scan on all mandibular premolars, and canines for anchorage (yellow arrows). **(b)** Placement of 13 aligners with intrusion of the incisors (blue arrows). Note the difference of height between canines and incisors, showing the amount of intrusion that had occurred. The next phase would intrude the canines (red arrows) with anchorage provided by vertical rectangular attachments on the mandibular premolars (yellow arrows). **(c)** Final situation after use of 22 aligners, with complete intrusion of mandibular canines and incisors and leveled curve of Spee.

Topic 16
Build up a "Speed Up"

Treatment:
- for addition to aligners to obtain improved occlusal pattern

The "Speed Up" is an additional device that a patient wears together with the aligners at night. The Speed Up is built in an individual laboratory process, described below, and can be used:
- in patients with a deep bite to increase the vertical force on the incisors, which can help to intrude them better and faster
- in patients who do not have perfect aligner fitting in the incisor area
- in patients with CMD and muscle pain and/or TMJ pain or in patients who develop peripheral pain syndromes

For incisor intrusion, the Speed Up needs to be checked with occlusal foil (preferred Bausch Progress 100). Contact points in posterior areas are ground to give a minimum of vertical support, leaving increased occlusal force at the incisors and canines.

If there is less than perfect aligner fitting in the incisor area, usually seen in the maxillary arch, there will be an increasing gap between the aligner and the incisor edge. Again here the thickness of the Speed Up helps to increase the pressure needed to obtain better anterior aligner fitment.

Maxillary and mandibular aligners can never create exactly equal supportive occlusion patterns on both sides and this can lead to CMD or TMJ pain. The Speed Up can be used to adjust contacts points to provide equal vertical support on both sides. The use of the Speed Up during the night can help to establish a more comfortable jaw alignment without precontacts on the aligners. Here, contact points of the Speed Up are checked with occlusal foil and excessive contacts are ground away to create symmetric contacts on the right and left premolar and molar area when the patient bites onto the aligners and Speed Up.

Fabrication of the Speed Up
An alginate impression is taken in the maxilla over the aligner (Fig 4-111a). Based on the ClinCheck superimposition, all the teeth that are planned to be moved are blocked out on the plaster cast and the laboratory technician blocks out the amount of space needed for the planned protrusion with blocker material. This ensures that the Speed Up will not interfere with the movements planned for the aligner action.

Using a thermoforming unit, the technician draws a Bioplast foil (Scheu) over the blocked-out plaster cast (Fig 4-111e,f). An anterior ramp is built onto the Bioplast aligner from maxillary canine to maxillary canine with the hot glue gun, which melts a transparent thermoforming material and enables it to be applied to the palatal anterior region (Fig 4-111g–i). This ramp can be smoothened with a metal burr. The final surface is obtained by drawing a second Bioplast foil over the aligner and the added ramp (Fig 4-111k).

Use of the Speed Up
Figure 4-112 shows the Speed Up in the maxilla over the aligner with occlusal contacts of the incisors in the closed mouth position (b). The contact points on the Speed Up can be checked with occlusal foil and then modified to improve occlusion by grinding. The patient is advised to wear the Speed Up at night together with the aligners.

TREATMENT OF DIFFERENT MALOCCLUSIONS WITH ALIGNERS 4

Fig 4-111 Fabrication of the Speed Up. **(a)** An alginate impression taken in the maxilla over the aligner. **(b)** The ClinCheck superimposition of the required movements. **(c,d)** Teeth that have planned movements are blocked out on the cast, as are the spaces needed for these movements. Here, the mesial aspects of teeth 12, 13 and 23, which are planned to be derotated and protruded, are blocked out (Blue Blokker, Scheu). **(e,f)** A thermoforming unit (Biostar/Scheu) is used to draw a Bioplast foil (Scheu) **(e)** over the blocked-out plaster cast **(f)**. **(g)** Hot glue gun. **(h)** Erkoflex stick-82 (Erkodent). **(i)** Placement of the thermoforming material over the palatal anterior region. **(j)** A ramp built up from canine to canine. **(k)** To obtain an optimal surface, a second Bioplast foil is drawn over the aligner and the added ramp.

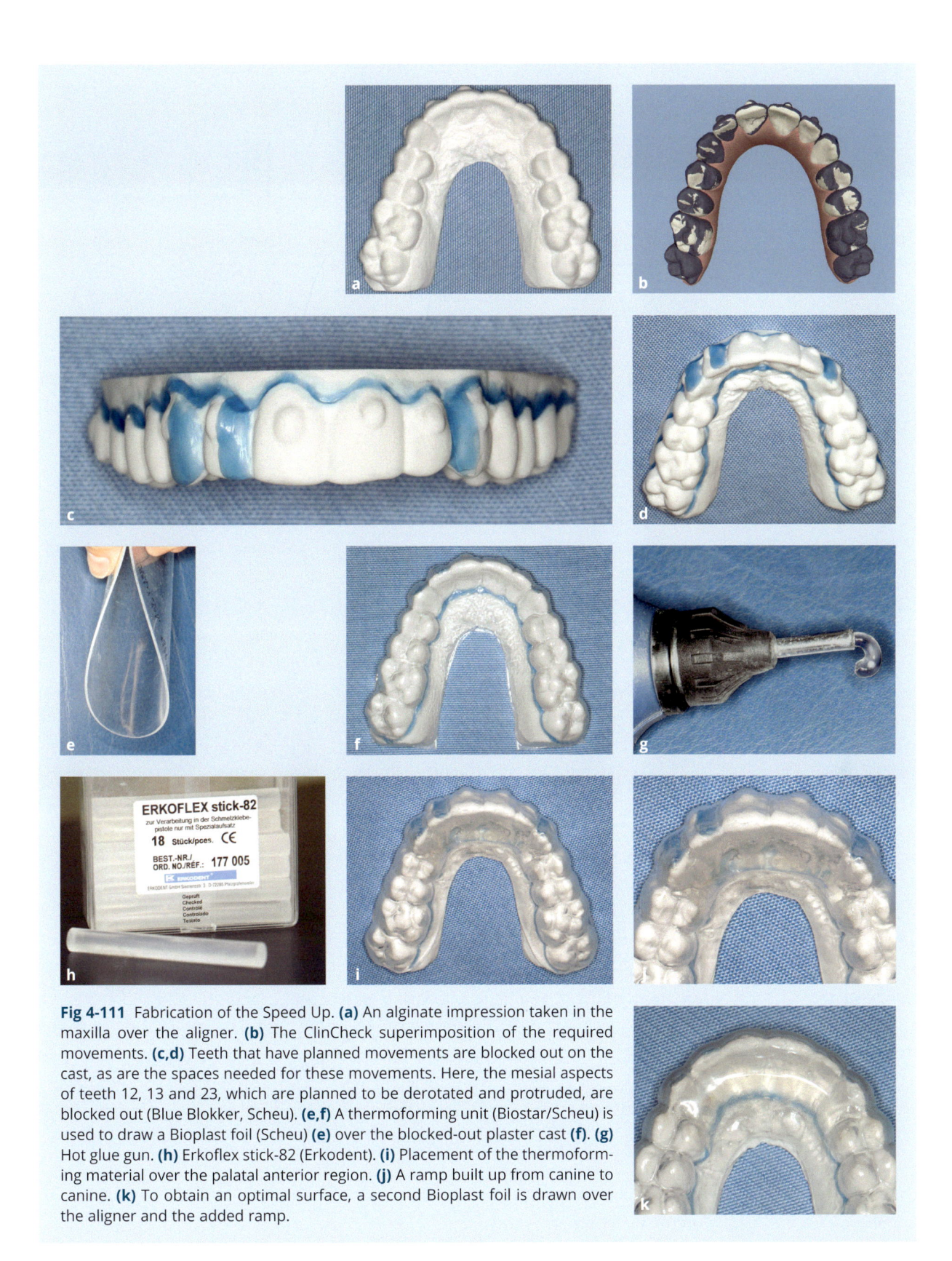

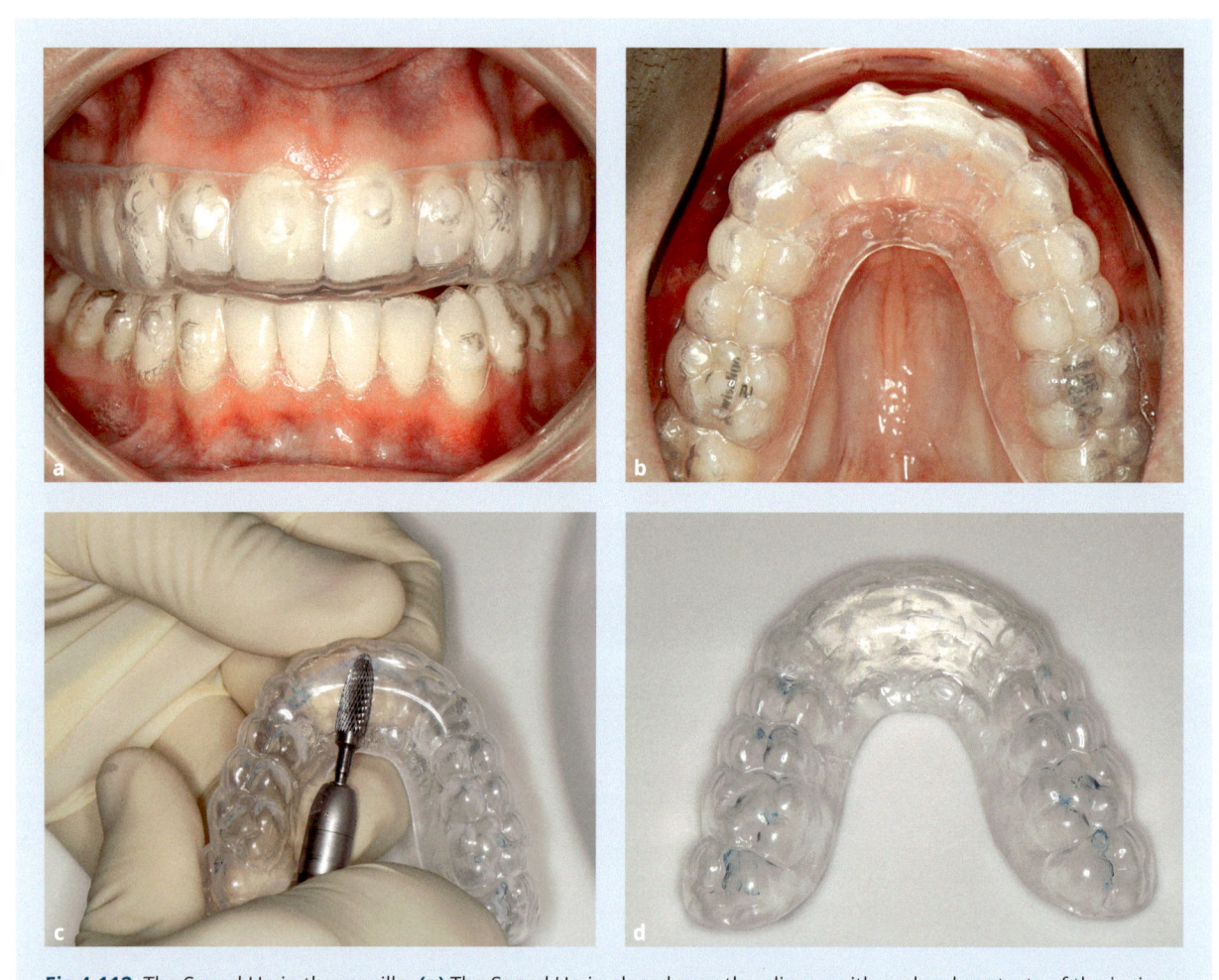

Fig 4-112 The Speed Up in the maxilla. **(a)** The Speed Up is placed over the aligner with occlusal contacts of the incisors in the closed mouth position. **(b)** Checking the contact points on the Speed Up using occlusal foil. **(c)** A metal handpiece (e.g. Komet H251GE) can be used to alter the occlusion to the required vertical support. **(d)** The final device.

Topic 17
Anterior open bite

Treatment:
- extrusion

Dentoalveolar open bites can be caused by speech disorders, oral habits, or mouth breathing due to enlarged lymphatic tissues or allergies. Positioning of the tongue during swallowing, speech, and rest plays an important role in the development of open bites, aside from any genetic predispositions. In such patients, consultation between orthodontist, otorhinolaryngologist, and myofunctional therapist becomes necessary before and during orthodontic treatment. For some time, it was not thought that extrusion could be achieved with the Invisalign technique, but the following case study will show that this can be successfully achieved.

Extruding an incisor by a tipping movement is easy to achieve but it takes more time to extrude one with absolute extrusion (Fig 4-113). Both movements can be performed with the Invisalign system and attachments.

This patient had an open bite from first molar to molar (Fig 4-114).

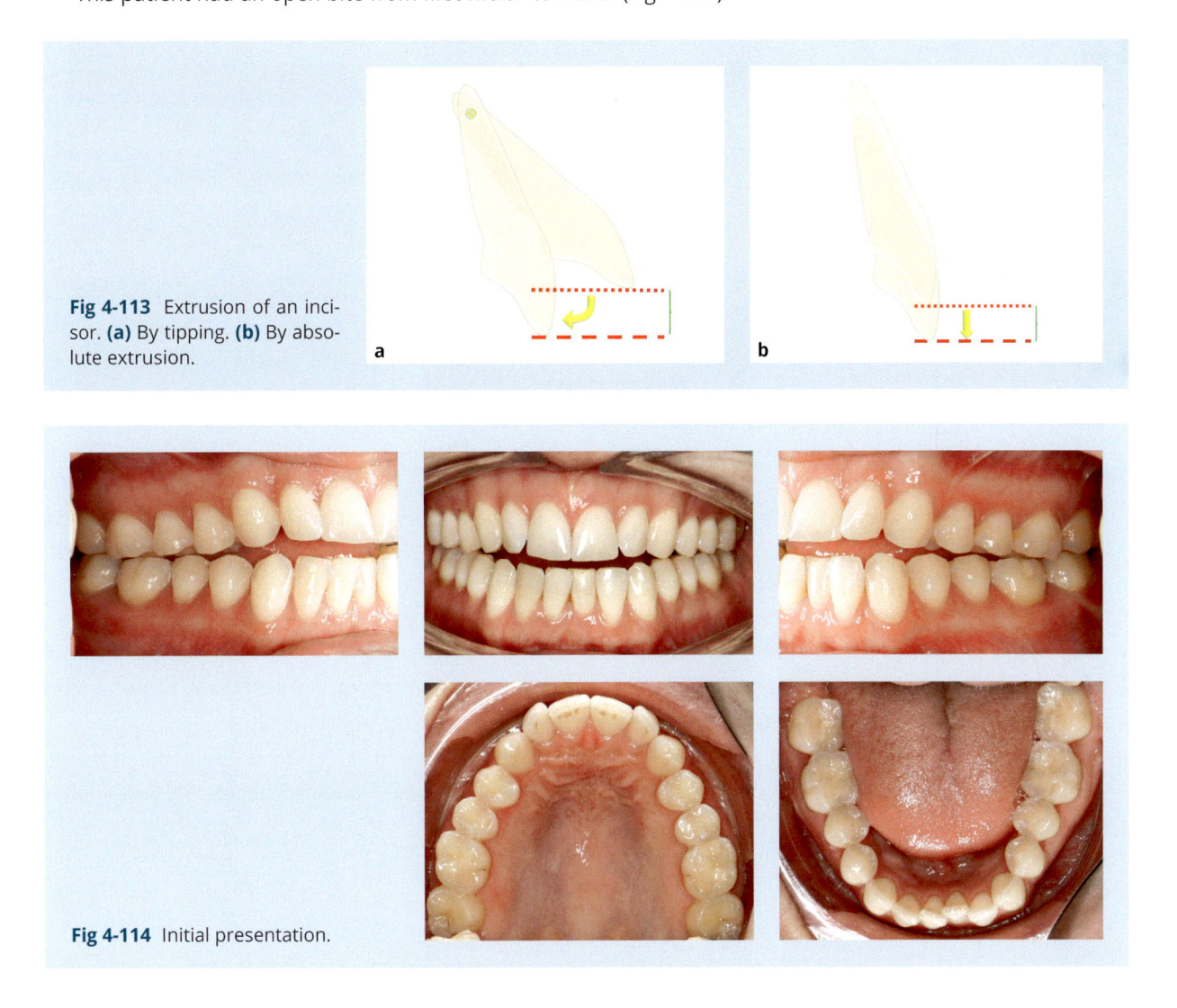

Fig 4-113 Extrusion of an incisor. **(a)** By tipping. **(b)** By absolute extrusion.

Fig 4-114 Initial presentation.

4 TREATMENT OF DIFFERENT MALOCCLUSIONS WITH ALIGNERS

Diagnosis:
- class I
- open bite from first molar to molar with reduced occlusal contact only on second molars
- mild crowding
- in static occlusion, exclusively contact points on second molars
- in dynamic occlusion, second molars lead to their single contact position in laterotrusion and protrusion.

Therapy:
- myofunctional therapy
- alignment of both arches
- extrusion of premolars, canines, and incisors in both arches with simultaneous intrusion of second molars to close the open bite.

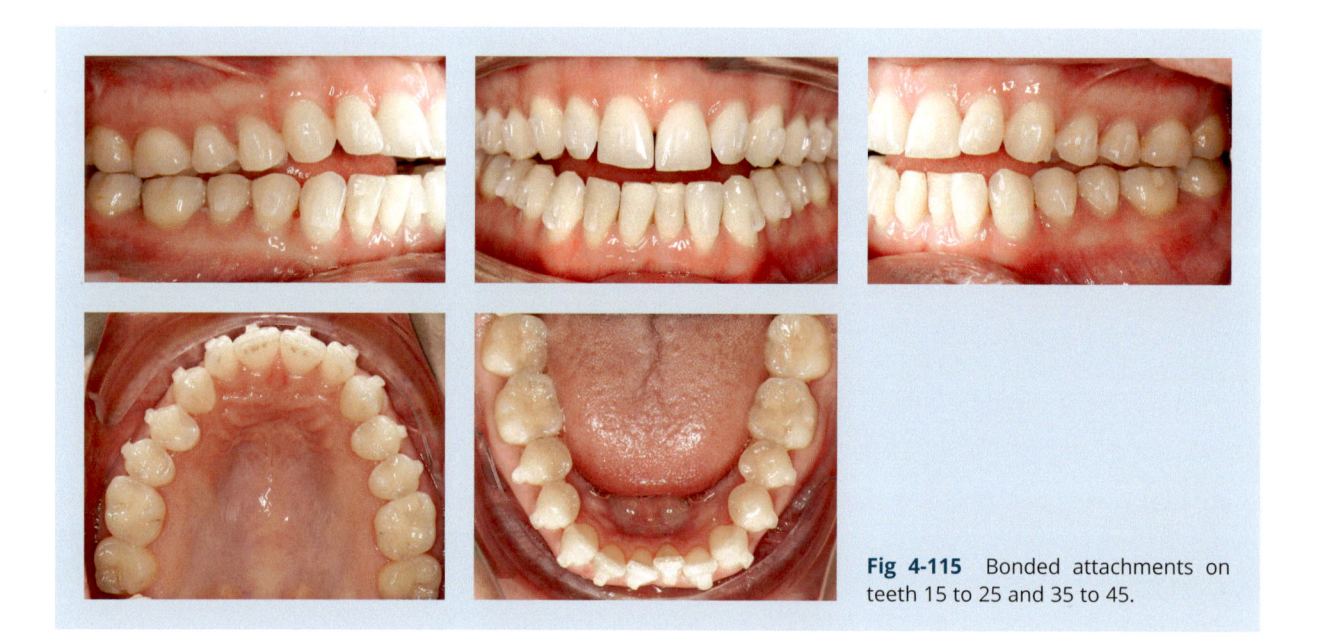

Fig 4-115 Bonded attachments on teeth 15 to 25 and 35 to 45.

Treatment

The patient underwent myofunctional therapy before Invisalign treatment started.

The treatment plan asked for attachments on teeth 15 to 25 and 35 to 45 (Fig 4-115). These attachments were bonded to achieve the extrusive movement of premolars into full contact with hard collision, as well as on canines and incisors to obtain a physiologic overbite and canine guidance.

Figure 4-116 shows the ClinCheck results. The first ClinCheck output was asked for 0.5 mm intrusion of the second molars and extrusion of first molars, premolars, canines, and incisors with 22 aligners. In the refinement, further extrusion of the maxillary canines and incisors with an additional 10 aligners was planned.

After 12 weeks of Invisalign treatment with aligner 6, tooth movement leading to closure of the anterior open bite was apparent, (Fig 4-117) and more so after the refinement phase (Fig 4-118).

Figures 4-119 to 4-121 show treatment progress. Retention with fixed lingual retainers in both arches was required.

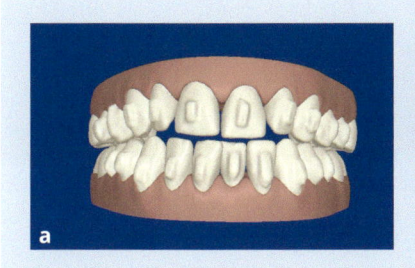

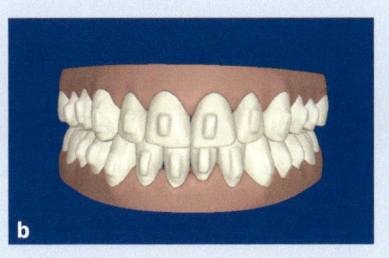

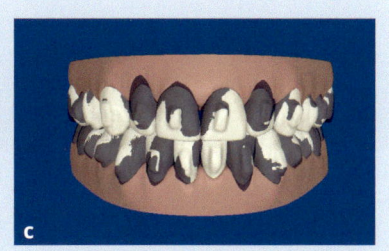

Fig 4-116 ClinCheck software results. **(a)** The initial situation. **(b)** Planned final result. **(c)** Superimposition of initial and final tooth positions (blue, initial tooth position; white, final tooth position).

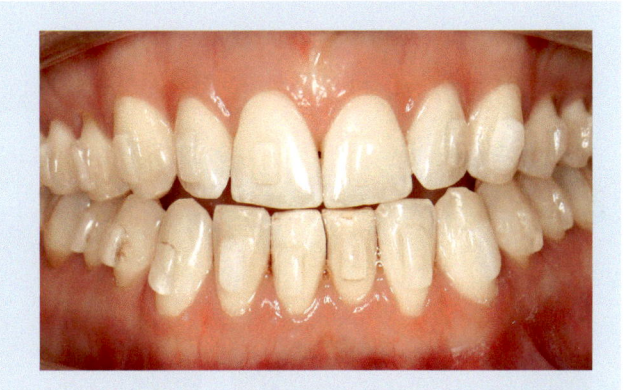

Fig 4-117 Result after 12 weeks.

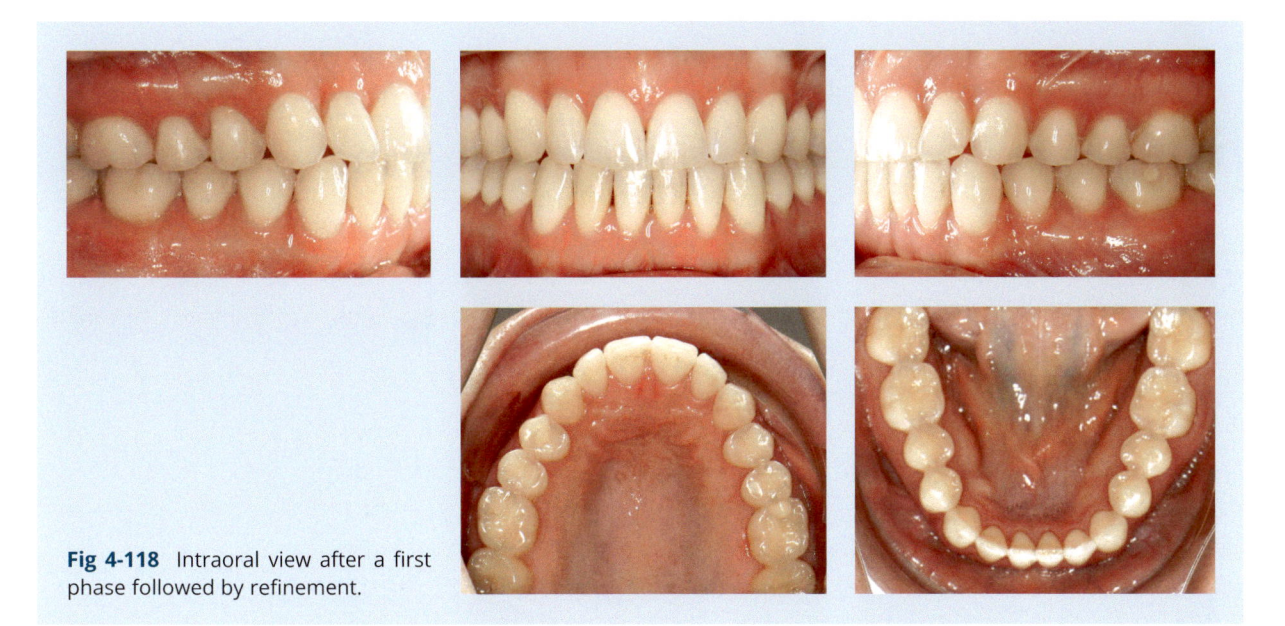

Fig 4-118 Intraoral view after a first phase followed by refinement.

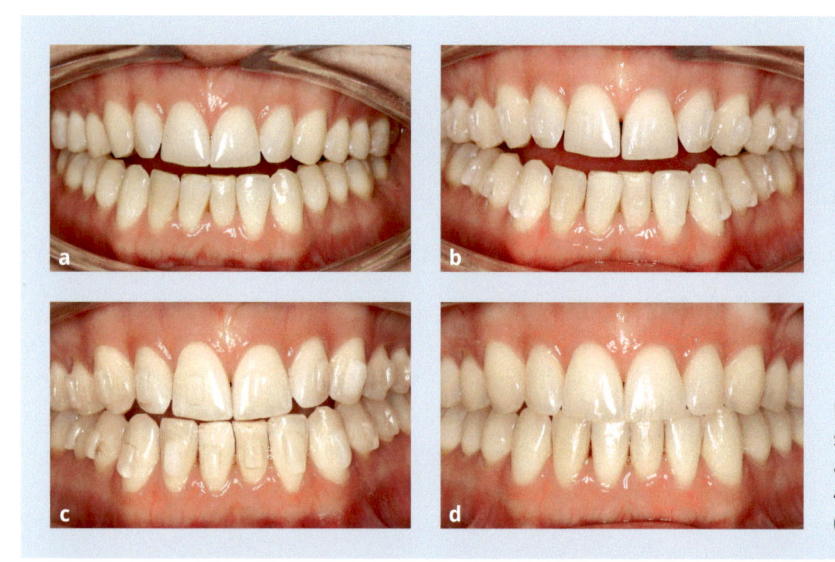

4 TREATMENT OF DIFFERENT MALOCCLUSIONS WITH ALIGNERS

Fig 4-119 Intraoral findings. **(a)** At start of treatment. **(b)** With bonded attachments on teeth 15 to 25, 35 to 45. **(c)** After 12 weeks of treatment. **(d)** Final result.

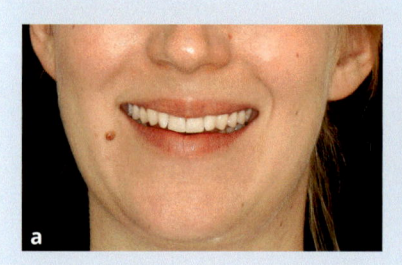

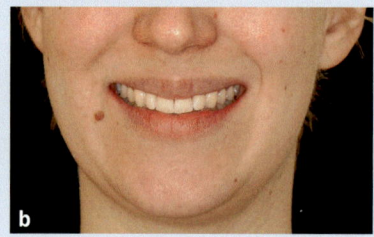

Fig 4-120 Extraoral initial **(a)** and final **(b)** views.

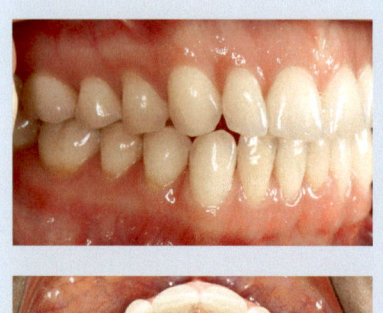

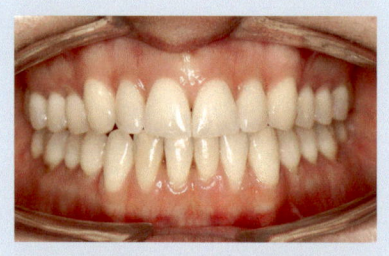

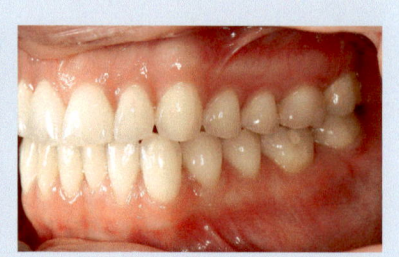

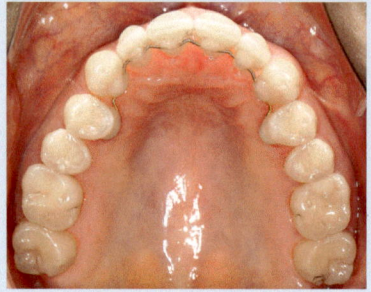

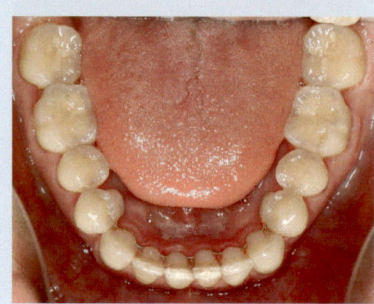

Fig 4-121 Intraoral views after 1 year of retention with fixed lingual retainers in both arches, showing a stable result.

Topic 18
Asymmetry of gingival height and crowding

Treatment:
- leveling of gingival height
- solving of crowding without extraction

The relationship of the gingival margins of maxillary incisors and canines is important for dentofacial esthetics and should be planned with precision from the beginning of a proposed treatment. The optimal position of the gingival margins of the central incisors is on an equal level to that of the canines, but more apical to that of the lateral incisors.

This patient showed no muscular or joint pain and no signs of problems with her TMJs. She asked for an esthetic treatment without extraction. The lip view showed microdontic maxillary lateral incisors (Fig 4-122).

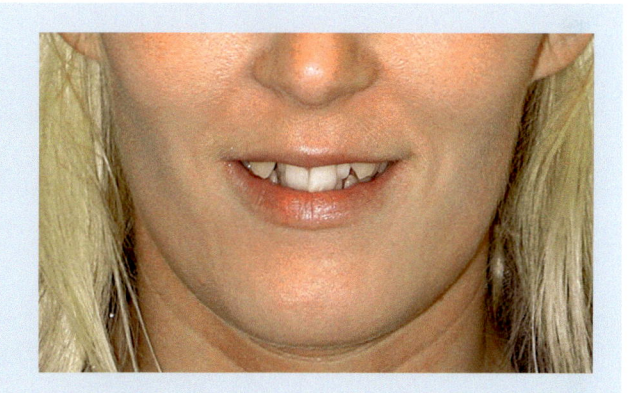

Fig 4-122 Initial presentation.

Diagnosis:
- class II
- severe rotations and crowding in the maxilla and mandible
- transversally constricted maxilla and mandible arch form
- unesthetic relationship of gingival levels of maxillary incisors and canines.

Therapy:
- alignment of the maxilla and mandible with IPR and transversal expansion
- solving of crowding without extraction
- leveling of the gingival height of maxillary incisors and canines for planned restoratives of teeth 12 and 22 after orthodontic treatment.

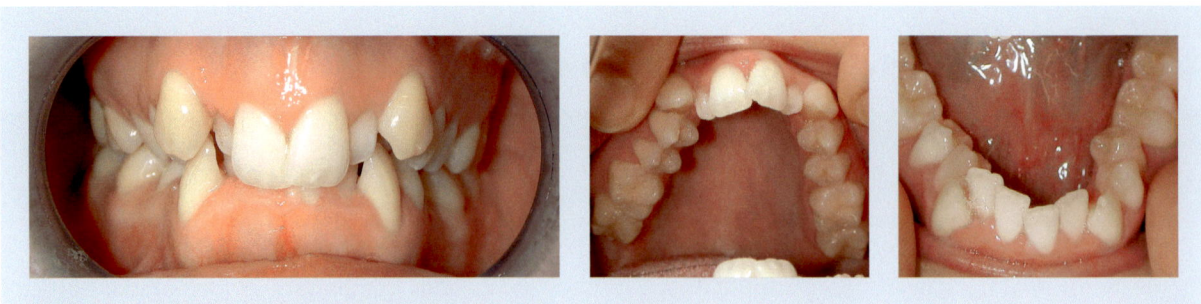

Fig 4-123 Intraoral views at start of treatment.

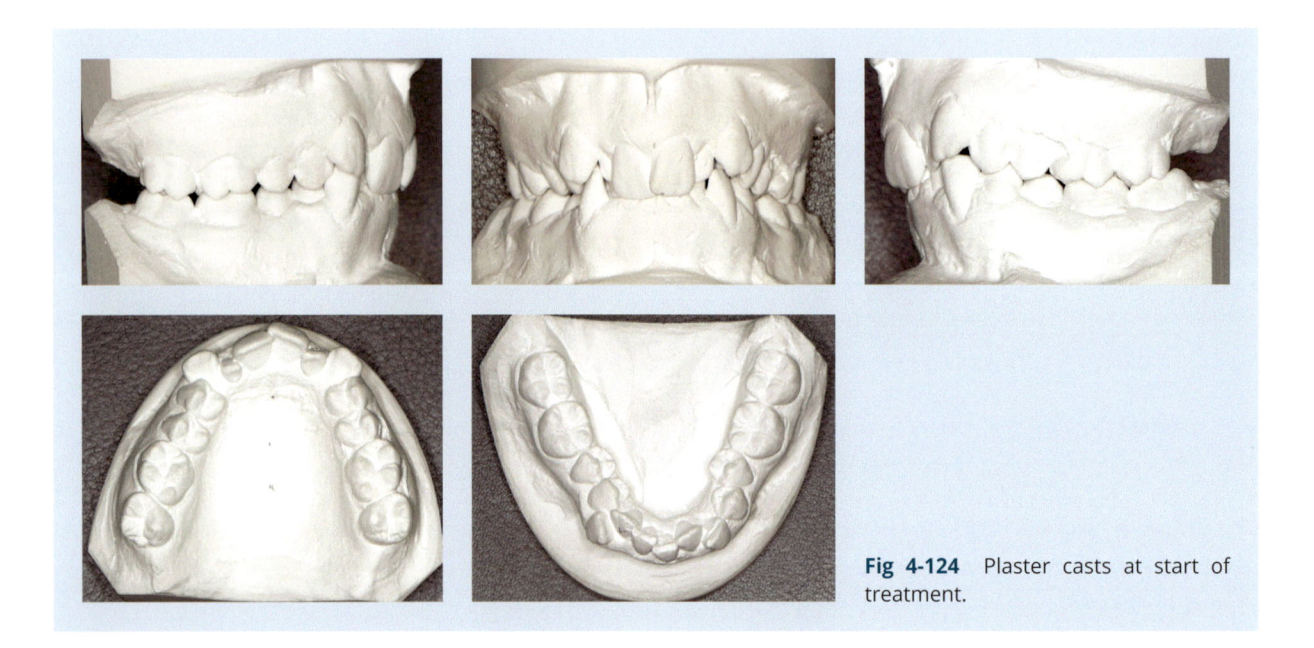

Fig 4-124 Plaster casts at start of treatment.

Treatment

The treatment initially dealt with the severe crowding and lack of space in both arches (Fig 4-123). Tooth 42 had almost contact with tooth 44, maintaining tooth 43 in a vestibular position, and the patient insisted on a non-extraction therapy. Maxillary and mandibular incisors were extruded, giving a dental deep bite. The gingival level of the incisors was much more caudal than the gingival level of the canines. The maxillary and mandibular arches were extremely narrow. The gingiva showed a stable morphotype.

Plaster casts confirmed the severe crowding and lack of space in both arches and the class II relationship (Fig 4-124).

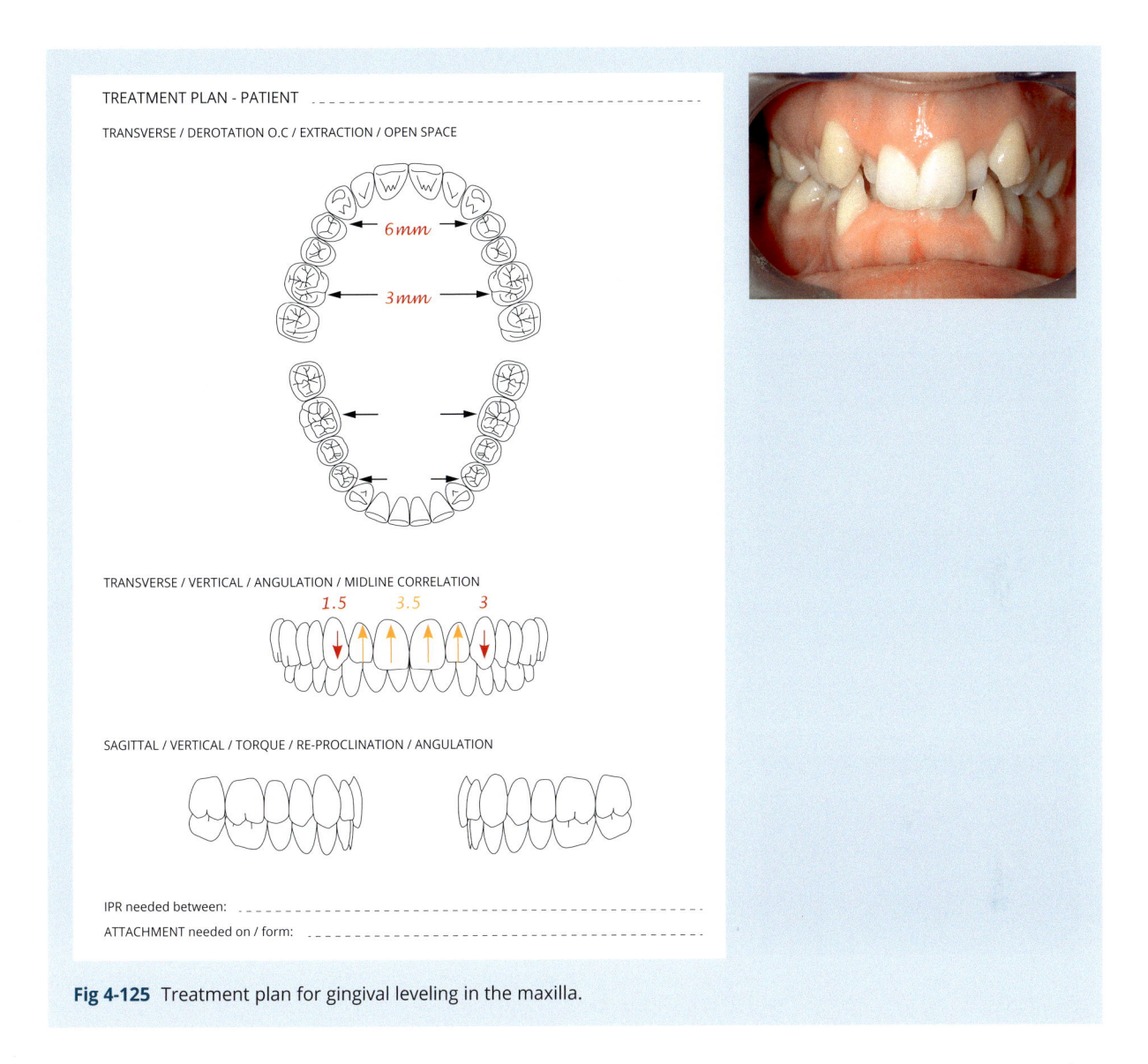

Fig 4-125 Treatment plan for gingival leveling in the maxilla.

The treatment plan for gingival management would optimize the uneven height of the gingival contour (Fig 4-125). It is important to describe the needed intrusion and extrusion of teeth in detail in the treatment plan with the finish in mind, including any overcorrection. In this patient, this was:
- 1.5 mm extrusion of tooth 13 + 0.5 mm overcorrection
- 3.0 mm extrusion of tooth 23 + 1 mm overcorrection
- 3.5 mm intrusion of maxillary incisors + 1 mm overcorrection.

The first phase was planned with 40 upper and 35 lower aligners. IPR was needed (Fig 4-126a) on maxillary canines and premolars and in the mandible distal of tooth 41 to mesial of 46. In this patient, ellipsoid attachments were used; however, if the G4 attachments had been available, even more precise tooth movements might have been possible.

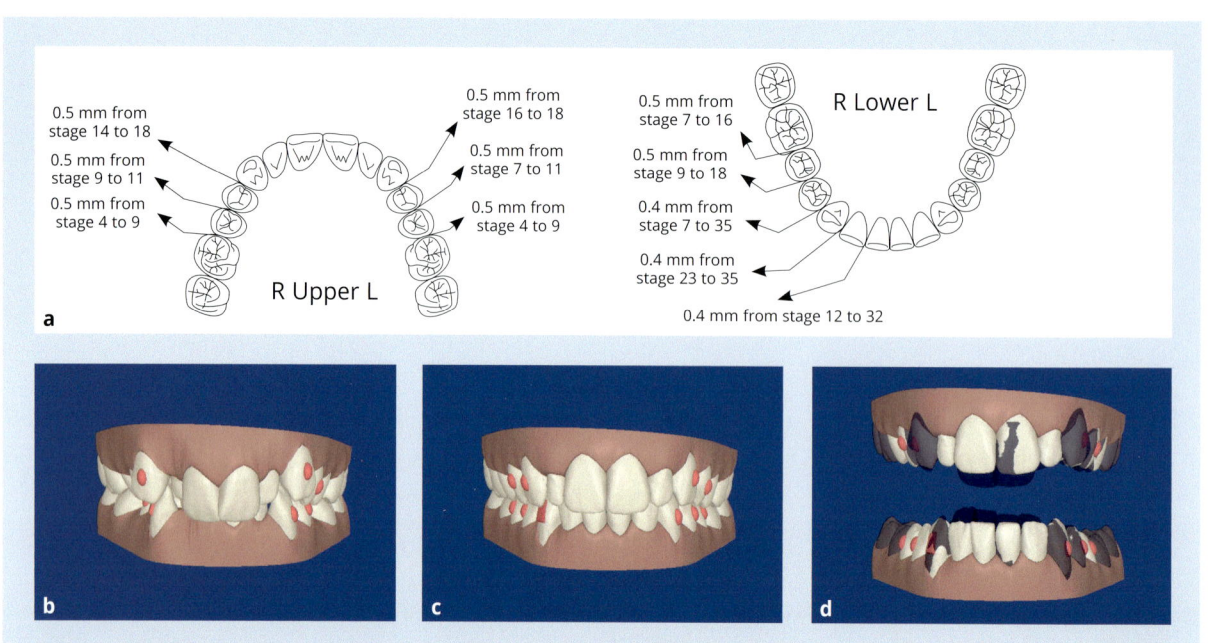

Fig 4-126 ClinCheck phase 1. **(a)** IPR chart. **(b)** Initial situation with attachments on maxillary and mandibular canines and premolars. **(c)** The planned result with aligned arches. **(d)** Superimposition shows the amount of intrusion intended in both arches (blue, initial tooth position; white, final tooth position).

Fig 4-127 ClinCheck superimposition shows tooth 42 with approximal contact to tooth 44 not 43.

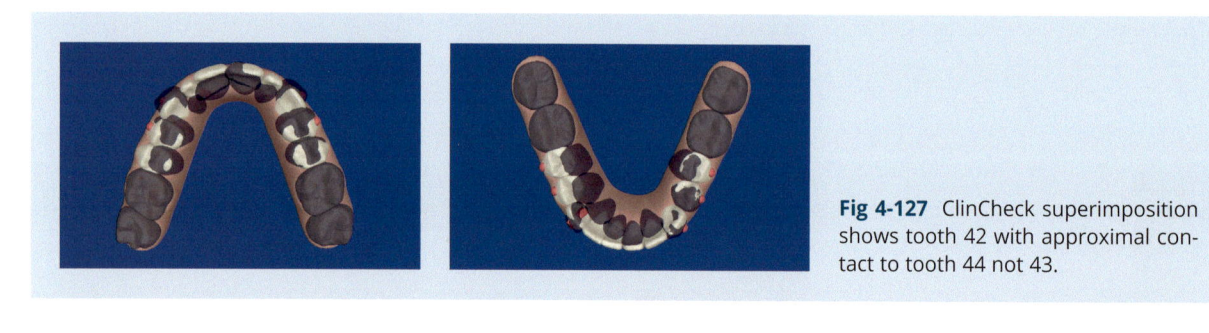

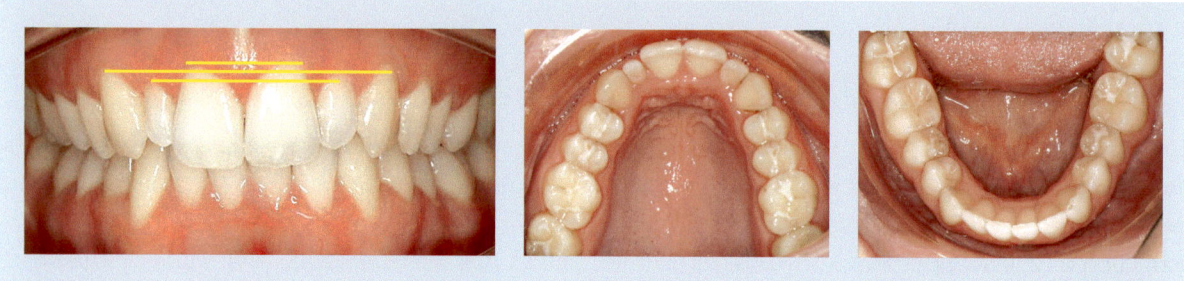

Fig 4-128 Final intraoral views showing well-aligned arches and esthetically aligned gingival contours of maxillary incisors in relation to canines.

The ClinCheck superimposition shows the position of tooth 42 with approximal contact to tooth 44 instead of 43 at the start of treatment (Fig 4-127). Tooth 43 was in a labial position without any approximal contact to 42. To solve the crowding, severe expansion with proclination and additional IPR was necessary. The patient declined multibracket therapy as well as extraction.

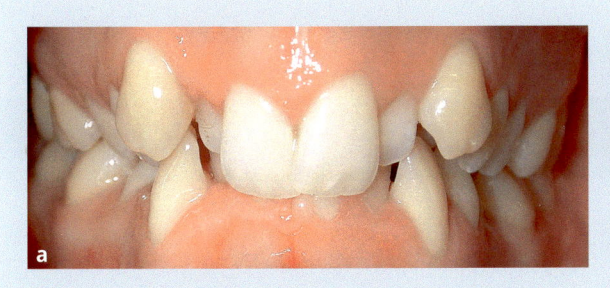

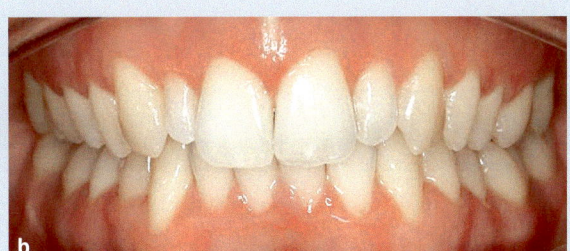

Fig 4-129 The initial **(a)** and final **(b)** intraoral views.

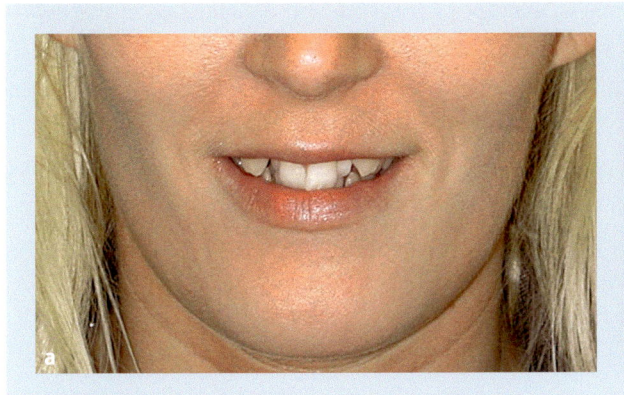

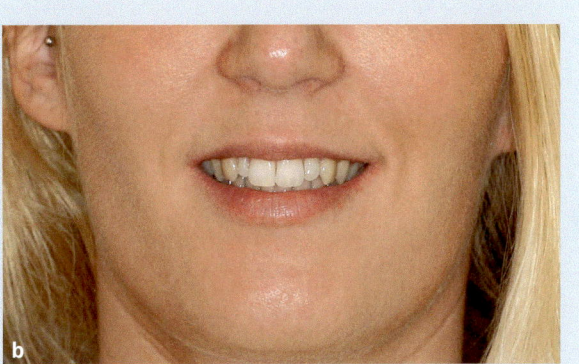

Fig 4-130 The initial **(a)** and final **(b)** extraoral views.

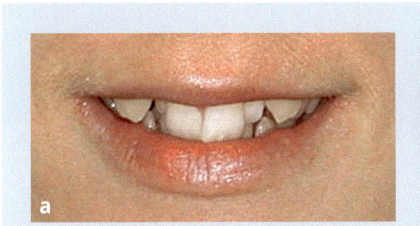

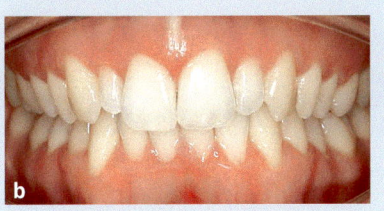

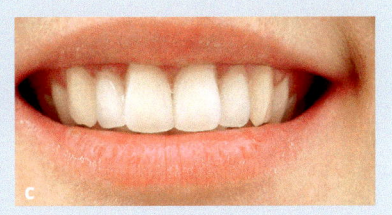

Fig 4-131 Course of treatment. **(a)** Extraoral lip view before orthodontic treatment. **(b)** Intraoral view at the end of treatment and before restoratives. **(c)** The end result with veneers on teeth 12 and 22.

Refinement in the maxillary arch included additional nine aligners for alignment of teeth 12 and 22 for later restoratives (veneers). A lifetime retention was necessary and this was clearly explained to the patient before treatment started.

The final intraoral pictures show well-aligned arches and esthetically aligned gingival contours of maxillary central and lateral incisors in relation to the canines (Fig 4-128).

Views at the start and end of treatment show the improved esthetic result, with a harmonious maxillary curve of teeth following the lower lip line. The overbite was improved; the mandibular incisors might have been intruded even slightly more (Figs 4-129 and 4-130). This provided a good basis for the restorative therapy with veneers on teeth 12 and 22 that had been planned with the dentist (Dr M Wendels, Cologne) right from the start of orthodontic treatment in the ClinCheck simulation.

Views during the course of treatment show the results achieved (Fig 4-131).

Topic 19
When to use interproximal enamel reduction

Treatment:
- use of IPR to create space for relief of crowding

Use of IPR is common both with fixed appliance treatment and Invisalign treatment. The technique has not resulted in increased caries risk (Jarjoura et al, 2006). Zachrisson et al (2011) found no evidence that proper mesiodistal enamel reduction within recognized limits and in appropriate situations would cause harm to the tooth or supporting structures. Zheng (2010) found that the severity of periodontal risks of orthodontic treatment can decrease, treatment duration is shortened, gingival esthetics improved, and the livespan of the dentition can be extended with IPR. There are a number of advantages of IPR (Zachrisson, 2008): it can be used to treat mild to moderate crowding, tooth size discrepancies, interdental recessions (black triangles) in adults, and reduction of approximal spaces after a significant bone loss. IPR is the method of choice to bring roots closer together and to bring the approximal contact more to apical, thus allowing papilla to fill out the space of a black triangle. IPR, carried out using extrafine diamond disks with air cooling followed by contouring and polishing, should always take place against the rotation to obtain a keystoning effect (keystoning procedure) (Barrer, 1975).

The IPR chart (Fillion, 1995) shows the maximum amount of possible IPR for the existing enamel size of the single tooth. Interdental enamel reduction according this protocol does not result in increased caries risk. Figure 4-132 shows a typical example.

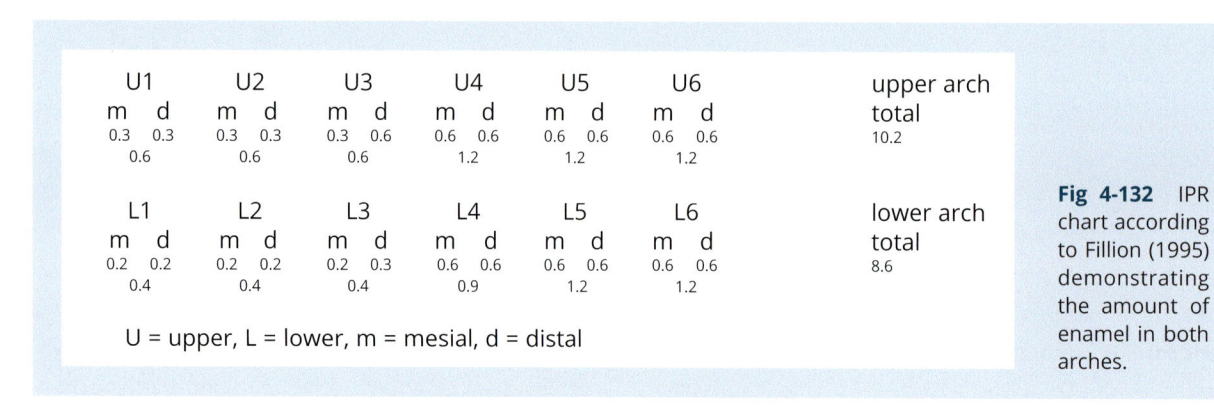

	U1		U2		U3		U4		U5		U6		upper arch total
	m	d	m	d	m	d	m	d	m	d	m	d	
	0.3	0.3	0.3	0.3	0.3	0.6	0.6	0.6	0.6	0.6	0.6	0.6	10.2
		0.6		0.6		0.6		1.2		1.2		1.2	

	L1		L2		L3		L4		L5		L6		lower arch total
	m	d	m	d	m	d	m	d	m	d	m	d	
	0.2	0.2	0.2	0.2	0.2	0.3	0.6	0.6	0.6	0.6	0.6	0.6	8.6
		0.4		0.4		0.4		0.9		1.2		1.2	

U = upper, L = lower, m = mesial, d = distal

Fig 4-132 IPR chart according to Fillion (1995) demonstrating the amount of enamel in both arches.

The IPR chart and the ClinCheck results should be checked at every appointment as the latter will simulate the IPR of the approximal surfaces. It is advisable to check that there is sufficient space for planned tooth movements in the ClinCheck software. When movements are impossible to perform because of approximal heavy contact, IPR will be necessary even if it is not advised by the ClinCheck IPR chart.

This topic covers two patients, with use of IPR with differing methods and times in relation to scans/impressions.

Patient 1
This first patient had moderate crowding in the mandibular arch (Fig 4-133).

Treatment
The treatment plan included IPR in the anterior of the mandibular arch to solve the moderate crowding. Initially separation from mesial 35 to mesial 45 was carried out for 1 day with interproximal elastics, which were inserted between teeth 41, 42, 43, and 44, according to the intraoral example shown in Figure 4-134. The fol-

Fig 4-133 Plaster casts showing tooth crowding.

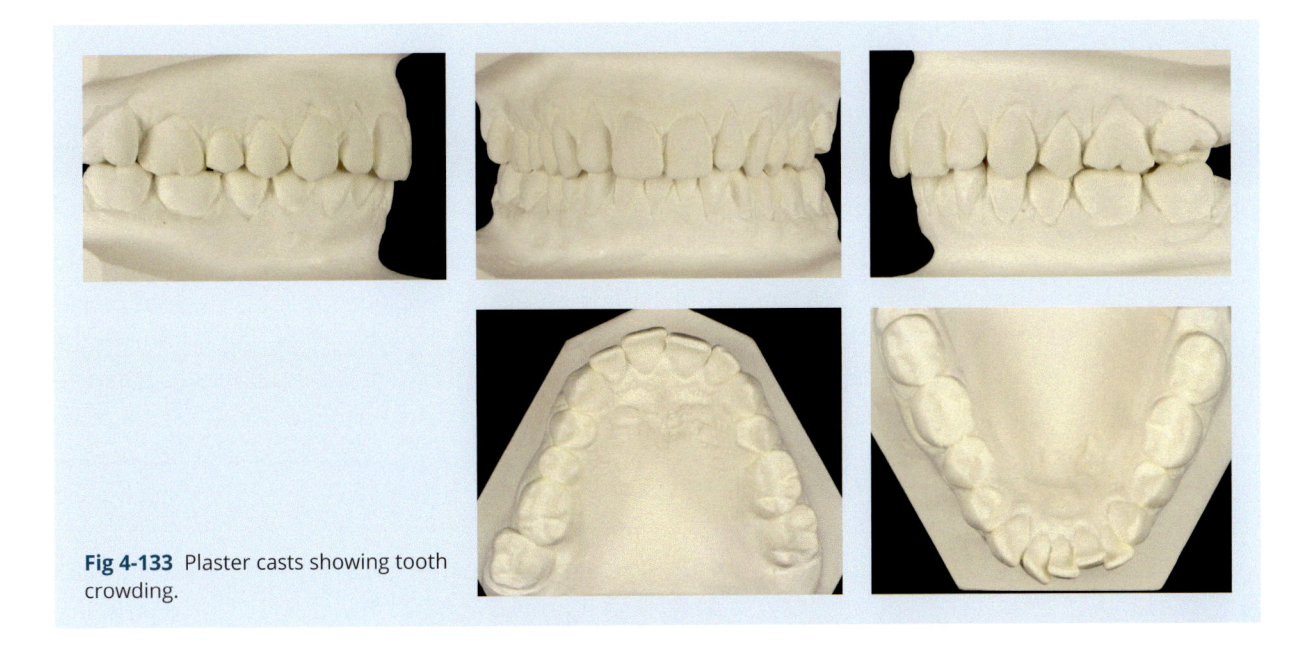

Fig 4-134 Start of treatment. **(a)** Elastics between the teeth 41, 42, 43, and 44. **(b)** Interproximal elastics have created sufficient interproximal space for IPR to be carried out with minimal damage to the soft tissues.

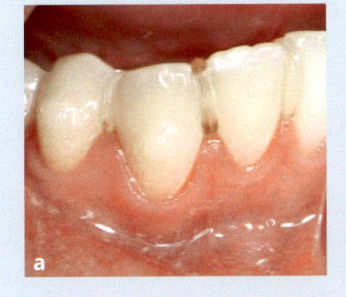

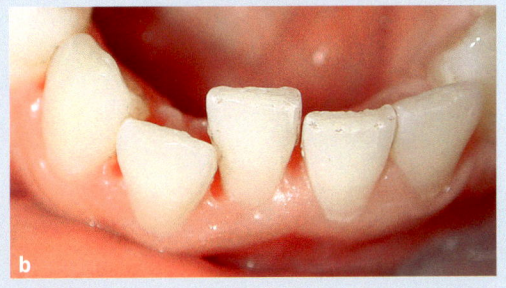

lowing day, the elastics were removed. The elastic forces help to create sufficient interproximal space to perform IPR. Because of the interproximal elastic position, the papilla is depressed and the interproximal enamel can be polished without injuring the interdental papilla or causing excessive bleeding. IPR was carried out from mesial 35 to mesial 45 before the scan/impression was taken (Fig 4-135). It is important to polish the surface of the reduced teeth precisely to obtain optimal smooth interproximal surfaces. A retention splint in the mandibular arch was necessary to maintain the gained spaces open until the first aligner was inserted. The patient wore the retention aligner only at night.

IPR can be carried out with a rotary disk instrument and tongue protection (Fig 4-136a,b) or an oscillating technique (Fig 4-136c). The enamel surfaces are polished after IPR (Fig 4-136d–f).

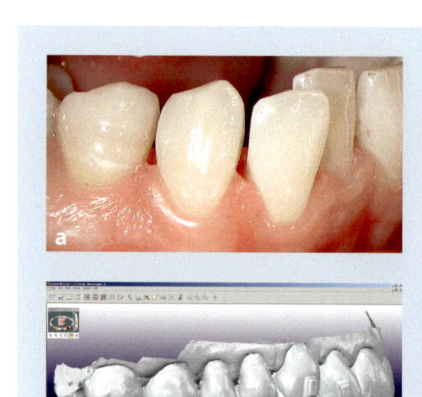

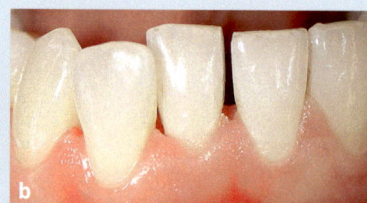

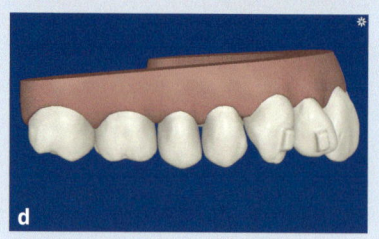

4 TREATMENT OF DIFFERENT MALOCCLUSIONS WITH ALIGNERS

Fig 4-135 After IPR. **(a,b)** The papilla is without injuries or bleeding. **(c,d)** A similar situation of pre-impression IPR on the upper right premolars in the scan and transferred into the ClinCheck software.

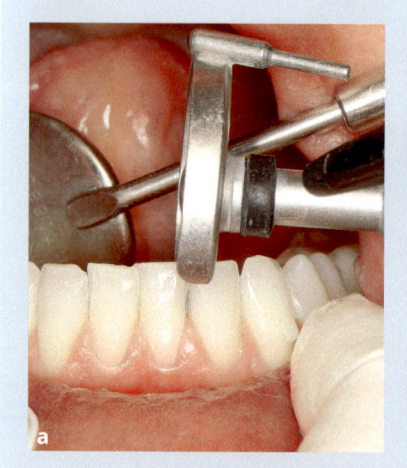

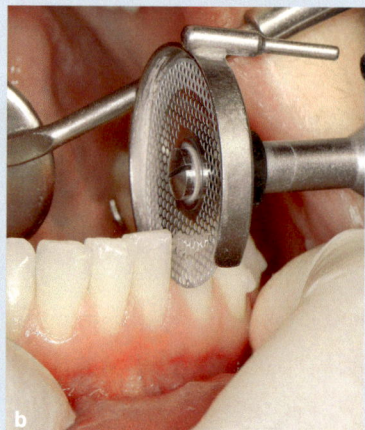

Fig 4-136 Performance of IPR. **(a,b)** Use of a rotary disk instrument with tongue protection on tooth 31. **(c)** The oscillating technique (e.g. using the Ortho-Strip System, Intensiv, Swiss Dental Products). **(d,e)** Polishing enamel surfaces with Sof-Lex disks (3M Espe) **(d)** followed by fluoride application **(e)**. **(f)** Manual polishing strips (Komet) in different sizes. **(g)** Finishing strips in two different sizes (3M Espe).

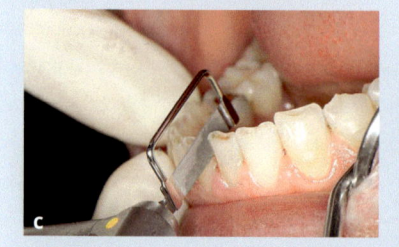

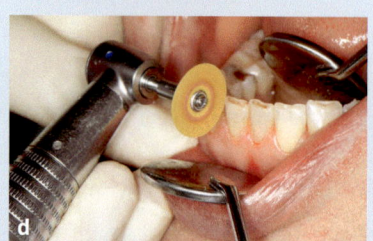

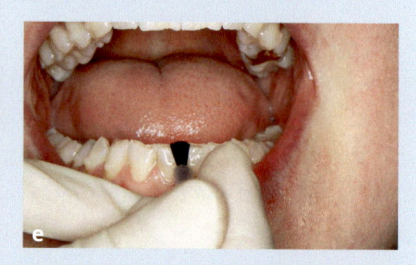

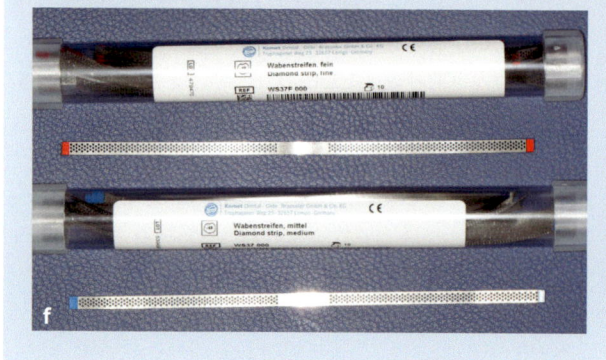

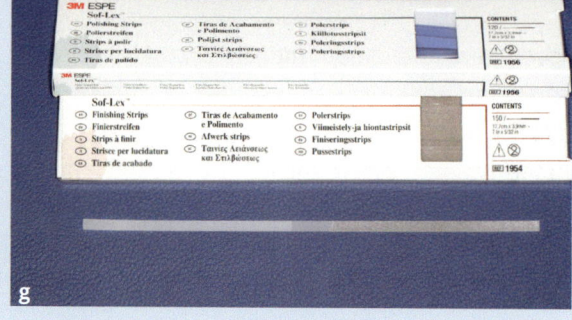

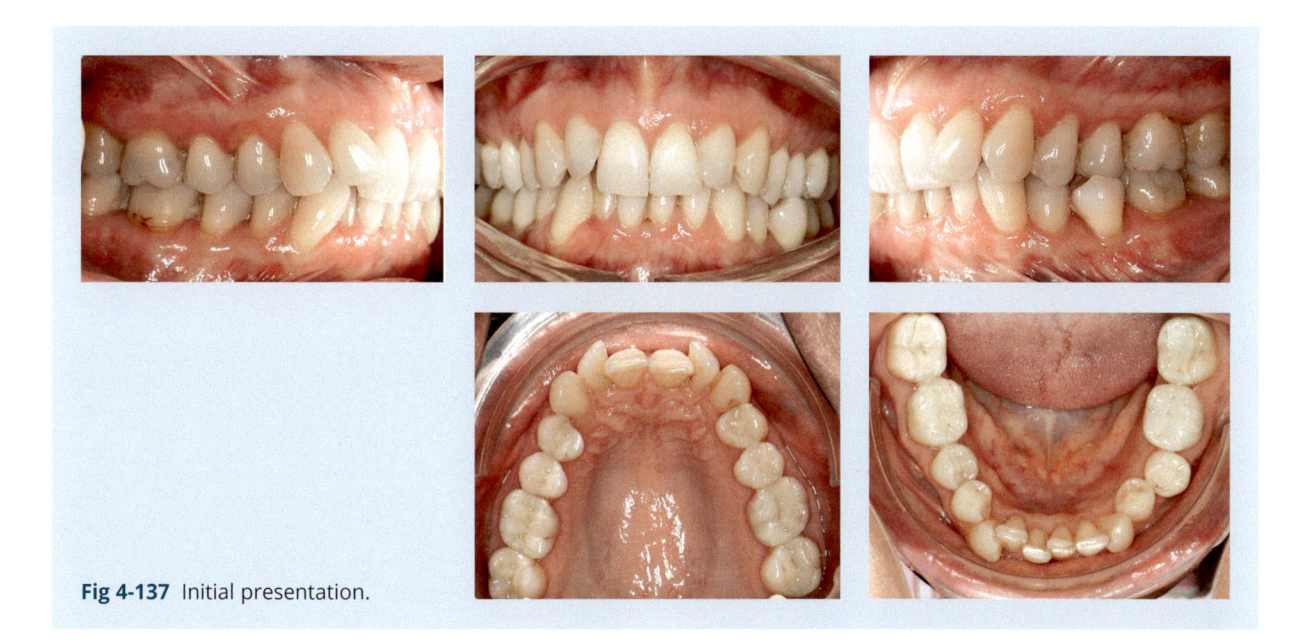

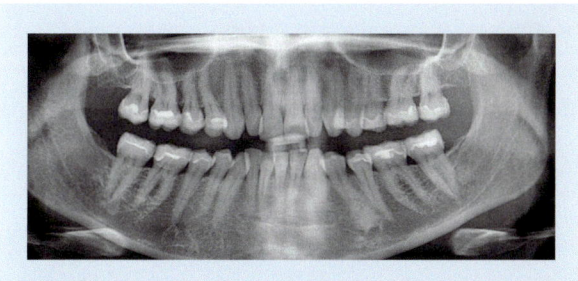

TREATMENT OF DIFFERENT MALOCCLUSIONS WITH ALIGNERS 4

Fig 4-137 Initial presentation.

Fig 4-138 Orthopantomography before treatment.

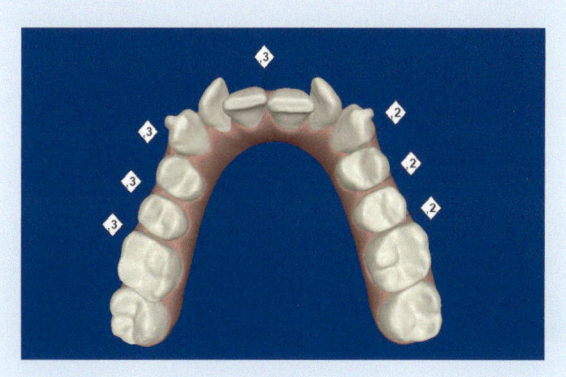

Fig 4-139 ClinCheck software showing the maxillary arch after IPR, showing spaces created mesial and distal of all maxillary premolars.

Patient 2

This adult had class II/2 relationship with crowding and rotations in both arches and a crossbite with teeth 25 to 35 (Fig 4-137). Orthopantomography showed periodontal stable bone with diverse fillings and crowns on maxillary and mandibular premolars and molars (Fig 4-138).

In this patient, performing IPR prior to the impressions/scans was the method of choice to gain an optimum of space for alignment and anchorage of the aligners on the teeth.

Treatment

The patient was treated with the Invisalign technique and IPR before impressions/scans were taken.

The treatment plan included the gaining of space in the maxillary and mandibular arches with excessive IPR on all restoratives with distalization to avoid extractions.

The ClinCheck software shows the maxillary arch after IPR in the premolar area performed prior to the impression to show the spaces created (Fig 4-139). The simulation of treatment showed even more need for IPR to obtain complete resolution of the anterior crowding and distalization into a full class I relationship.

Fig 4-140 Intraoral views after treatment.

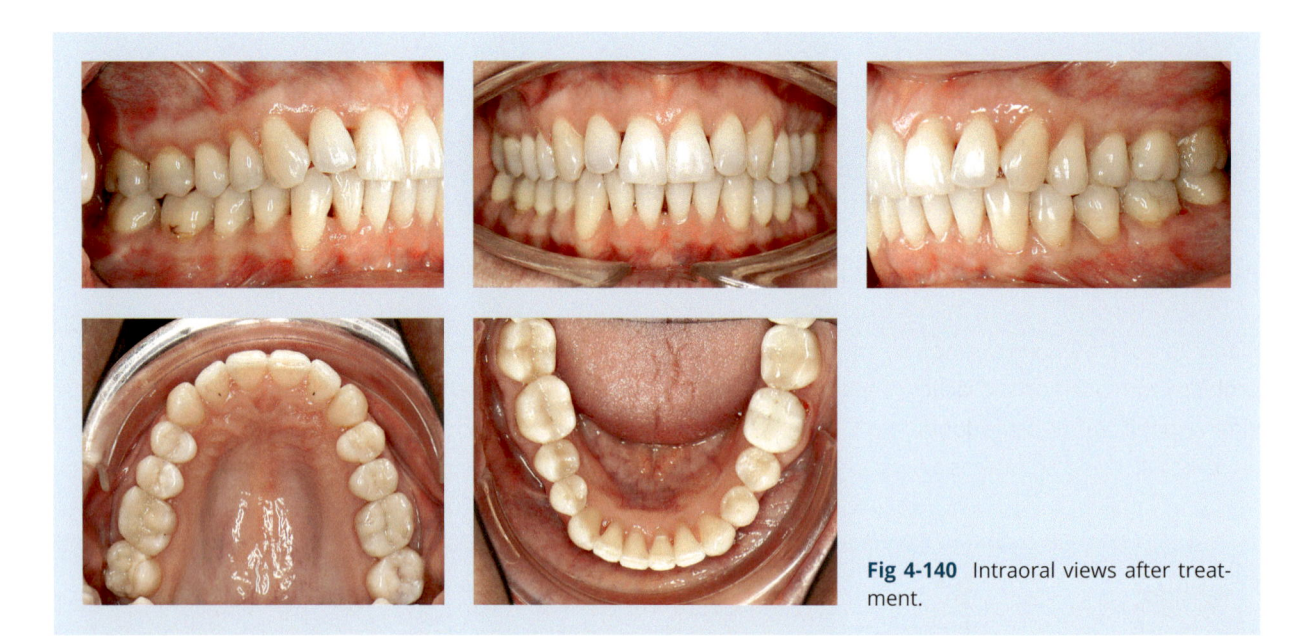

Figure 4-140 shows the final result after treatment with the Invisalign system. All gaps created by excessive IPR on the restoratives had been closed, and distalization of premolars and canines into a class I relationship was achieved. Crossbite of tooth 35 to 25 was solved and a physiologic anterior relationship created.

Topic 20
Mandibular crowding: Extraction of a mandibular incisor

Treatment:
- closure of the extraction space
- root movement
- papilla management

Extraction of a mandibular incisor is a highly predictable treatment option with the Invisalign system. The major problem with such an extraction, regardless of the orthodontic technique used, is the possibility of loss of the gingiva papilla after orthodontic treatment.

This patient had rotations and crowding in the maxillary and mandibular arch, as well as a deepbite (Fig 4-141).

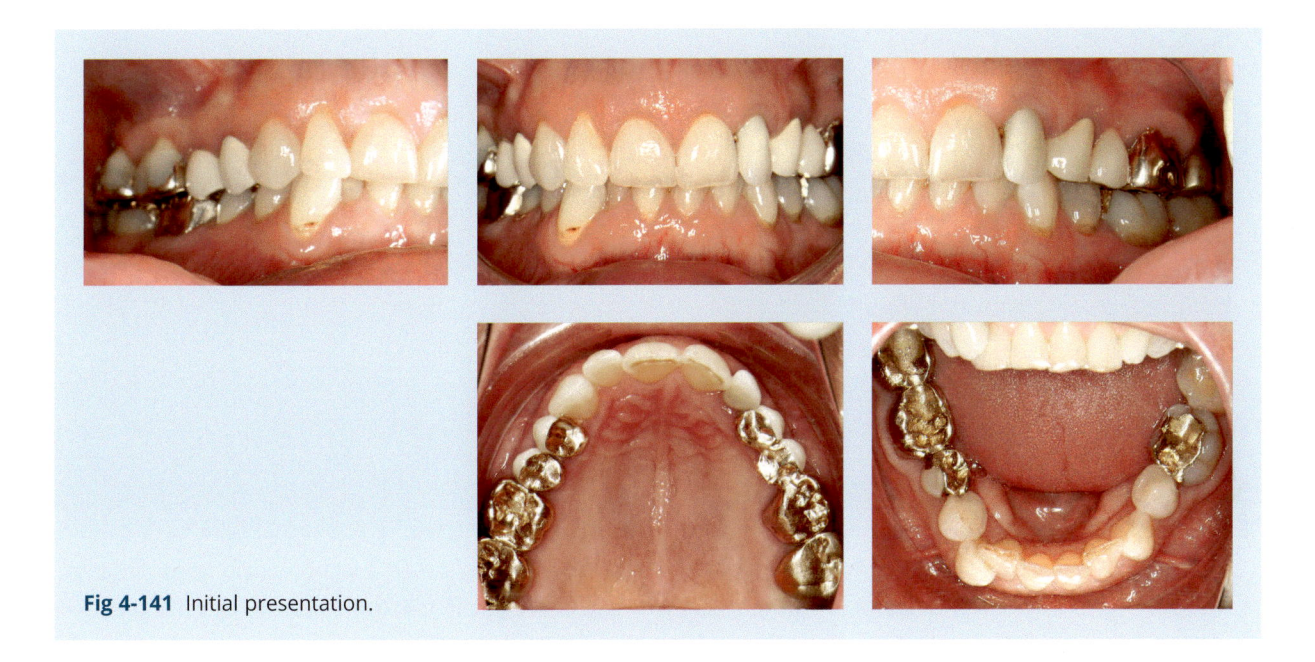

Fig 4-141 Initial presentation.

Diagnosis:
- class I
- rotation and crowding in the maxillary and mandibular arch
- missing tooth 23 with space closure and prothetics
- deep bite
- severe abrasion from incisor contacts.

Therapy:
- alignment of the maxilla and mandible
- extraction of tooth 42
- create a physiologic overjet.

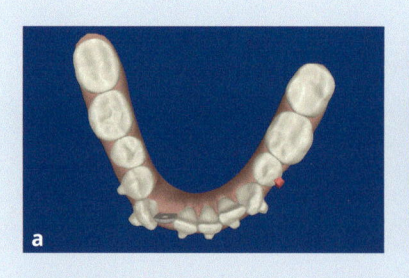

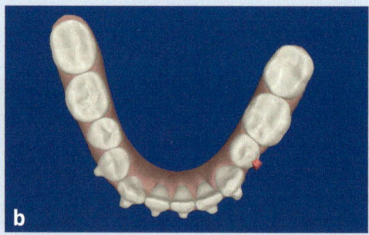

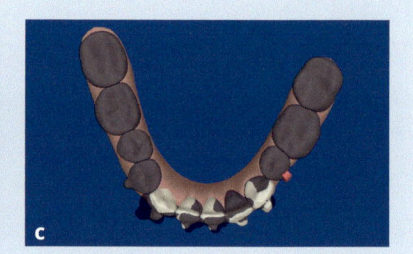

4 TREATMENT OF DIFFERENT MALOCCLUSIONS WITH ALIGNERS

Fig 4-142 ClinCheck software results. **(a)** Initial situation. **(b)** Planned final situation. **(c)** Superimposition with planned tooth movements (blue, initial tooth position; white, final tooth position).

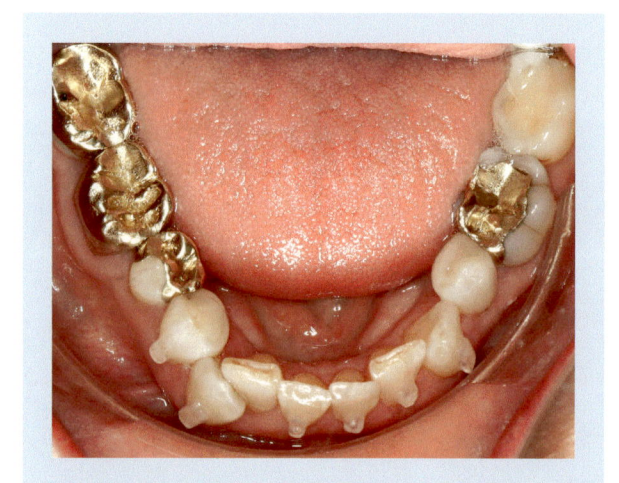

Fig 4-143 Tooth 42 for extraction.

Treatment

The extraction of tooth 42 was planned and approved by the patient. If extraction is going to be part of a treatment plan including Invisalign treatment, it is advisable to perform the impression/scan first with all teeth present and set up the ClinCheck virtual end-result as usual. Once the final simulated result is satisfying, the extraction can occur shortly before inserting the first aligners.

The ClinCheck simulation of the first phase showed 21 aligners, with an additional four in the refinement (Fig 4-142). In order to obtain a bodily movement of the teeth into the extraction space and to avoid tipping of the crowns, it is important to take particular care both during movement of the crowns and in bringing together the roots during the space closure. The tooth to be extracted (in this case tooth 42; Fig 4-143) is removed in the virtual ClinCheck simulation, but the extraction is not performed until the aligners are ready for use. Once this point is reached, the patient is advised to get the tooth extracted by the dentist or oral surgeon. Aligner treatment can begin 1 day after extraction with placement of the first aligners. This ensures that orthodontic movement is commenced with optimal bone conditions.

After Invisalign treatment, there has been bodily axial movement of the mandibular incisors into the extraction space (Fig 4-144). Mandibular and maxillary incisors show severe enamel abrasions from the initial malocclusion.

The mandibular incisor extraction occurred without loss of gingiva papilla (Fig 4-145), and together with the Invisalign treatment successfully relieved the crowding in the mandible (Fig 4-146).

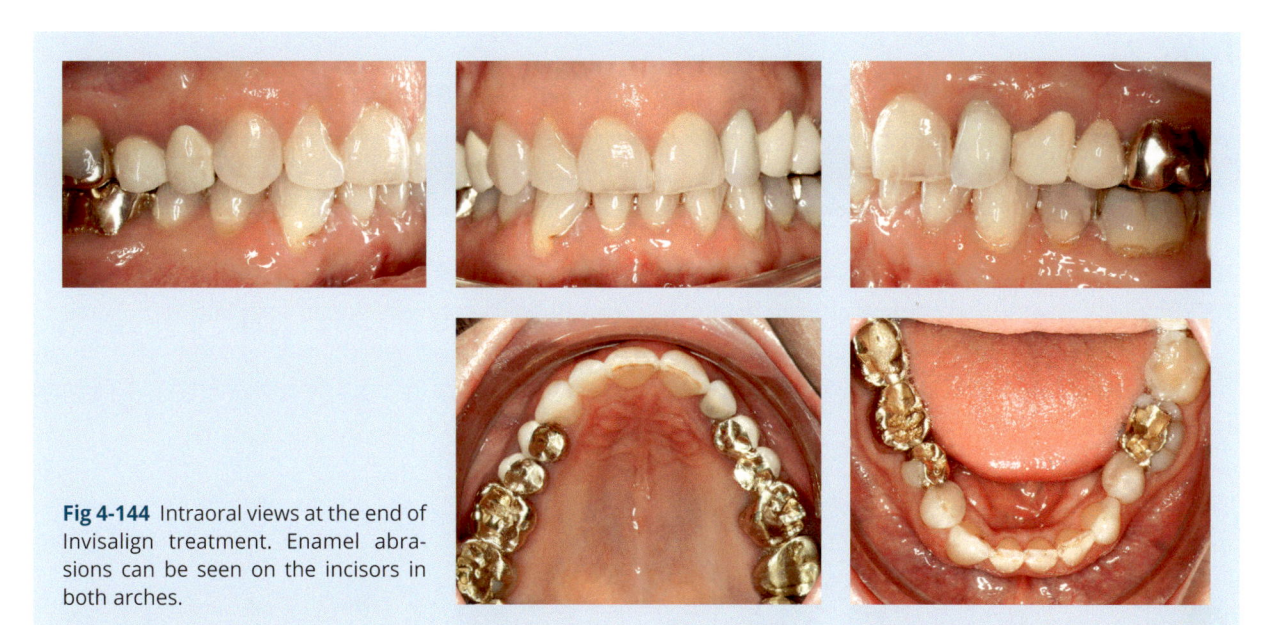

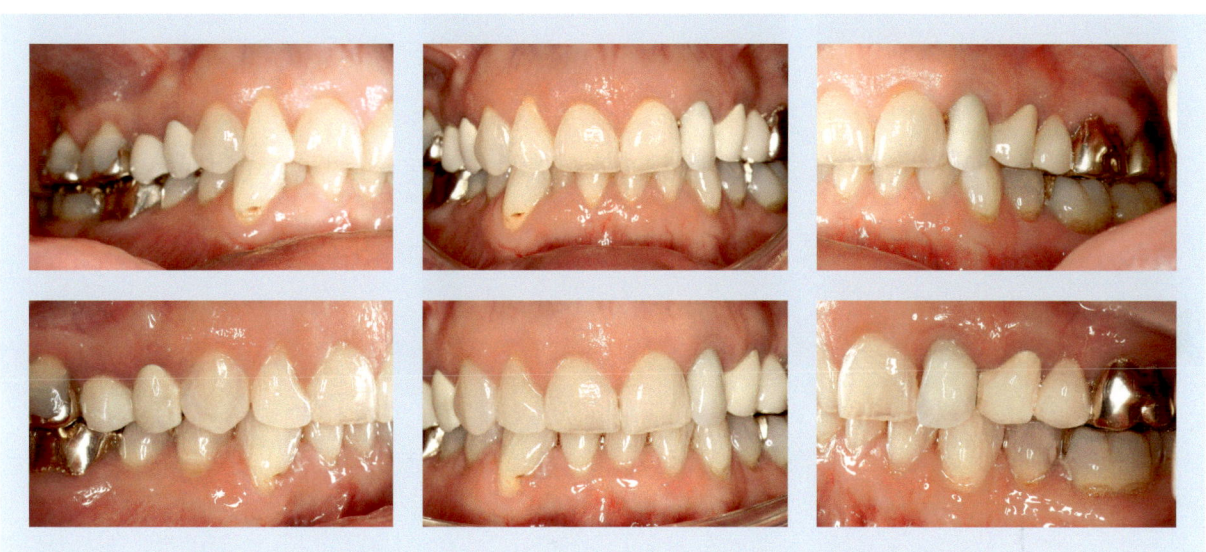

TREATMENT OF DIFFERENT MALOCCLUSIONS WITH ALIGNERS 4

Fig 4-144 Intraoral views at the end of Invisalign treatment. Enamel abrasions can be seen on the incisors in both arches.

Fig 4-145 Initial **(top)** and final **(bottom)** views showing that extraction did not lead to loss of gingiva.

Fig 4-146 The initial **(a)** and final **(b)** intraoral views showing relief of the crowding.

121

Topic 21
Bialveolar protrusion: Extraction of a mandibular incisor

Treatment:
- extraction of a mandibular incisor to create overjet for maxillary incisor retraction

Bialveolar protrusion makes lip closure difficult and often incisors tend to show with insufficient lip closure. In these patients, a retraction of maxillary and mandibular incisors is necessary to obtain complete lip closure.

This patient has a bialveolar lip protrusion with insufficient lip closure and showing of tooth 21. She has increased overjet with protrusion of tooth 21, narrow arches, and crowding in class I relationship (Figs 4-147 and 4-148).

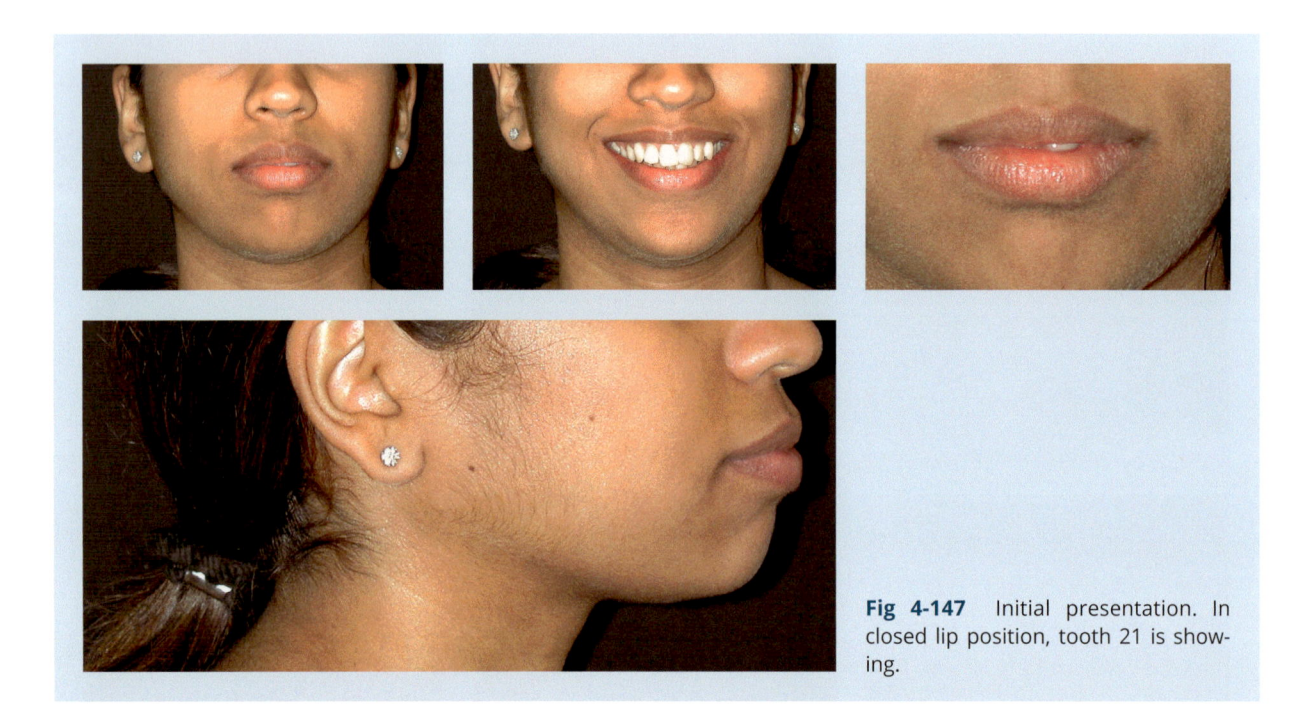

Fig 4-147 Initial presentation. In closed lip position, tooth 21 is showing.

Diagnosis:
- insufficient lip closure
- increased overjet with protrusion of tooth 21
- narrow arches
- crowding in class I relationship.

Therapy:
- extraction of tooth 31 to gain space
- alignment and retraction of mandibular anterior teeth
- retraction of maxillary incisors.

Treatment

The planned treatment was not to extract premolars but to extract tooth 31 to gain sufficient space to align and retract the mandibular anterior teeth. This would provide enough space to retract the maxillary incisors (Fig 4-149).

Figure 4-150 shows the intraoral situation with aligner 12 with good development of healthy gingiva papilla in the extraction site. This matched the planned situation in the ClinCheck software.

TREATMENT OF DIFFERENT MALOCCLUSIONS WITH ALIGNERS 4

Fig 4-148 Initial intraoral views.

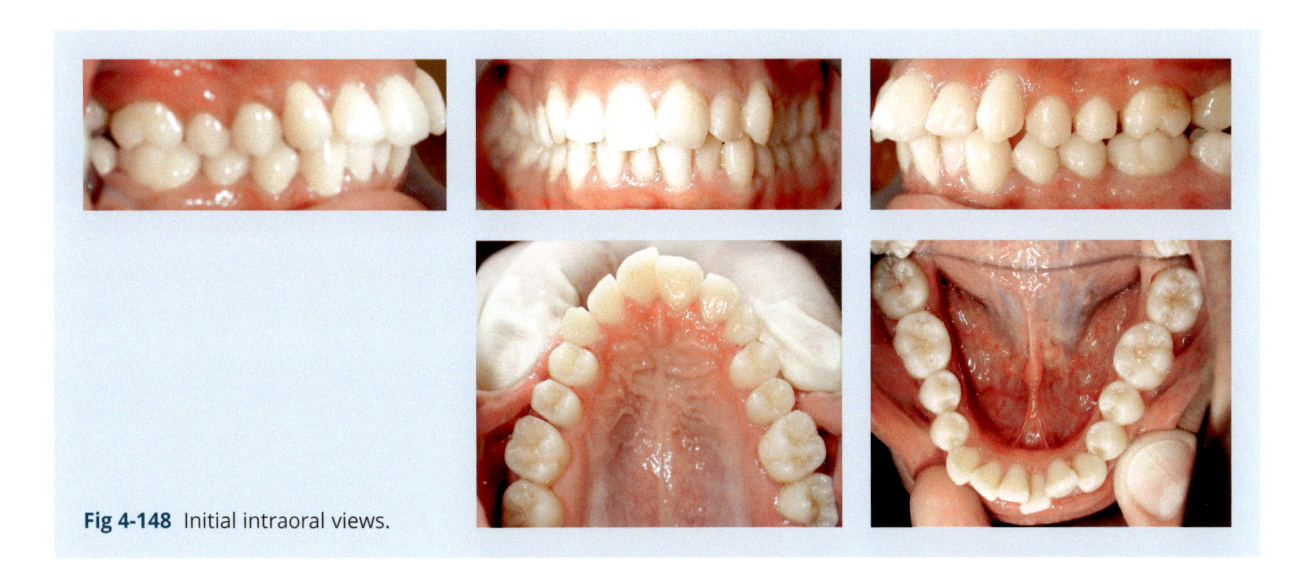

Fig 4-149 ClinCheck software results showing the superimposition of initial (blue) and final (white) tooth positions.

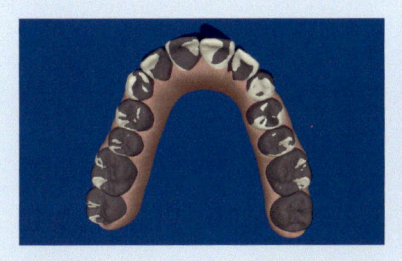

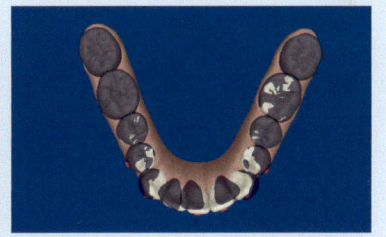

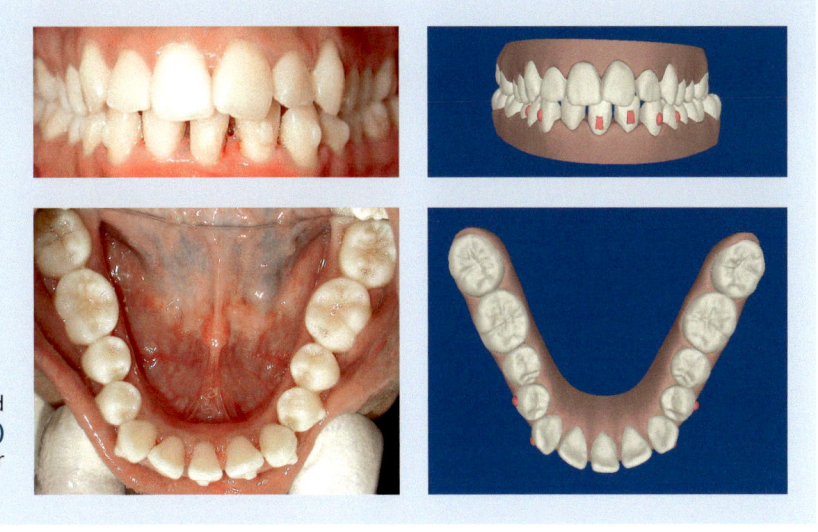

Fig 4-150 Intraoral views **(left)** and ClinCheck software images **(right)** showing placement of aligner 12 after extraction.

123

Fig 4-151 Final intraoral views.

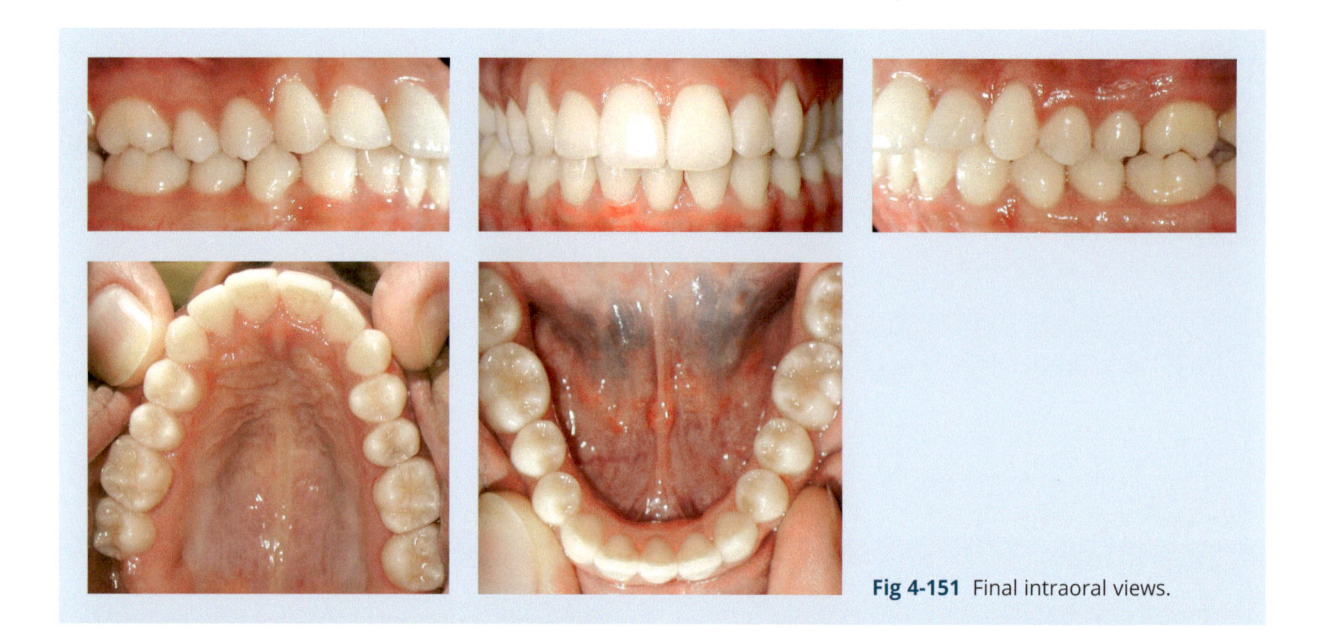

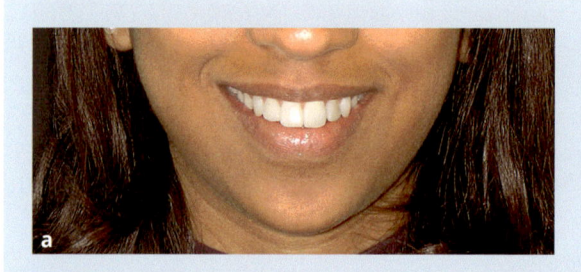

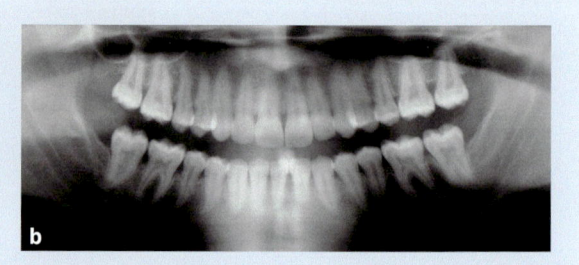

Fig 4-152 Final frontal view showing smile (a). Orthopantomograph showing parallel incisor roots (b).

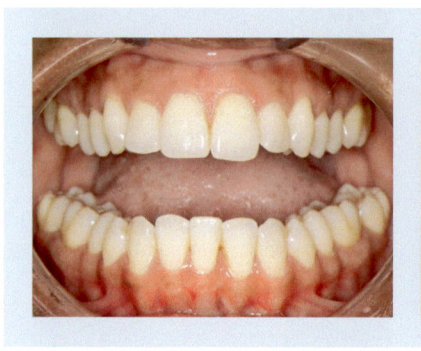

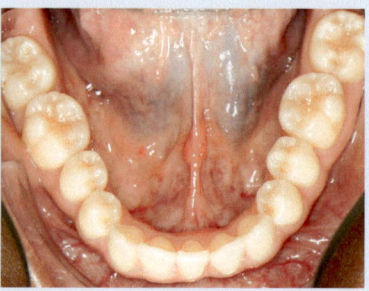

Fig 4-153 Intraoral views of the lower arch in detail with a stable result 9 years after orthodontic treatment.

At the end of treatment, there is a stable class I occlusion with a physiological overbite and a "Shim-stock foil" open overjet. In full smile, there is a harmonious relation of the maxillary dentition, which follows the lower lip curve (Figs 4-151 and 4-152). Orthopantomography shows parallel mandibular incisor roots with a physiologic bone situation between the roots (Fig 4-152).

Topic 22
Crowding in the lower arch with crossbite: Extraction of lower second premolars

Treatment:
- extraction of lower second premolars

This patient has maxillary teeth 13, 23 and 27 missing, severe crowding in the mandibular arch plus lingually tipped second premolars (Fig 4-154). There is some periodontal disease.

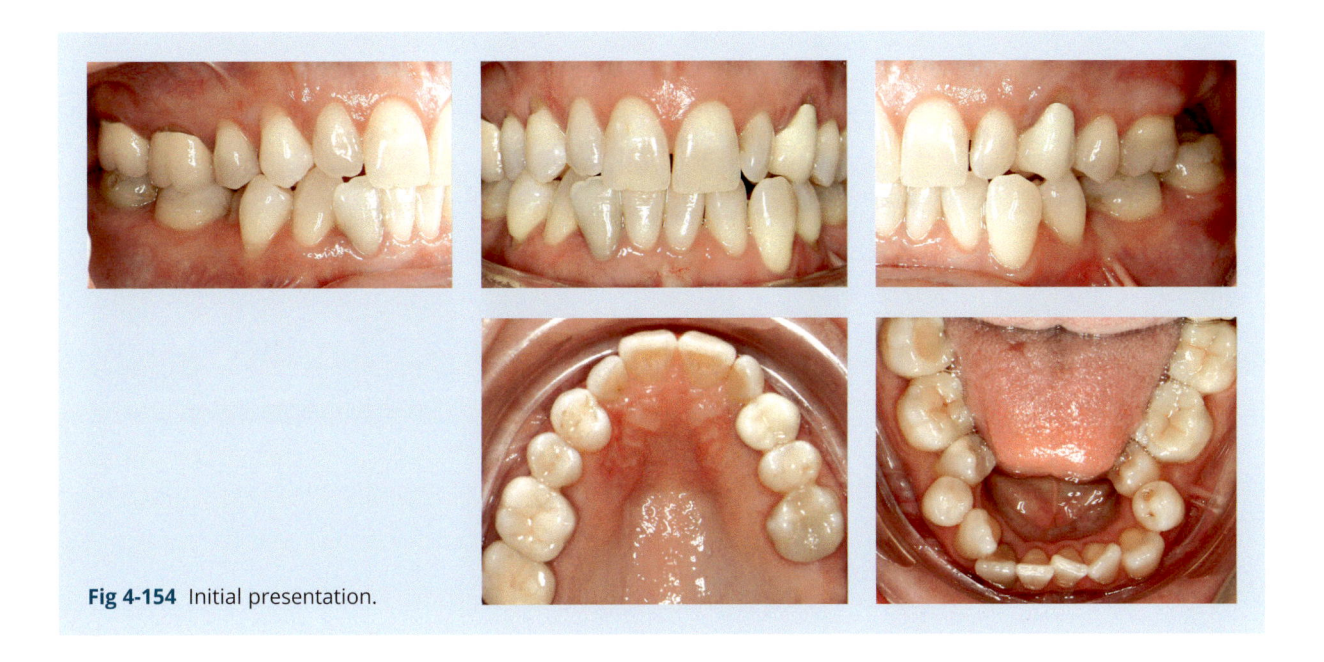

Fig 4-154 Initial presentation.

Diagnosis:
- missing upper canines
- severe crowding in the mandibular arch
- missing upper canines and tooth 27
- crossbite.

Therapy:
- periodontal treatment
- extraction of mandibular second premolars.

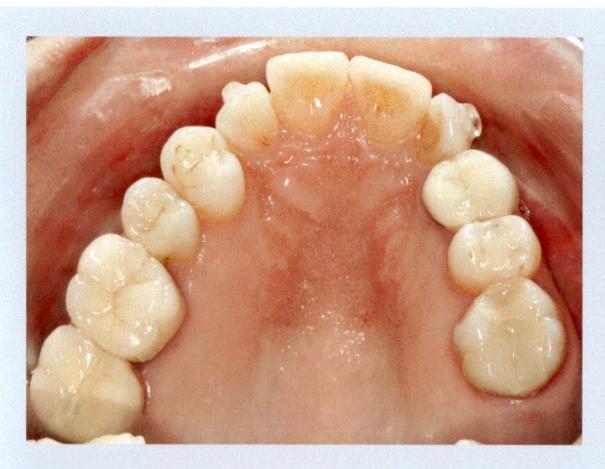

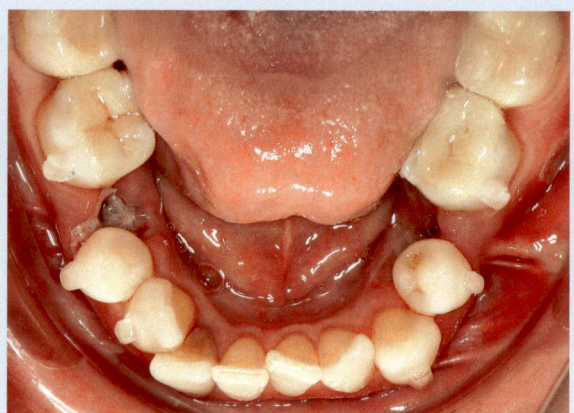

Fig 4-155 Intraoral views showing the extraction site 35, 45.

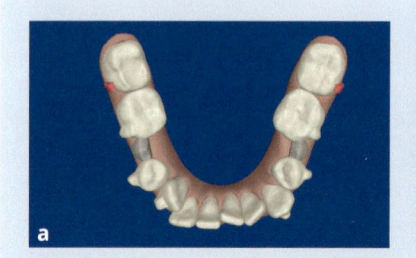

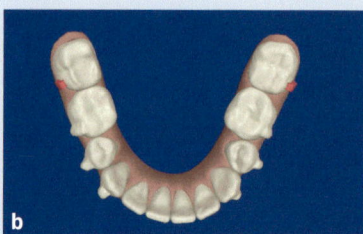

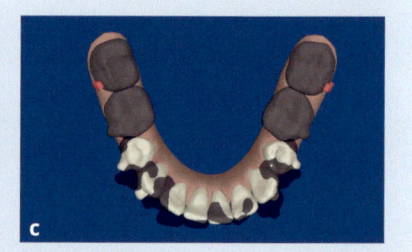

Fig 4-156 ClinCheck software results. **(a)** Virtually extracted teeth 35 and 45 and inserted pontics for these teeth. Vertical rectangular attachments have been bonded on all mandibular molars, first premolars, and canines to permit maximum anchorage during the space closure. **(b)** Planned final result. **(c)** Superimposition of initial and final views (blue, initial tooth position; white, final tooth position).

Treatment

After periodontal treatment, the gingiva was in a stable condition but with some recessions in the premolar region.

Invisalign treatment was started the day after the extraction of teeth 35 and 45 (Fig 4-155), which only occurred once the aligners had arrived for use. The planned tooth movements included distalization of mandibular first premolars, canines, and incisors into the extraction space and maximum anchorage of the mandibular first and second molars. Rectangular attachments were bonded on all mandibular molars, first premolars, and canines to permit maximum anchorage during space closure (Fig 4-156). In most cases, ClinCheck software helps in deciding if extractions are needed for orthodontic treatment. Several possible solutions to a problem can be requested in order to make the best decision for the patient, for example whether to extract teeth.

Figure 4-157 shows the final result. There is improved esthetic appearance but the maxillary canines are missing and in this area the arch could be a little more prominent. There is sufficient occlusion with vertical support without the missing canines. The maxillary lateral incisors are very small and the smile esthetic could be improved by increasing their size with restoratives. The patient was transferred to the dentist for further restoratives and new prosthetics.

Figure 4-158 shows the changes achieved with the treatment.

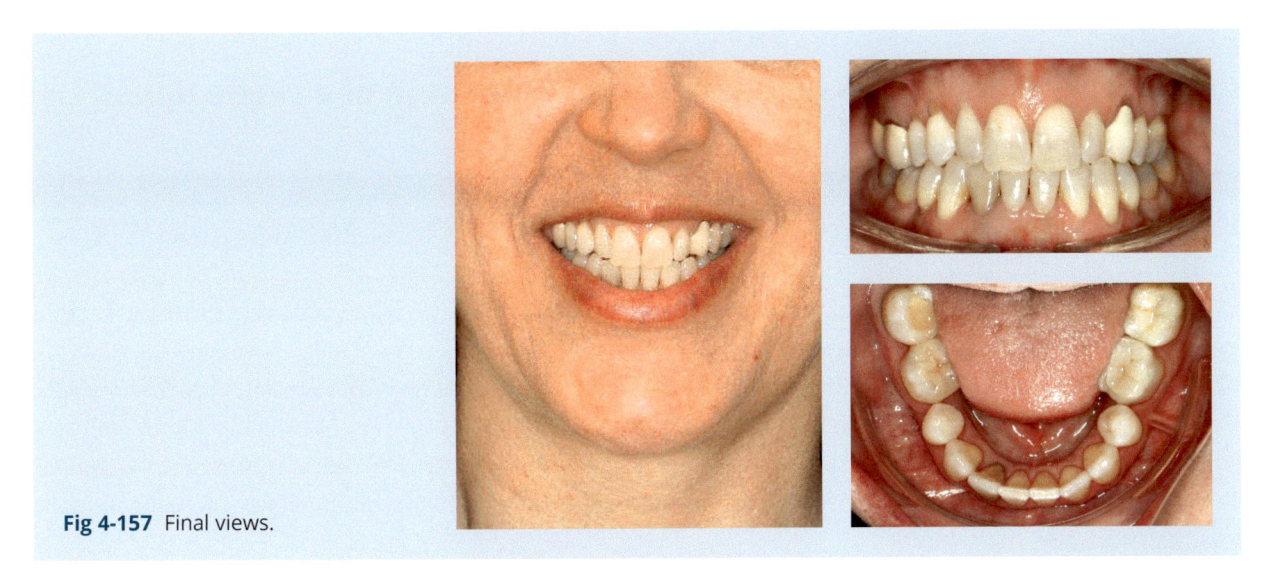

TREATMENT OF DIFFERENT MALOCCLUSIONS WITH ALIGNERS 4

Fig 4-157 Final views.

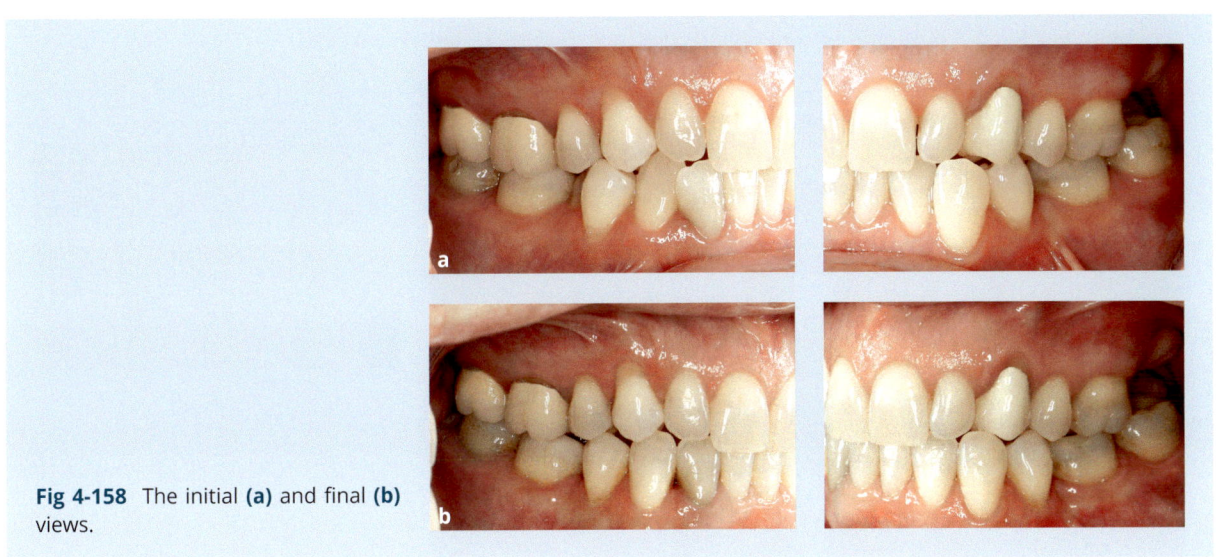

Fig 4-158 The initial (a) and final (b) views.

Topic 23
CMD with unilateral class II relationship: Extraction of a single upper premolar

Treatment:
- extraction of a single premolar

In a unilateral class II relationship, extraction of only one premolar might be a favorable way to create a stable intercuspation on both sides, particularly if the premolar has a crown or a bigger filling. In this special situation, it is important to examine if the asymmetric class II in habitual intercuspation is also present in centric relation. If there is any doubt, particularly when disorders of the craniomandibular or musculoskeletal system are present, functional analysis followed by occlusal splint therapy is the right choice before orthodontic treatment begins (see Chapter 1). The occlusal splint helps to determine the correct centric relation for future orthodontic treatment (see also Topic 48).

This patient has reclined and extruded maxillary and mandibular incisors and a deep bite, She has a class II relationship on the right side, and crowding and rotations in both arches (Fig 4-159).

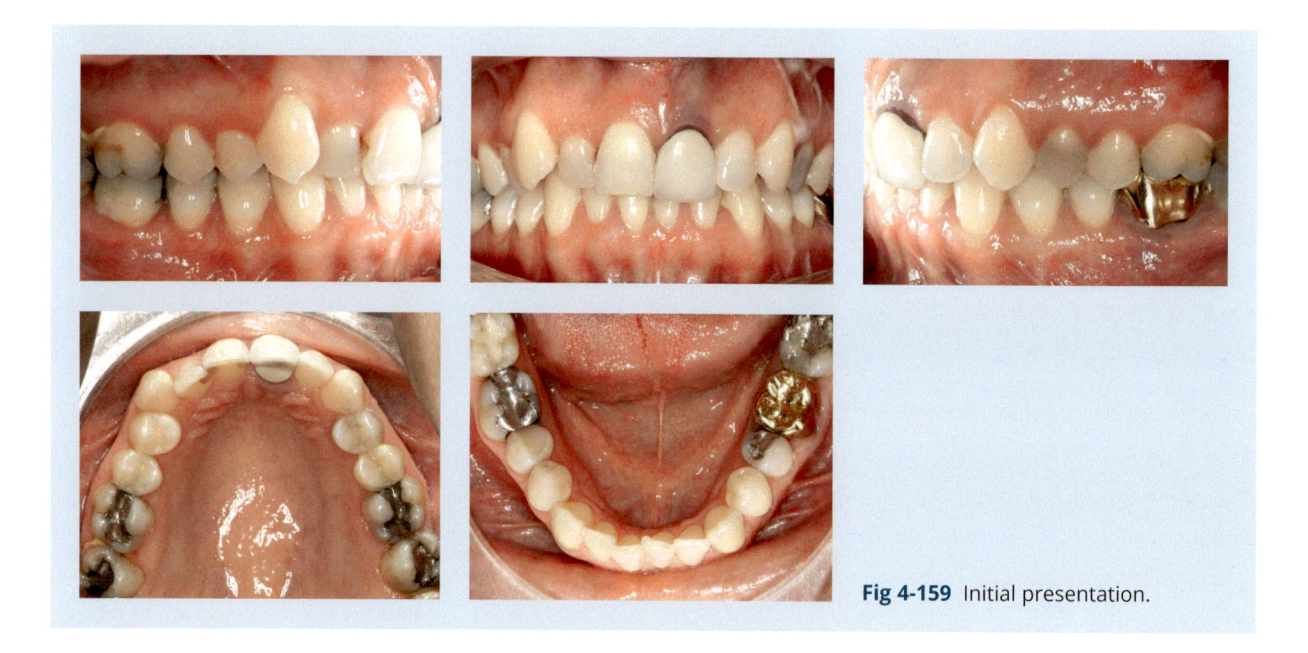

Fig 4-159 Initial presentation.

Diagnosis:
- prosthodontics and restorations needing treatment
- reclined and extruded maxillary and mandibular incisors
- deep bite with incisor contacts
- dorsal shift from centric to habitual occlusion 0.5 mm
- class II relationship on the right side
- crowding and rotations in both arches.

Therapy:
- extraction of tooth 14 and Invisalign treatment
- restorative and prosthetics after orthodontic treatment.

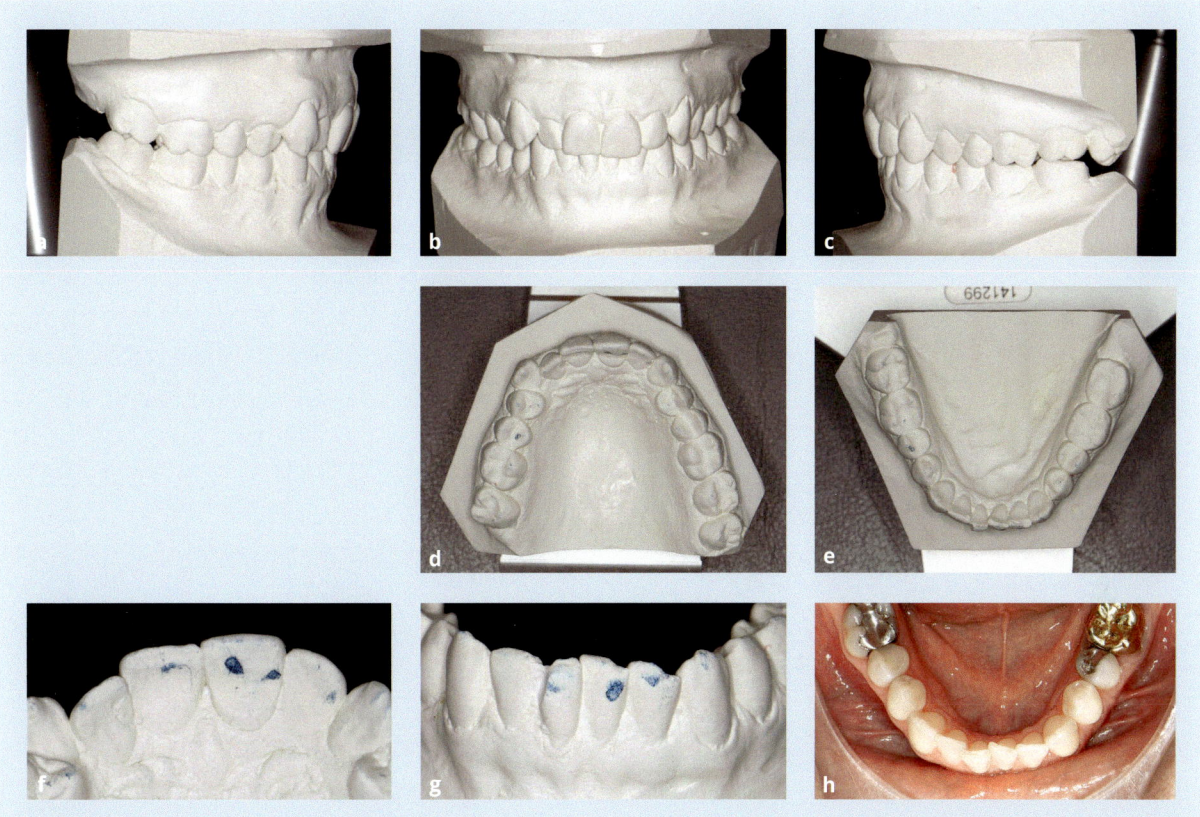

Fig 4-160 Initial occlusion and tooth abrasion. **(a–e)** Articulated plaster casts showing exclusively contacts on tooth 15 to 45 and contacts on all incisors at the beginning of the treatment. **(f,g)** Plaster casts showing enamel abrasion. **(h)** Intraoral view showing enamel abrasion.

Treatment

Before Invisalign treatment was started, the dentist changed the crown on tooth 21 into a long-term provisional crown.

The articulated plaster casts show exclusively contacts on tooth 15 to 45 and contacts on all incisors at the beginning of the treatment (Fig 4-160a-d). The left side showed no contacts at all for canines, premolars, and molars. Tooth 18 was planned for later extraction. In such a situation, with retracted maxillary incisor position and deep bite, the mandibular arch cannot be positioned more anterior with an occlusal splint. Enamel abrasion from the heavy occlusal contacts of the incisors has led to traumatizing enamel defects and can result in a lack of posterior support and compression in the TMJ (Fig 4-160e–h).

In patients with acute CMD or pain, orthodontic treatment is usually started with fixed occlusal splints in order to enhance the vertical condyle position. Orthodontic treatment follows the course described for other topics covering treatment of craniomandibular dysfunctions. In this patient, it was decided to start right away with orthodontic treatment to solve the traumatizing occlusal contact of the incisors. To obtain major intrusion of the incisors, a Speed Up can be helpful and will also help to obtain a balanced anterior and bilateral posterior relationship at night (see Topic 16).

Before the treatment plan was transmitted online to Align, the whole treatment was outlined in the planning chart to end with a physiologic overjet of 0.5 mm (Fig 4-161).

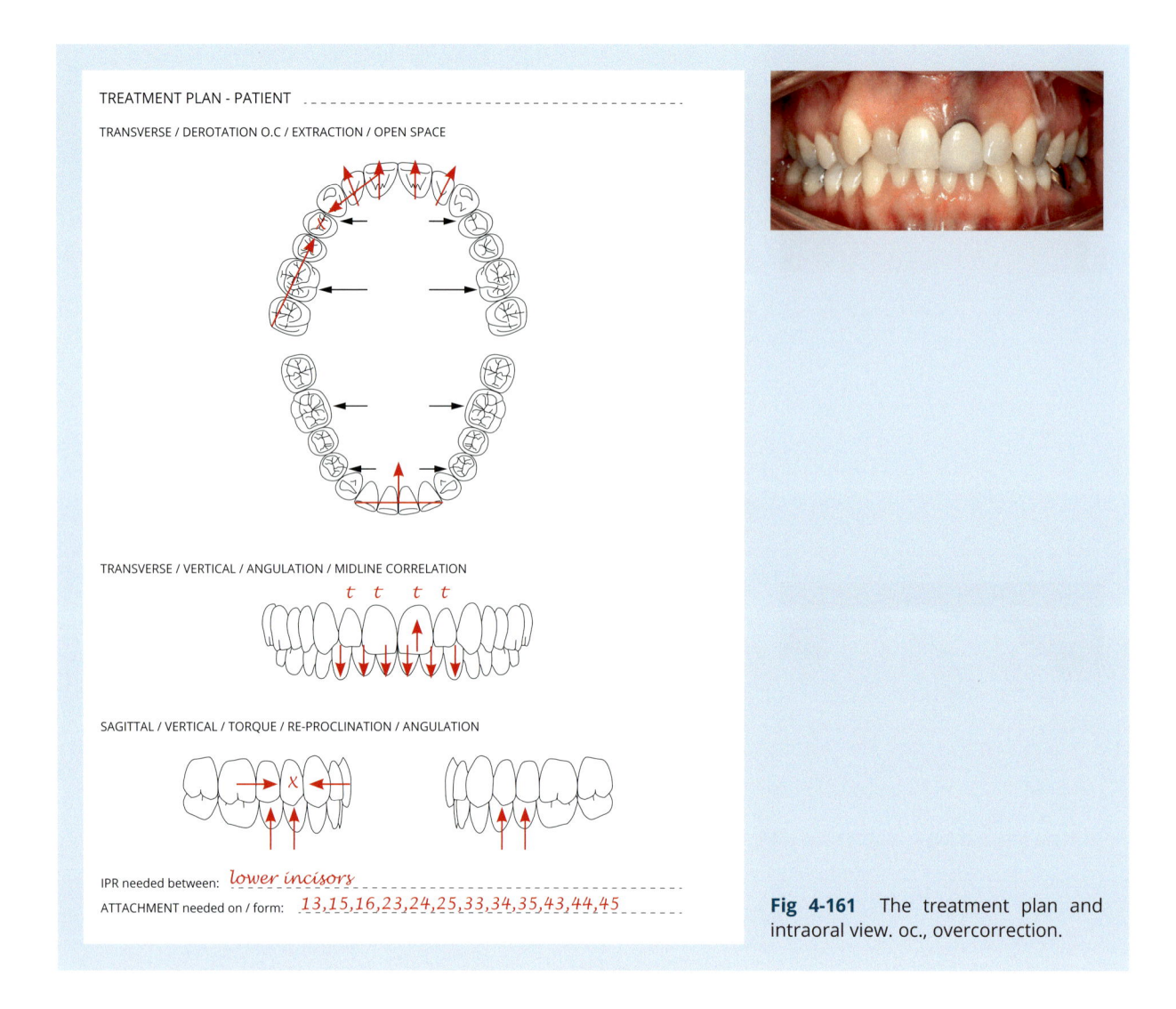

4 TREATMENT OF DIFFERENT MALOCCLUSIONS WITH ALIGNERS

Fig 4-161 The treatment plan and intraoral view. oc., overcorrection.

- extraction of tooth 14
- mesialization of teeth 15, 16, and 17 with root movement to anterior
- distalization of tooth 13, followed by incisors
- lingual root torque of maxillary incisors, attachments for anchorage on teeth 13 and 23
- retraction and alignment of mandibular incisors with IPR
- intrusion of mandibular incisors and canines, as well as of tooth 21 to obtain equal gingival height as tooth 11
- 0.4 mm extrusion of mandibular premolars.

Invisalign therapy was started with bonding of attachments, 33 aligners in the maxillary and 20 in the mandibular arch (Fig 4-162) before the oral surgeon extracted tooth 14. The patient started with aligner wear immediately after the extraction.

The IPR chart (Fig 4-163a) shows the amount of approximal reduction needed in the maxillary and mandibular arches. The ClinCheck software shows the planned treatment (Fig 4-163b–d).

The final result shows a stable occlusion on the right side in a full class II molar relationship with all posterior teeth in contact (Fig 4-164). Due to the mesializing movement, the molar crown of tooth 16 has tipped slightly to mesial, but the occlusion of 16 to 46

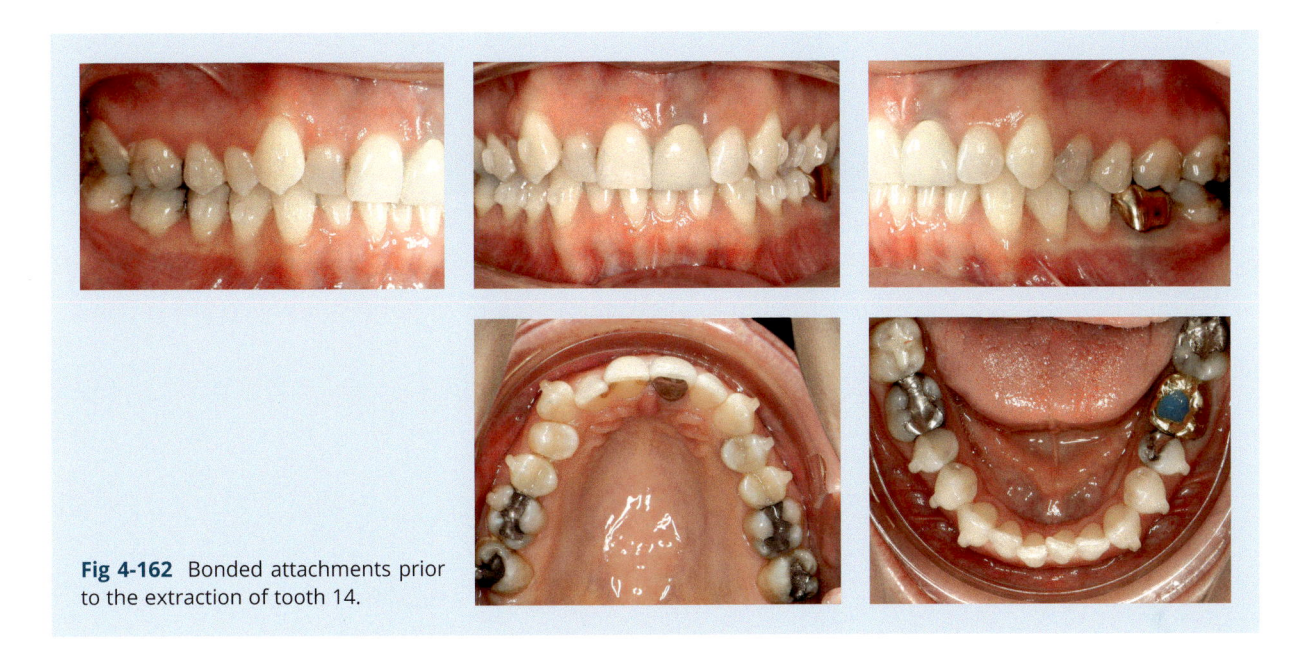

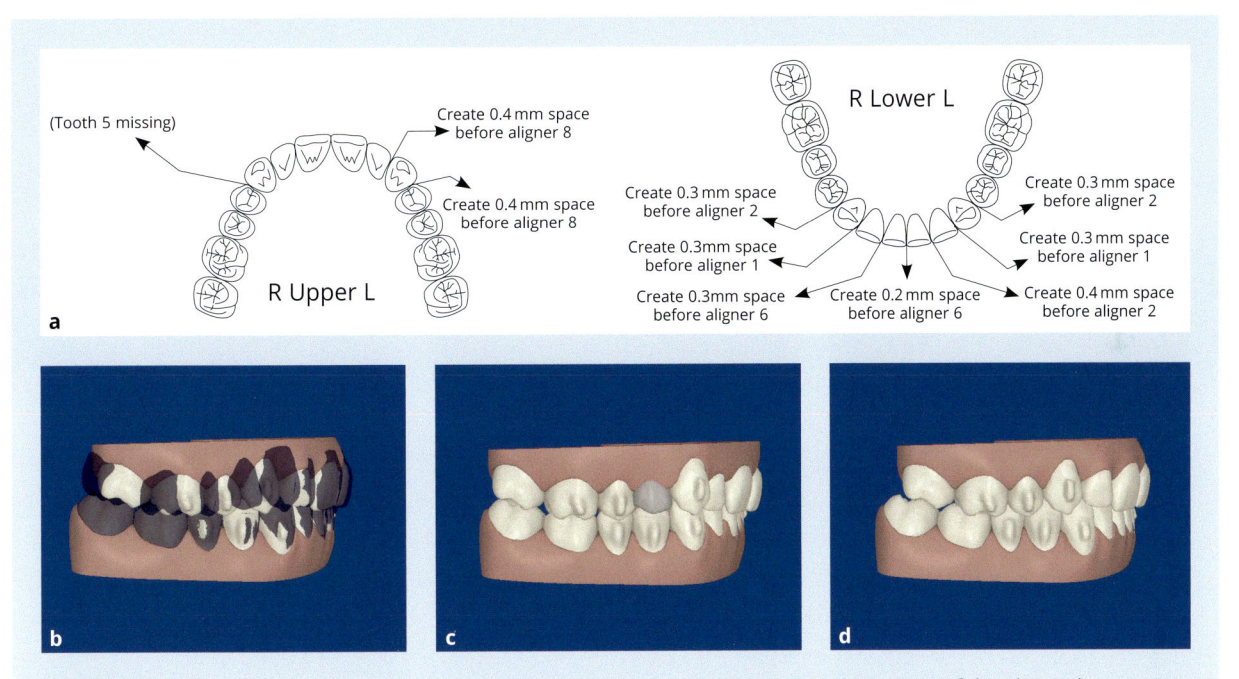

Fig 4-162 Bonded attachments prior to the extraction of tooth 14.

Fig 4-163 Treatment planning. **(a)** IPR chart. **(b-d)** ClinCheck results showing superimposition of the planned movement of the right side **(b)**; the starting point with a pontic for the extracted tooth 14 **(c)**; and the planned final situation of the right side after space closure **(d)**. Blue, initial tooth position; white, final tooth position.

4 TREATMENT OF DIFFERENT MALOCCLUSIONS WITH ALIGNERS

Fig 4-164 Final views.

Fig 4-165 Remounted plaster casts after treatment showing open incisor area (as shown with Shimstock foil) and full contact (blue) of premolars and molars with canine guidance (red).

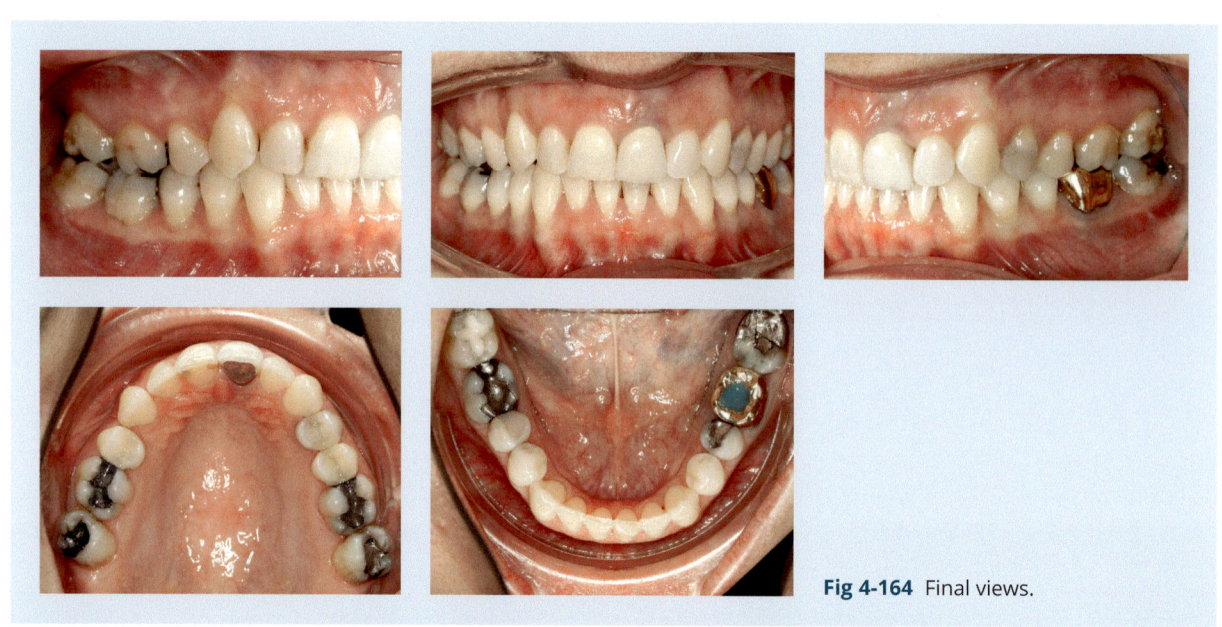

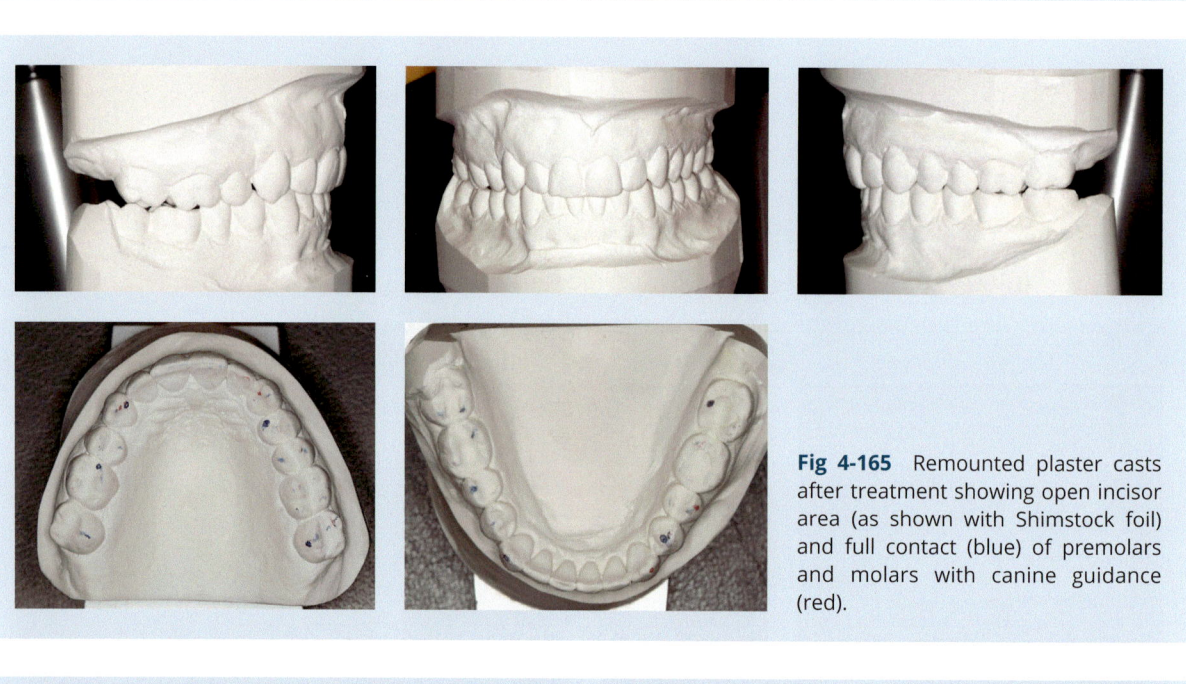

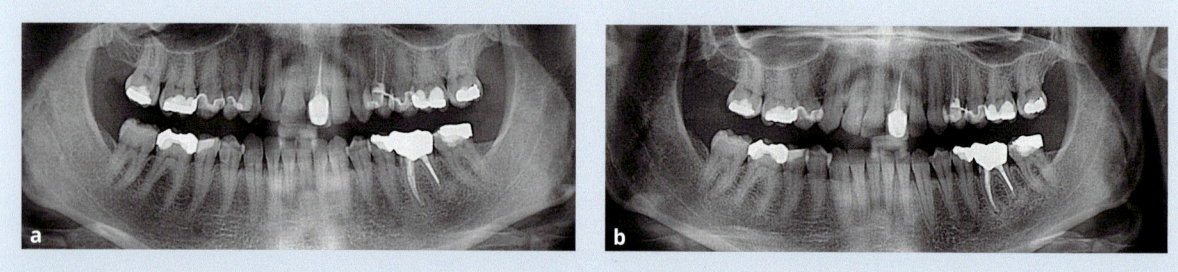

Fig 4-166 Initial **(a)** and final **(b)** orthopantomography with need for new endodontic supply.

Fig 4-167 Initial (a,c) and final (b,d) views.

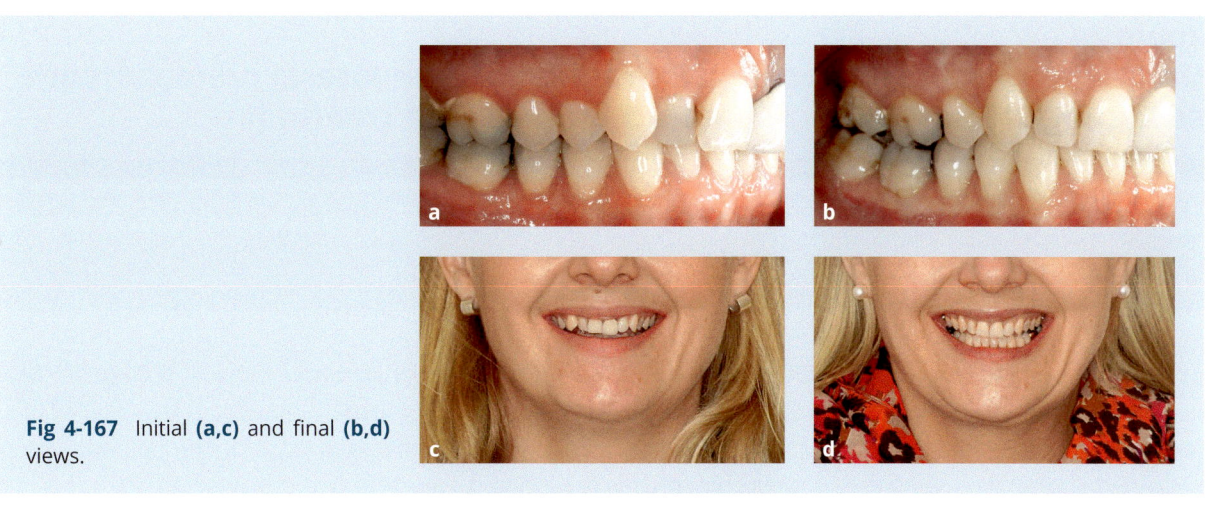

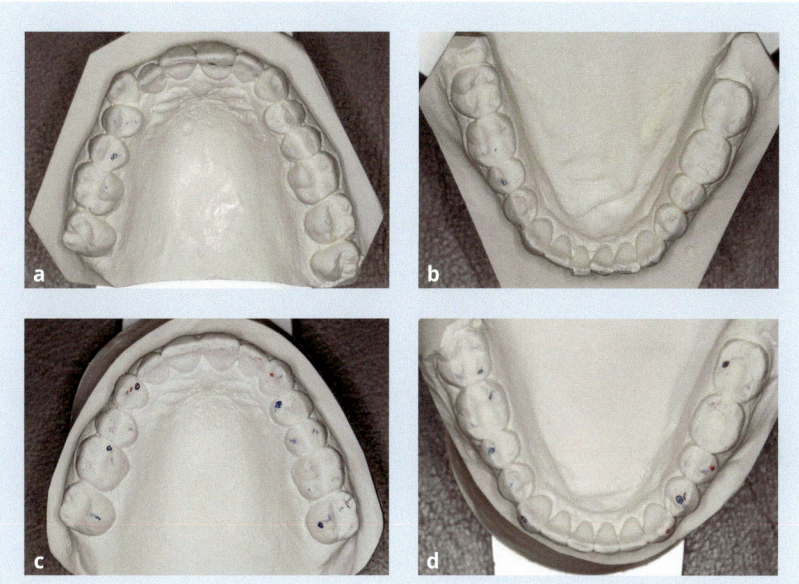

Fig 4-168 Initial (a,b) and final (c,d) plaster casts showing the final stable centric relation with canine guidance.

is sufficient to allow an optimal rebuilding with restoratives by the dentist.

The remounted plaster casts after Invisalign treatment demonstrate a "Shimstock open" incisor area and full contact of premolars and molars with canine guidance, as tested with Shimstock foil (Fig 4-165). Orthopantomography shows the tooth movements achieved (Fig 4-166). Tooth 15 shows a slightly mesial tipped crown position, which might have been less if the G6 features for premolar extraction had been available at the time. Endodontic revision of tooth 36 will be required.

Views before and after orthodontic treatment (Fig 4-167) confirm the results seen on the final plaster casts (Fig 4-168). There was an improved smile line, with the maxillary incisors harmonically following the lower lip line (Fig 4-167c,d). The heavy occlusal contacts in the incisor area and only one single posterior contact on teeth 15 to 45 had been removed, leaving a stable centric relation with canine guidance. The slight tipping of teeth 13 and 15 into the extraction space can be seen. However, the mesial inclination does not lead to occlusal restriction. The use of more torque on the maxillary incisors with power ridges might have allowed a better anterior relationship and esthetics to be achieved. The final situation represents an optimal starting point for the future restorative procedures.

Topic 24
Unilateral class II relationship: Extraction of a unilateral premolar with sectional fixed mechanics followed by Invisalign treatment

Treatment:
- extraction
- sectional fixed mechanics
- Invisalign treatment

In some patients, it is easier to start with sectional fixed mechanics if premolar extraction is required. Fixed mechanics for several weeks with distalization of the canine into the extraction space allows optimal canine root angulation and opens up space distally of the lateral incisors, which allows a subsequent aligner to grip to the complete canine crown, thus increasing control during canine distalization (Fig 4-169). An alternative is described in Topic 63.

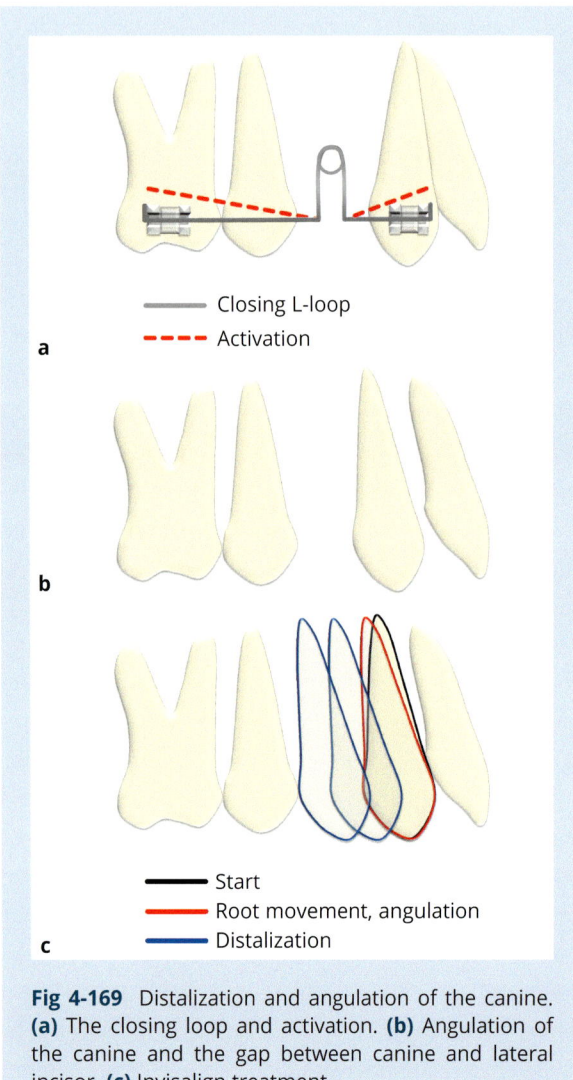

Fig 4-169 Distalization and angulation of the canine. **(a)** The closing loop and activation. **(b)** Angulation of the canine and the gap between canine and lateral incisor. **(c)** Invisalign treatment.

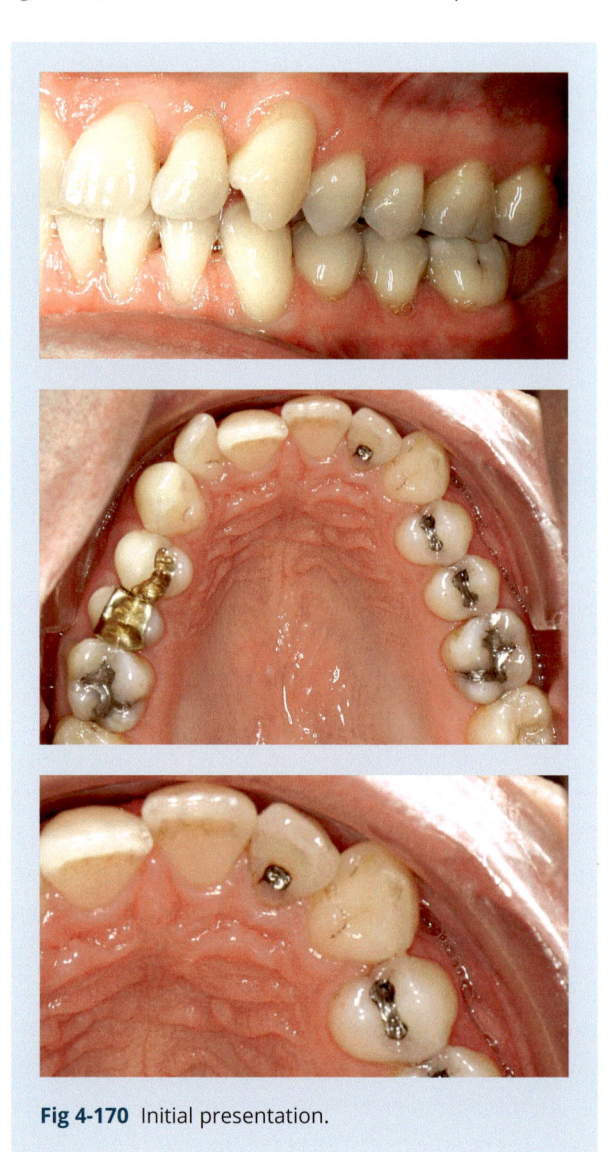

Fig 4-170 Initial presentation.

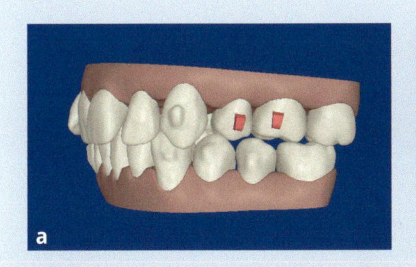

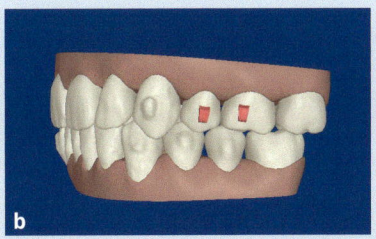

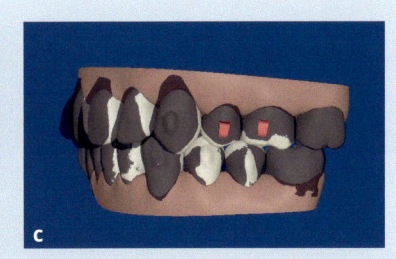

TREATMENT OF DIFFERENT MALOCCLUSIONS WITH ALIGNERS 4

Fig 4-171 ClinCheck software results. **(a)** Initial situation after pretreatment with the partial fixed appliance. **(b)** Final planned situation. **(c)** Superimposition to show the planned tooth movements (blue, initial tooth position; white, final tooth position).

This patient is class II/2, with a class I relationship on the right and a class II relationship on the left plus crowding and a midline deviation (Fig 4-170).

Diagnosis:
- class II/2 with class I relationship on the right and class II relationship on the left
- crowding
- midline deviation
- missing antagonist of tooth 27.

Therapy:
- extraction of tooth 24
- sectional fixed mechanics on teeth 23, 25, 26
- Invisalign treatment.

Treatment

After pretreatment with the partial fixed appliance, attachments were bonded and also vertical conventional attachments were added to obtain maximum anchorage on teeth 23, 25, and 26 during the space closure (Fig 4-171). In total 29 aligners were used.

Views during the course of the treatment show the highly predictable results achieved with the combination of sectional mechanics and the Invisalign technique (Fig 4-172). It is definitely possible to start earlier with the Invisalign system than the several months chosen here. A gap opening of 1.5 mm between the lateral incisor and the canine is perfect for commencing with the aligner treatment. Here the canine was distalized more than 3 mm into the extraction space to create the optimal space distally of tooth 22, so that the aligner could get a good grip of the whole canine crown and even the lateral incisor crown.

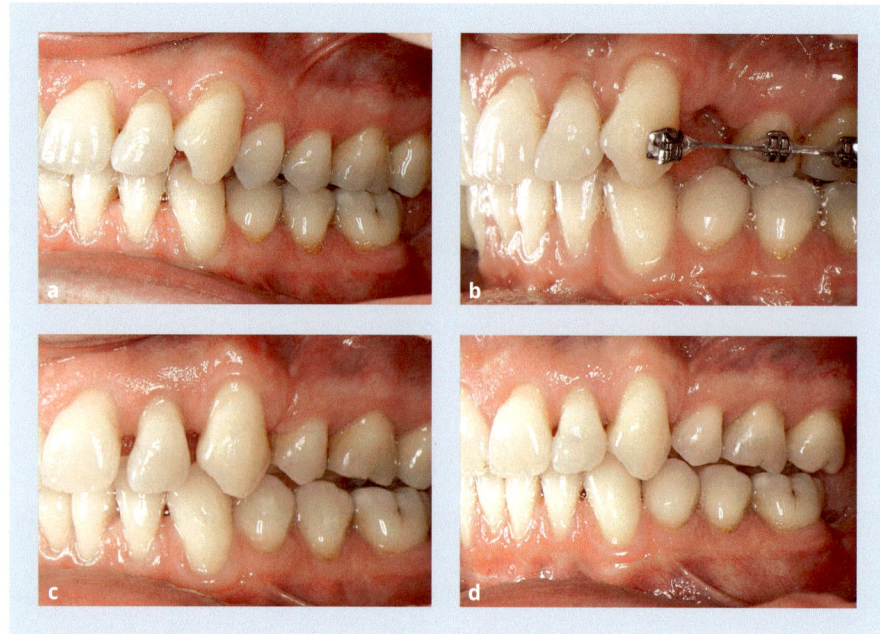

Fig 4-172 Treatment progression. **(a)** Initial findings with class II relationship and severe mesial angulation of tooth 23. **(b)** Pretreatment with a sectional fixed appliance after extraction of tooth 24. **(c)** Invisalign treatment started after several months of pretreatment. **(d)** Final situation on the left side with a physiologically angulated canine in a one tooth to two teeth relationship.

An alternative to the pretreatment with partial fixed appliance followed by the Invisalign treatment is described also in chapter 63, Fig 4-568 to 4-581.

Topic 25
Bialveolar protrusion: Extraction of four premolars
(Treatment performed by Dr Kenji Ojima, Tokyo, Japan)

> **Treatment:**
> - extraction of upper and lower premolars

In patients with severe crowding and a need for tooth alignment, tooth extraction is sometimes inevitable. While solving the crowding is easier with the major amount of space offered by extractions, treatment can become even more difficult. The strategy to control tooth movement with the Invisalign system after extraction of four premolars should consider:
- exact knowledge of the characteristics of the aligner
- anchorage control
- staging
- selection of the attachments
- combination of Invisalign treatment with elastics
- timing of refinement
- techniques of recovery.

In patients with premolar extractions, it is necessary to use class II elastics (Fig 4-173). Force is applied and transferred onto the maxillary arch with the elastics, leading to strengthening of the anchorage of the maxillary molars. In addition, elastics help to avoid a bowing effect. The elastics can be worn from a precision cut or a hook directly bonded onto the maxillary canines.

The patient described here has severe crowding of the maxillary and mandibular anterior arches (Fig 4-174).

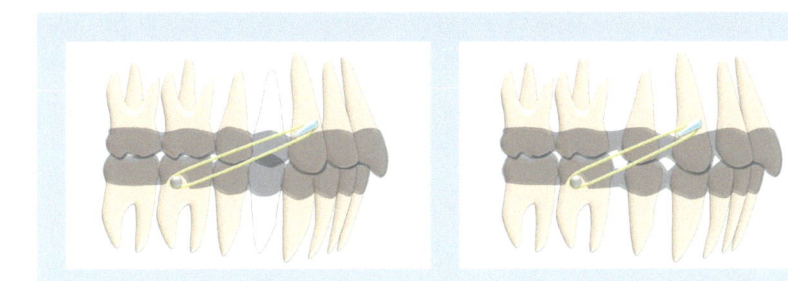

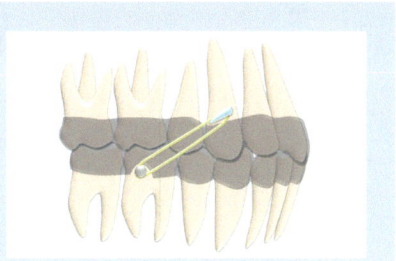

Fig 4-173 Class II elastics for patients with premolar extractions.

Diagnosis:
- bialveolar protrusion
- class II relationship
- severe crowding of the maxillary and mandibular anterior arches
- severe rotation of tooth 21.

Therapy:
- extraction of teeth 14, 24, 34, and 44
- class II elastics
- closure of all extraction spaces
- obtain class I relationship with physiologic overbite and overjet.

Fig 4-174 Initial presentation.

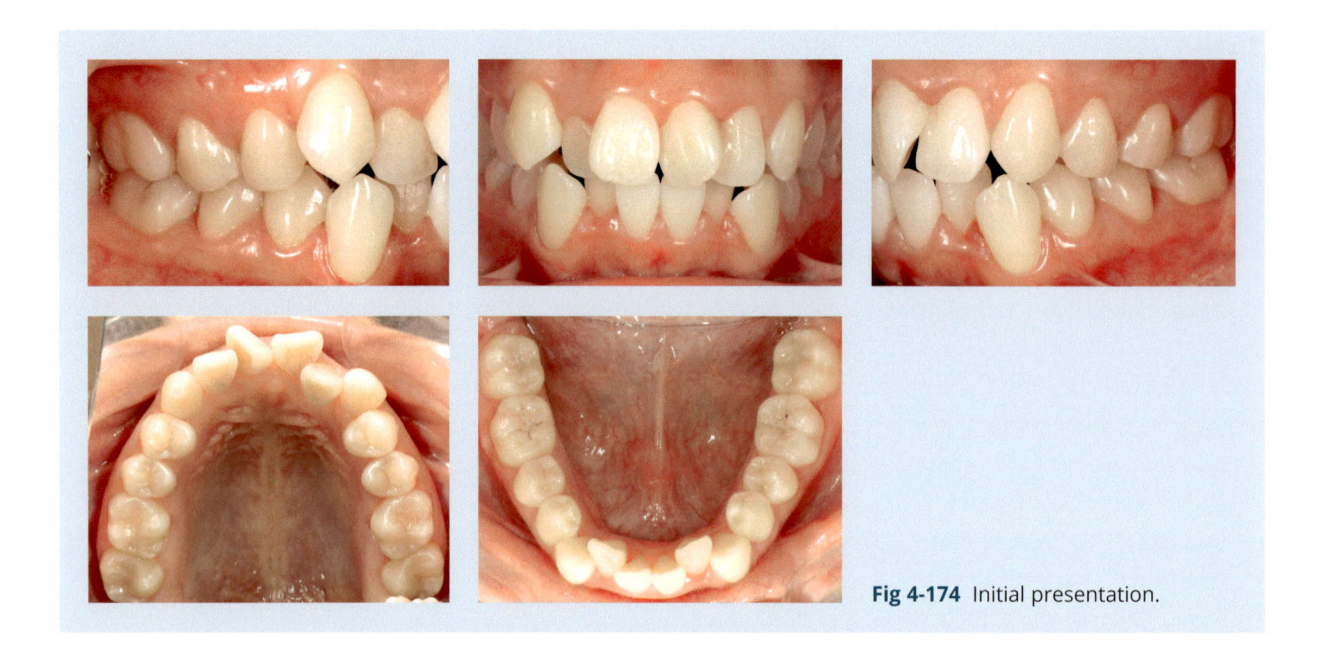

Treatment

Treatment commenced with extraction of all first premolars (Fig 4-175) before before inserting vertical rectangular attachments on 12 teeth. Hooks were placed on teeth 13 and 23 and metal buttons on teeth 36 and 46 for class II elastics. Directly bonded hooks on canines were chosen to obtain major force on the canines in direction of "desorption." This force helps to maintain optimal fitting of the aligners and, therefore, optimal tooth control.

Retraction of maxillary and mandibular canines and the alignment of maxillary and mandibular anterior teeth was achieved without loss of anchorage at molars and second molars. With the distalization of the canines, it is important to maintain the root position distally. A bowing effect can be avoided with slow staging. Further use of aligners (Fig 4-175c–e) followed by assessment with fresh impressions confirmed that an additional refinement was needed for further angulation and torque of the incisors; this used an additional 13 aligners.

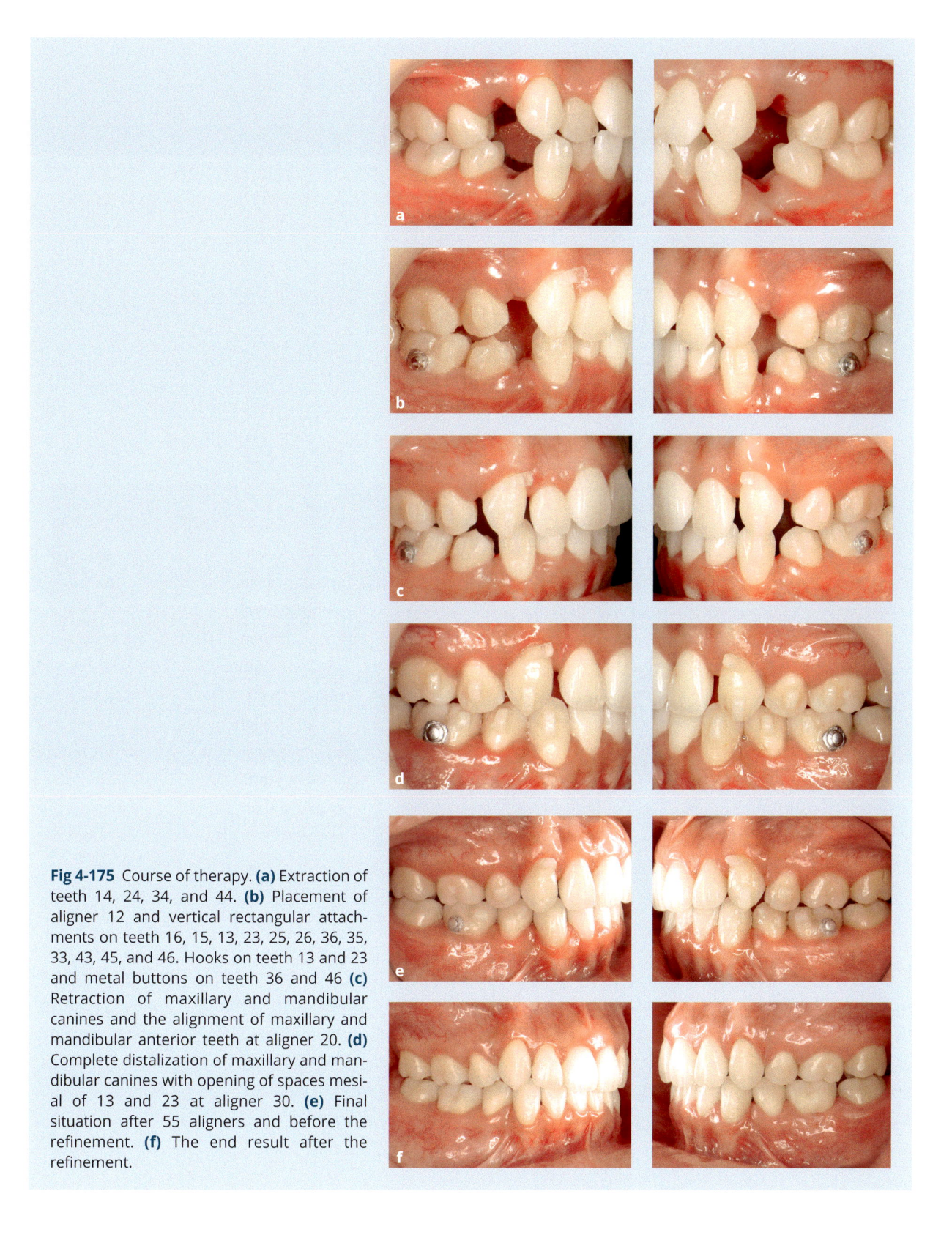

Fig 4-175 Course of therapy. **(a)** Extraction of teeth 14, 24, 34, and 44. **(b)** Placement of aligner 12 and vertical rectangular attachments on teeth 16, 15, 13, 23, 25, 26, 36, 35, 33, 43, 45, and 46. Hooks on teeth 13 and 23 and metal buttons on teeth 36 and 46 **(c)** Retraction of maxillary and mandibular canines and the alignment of maxillary and mandibular anterior teeth at aligner 20. **(d)** Complete distalization of maxillary and mandibular canines with opening of spaces mesial of 13 and 23 at aligner 30. **(e)** Final situation after 55 aligners and before the refinement. **(f)** The end result after the refinement.

4 TREATMENT OF DIFFERENT MALOCCLUSIONS WITH ALIGNERS

Fig 4-176 ClinCheck software results. **(a)** Initial situation. **(b)** Start of canine distalization. **(c)** Closure of the extraction space. **(d)** Final situation.

Fig 4-177 Intraoral pictures showing full class I relationship with correct midlines and a physiologic overjet and overbite.

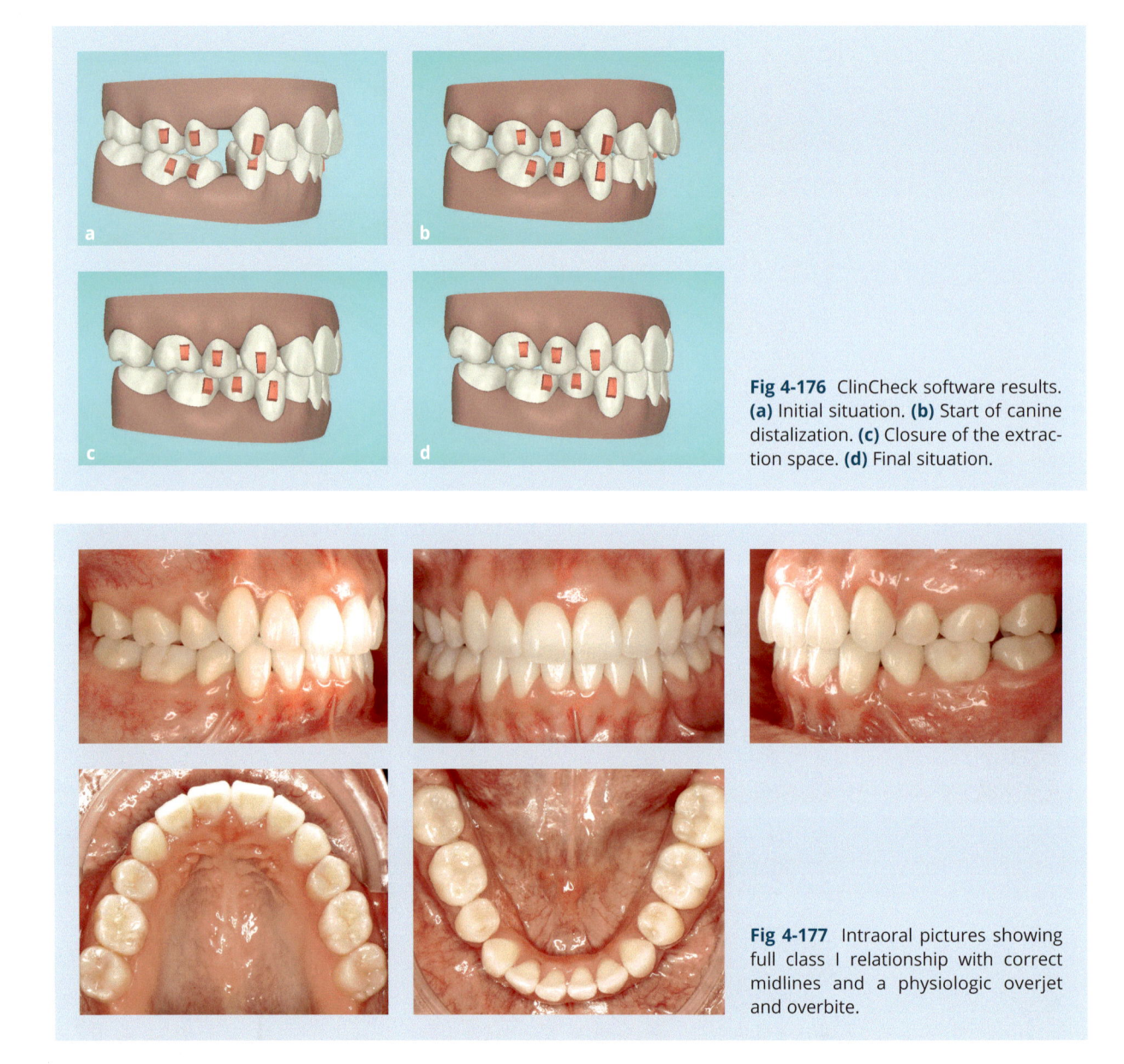

Figure 4-176 shows the ClinCheck software results.

Final views show the success of the treatment (Figs 4-177 and 4-178). Both sides showed class I canine guidance, and there was a physiologic overjet and overbite. Maxillary and mandibular anterior teeth have been aligned and all extraction spaces have been completely closed. Molars and second premolars show posterior contact in a stable class I relationship. Lip closure is more competent without forced muscle tension of muscularis mentalis. The extraoral lateral profile has been improved.

Radiography shows the change in tooth position during treatment (Fig 4-179).

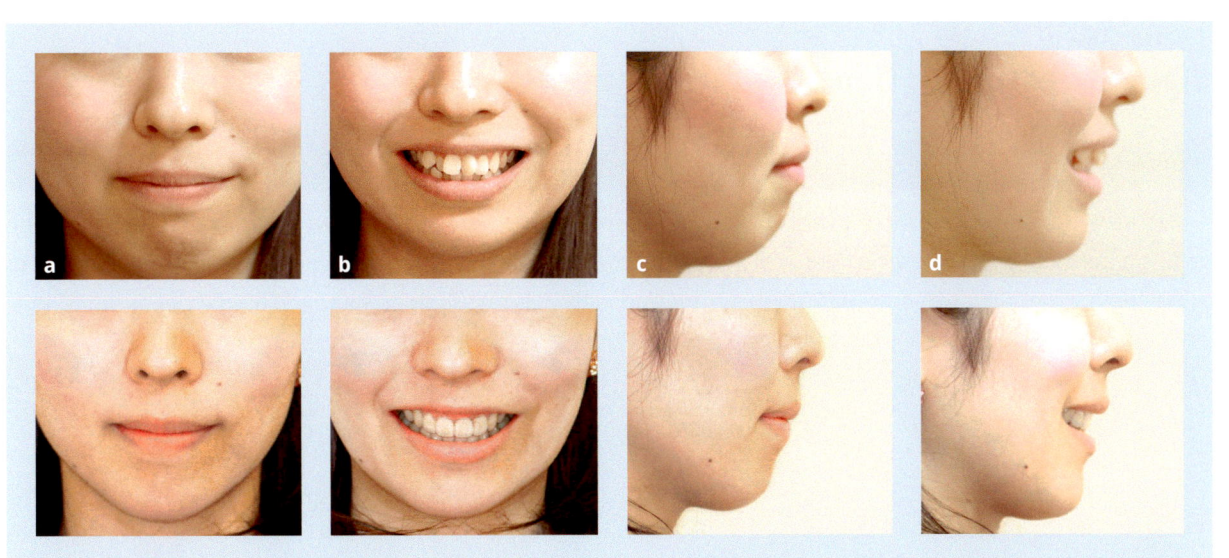

Fig 4-178 Comparison of lip closure **(a)**, extraoral smile **(b)**, and profile views **(c,d)** before **(upper)** and after **(lower)** treatment with a four premolar extraction.

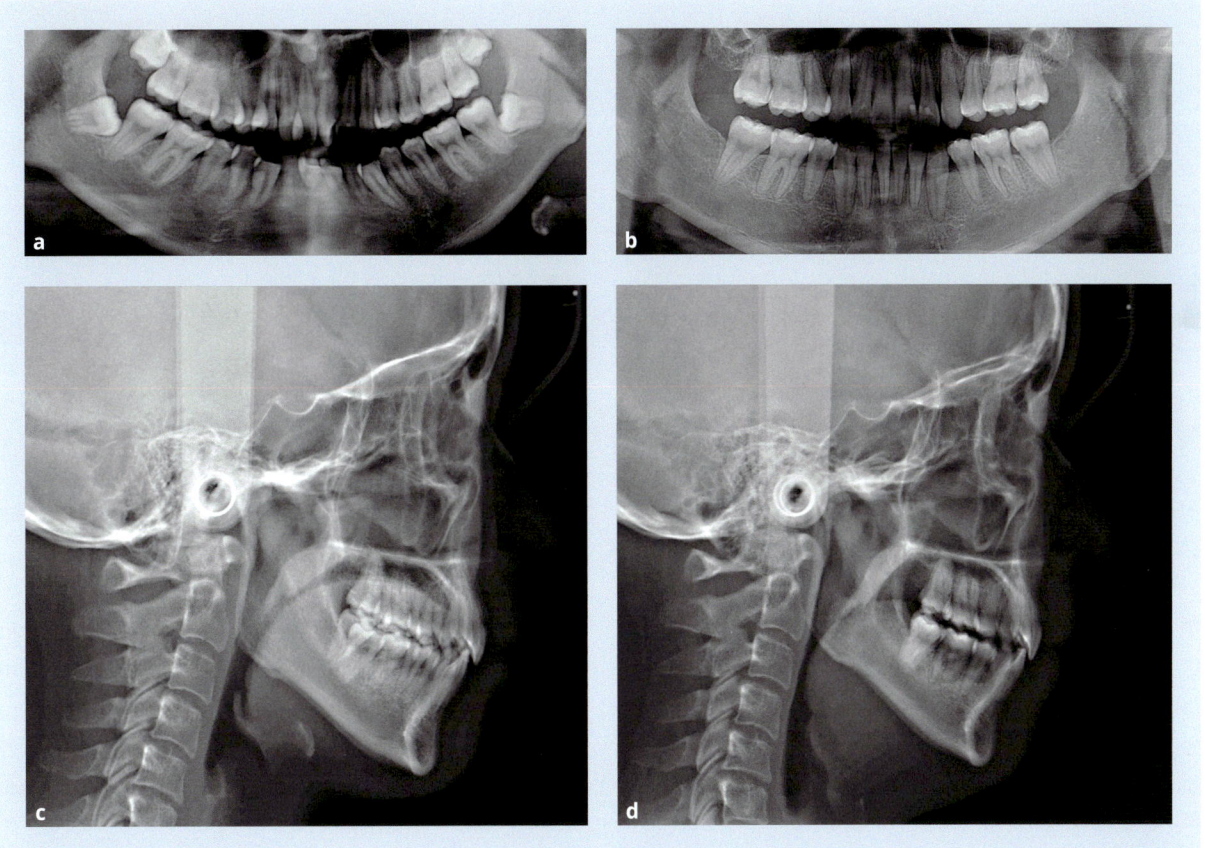

Fig 4-179 Radiography. **(a)** Initial orthopantomogram with all wisdom teeth in situ. **(b)** Orthopantomogram after extraction of all third molars and first premolars with complete space closure. The roots are parallel in both arches. **(c)** Lateral radiography at the beginning of treatment. **(d)** Lateral radiography after retraction of anterior teeth in both arches into the extraction spaces.

Topic 26
Class II treatment: General considerations

The combined treatment of a skeletal class II in the growing patient as well as a combination with surgery in an adult can be performed with the Invisalign system.

Figure 4-180 shows the force effects occurring when teeth are moved. Because exertion of a force by one body on another generates an equal and opposite reaction, anchorage is needed whenever force is used to move teeth. Particularly when distalization is required with the Invisalign system, anchorage needs to be provided with class II elastics to avoid undesired mesial counterforces.

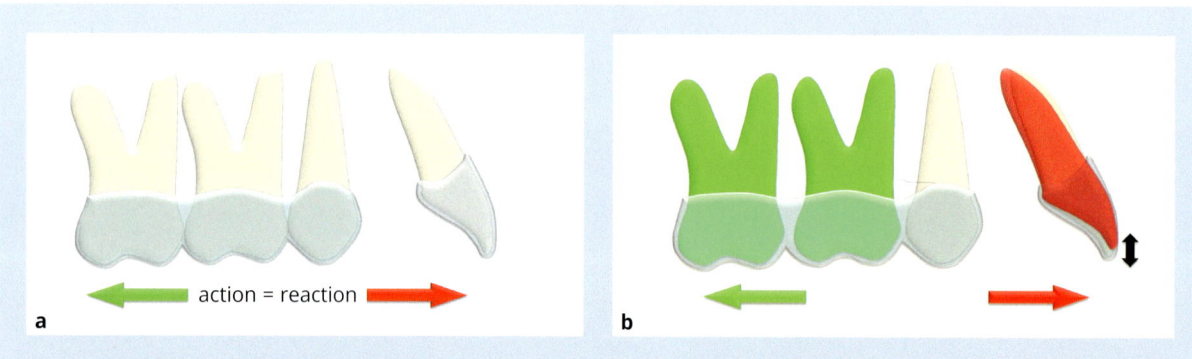

Fig 4-180 Tooth movements under force. **(a)** A force exerted by one body on another generates an equal and opposite reaction (Newton´s third law). **(b)** Loss of anchorage can lead to anterior proclination and relative intrusion of a tooth.

Loss of anchorage may manifest with anterior proclination, resulting in a relative intrusion of the maxillary incisors; this will hamper the fitting of an aligner in this region. Attachments on the maxillary incisors at the start of the distalization of maxillary canines may be helpful for major anchorage.

In almost all patients with class II relationship and planned distalization in the maxillary arch, we use class II elastics from a clear hook on the maxillary canine to a bonded button on the mandibular first molar (Fig 4-181a,b). To avoid rotation of the canine under the force of the elastics, an attachment is placed on the canine. The crystal-clear plastic hook is sandblasted and then coated with bonding agenol for acrylic resins (e.g. Perlibond, Scheu Dental) to ensure an optimal adhesion.

An alternative approach is to order a precision cut (elastic hook) directly in the aligner for the elastic wear. A button cut-out for bonded hooks or buttons can be requested in the opposite arch (Fig 4-182).

Figure 4-183 shows an elastic in position with the aligner.

Based on our experience, it is best to use the following procedure to treat class II relationships:

1. Start exclusively with the single distalization of the second molar.
2. When the second molar is distalized 50%, start distal movement of the first molar.
3. Start premolar distalization when the second molar has reached its final position.
4. Start canine distalization when the first molar has reached its final position. Attachments on 12, 11, 21, and 22 can help to obtain major anchorage when the canine starts distalization.

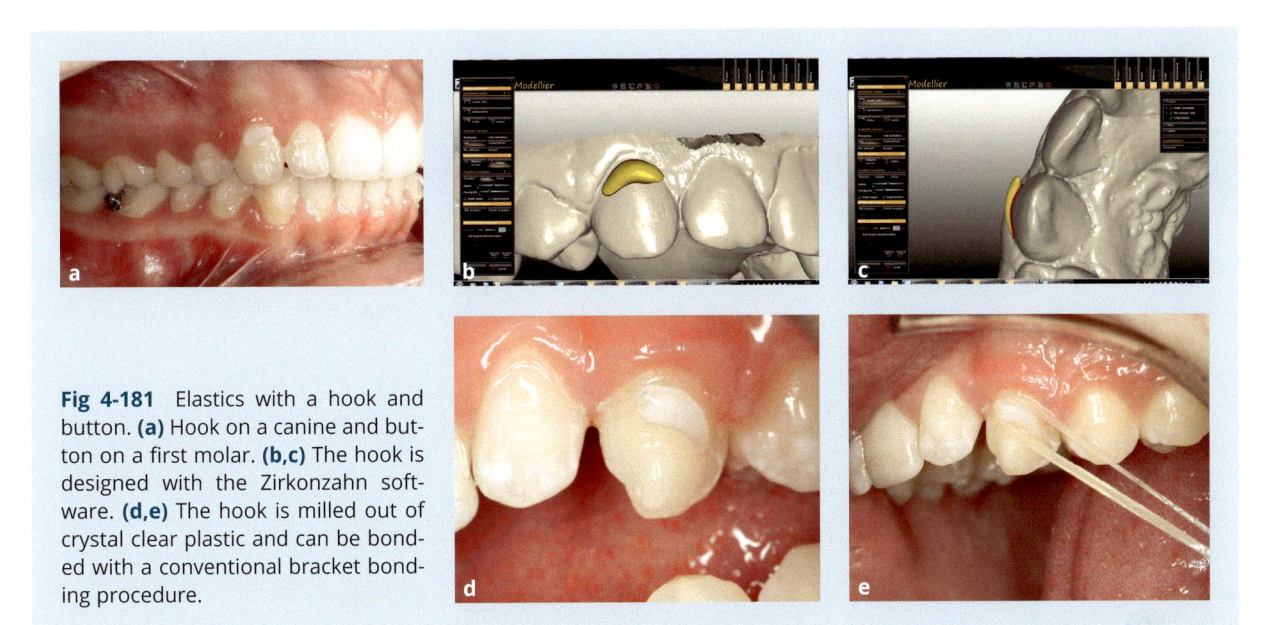

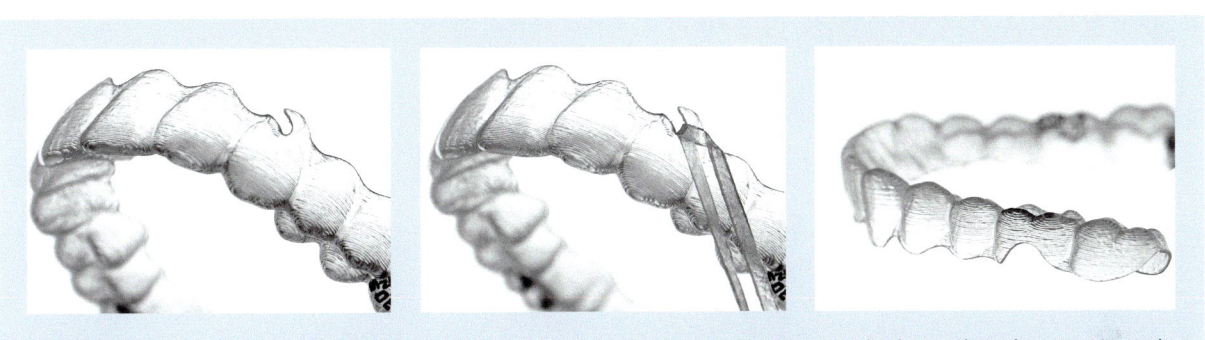

TREATMENT OF DIFFERENT MALOCCLUSIONS WITH ALIGNERS 4

Fig 4-181 Elastics with a hook and button. **(a)** Hook on a canine and button on a first molar. **(b,c)** The hook is designed with the Zirkonzahn software. **(d,e)** The hook is milled out of crystal clear plastic and can be bonded with a conventional bracket bonding procedure.

Fig 4-182 A precision cut (elastic hook) in an aligner for the elastic. A button cut-out can also be made in the opposite arch.

The patient is asked to wear the elastic only at night during the movement of the second molar, but to wear it for an additional 3 hours during the day with the start of movement of the first molars. The patient is also advised to wear the elastics during the night for at least 3 months after active treatment is completed.

The force of the class II elastics for anchorage should be a maximum of 100 g for class II and a maximum of 80 g for class III.

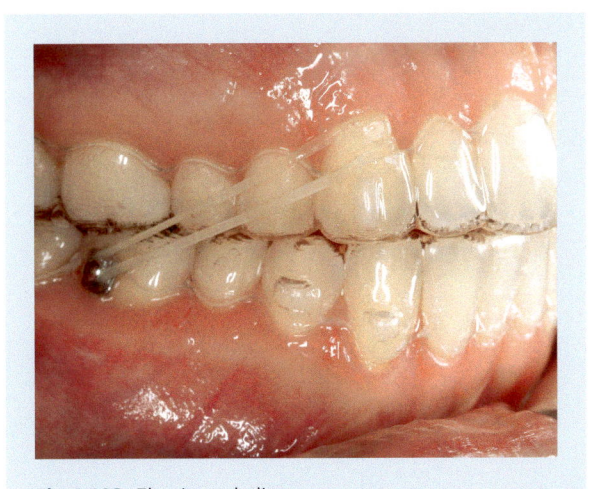

Fig 4-183 Elastic and aligner.

Topic 27
Class II with highly erupted upper canines

Treatment:
- Distalization with the Invisalign system and class II elastics

This patient had a class II relationship, crowding, and rotations in both arches, and highly erupted maxillary canines (Fig 4-184).

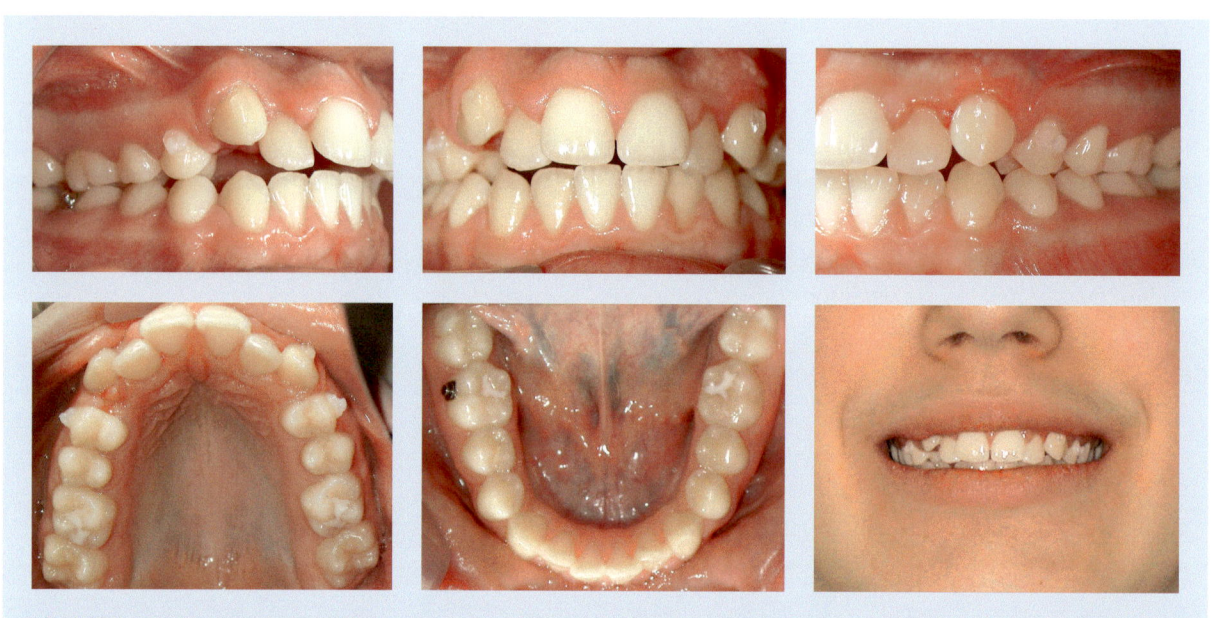

Fig 4-184 Initial presentation with buttons and hooks placed (button on tooth 36 came off prior to picture taking and needed to be rebonded).

Diagnosis:
- class II relationship
- crowding and rotations in the maxillary and mandibular arches
- frontal open bite
- highly erupted tooth 13 more than 23.

Therapy:
- myofunctional therapy
- distalization in the maxillary arch with class II elastics
- alignment of the maxilla and mandible
- extrusion of the highly erupted teeth 13 and 23.

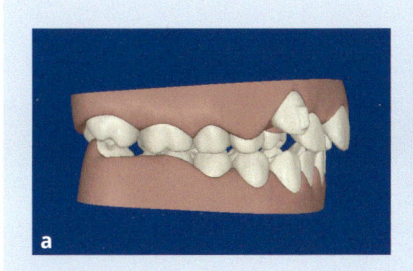

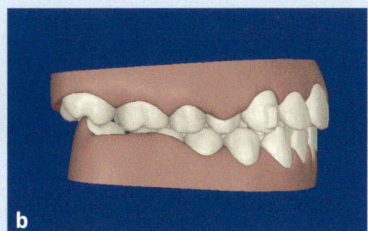

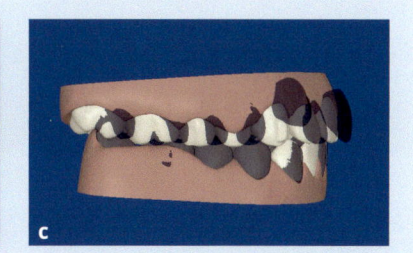

Fig 4-185 ClinCheck software results. **(a)** Initial situation on the right side. **(b)** Planned final situation. **(c)** Superimposition to show planned movements (blue, initial tooth position; white, final tooth position).

Treatment

At the start of treatment, vertical rectangular attachments were placed on maxillary canines for extrusion, as well as hooks on teeth 14 and 24 and buttons on teeth 36 and 46 for class II elastic wear.

ClinCheck software was used for planning, with 51 aligners in the first phase (Fig 4-185). Because of the large number of aligners, the patient was advised to change these every 10 instead of 14 days.

Figure 4-186 shows the course of therapy. The transparent plastic hook on the maxillary first premolars was replaced with a metal hook. The bonding stability has since increased for transparent hooks fabricated in the laboratory (see Topic 26), and in most cases metal hooks are not needed. Once the molars and premolars were in a full class I relationship, attachments were added to the maxillary and lateral incisors for major anchorage during the upcoming distalization. After the first aligner phase, refinement occurred as tooth 13 still needed some extrusive movement to end up in sufficient canine guidance and there was still some rotation of the mandibular anterior teeth to correct.

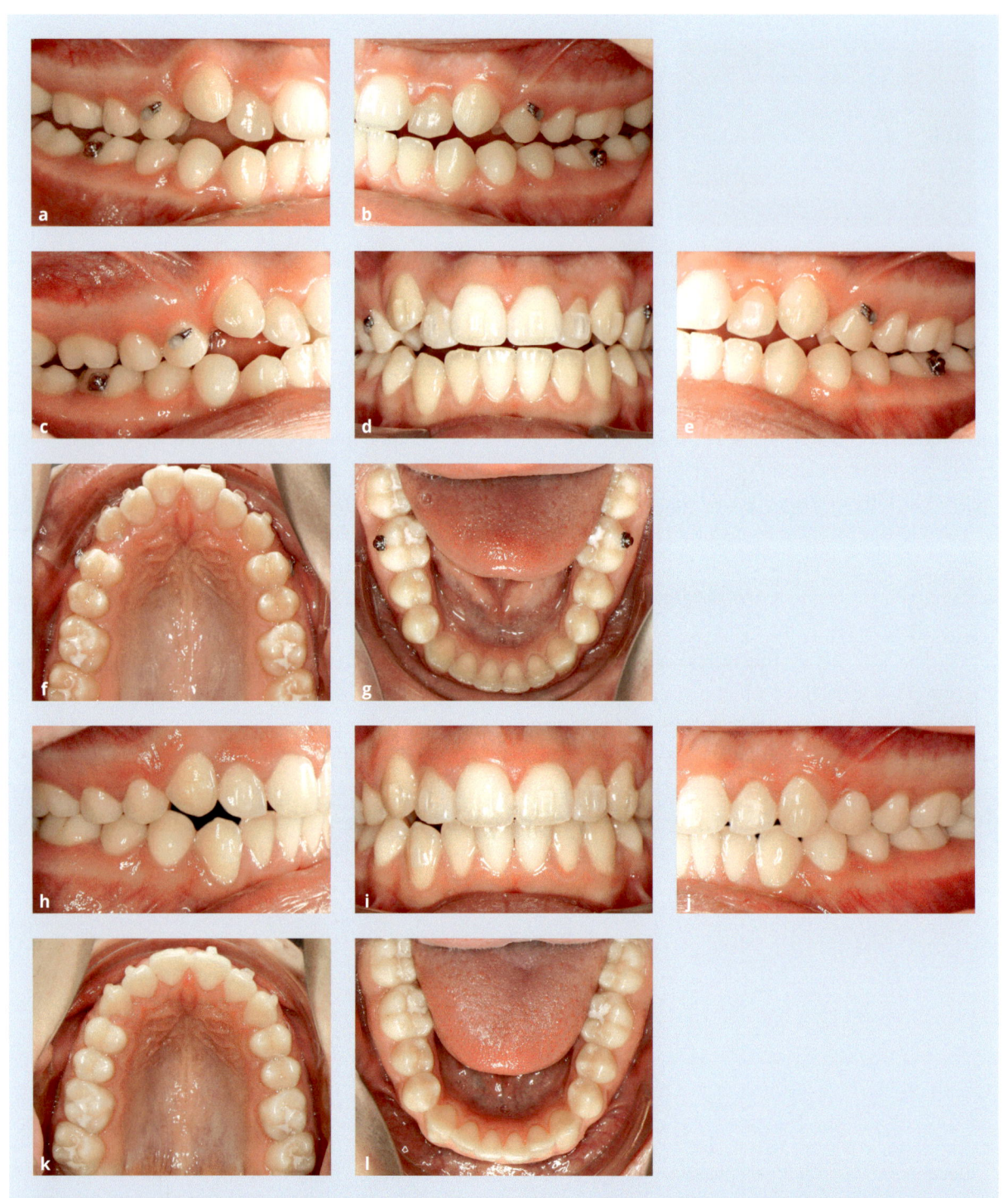

4 TREATMENT OF DIFFERENT MALOCCLUSIONS WITH ALIGNERS

Fig 4-186 Course of therapy. **(a,b)** Aligner 13 stage and a metal hook on the maxillary first premolars. **(c–g)** Molars and premolars in a full class I relationship. Attachments added to the maxillary and lateral incisors. **(h–l)** After the first phase of aligners and the beginning of refinement.

Fig 4-187 No decalcification, white spots, or root resorption can be seen at the end of orthodontic treatment.

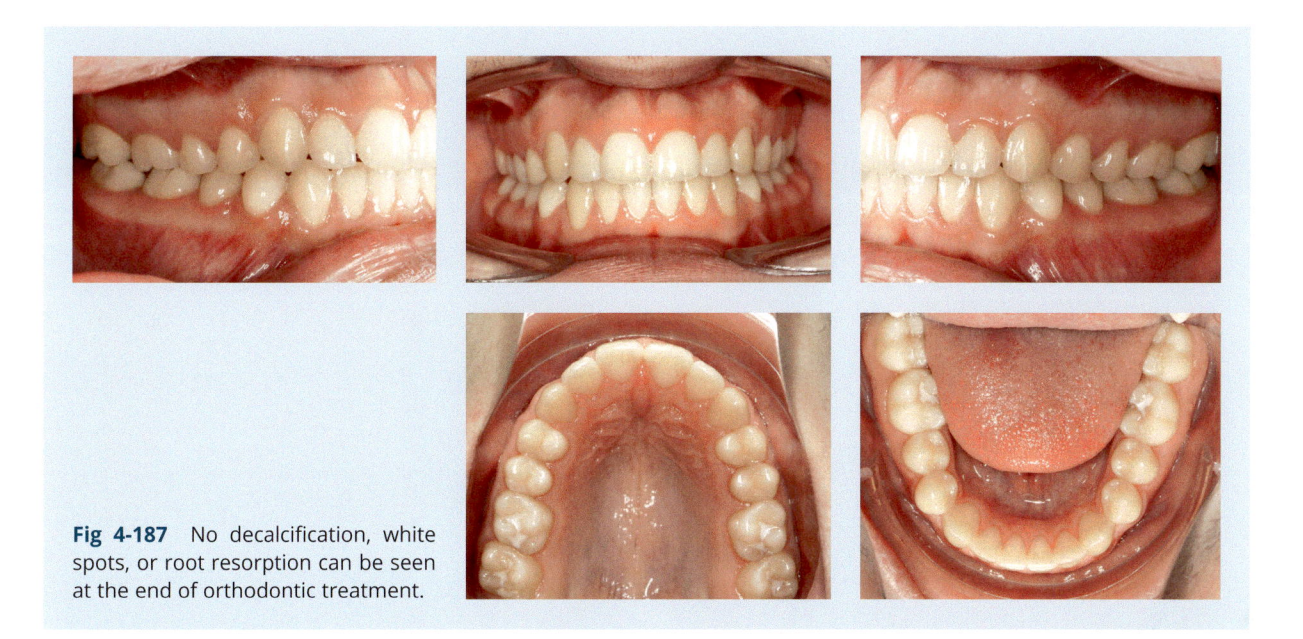

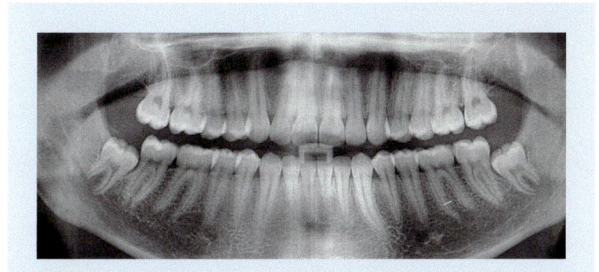

Fig 4-188 Final orthopantomography.

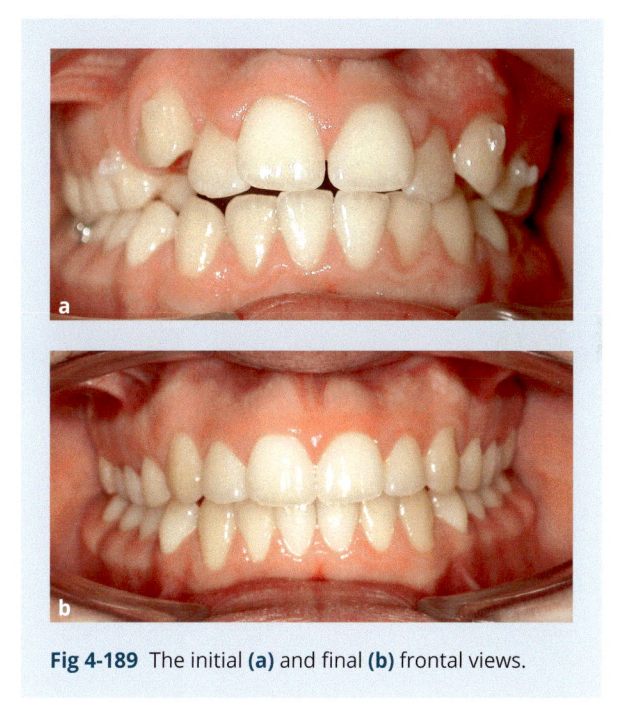

Fig 4-189 The initial (a) and final (b) frontal views.

Because of the minimal invasive Invisalign treatment, the patient showed no decalcification, white spots, or root resorptions at the end of orthodontic treatment (Fig 4-187). The final orthopantomogram showed no pathologic findings (Fig 4-188). Extraction was advised for teeth 38 and 48.

Comparison of initial and final views confirmed the success of treatment, with extruded teeth 13 and 23, distalization, and a physiologic anterior relationship. The smile esthetics had been improved, with the maxillary dentition following harmonically the lower lip curve (Figs 4-189 to 4-191).

Fig 4-190 The initial (a) and final (b) occlusion.

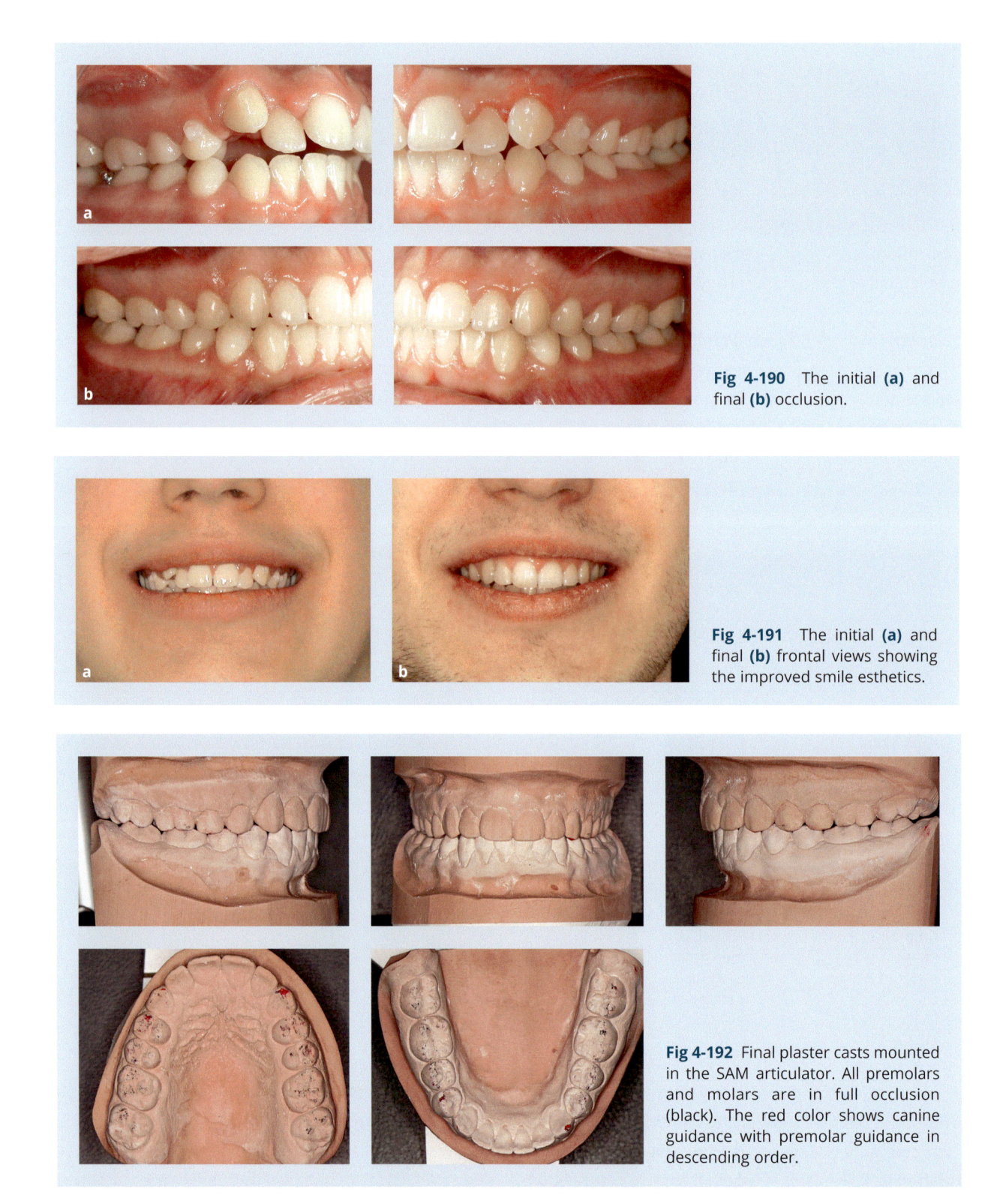

Fig 4-191 The initial (a) and final (b) frontal views showing the improved smile esthetics.

Fig 4-192 Final plaster casts mounted in the SAM articulator. All premolars and molars are in full occlusion (black). The red color shows canine guidance with premolar guidance in descending order.

The final plaster casts mounted in the SAM articulator show the premolars and molars in full occlusion, with canine guidance and premolar guidance in descending order (Fig 4-192).

Topic 28
Class II/2 treatment

Treatment:
- distalization with the Invisalign system and class II elastics
- power ridges on maxillary central incisors for torque

Castroflorio et al (2013) demonstated that the torque produced with the Invisalign system using power ridges is predictable (see Fig 4-193). They stated:

Invisalign represents a good alternative for control of upper-incisor root torque. Aligners offer customized prescriptions with none of the disadvantages related to bracket design and positioning or to tooth morphology. Although previous reports have demonstrated the limited ability of thermoplastic appliances to control root-tipping movements and to establish root control comparable to that of fixed appliances, our preliminary study of power ridges demonstrates that when a torque correction of about 10° is required, torque loss is negligible. Therefore, it is possible that aligners with power ridges may provide better control of the upper incisors than can be achieved with a preadjusted system, at least in some prescriptions.

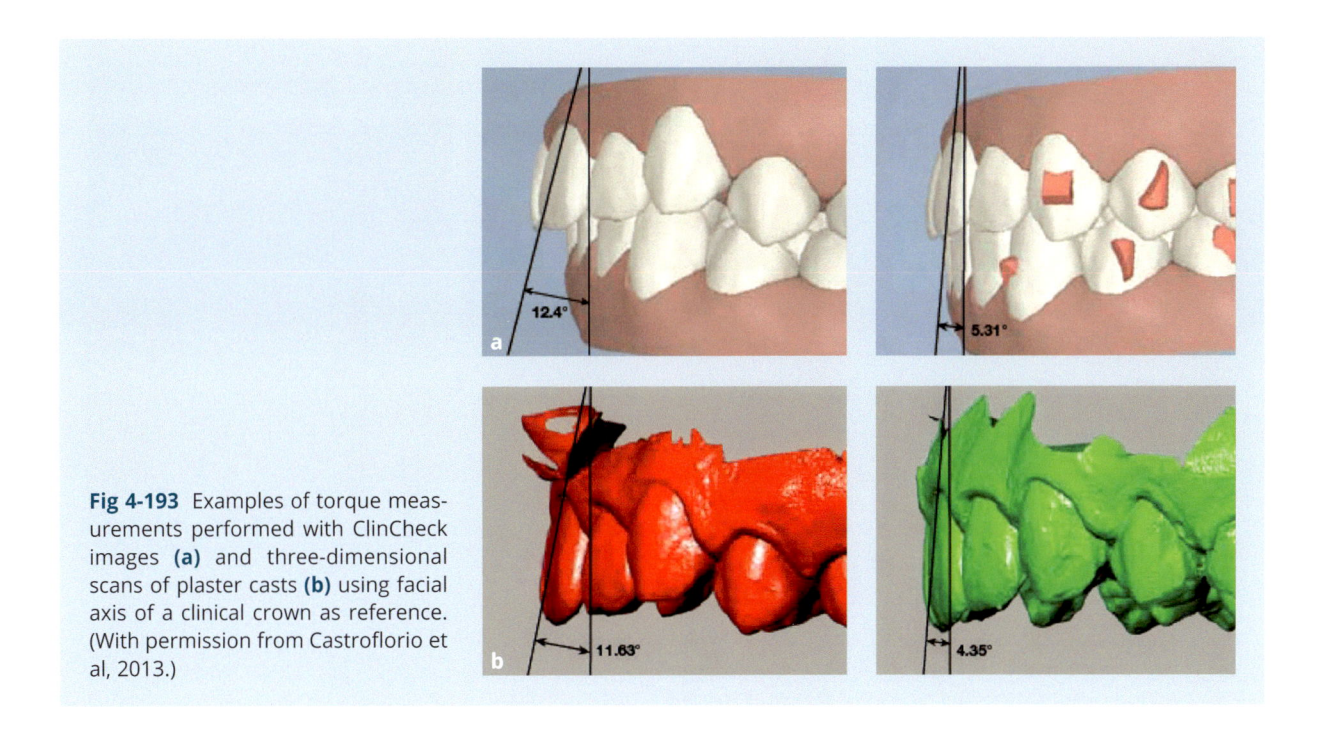

Fig 4-193 Examples of torque measurements performed with ClinCheck images **(a)** and three-dimensional scans of plaster casts **(b)** using facial axis of a clinical crown as reference. (With permission from Castroflorio et al, 2013.)

This patient had a bilateral class II relationship, reclined teeth 11 and 21, extruded tooth 21 more than 11, mild crowding, and a dental deep bite (Fig 4-194). He had an esthetic profile with a harmonious maxillary arch in relation to the width of the lips (transverse direction) (Fig 4-195). Orthopantomography showed that teeth 36 and 46 had older composite resin fillings with defects and missing buccal cusps (Fig 4-196).

4 TREATMENT OF DIFFERENT MALOCCLUSIONS WITH ALIGNERS

Fig 4-194 Initial intraoral presentation.

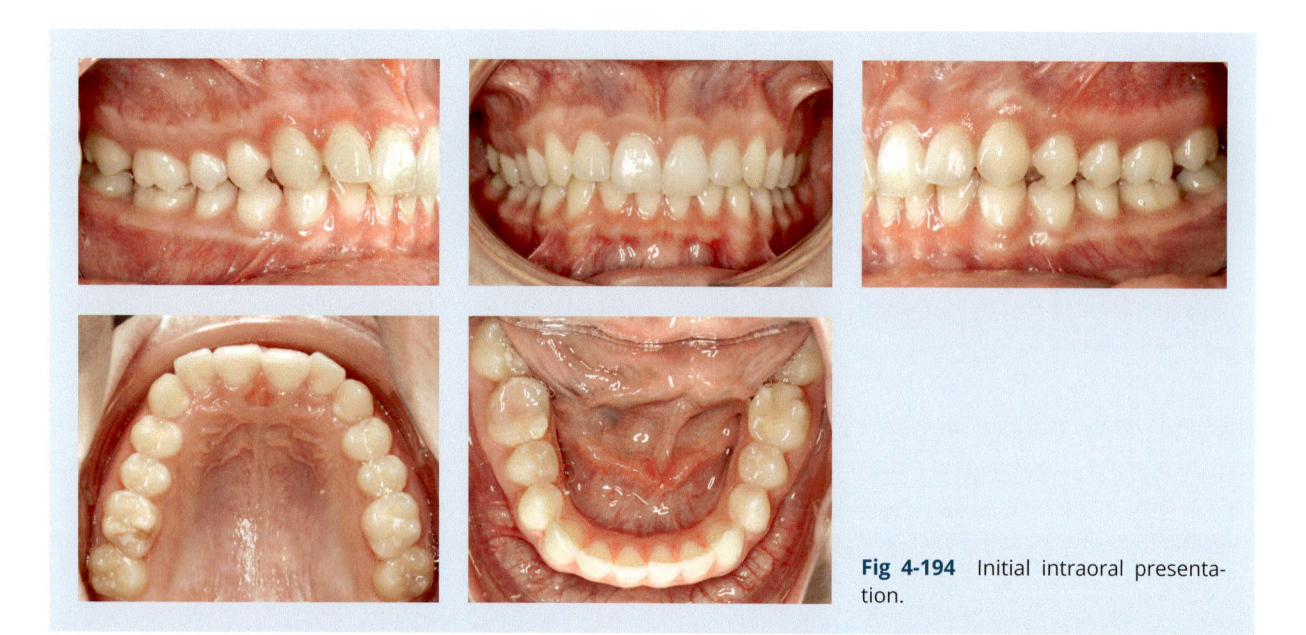

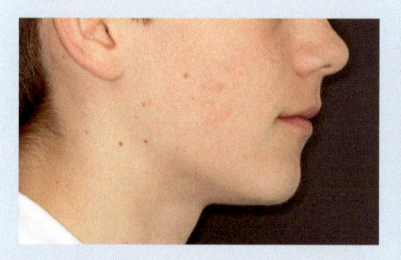

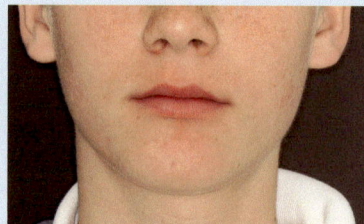

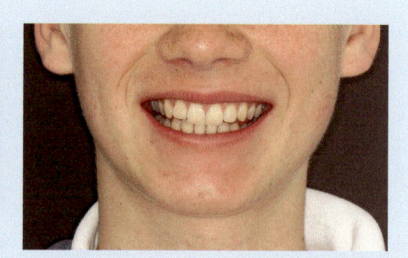

Fig 4-195 Initial extraoral presentation.

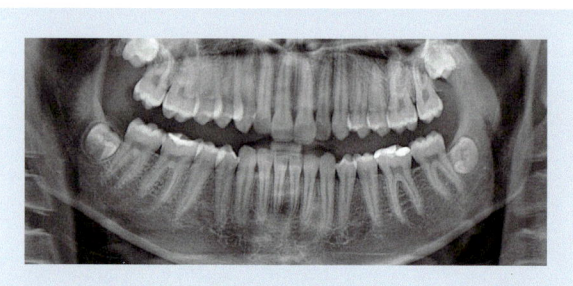

Fig 4-196 Initial orthopantomography.

Diagnosis:
- older insufficient fillings
- bilateral class II relationship
- reclined teeth 11 and 21, tooth 21 more extruded than 11
- mild crowding
- dental deep bite.

Therapy:
- extraction of wisdom teeth
- Invisalign treatment with distalization in the upper arch, class II elastics for anchorage and power ridges on upper central incisors
- renewal of insufficient fillings.

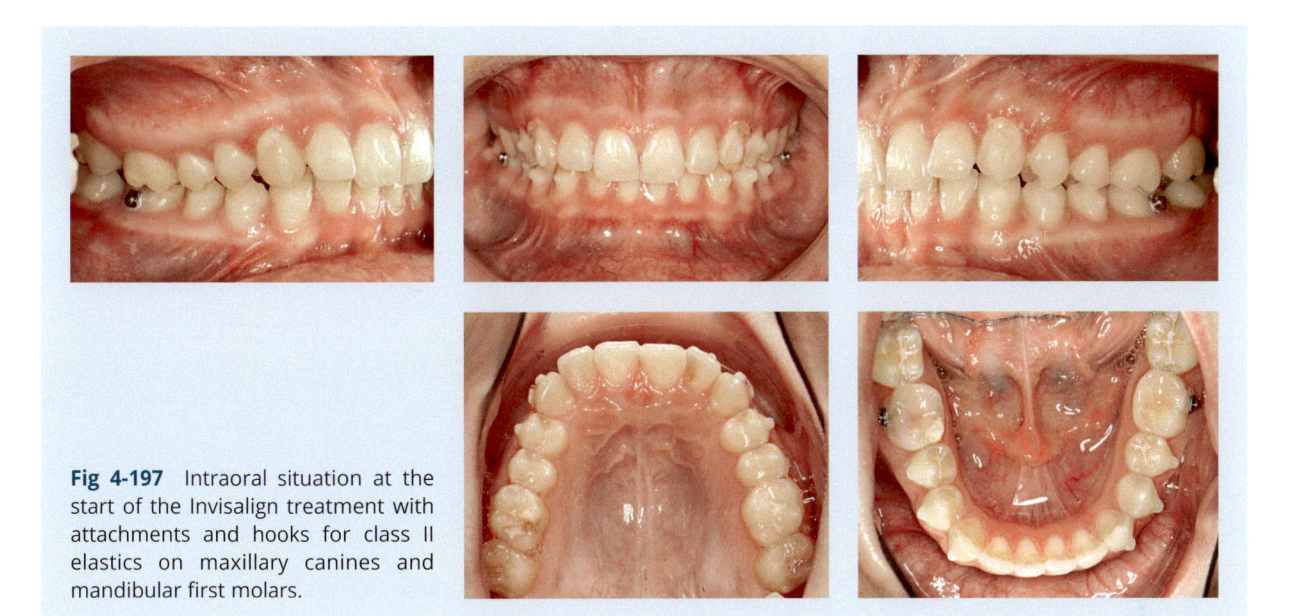

TREATMENT OF DIFFERENT MALOCCLUSIONS WITH ALIGNERS 4

Fig 4-197 Intraoral situation at the start of the Invisalign treatment with attachments and hooks for class II elastics on maxillary canines and mandibular first molars.

Fig 4-198 ClinCheck showing power ridges for torque on maxillary central incisors on teeth 11 and 21, as well as on mandibular central incisors 31 and 41 (blue lines in the ClinCheck software list on the right side).

Treatment

The older damaged composite resin fillings were planned to be renewed after orthodontic treatment. The patient was referred to the oral surgeon for extraction of all wisdom teeth.

To obtain maximum torque on the maxillary central incisors, power ridges were added on teeth 11 and 21 over the whole treatment time. To achieve optimal force application, hooks for class II elastics were placed on maxillary canines and mandibular first molars (Fig 4-197).

The first treatment phase consisted of 48 aligners. To reduce the overall treatment time, the patient was advised to change the aligners every 10 instead of 14 days. Changing of the aligner wearing time should not be prescribed without sufficient expertise with the Invisalign system.

Power ridges for torque on maxillary central incisors were planned for teeth 11 and 21, as well as for mandibular central incisors 31 and 41 (Figs 4-198 and 4-199). Attachments on maxillary lateral incisors and canines were bonded for additional anchorage to apply the torque.

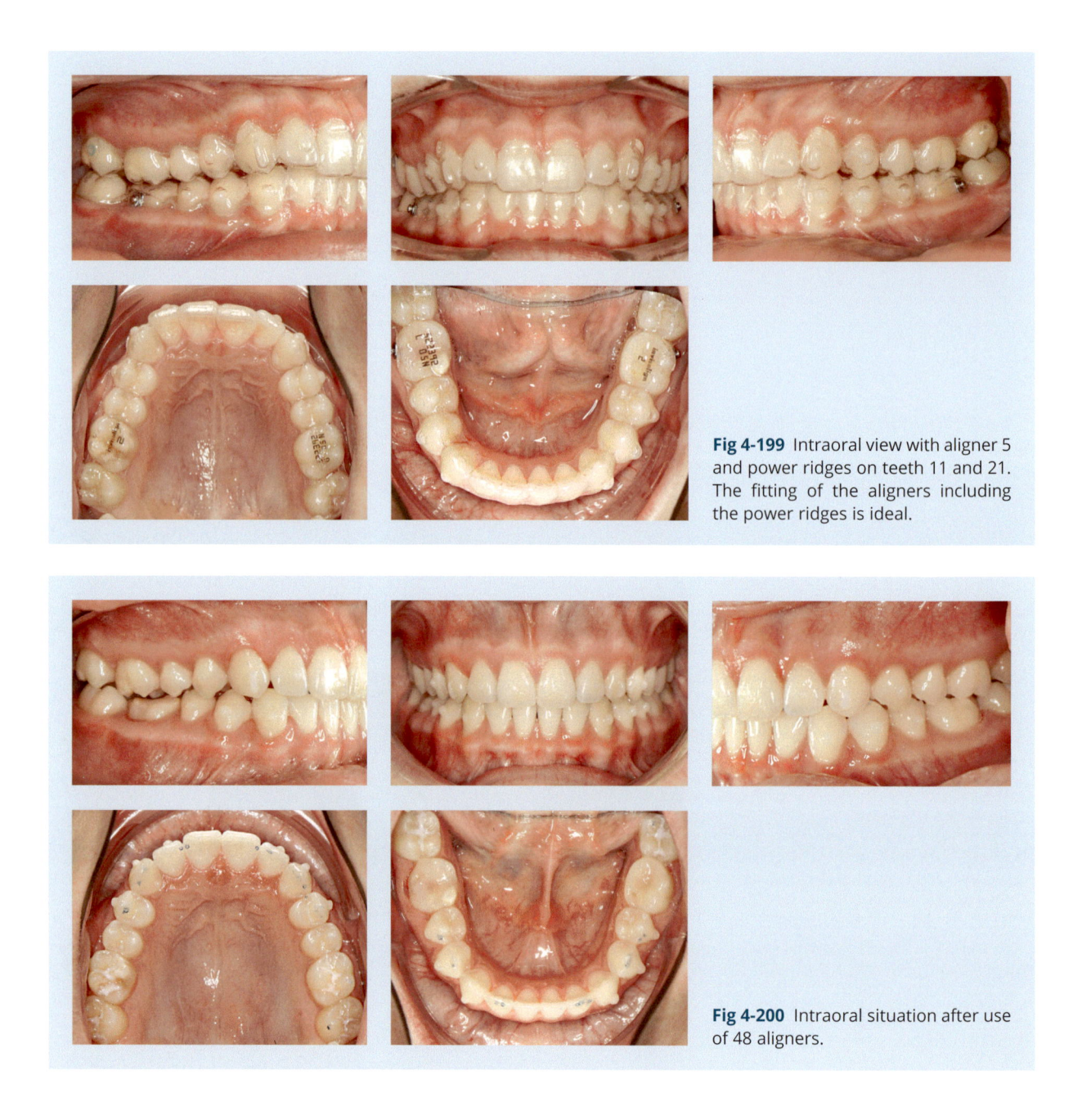

Fig 4-199 Intraoral view with aligner 5 and power ridges on teeth 11 and 21. The fitting of the aligners including the power ridges is ideal.

Fig 4-200 Intraoral situation after use of 48 aligners.

After use of 48 aligners (Fig 4-200), scans were taken for an additional refinement to obtain posterior occlusion and to solve anterior contacts (Fig 4-201). Teeth 36 and particularly 46 were not planned for extrusion as new restoratives would be placed.

Figure 4-202 shows the intraoral situation with last aligner of the first phase in place. The aligners show perfect fitting. The planned refinement included nine aligners with three overcorrection aligners. Power ridges were placed on teeth 11 and 21 (Fig 4-203). The last aligners of the first phase after 17 months of treatment time showed good fit; the gingiva was without irritation or inflammation, and the attachments fully captured by the aligners.

TREATMENT OF DIFFERENT MALOCCLUSIONS WITH ALIGNERS 4

Fig 4-201 Intraoral views and ClinCheck software results. **(a)** Initial intraoral view. **(b)** Initial ClinCheck image. **(c)** Final planned situation in the ClinCheck software. **(d)** Final intraoral view after 17 months of treatment time and before refinement.

Fig 4-202 Intraoral view with last aligner of the first phase in situ showing perfect fitting.

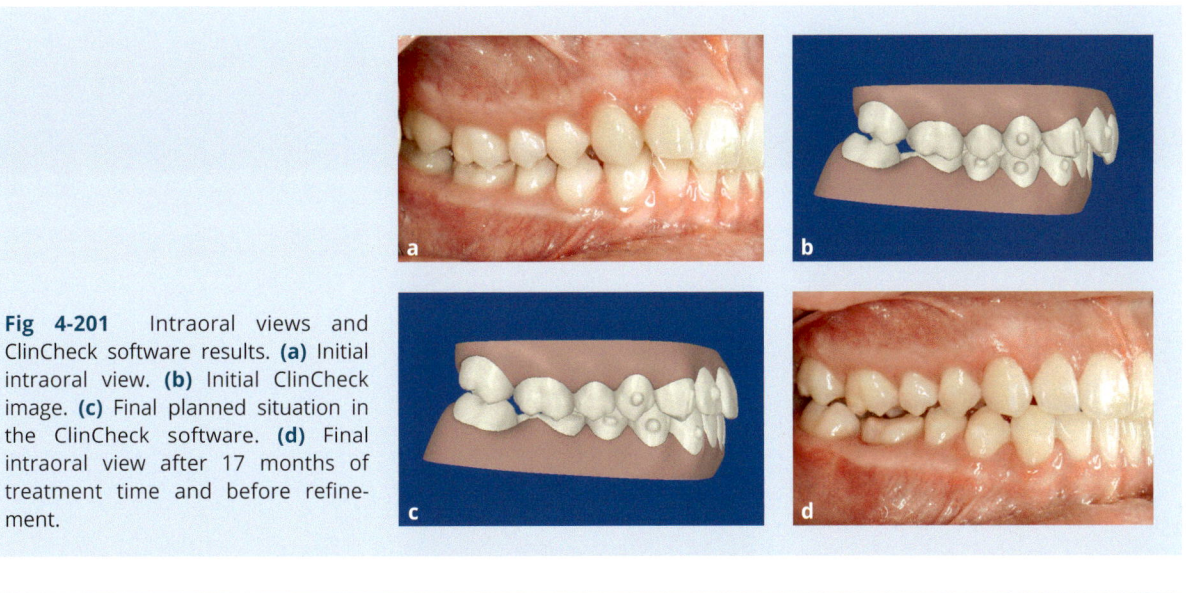

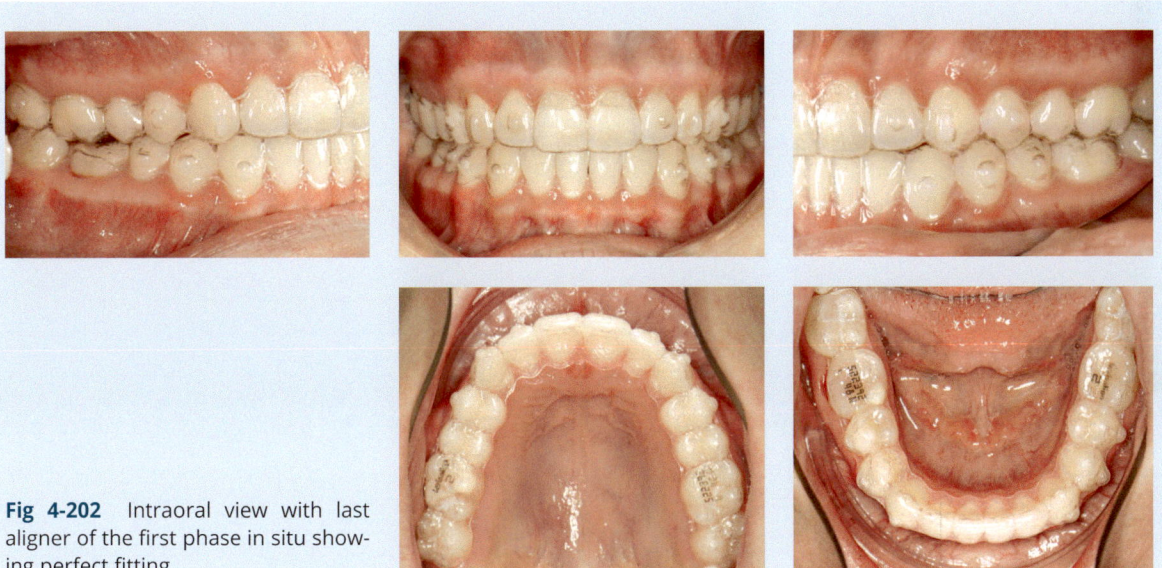

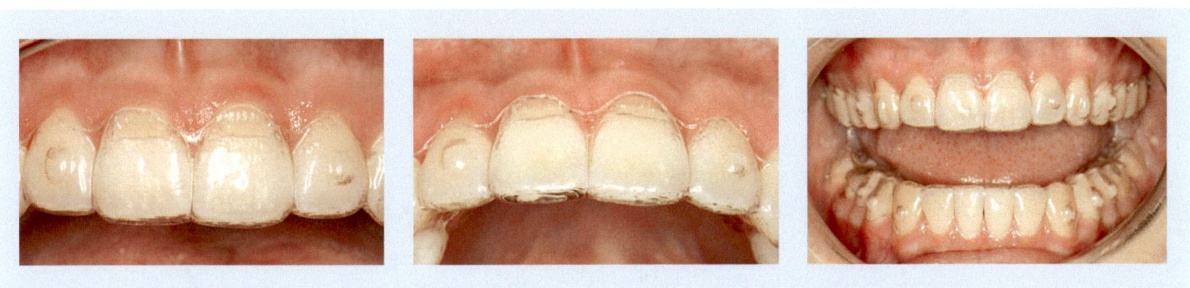

Fig 4-203 Detailed view of the power ridges on teeth 11 and 21 with last aligner of the first phase.

153

4 TREATMENT OF DIFFERENT MALOCCLUSIONS WITH ALIGNERS

Fig 4-204 Final intraoral views.

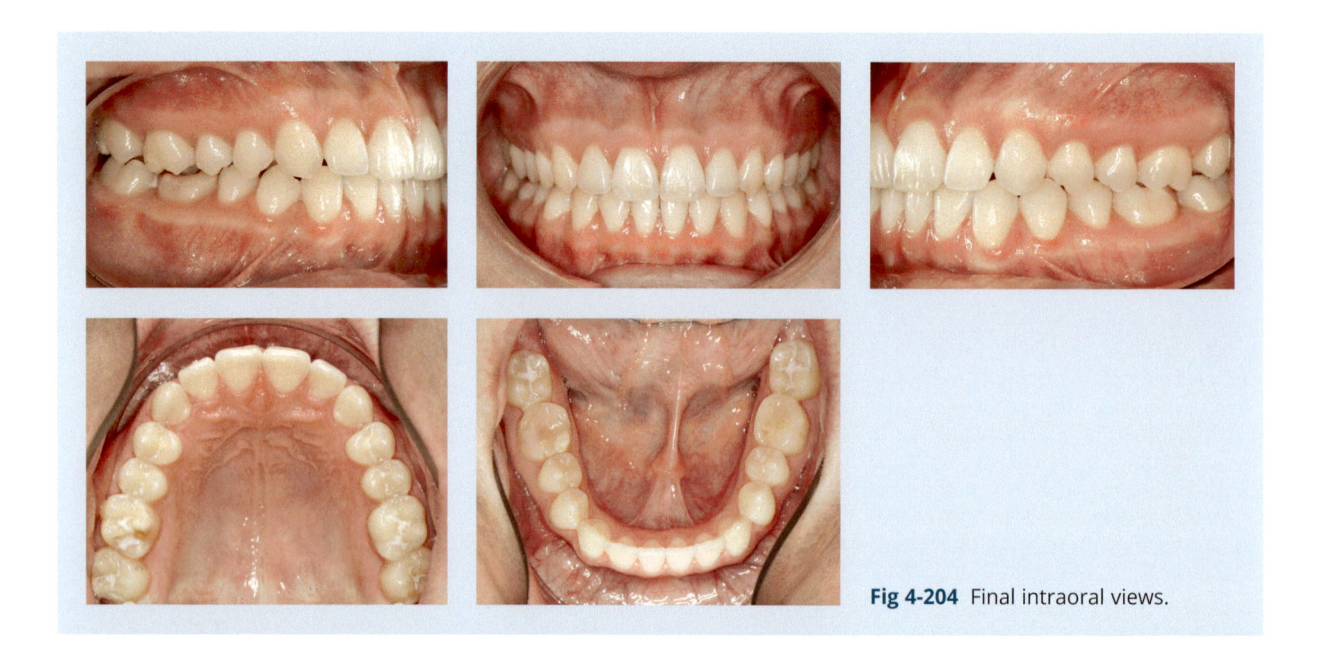

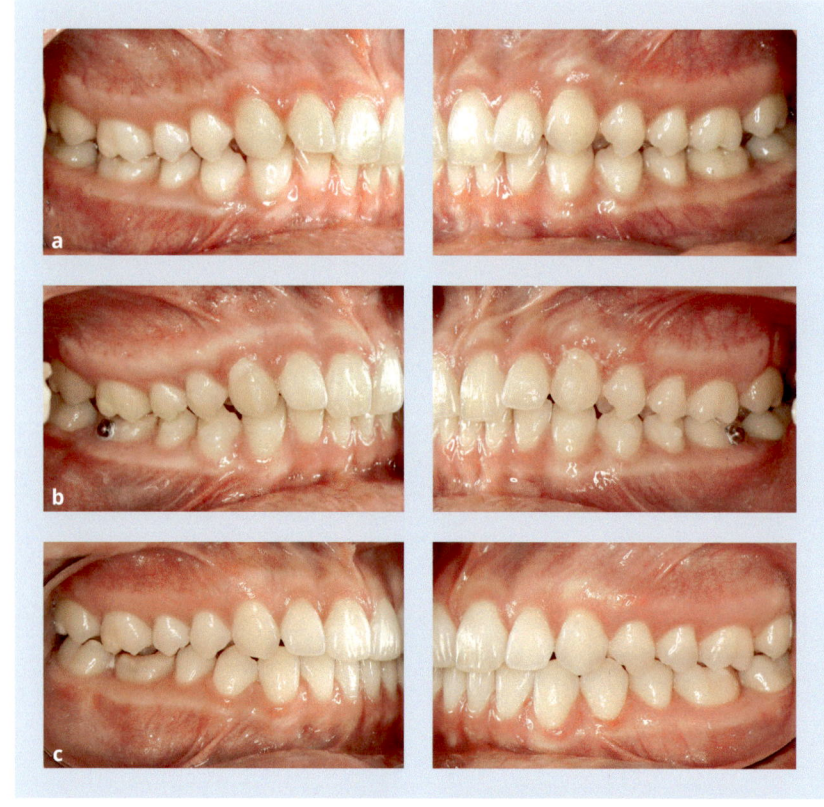

Fig 4-205 The initial **(a)**, start of Invisalign treatment with attachments, hooks, and buttons for class II elastics **(b)**, and final views **(c)**.

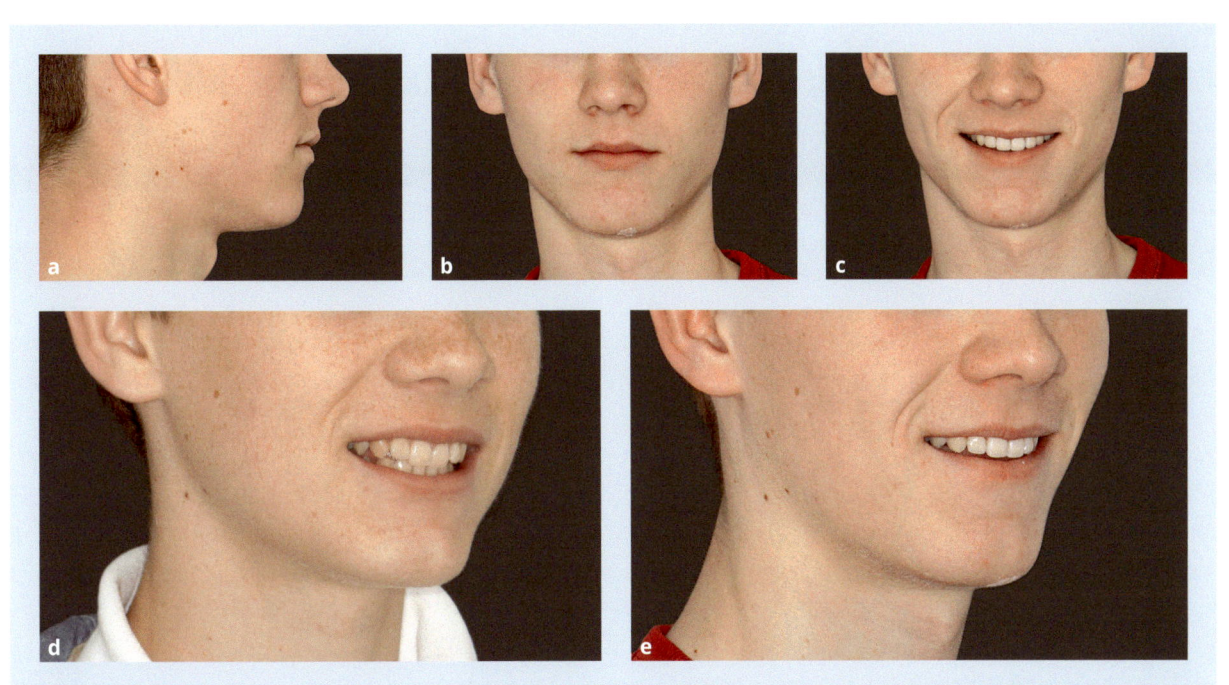

Fig 4-206 Final external views. **(a–c)** Facial lateral and frontal views. **(d,e)** Lateral smile before **(d)** and after **(e)** treatment.

After Invisalign treatment, there is a class I relationship, functional anterior relationship, and canine guidance. Teeth 36 and 46 were planned for new restoratives from the start (Fig 4-204).

Figure 4-205 shows the treatment course to class I and a functional anterior relationship. At this point the patient was transferred for new restoratives on teeth 36 and 46. Extraoral findings at the end of treatment are shown in Figure 4-206. The retruded maxillary anterior teeth have been torqued and the lower lip line follows harmonically the line of maxillary incisors.

4 TREATMENT OF DIFFERENT MALOCCLUSIONS WITH ALIGNERS

Topic 29
Class II pretreatment with Carrière distalizer in a teenager with all permanent teeth erupted

Treatment:
- treatment with Carrière distalizer
- Invisalign system

To limit extractions and to turn a difficult class II occlusion into a simpler class I occlusion, we often start orthodontic treatment with a Carrière distalizer (Carriere motion appliance, Ortho Organizer, ODS) followed with Invisalign as soon as the class I relationship is obtained.

The Carrière distalizer is a direct bonded appliance with anchorage on the maxillary canines and first molars. Metal buttons are used to support class II elastics and a splint in the mandibular arch provides retention and anchorage for the forces generated (Fig 4-207). The appliance distalizes the maxillary posterior segment as a block with simultaneous derotation and uprighting of the maxillary first molars into perfect occlusion. Using this appliance at the beginning of treatment when there are no competing forces in the mouth allows distalization of the molars and premolars of 3–6 mm, on average.

This 14-year-old patient had a full class II occlusion on the right side and a less pronounced class II on the left (Fig 4-208).

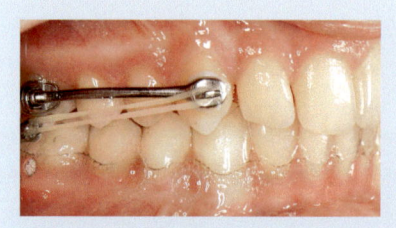

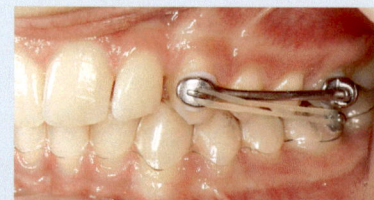

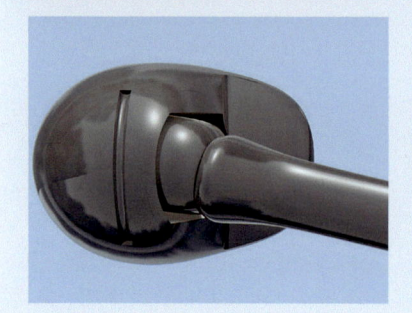

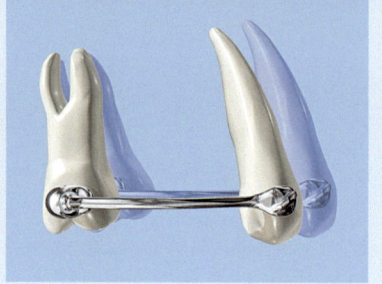

Fig 4-207 Intraoral situation with inserted Carrière distalizer on upper canines and first molars, bonded buttons on teeth 36 and 46 with an additional removable aligner in the lower arch for anchorage.

Diagnosis:
- class II relationship
- reclined maxillary incisors
- extruded mandibular canines and incisors
- excessive mandibular curve of Spee
- deep bite.

Therapy:
- distalization using Carrière distalizer
- Invisalign treatment.

TREATMENT OF DIFFERENT MALOCCLUSIONS WITH ALIGNERS 4

Fig 4-208 Initial presentation.

Fig 4-209 Intraoral situation in class I relationship at the end of distalization with the Carrière distalizer and the start of the Invisalign treatment.

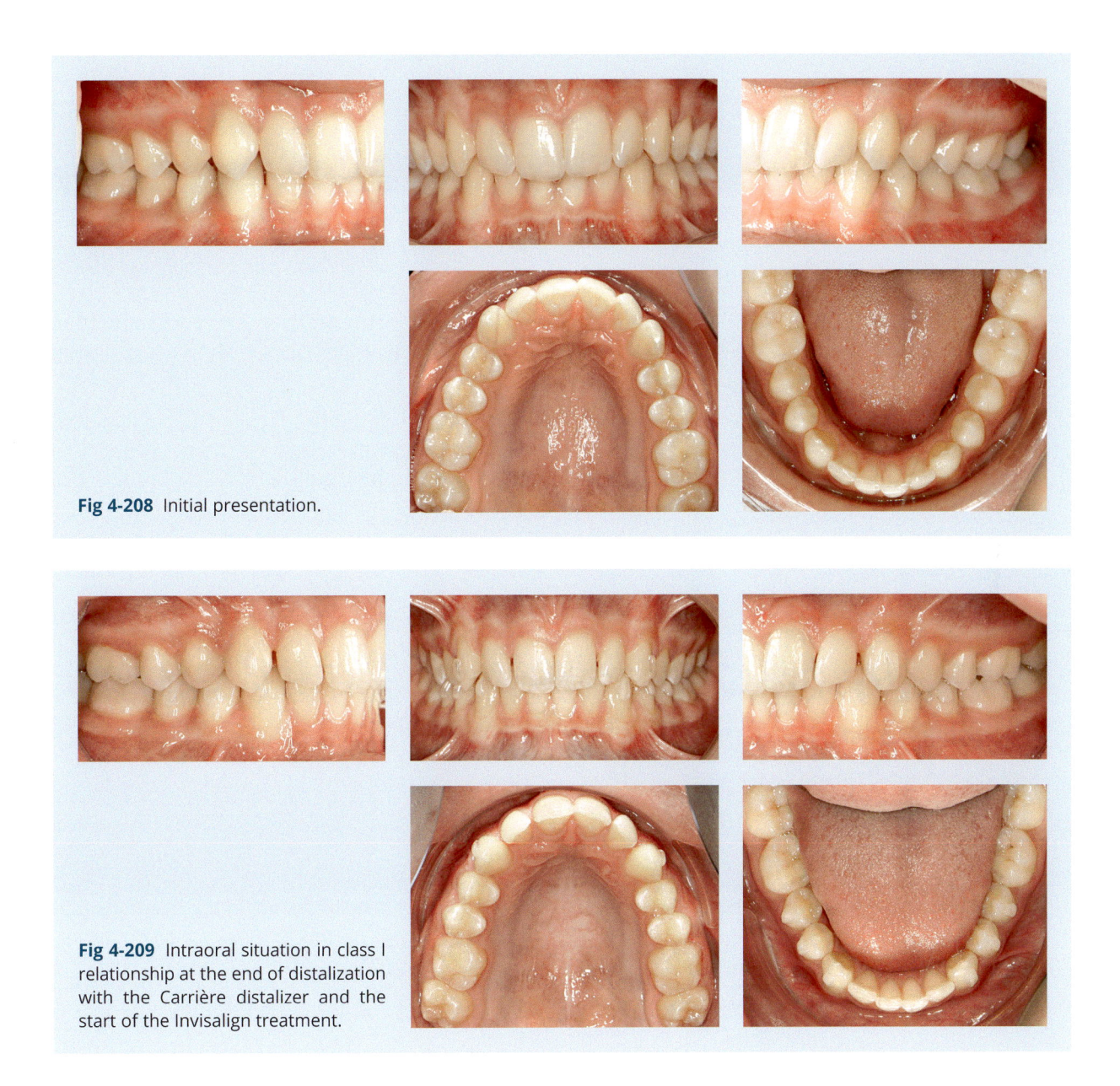

Treatment

Treatment was started with the Carrière distalizer, as described above. A retention aligner (Lamitec, Hinz Dental) was used to avoid undesired tipping of the mandibular incisors. The patient was asked to wear the elastic full-time and the retention aligner for anchorage at night. Once a class I relationship was achieved, after 14 weeks (Fig 4-209), Invisalign therapy was commenced with retention of the elastics at night until the first aligners were set in. It is recommended that elastics are worn at night also during Invisalign treatment to avoid any relapse. Buttons and hooks on the maxillary canines and mandibular molars, or precision cuts in the aligners, are incorporated to allow continued use of the elastics.

Fig 4-210 Final occlusion in class I relationship.

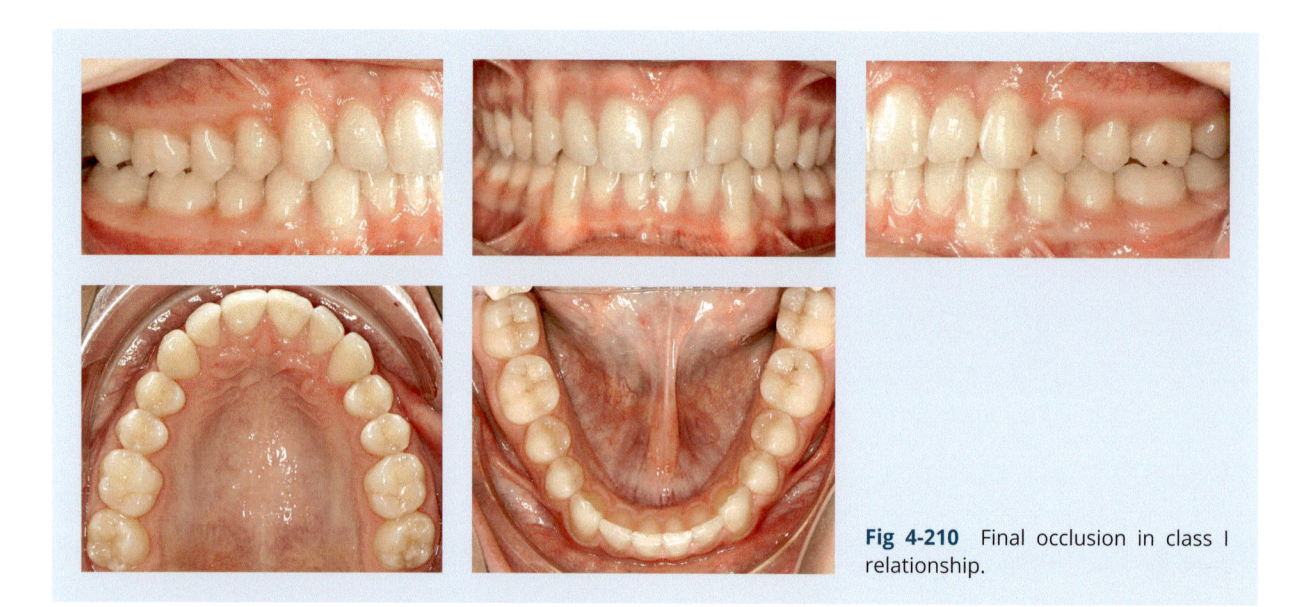

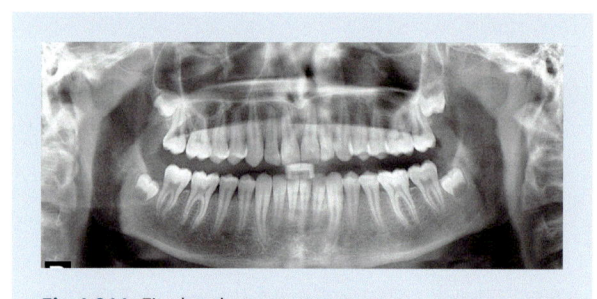

Fig 4-211 Final orthopantomogram.

The final occlusion in class I relationship, with full occlusal contacts on premolars and molars and canine guidance, is shown in Figure 4-210. The overbite and overjet are in a physiologic relation. Orthopantomography shows the distalized teeth in the maxillary arch (Fig 4-211). Teeth 18, 28, 38, and 48 were recommended for extraction.

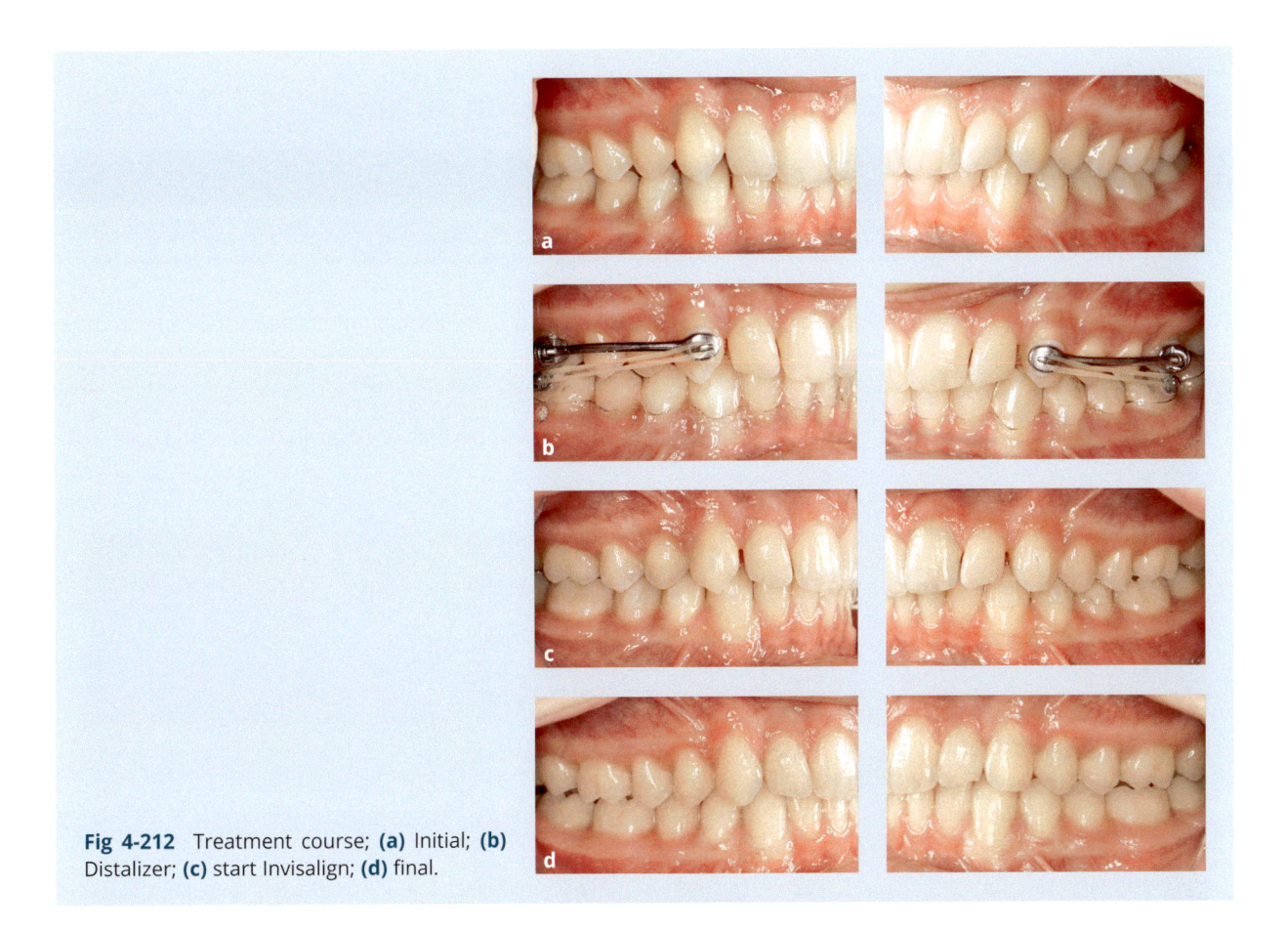

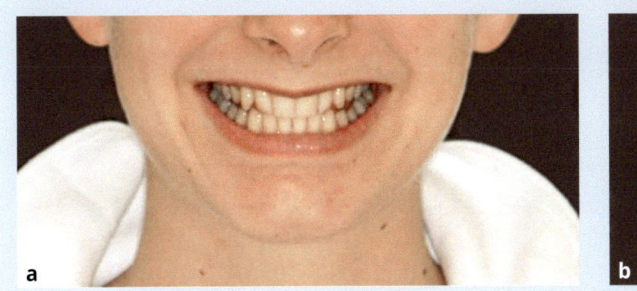

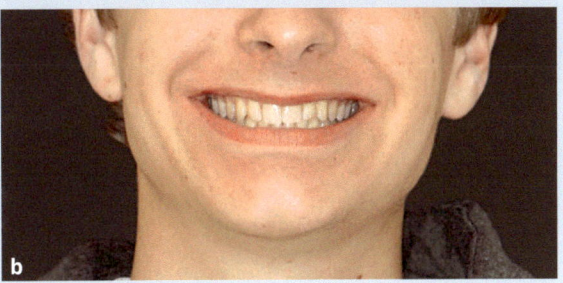

Fig 4-212 Treatment course; **(a)** Initial; **(b)** Distalizer; **(c)** start Invisalign; **(d)** final.

Fig 4-213 The initial **(a)** and final **(b)** views show the significant esthetic improvement.

Figure 4-212 shows the course of treatment. The unstable class II relationship and the dental deep bite with traumatizing incisor contacts was successfully treated with the combination of the Carrière distalizer and the Invisalign system. The narrow maxillary arch has been transversally widened and the initial buccal corridor is now filled with teeth, which leads to a significant esthetic improvement (Fig 2-213).

Topic 30
Class II pretreatment with Carrière distalizer in an adult

Treatment:
- Carrière distalizer
- Invisalign system

Pretreatment with the Carrière distalizer followed by Invisalign can also be used in adults provided there is good patient compliance. However, pretreatment takes more time in adults (5–7 months) than in teenagers (3–4 months).

This adult had a class II relationship with crowding in both arches and reclined maxillary incisors (Fig 4-214).

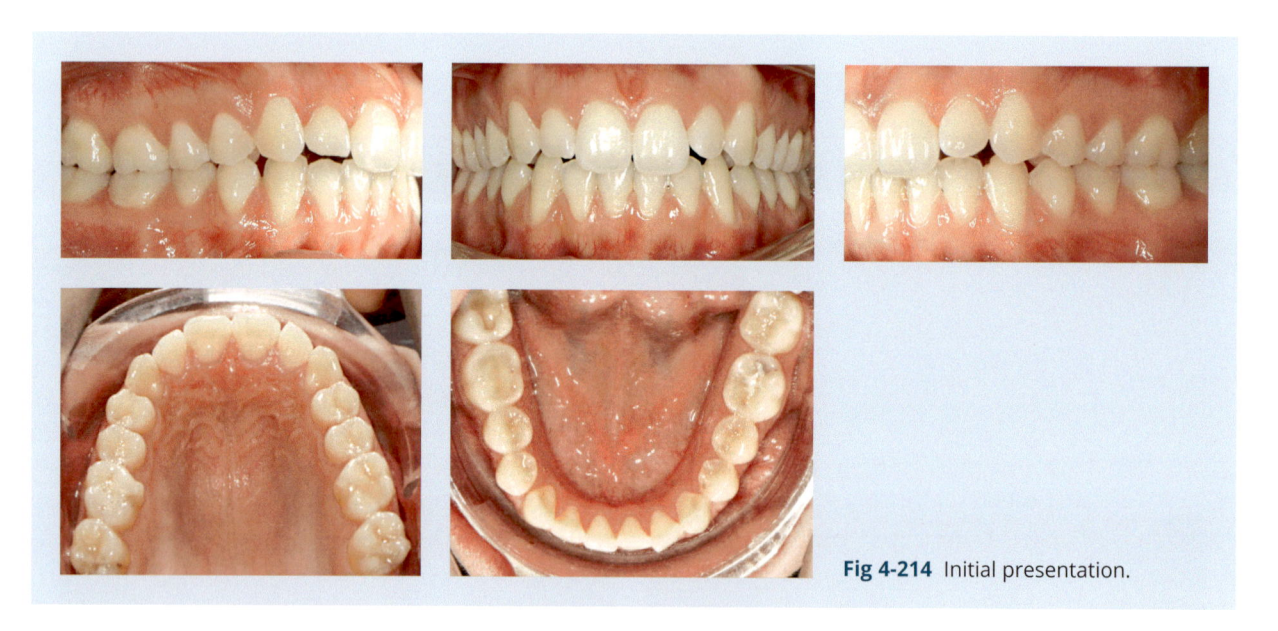

Fig 4-214 Initial presentation.

Diagnosis:
- class II relationship
- reclined maxillary incisors
- crowding in both arches
- open bite tendency.

Therapy:
- distalization using the Carrière distalizer
- Invisalign treatment.

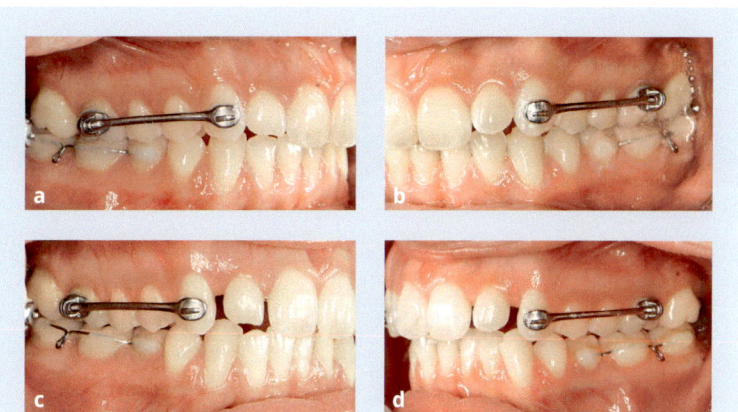

TREATMENT OF DIFFERENT MALOCCLUSIONS WITH ALIGNERS 4

Fig 4-215 Carrière distalizer. **(a,b)** Distalizer in place with a partial wire and hook on both sides on the second premolars and molars in the mandibular arch. **(c,d)** After 6 months, spaces have opened mesial and distal of the maxillary incisors and a class I relationship has been established on both sides.

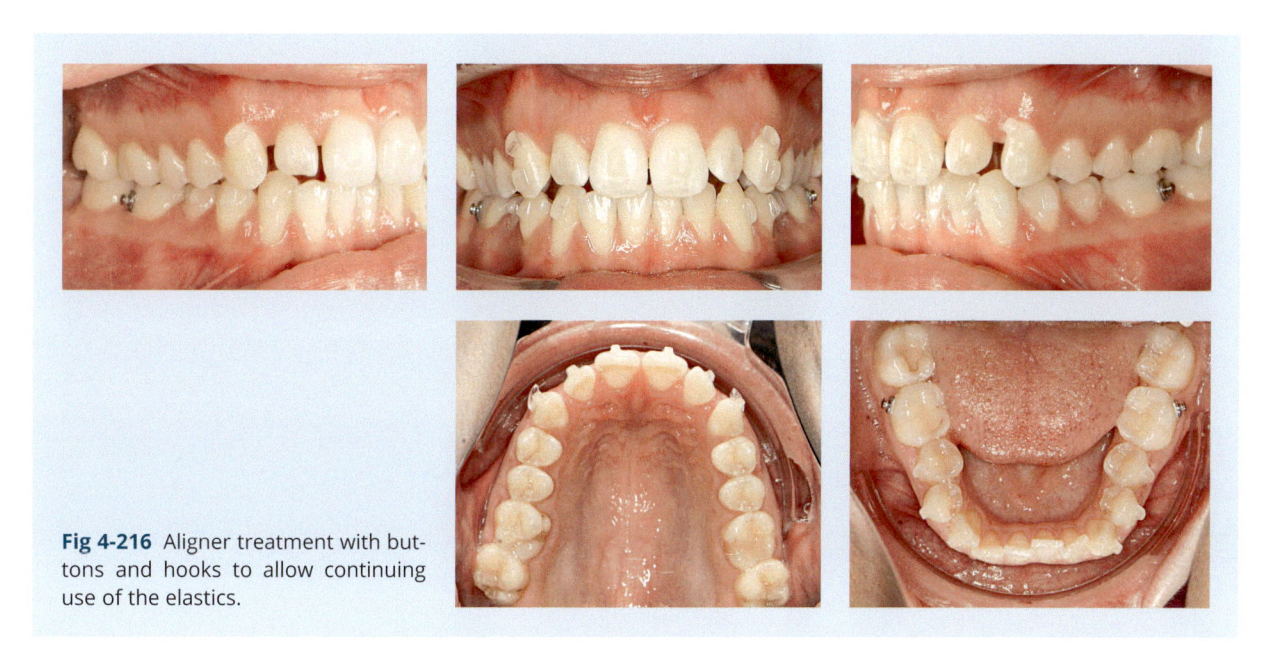

Fig 4-216 Aligner treatment with buttons and hooks to allow continuing use of the elastics.

Treatment

The Carrière distalizer was inserted as described in Topic 29. In addition, a partial wire with an inserted hook was fixed on both sides of the second premolars and molars in the mandibular arch (Fig 4-215). Additionally, the patient wore a removable aligner (Lamitec, Hinz Dental) in the mandible to avoid undesired tipping of the mandibular anterior teeth under the elastic force. After 6 months of permanent elastic wear, spaces had opened mesial and distal of the maxillary incisors and a class I relationship had been established on both sides (Fig 4-215c,d).

After 6 months of distalization, both distalizers and archwires were removed and Invisalign treatment was started. For retention, the patient wore removable retention aligners (vacuum-formed splints) in both arches until the first Invisalign aligners were set in. Buttons and hooks on the maxillary canines and mandibular molars, or precision cuts in the aligners, allowed elastics use during aligner treatment (Fig 4-216).

After 9 months of aligner treatment (Fig 4-217), impressions/scans were taken to decide on refinement and solve the remaining crowding in the mandibular anterior.

4 TREATMENT OF DIFFERENT MALOCCLUSIONS WITH ALIGNERS

Fig 4-217 Intraoral view after 9 months of aligner treatment.

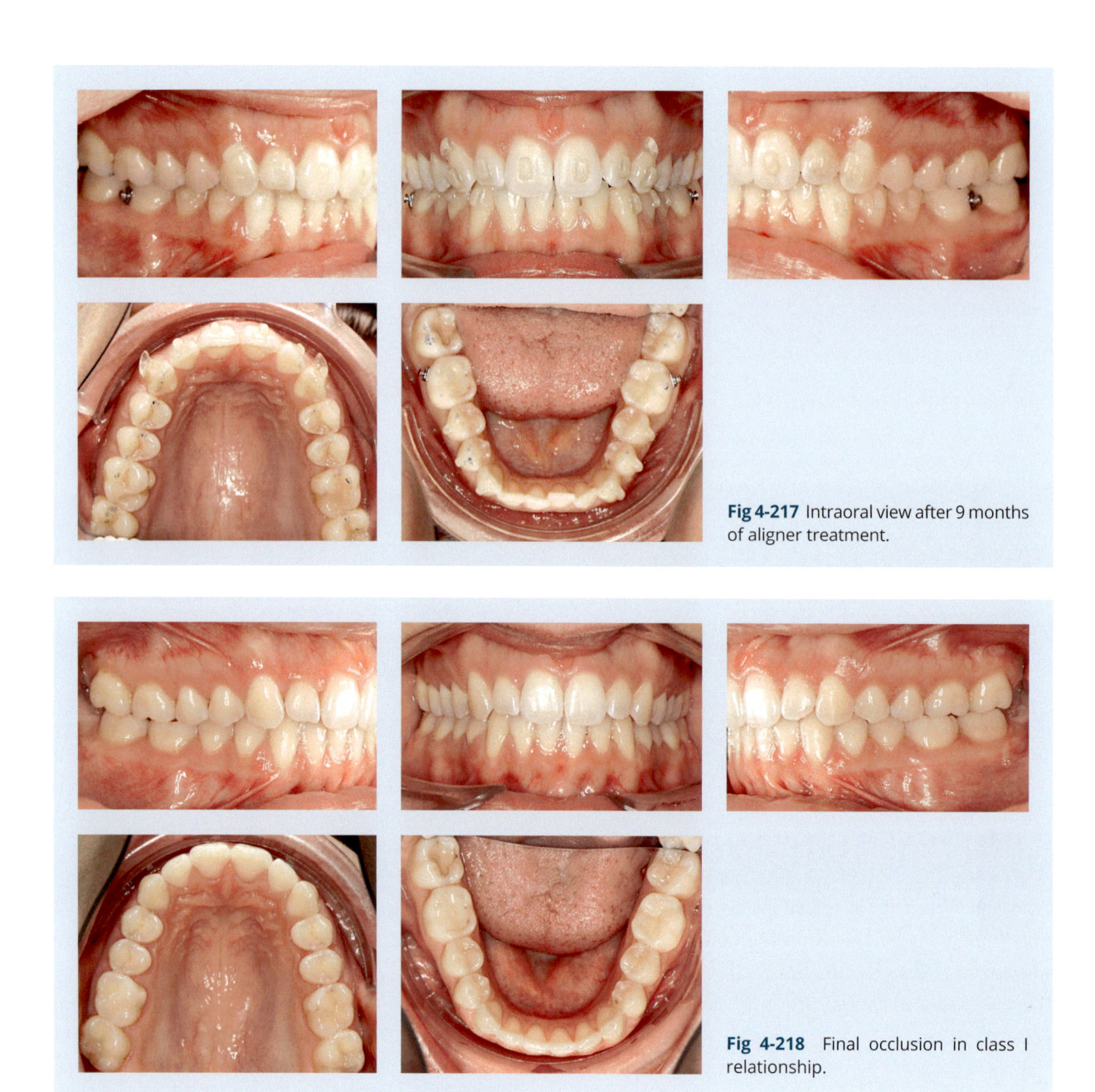

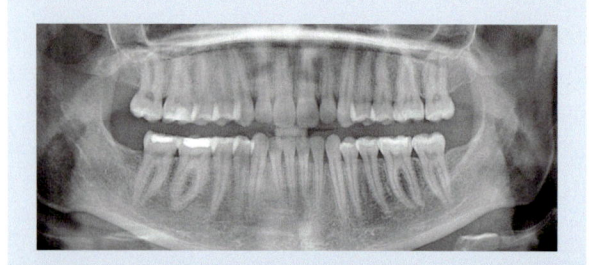

Fig 4-218 Final occlusion in class I relationship.

Fig 4-219 Final orthopantomogram.

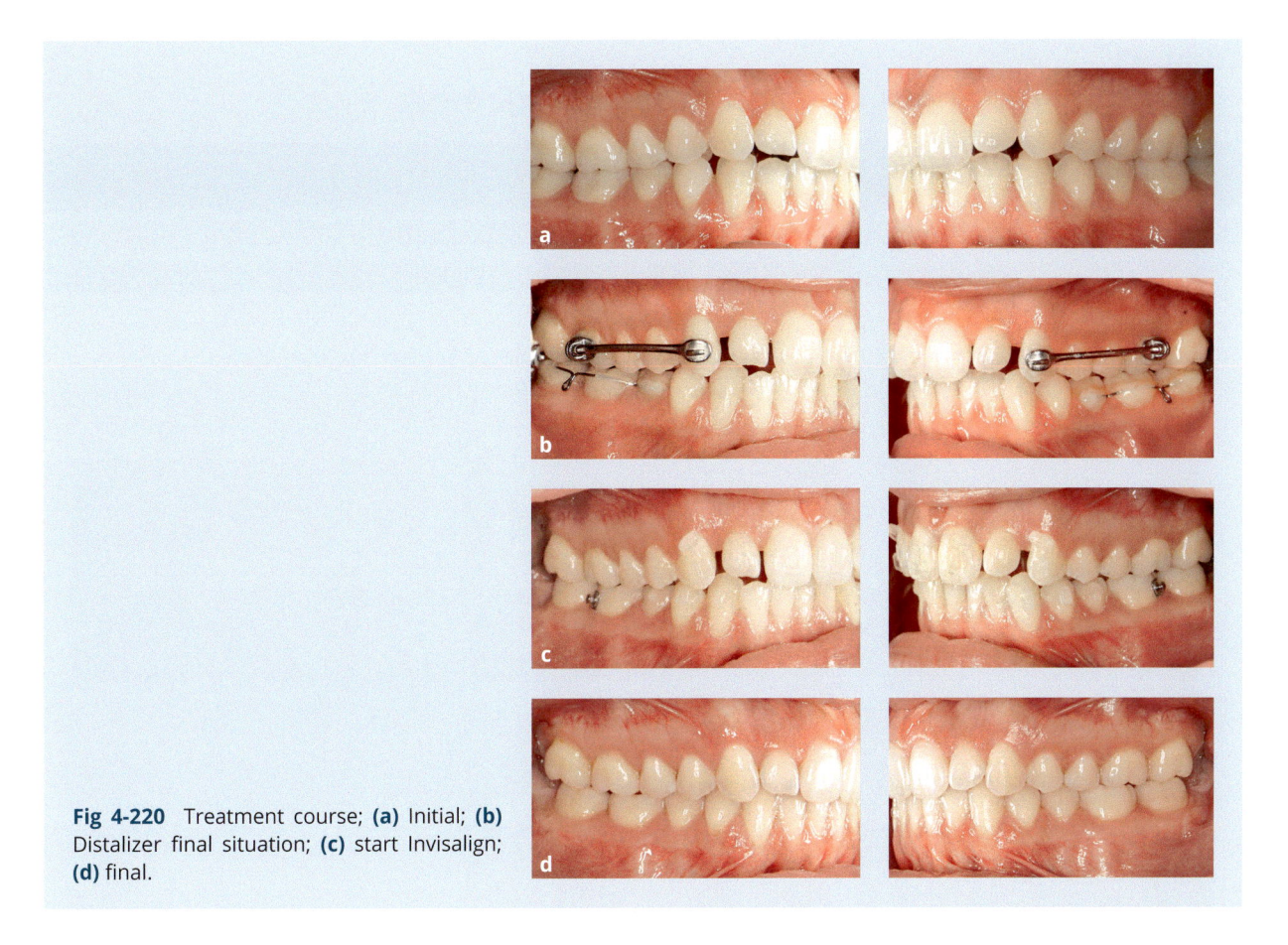

Fig 4-220 Treatment course; **(a)** Initial; **(b)** Distalizer final situation; **(c)** start Invisalign; **(d)** final.

At the end of treatment, which took 2 years in total (6 months for distalizer treatment and 1.5 years for Invisalign treatment), occlusion in a class I relationship, full occlusal contacts on premolars and molars, and canine guidance had been achieved (Fig 4-218). The overbite and overjet are in physiologic relation. Orthopantomography shows the distalized teeth with parallel root position in the maxillary arch (Fig 4-219).

Figure 4-220 shows the course of treatment. The unstable initial class II relationship was successfully treated.

Topic 31
Craniomandibular disorder and class II relationship

Treatment:
- distalization
- Invisalign treatment
- prosthodontics

This patient presented with headaches, back pain, and a craniomandibular disorder (Fig 4-221).

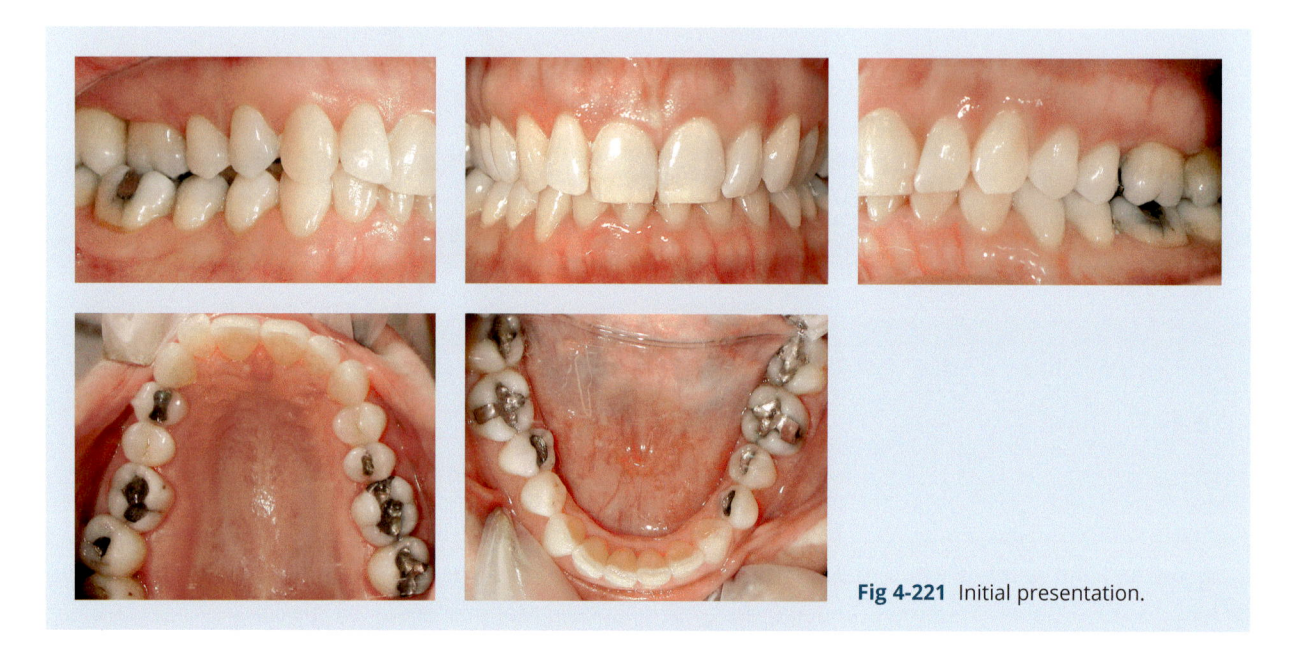

Fig 4-221 Initial presentation.

Diagnosis:
- class II
- crowding and rotations in the maxillary and mandibular arches
- loss of posterior height with anterior contact
- reclined position of teeth 11 and 21
- crossbite 16 to 46
- CMD and pain (headache, back pain).

Therapy:
- removable splint therapy
- Invisalign treatment
- adjacent restoratives.

Treatment
Treatment started with a removable splint in the mandibular arch, and interdisciplinary manual and physical therapy for 6 months. After a pain-free situation had been achieved, orthodontic treatment started to solve the class II relationship, the crossbite, and the anterior contact caused by the dental deep bite. This was required before restorative therapy could be undertaken.

Planning was based on mounted plaster casts in the SAM articulator, which showed an unstable occlusion with an incisor contact which restricted the mandible in a distal position. There was no lack of posterior support (Fig 4-222).

Fig 4-222 Plaster casts in the articulator.

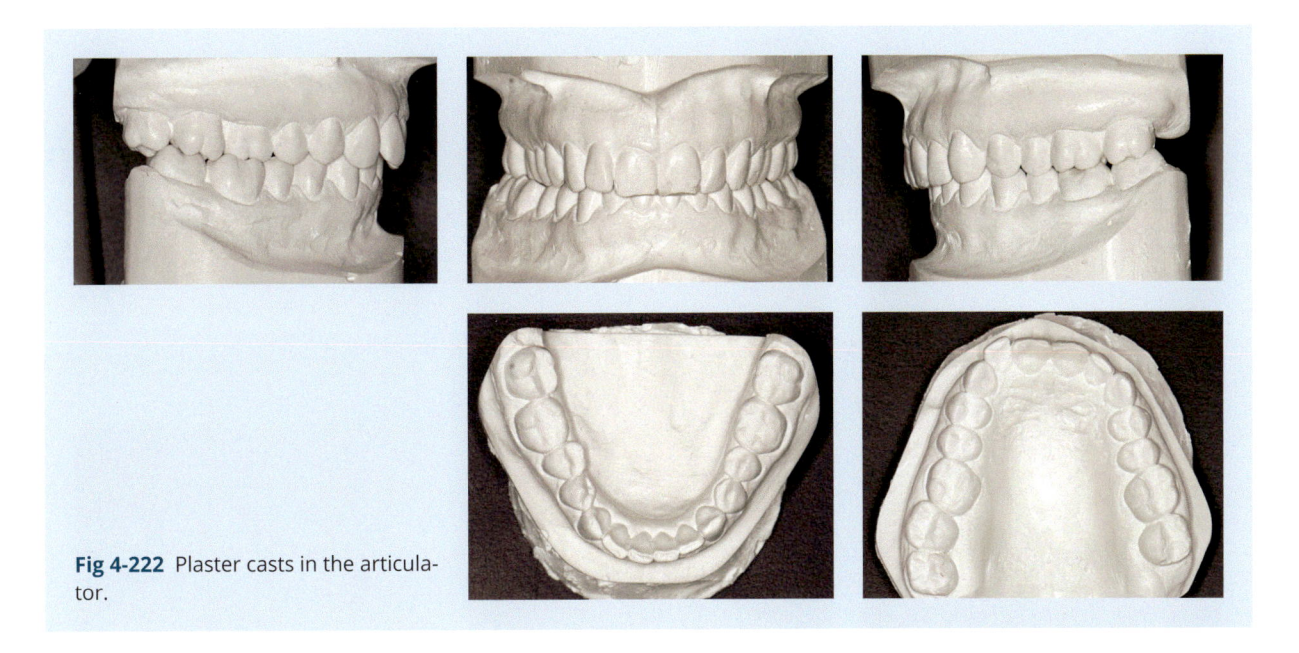

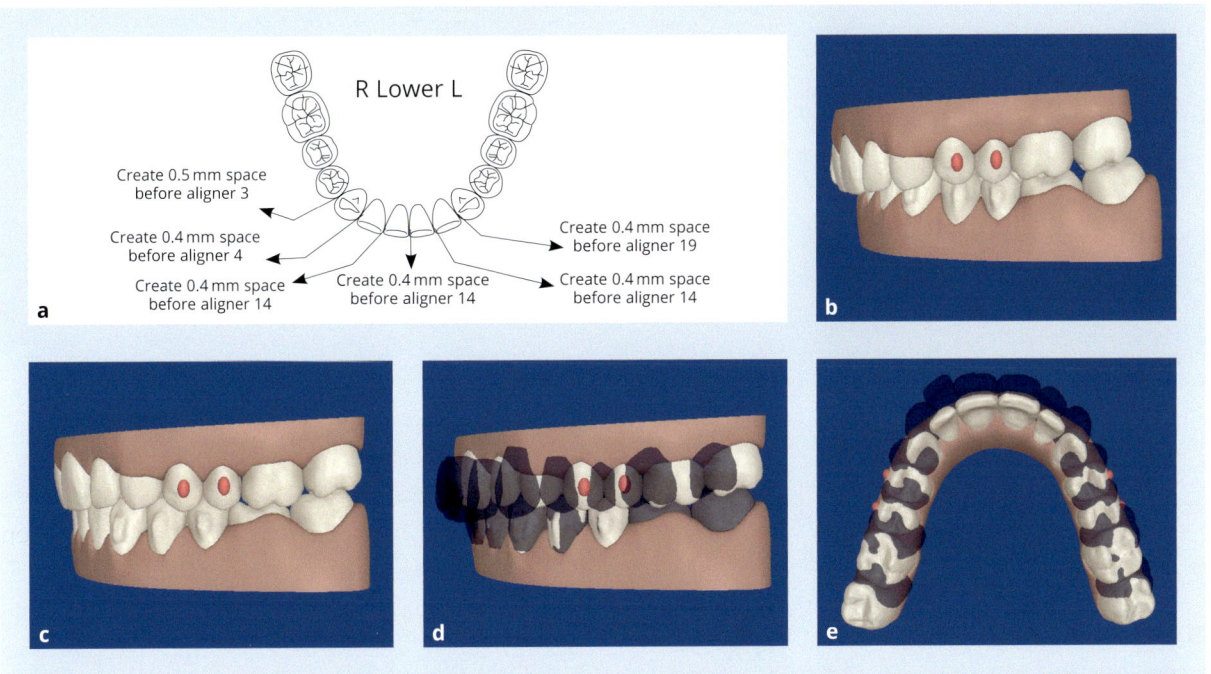

Fig 4-223 ClinCheck software results. **(a)** IPR chart. **(b)** Initial left side with attachments in both arches and lifted gingival levels for buttons. **(c)** Planned final result. **(d,e)** Superimposition of initial and final views to show the planned movements (blue, initial tooth position; white, final tooth position).

ClinCheck software was used to plan tooth movements (Fig 4-223). The gingival levels were raised on maxillary canines and mandibular first molars to allow placement of buttons and hooks. The plan used 62 aligners to achieve the required distalization.

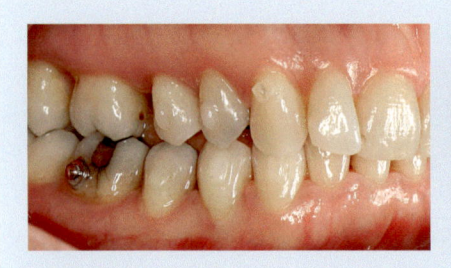

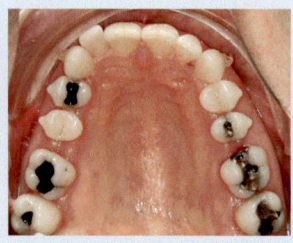

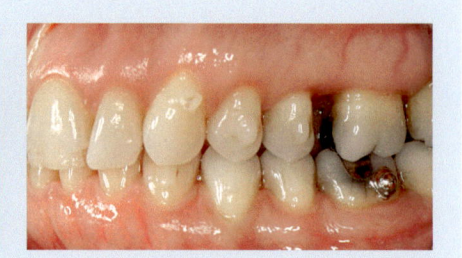

4 TREATMENT OF DIFFERENT MALOCCLUSIONS WITH ALIGNERS

Fig 4-224 Intraoral pictures at the start of distalization of the premolars.

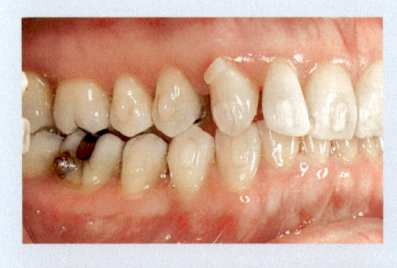

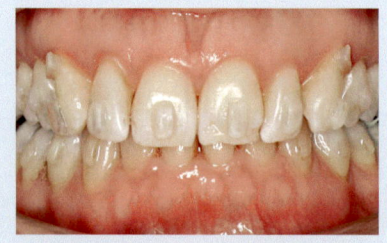

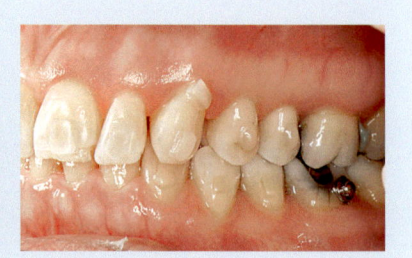

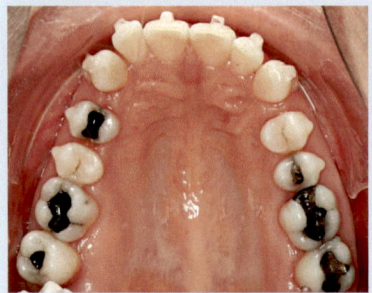

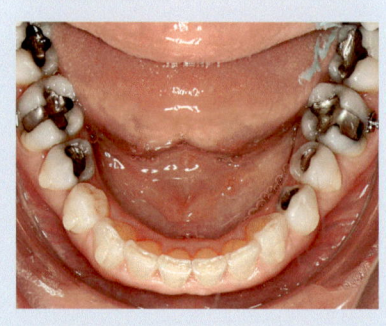

Fig 4-225 Intraoral pictures after distalization of the second premolars. Additional rectangular attachments have been added to maxillary incisors and canines for major anchorage.

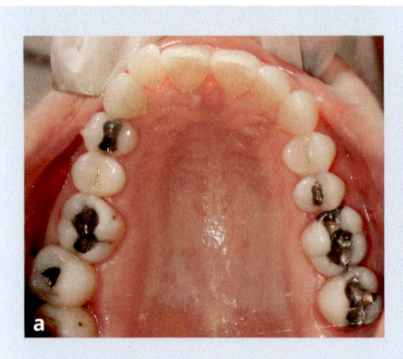

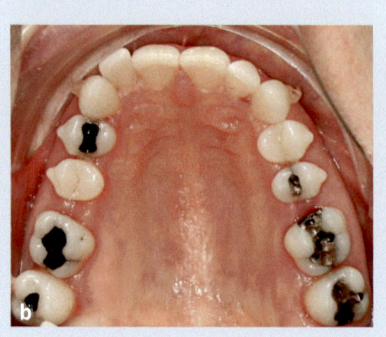

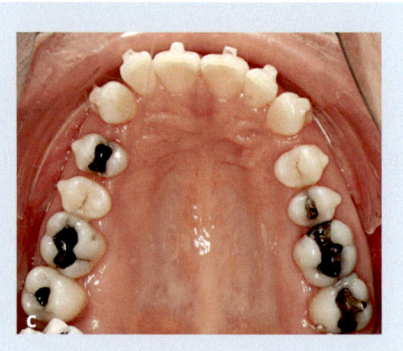

Fig 4-226 Course of distalization in the maxillary arch. **(a)** Initial situation. **(b)** Molars distalized and start of distalization of premolars. **(c)** Distalized premolars and start of distalization of canines and incisors.

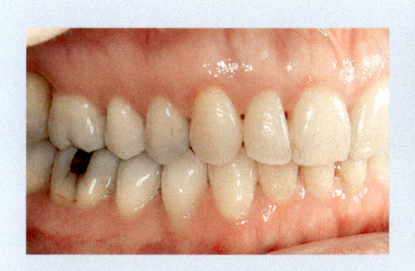

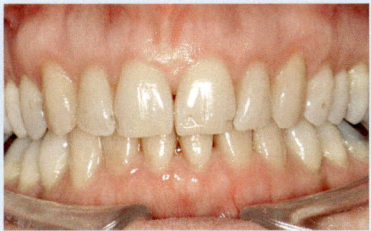

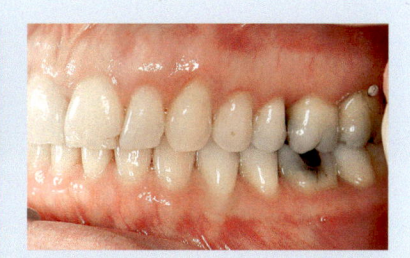

Fig 4-227 Final views after orthodontics.

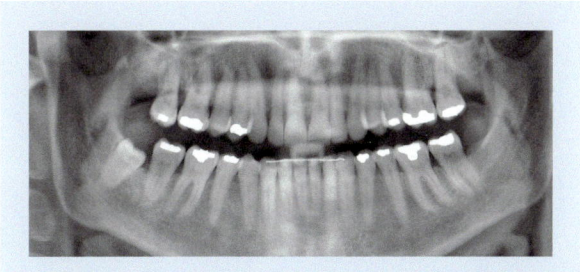

Fig 4-228 Orthopantomography shows root parallelism and bodily distalization of the maxillary dentition.

The distalization was planned to start with the second molars followed by first molars; distalization of the premolars started after the distalization of the second molars had finished (see Topic 26). Figure 4-224 shows the situation just before distalization of the premolars begins. Both maxillary canines have bonded hooks for class II elastics, which helps to avoid undesired rotation of canines.

After distalization of the second premolars, distalization of the canines occurred (Fig 4-225). With the distalization of the canines, additional rectangular attachments were added to the maxillary incisors as well as on canines to obtain anchorage (see distalization scheme, Fig 4-226).

Treatment resulted in a class I relationship, with solving of the crossbite and reduction of the dental deep bite (Figs 4-227 and 4-228). There was sufficient overjet and a physiologic dynamic occlusion. The availability of power ridges now can help to obtain more torque for incisors, which might have helped here.

Wisdom tooth 48 was advised for extraction. Teeth 33 to 43 have a bonded lingual fixed retainer.

Six months after completion of orthodontic treatment, restorative, esthetic, and prosthodontic treatment commenced with the correction of the maxillary incisors (Dr W Boisserée, Cologne; dental technician M. Läkamp, Ostbevern). For esthetic reasons, the enamel defects were reshaped with Enamel plus HFO (Vanini). The preparation and provisory restoratives used were GDexactoCore (George Dental) (Fig 4-229).

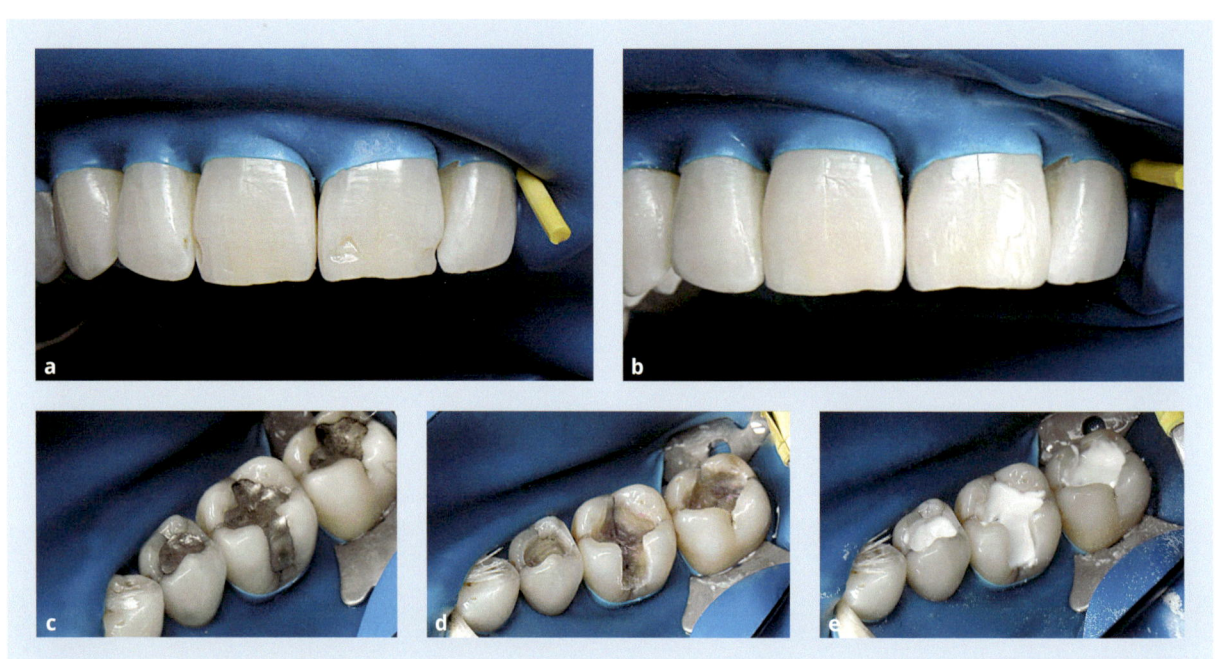

Fig 4-229 Planned restorative work. **(a,b)** Enamel defects to be reshaped with Enamel plus HFO (Vanini) supported by rubber dam technique. **(c)** Initial view with amalgam fillings. **(d)** Excavation of the teeth with the amalgam fillings. **(e)** Fillings using snow-white dentin adhesive **(e)** GDexactoCore (George Dental).

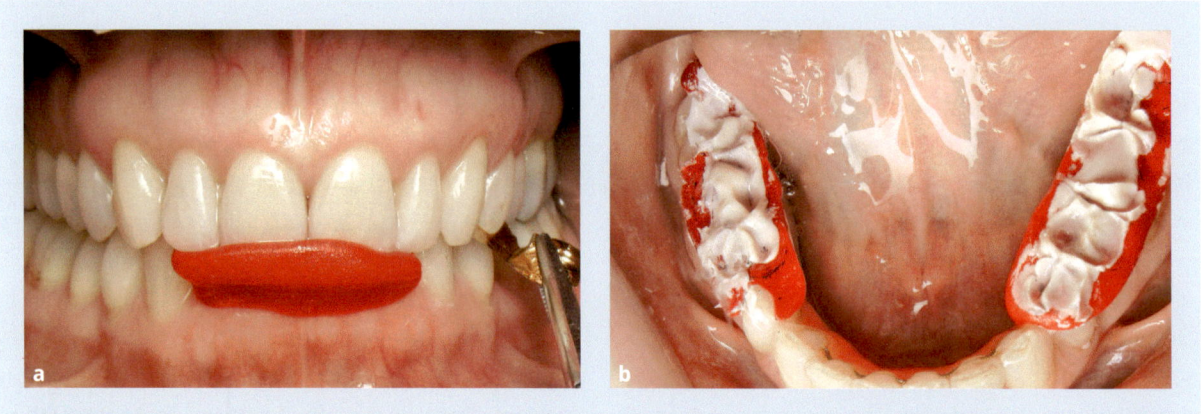

Fig 4-230 Reference bite registration to ensure maintenance of the therapeutic centric relation. **(a)** Reference bite (GC Pattern Resin) for fixation of the correct posterior support using Shimstock foil in the posterior region, where the foil must be held by the posterior occlusion. **(b)** Posterior bite registration carried out with the anterior reference bite in situ.

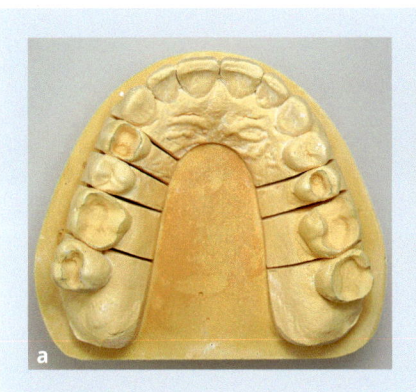

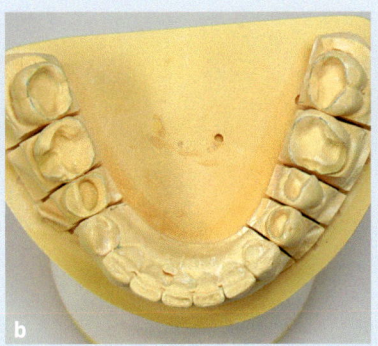

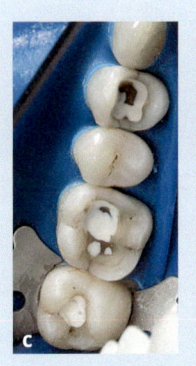

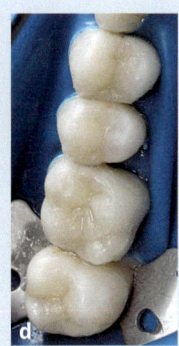

Fig 4-231 Restorative preparation. **(a,b)** Plaster casts for both arches. **(c)** Maxillary molars and premolars prepared for the insertion of the restoratives (IPS e.max; Ivoclar). **(d)** Final result.

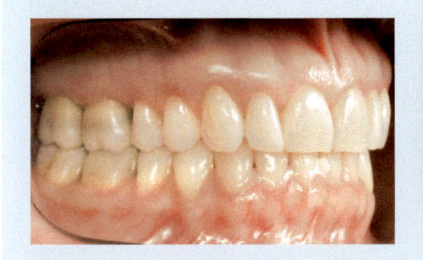

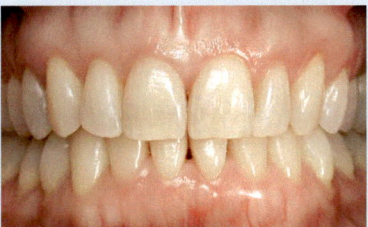

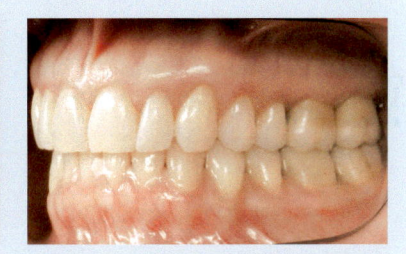

Fig 4-232 The final intraoral views.

Control was assessed with Shimstock foil in the posterior region: the foil must be held by the posterior occlusion. An important point for restorative and prosthodontic treatment is to keep the three-dimensional relationship of the mandibular and maxillary dentition in therapeutic centric relation. A reference bite is used to reproduce this relationship in the same pain-free position the patient had after Invisalign treatment. Similarly, a posterior bite registration is carried out with the anterior reference bite in place (Fig 4-230). The posterior bite registration is completed with Super-T (American Dental Systems) to improve the details.

Plaster casts mounted in SAM articulator were used to prepare the restoratives (Fig 4-231).

Figures 4-232 and 4-233 show the final treatment result. The dental deep bite has been changed into a physiologic overbite. The maxillary arch has been transversally expanded and the crossbite of tooth 16 to 46 has been corrected. (Fig 4-234).

Comparison of the lateral situation before and after the interdisciplinary treatment shows that the dental deep bite and the crossbite have been solved and there is a stable class I relationship.

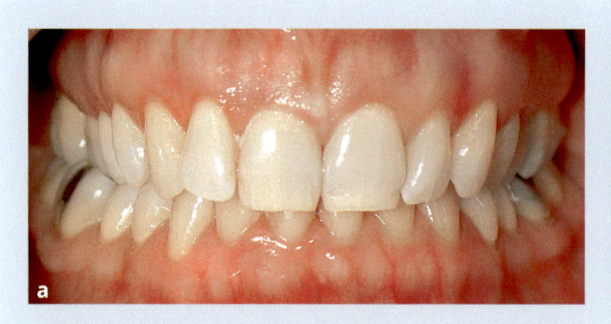

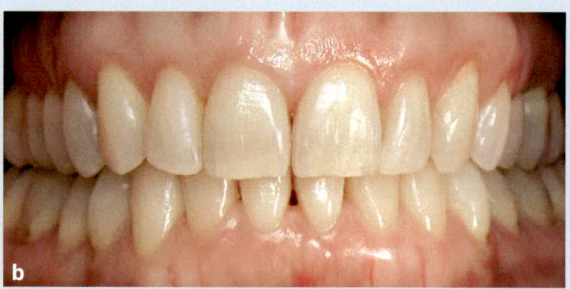

4 TREATMENT OF DIFFERENT MALOCCLUSIONS WITH ALIGNERS

Fig 4-233 The initial (a) and final (b) anterior situations.

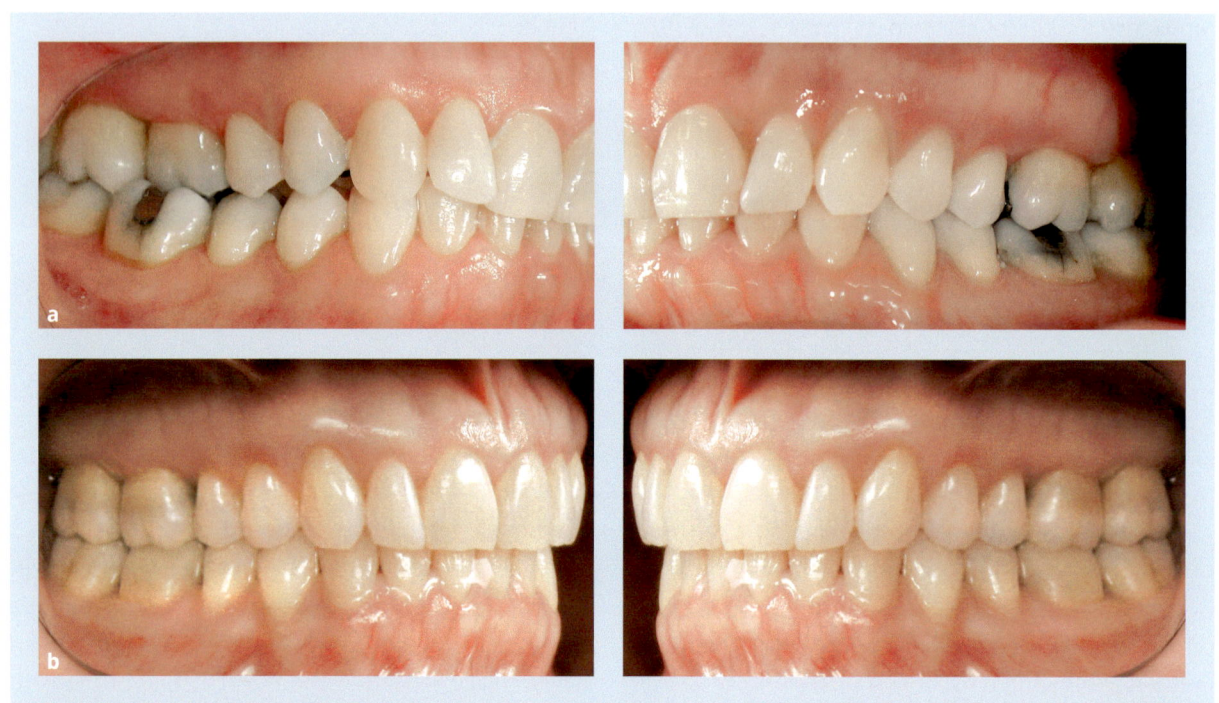

Fig 4-234 The initial (a) and final (b) lateral views.

Topic 32
Class II with open bite

Treatment:
- distalization
- anterior extrusion

The Invisalign system can be used in combination with class II elastics for distalization with anterior extrusion in patients with open bites and class II relationship.

This patient has a class II relationship, crowding, and an anterior open bite (Fig 4-235). Due to a former fixed appliance treatment alio loco the patient showed decalcifications on multiple teeth.

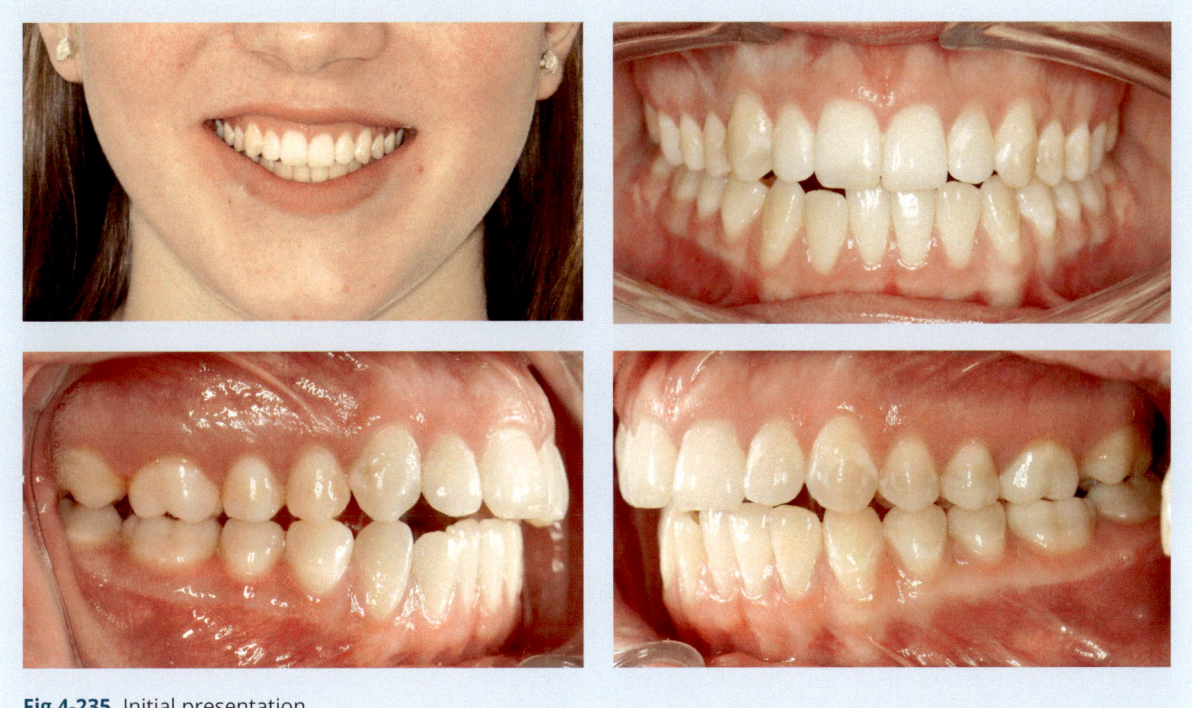

Fig 4-235 Initial presentation.

Diagnosis:
- class II
- anterior open bite
- crowding
- decalcification from use of a fixed appliance alio loco.

Therapy:
- myofunctional therapy
- Invisalign system in combination with class II elastics.

4 TREATMENT OF DIFFERENT MALOCCLUSIONS WITH ALIGNERS

Fig 4-236 Mounted plaster casts show in centric static occlusion contact points (black) only on the premolars and left canines.

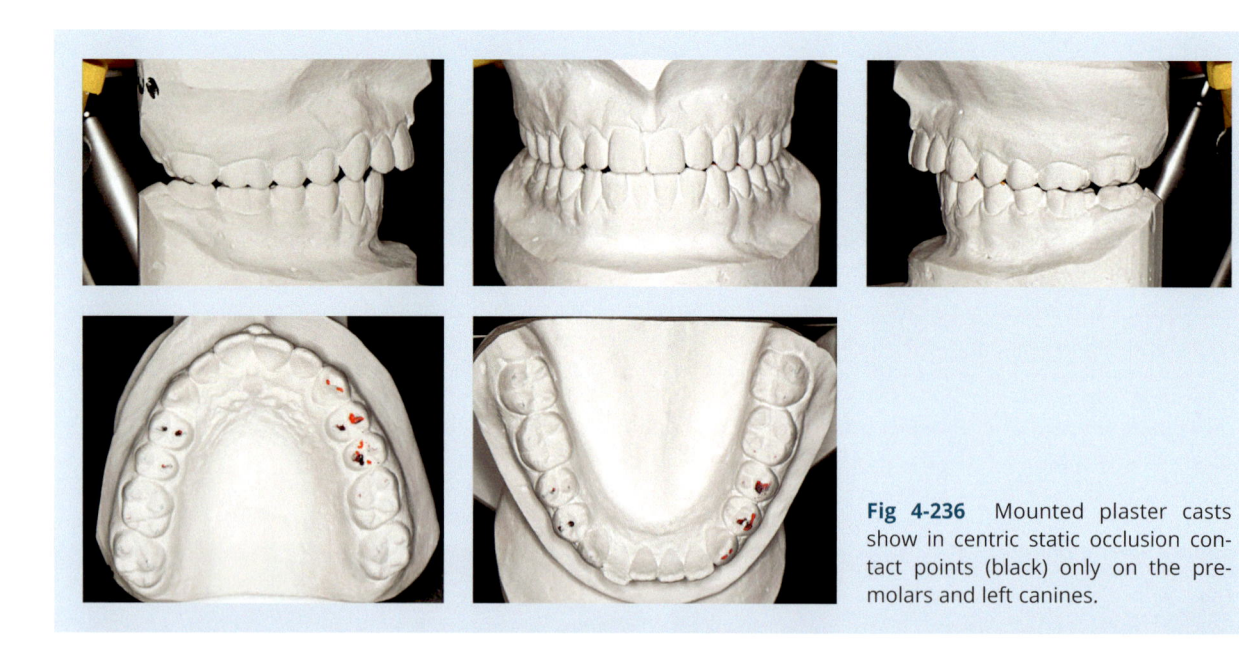

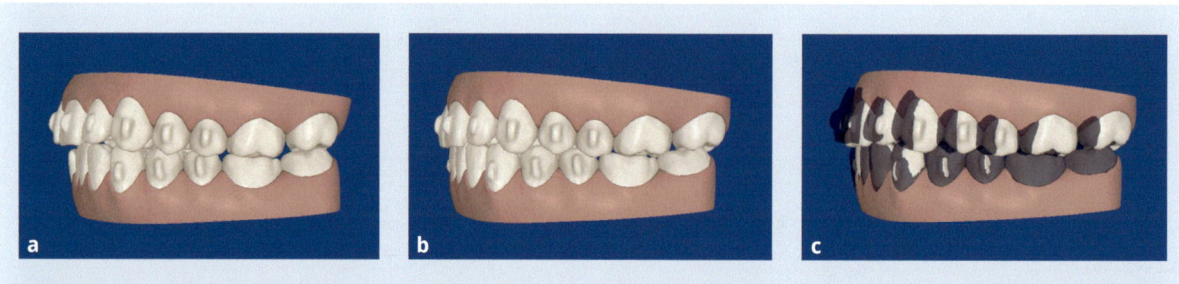

Fig 4-237 ClinCheck software results. **(a)** Initial situation. **(b)** Final planned outcome. **(c)** Superimposition showing the planned movements (blue, initial tooth position; white, final tooth position).

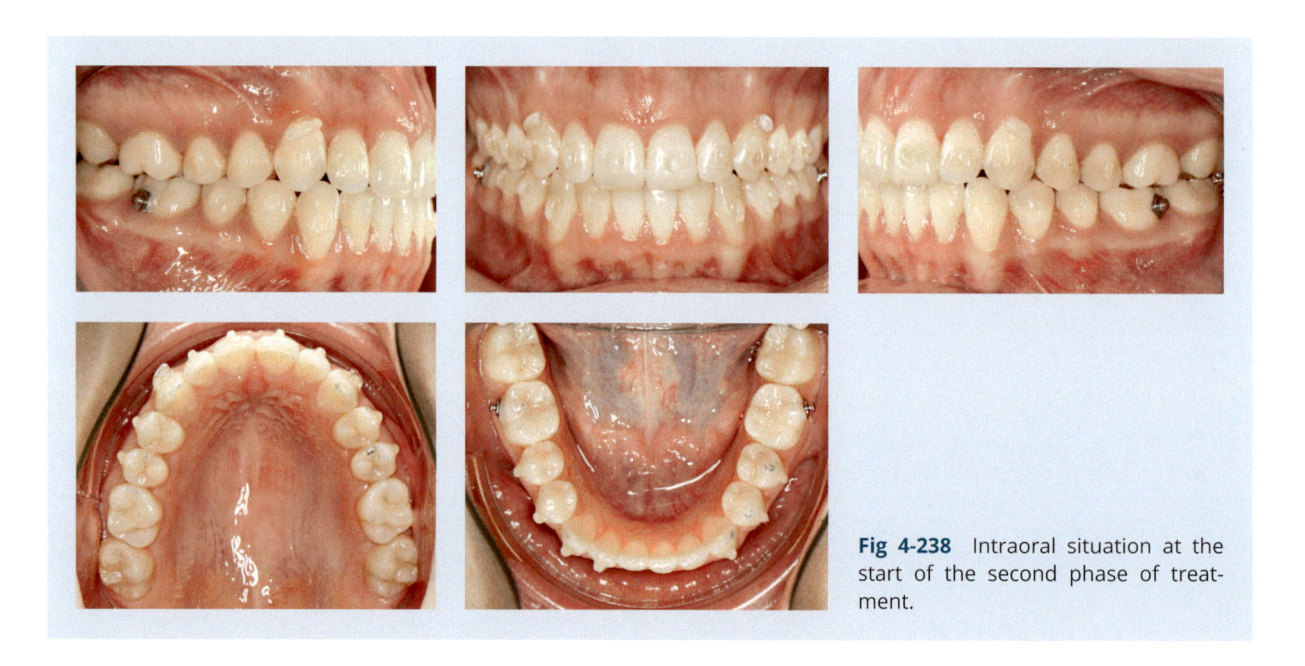

Fig 4-238 Intraoral situation at the start of the second phase of treatment.

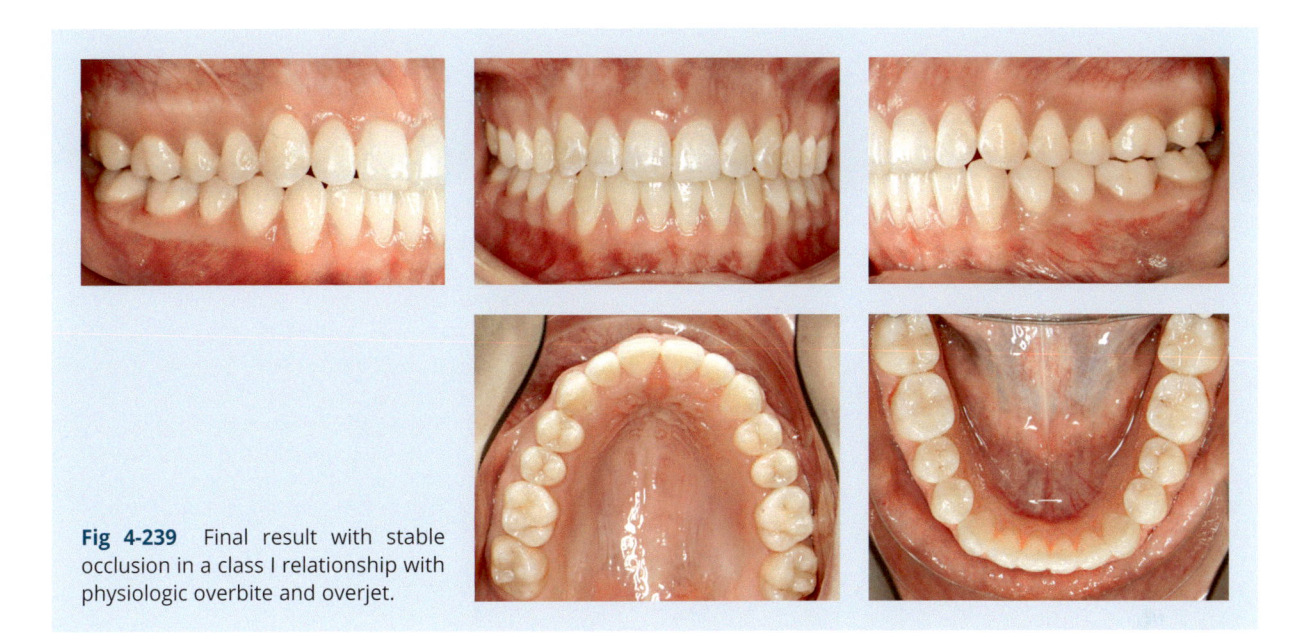

Fig 4-239 Final result with stable occlusion in a class I relationship with physiologic overbite and overjet.

Treatment

The patient underwent myofunctional therapy before the start of the Invisalign treatment and within the first month of orthodontic treatment.

Mounted plaster casts showed centric static occlusion contact only on the premolars and left canines (Fig 4-236). Scanning transferred this occlusal pattern into the ClinCheck software (Fig 4-237). The first phase planned distalization with 30 aligners in the maxillary arch to obtain a class I relationship and close the open bite with extrusion of the maxillary incisors (Fig 4-238). Particularly in an open bite requiring extrusion, it is better to use a slower staging with reduced force from aligner to aligner, as this gives predictable results.

The second phase of treatment used an additional six refinement aligners. IPR of 0.2 mm from mesial 33 to mesial 43 created more space to retract the mandibular incisors and extruded the canines and premolars into full occlusal contact (hard collision).

The final result shows a stable occlusion in a class I relationship with physiologic overbite and overjet (Fig 4-239). The maxillary and mandibular arches are aligned harmonically.

Remounting of maxillary and mandibular plaster casts into the SAM articulator in centric relation shows the contact points in static centric occlusion and canine guidance in dynamic occlusion. This mounting at the end of the treatment can provide information about the occlusion to determine if a refinement or tooth reshaping is necessary. Static and dynamic occlusion was also assessed intraorally with articulating paper (Bausch Arti-Fol, 8 μm; Bausch, Cologne).

Fig 4-240 Remounting of maxillary and mandibular plaster casts into the SAM articulator in centric relation shows the contact points in static centric occlusion (blue) and the canine guidance in the dynamic occlusion (red).

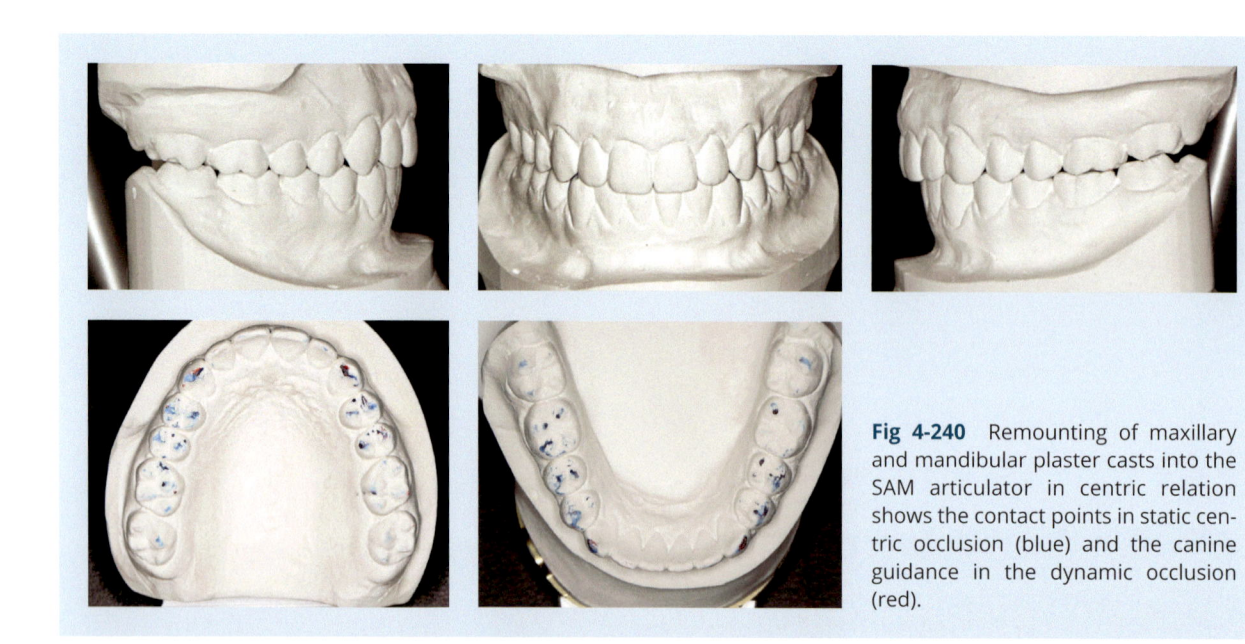

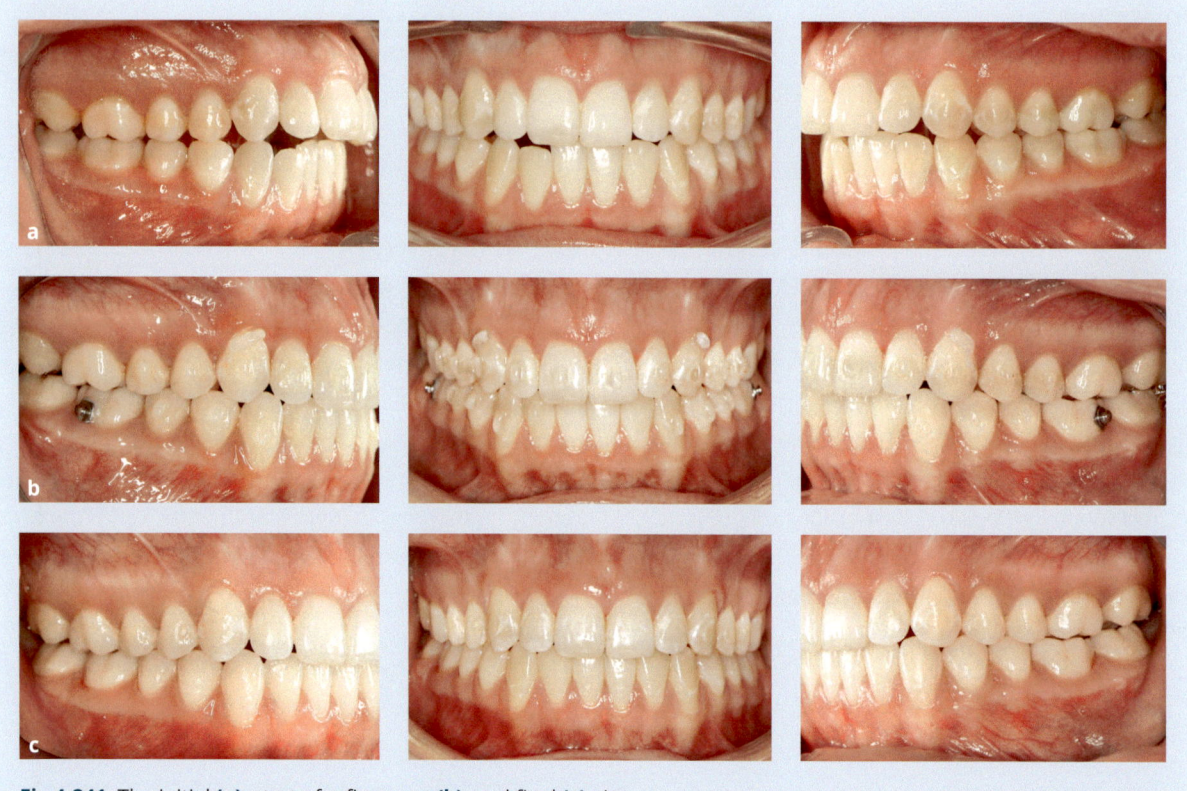

Fig 4-241 The initial (**a**), start of refinement (**b**), and final (**c**) views.

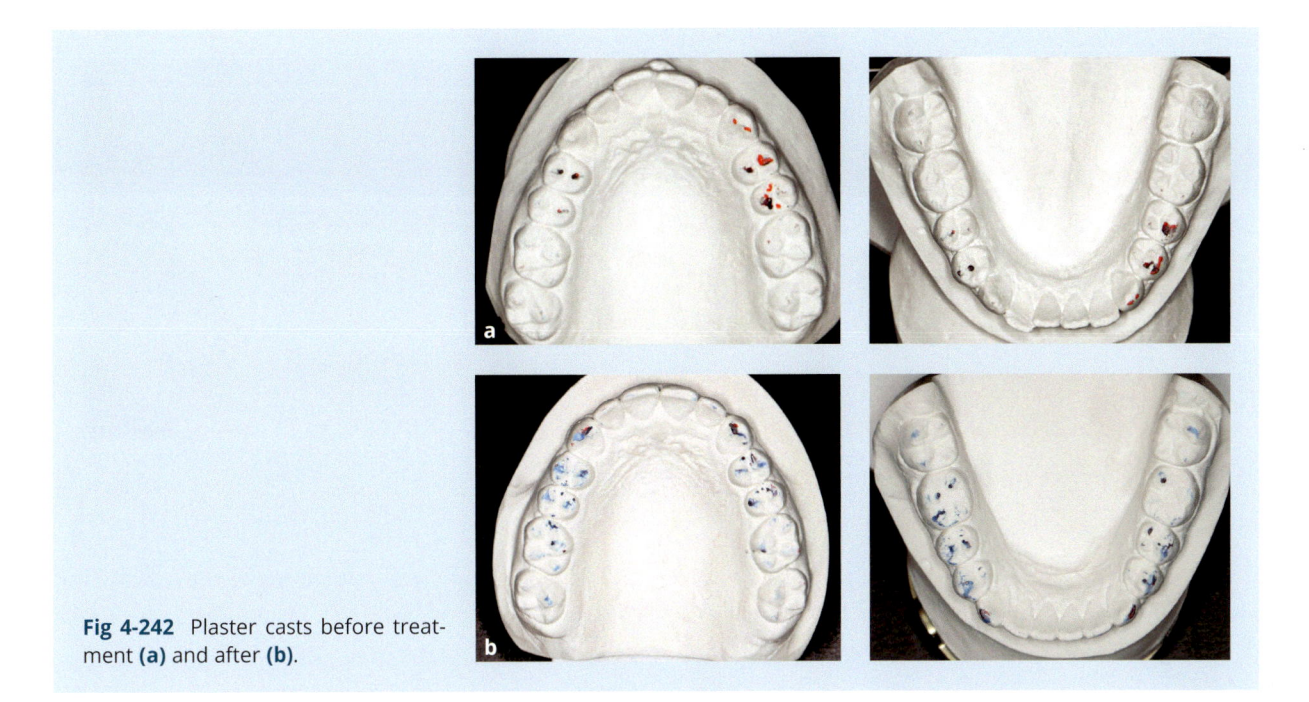

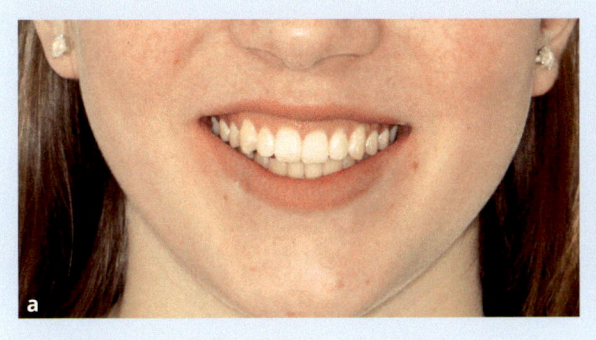

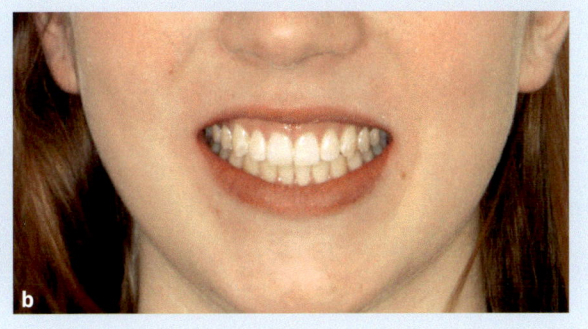

Fig 4-242 Plaster casts before treatment **(a)** and after **(b)**.

Fig 4-243 Lip view before **(a)** and after **(b)** treatment.

If tooth reshaping is required, it is advisable to do a preliminary elimination of precontacts on the mounted plaster casts prior to grinding on the natural teeth.

The course of treatment is shown in Figures 4-240 to 4-243. At the end of treatment, there is a symmetric maxillary arch following harmonically the lower lip curve.

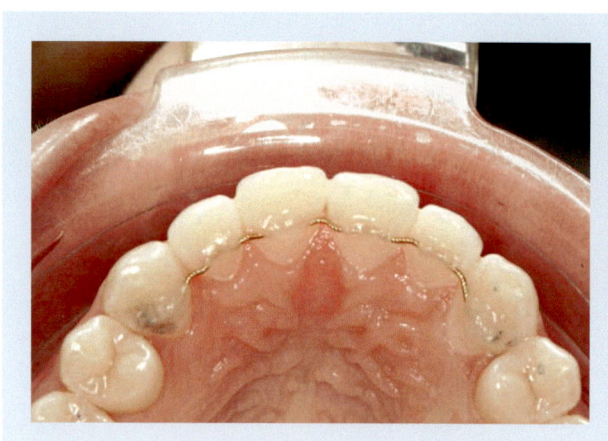

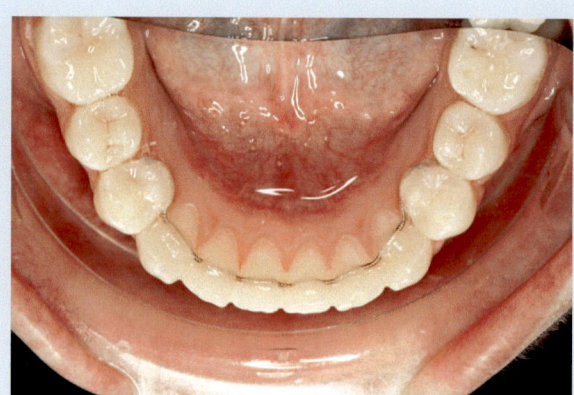

Fig 4-244 Fixed maxillary (3-3) and mandibular (4-4) retainers.

Retention was ensured with fixed maxillary (3-3) and mandibular (4-4) retainers (Fig 4-244). While the latter can be used for a substantial period, the maxillary retainer might lead to blocking of the maxilla and thus osteopathic symptoms. Consequently, the maxillary retainer should only be used for a limited time.

Topic 33
Class III relationship and tongue dysfunction

Treatment:
- Invisalign system
- non-surgical procedure

In growing patients with a class III relationship, we usually start the treatment with a Frankel appliance as soon as the permanent mandibular incisors have erupted. In adults with a sufficient class III relationship, combined orthodontics and orofacial surgery is usually needed (see Topic 46). However, in patients with little skeletal dysgnathia, orthodontic treatment alone is possible, for example using anchorage in the posterior area of the mandible with miniscrews for class III elastics (Lin et al, 2010; Jing et al, 2013; Melson et al, 2014). Many patients with a class III relationship also have a tongue dysfunction and may need myofunctional therapy prior to any orthodontic treatment.

This patient had molars in class III relationship, anterior crossbite, and tongue dysfunction (Figs 4-245 and 4-246). Ricketts analysis gave the following values:

- facial depth: 82.6 degrees
- facial axis: 89.7 degrees
- facial posterior height: 93.0 mm
- mandible body length: 101.4 mm.

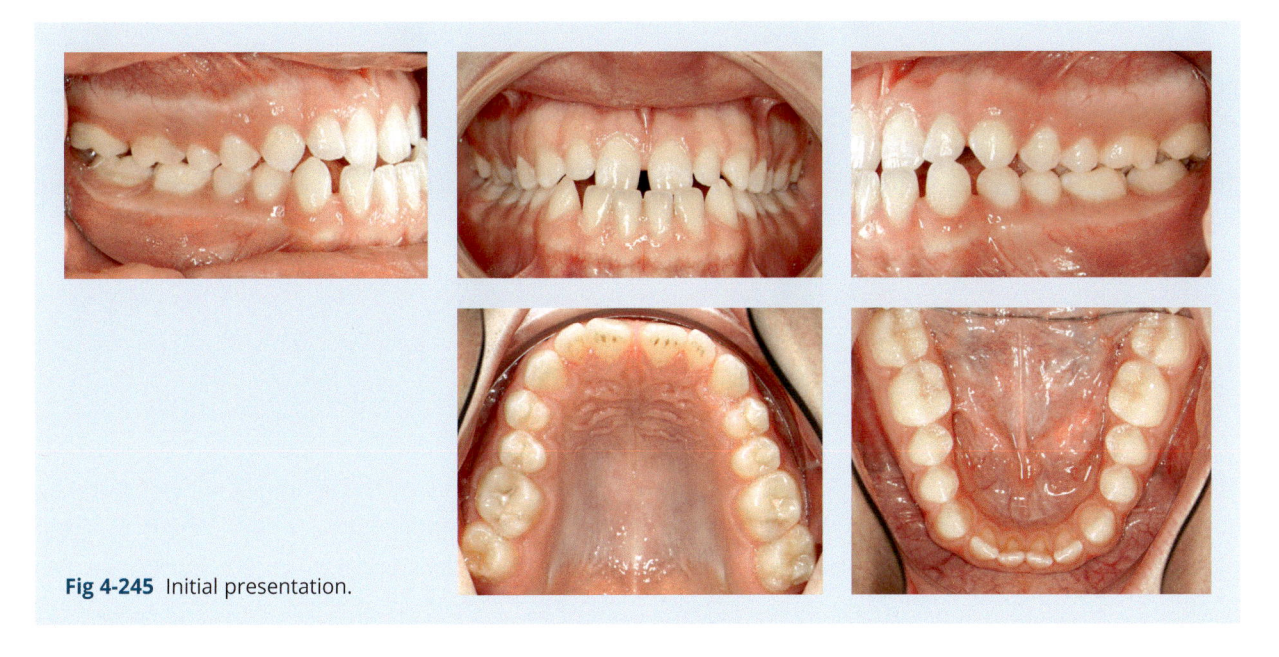

Fig 4-245 Initial presentation.

Diagnosis:
- molars in class III relationship, left more than right
- anterior crossbite
- spaces
- tongue dysfunction.

Therapy:
- myofunctional therapy
- Invisalign treatment with class III elastics.

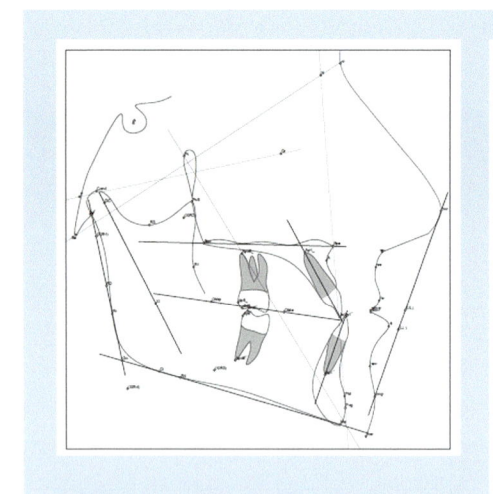

Fig 4-246 Initial analysis of the lateral cephalogram showing class III relationship with anterior crossbite.

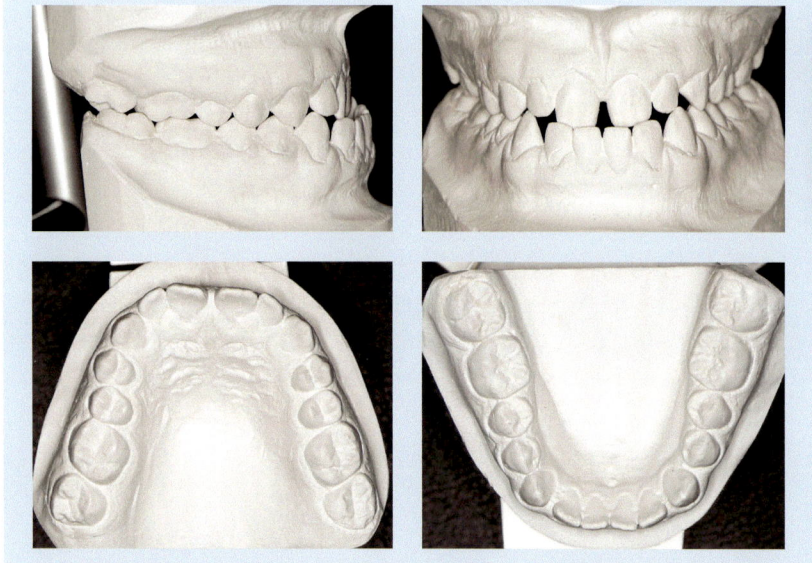

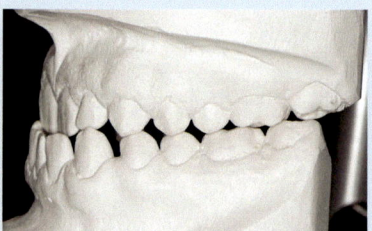

Fig 4-247 Mounted plaster casts at the start of treatment.

Treatment

The wisdom teeth were removed before starting orthodontic treatment. Mounted plaster casts confirmed the class III molar relationship, anterior crossbite, and spaces and rotations in the anterior region in both arches (Fig 4-247).

Rectangular attachments were used (prior to G4 launch) with bonded transparent plastic hooks on teeth 33 and 43, and metal buttons on teeth 16 and 26 for class III elastics (maximum force 80 g; Fig 4-248). A hook bonded directly to the canines should always be used in combination with an attachment to avoid undesired rotations under the direct elastic force. The treatment plan included distalization in the mandibular arch of almost 2 mm into a full class I relationship. The anterior teeth were planned for retraction of 5 mm. If treatment is planned with mandibular molar distalization of more than 2–3 mm, additional anchorage with miniscrews is necessary to obtain a highly predictable result.

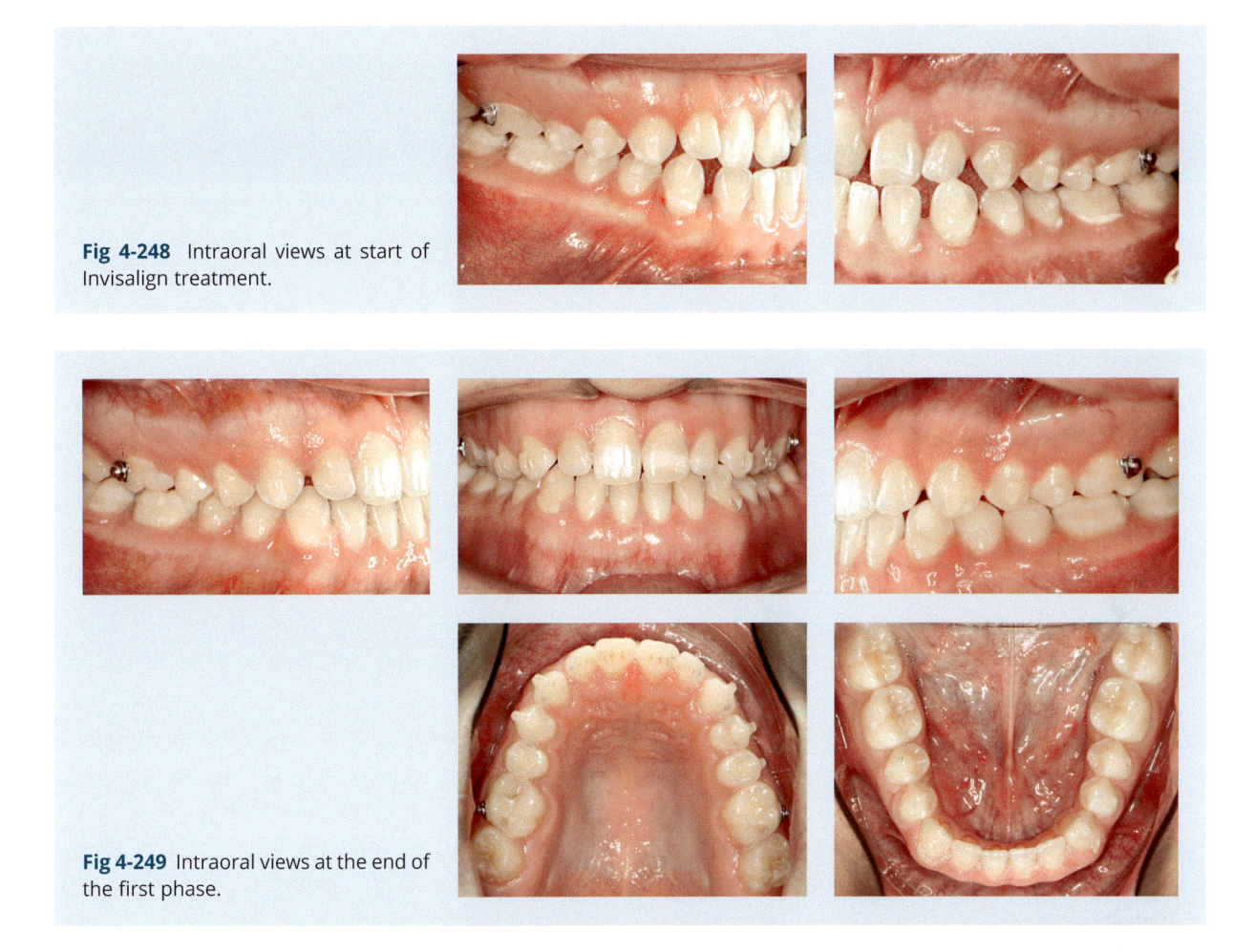

Fig 4-248 Intraoral views at start of Invisalign treatment.

Fig 4-249 Intraoral views at the end of the first phase.

Fig 4-250 The ClinCheck software shows the initial situation at the start of the second phase.

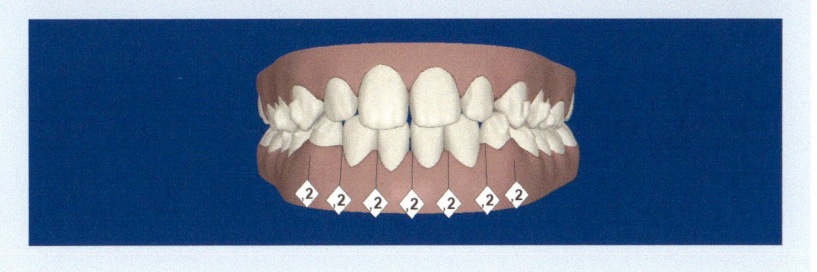

The first phase used 8 maxillary and 34 mandibular aligners. At the end of this phase, the first molars were in a full class I relationship and the maxillary first molar was in an optimal position, with a deep position of the distobuccal cusp onto approximal contact between the mandibular first and second molar and with an occlusal contact on the marginal ridge (Fig 4-249). This particular aspect is important for stable interdigitation and therefore the end-result of orthodontic treatment (Ricketts, 1998).

The ClinCheck software shows the situation at the start of the second phase (Fig 4-250), which included 19 refinement aligners. Additional IPR of 0.2 mm on each tooth was necessary from mesial 34 to mesial 44, plus power ridges on maxillary and mandibular incisors to obtain more torque of anterior teeth and

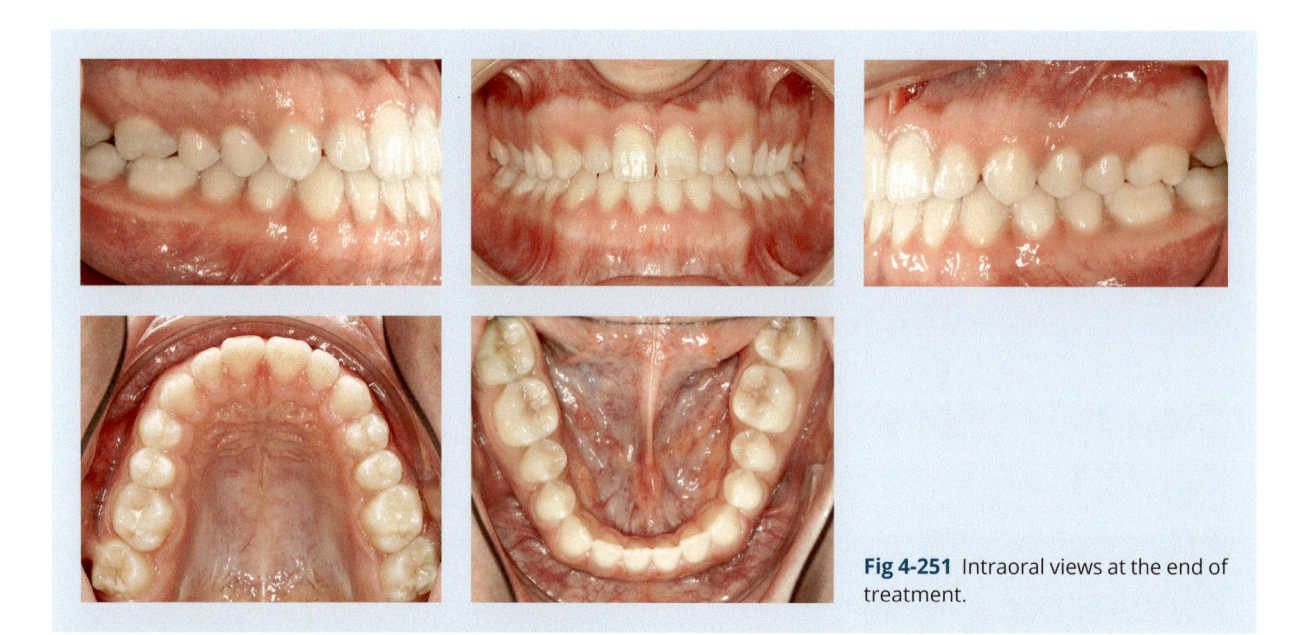

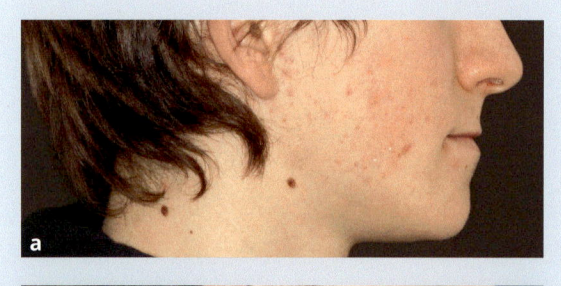

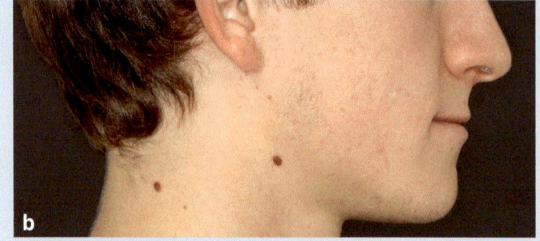

Fig 4-251 Intraoral views at the end of treatment.

Fig 4-252 Profile views before (a) and after (b) treatment.

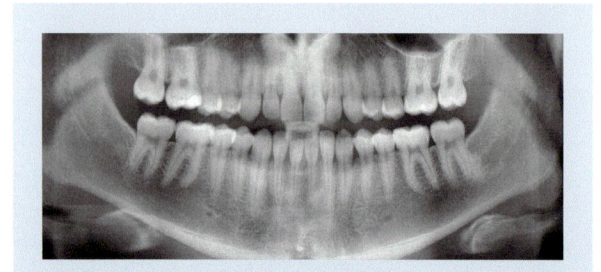

Fig 4-253 Final orthopantomogram.

improve the anterior relationship. At the end of treatment, the mandibular anterior teeth had been retracted, the anterior crossbite was resolved, and a physiologic anterior tooth relationship was achieved. There was a class I relationship on both sides (Figs 4-251) The extraoral profile showed improved harmonics of the lower face (Fig 4-252). Orthopantomography showed no pathology (Fig 4-253).

Ricketts analysis of the final lateral cephalogram showed improved values (Fig 4-254) and mounted casts confirmed this (Fig 4-255).

For retention, the patient was advised to wear an occlusal splint in the maxillary arch (Fig 4-256). The mandibular arch was retained with a lingual fixed retainer from 33 to 43. Figure 4-256 shows the intraoral situation after 1 year of retention with a stable result.

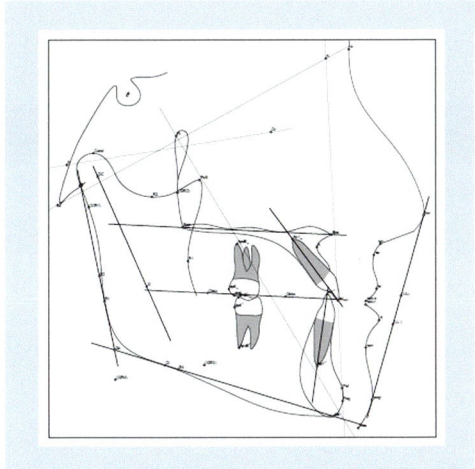

Fig 4-254 Ricketts analysis of the final lateral cephalogram.

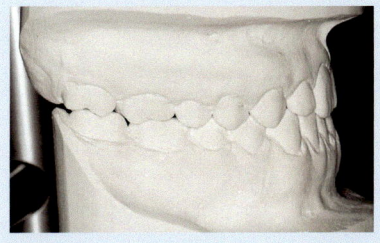

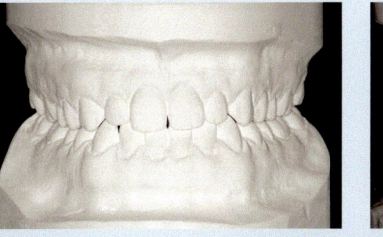

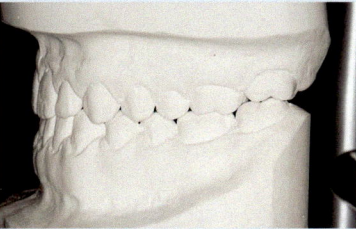

Fig 4-255 Mounted plaster casts showing a class I molar relationship, anterior physiologic anterior relationship, and harmonically aligned arches with equal posterior occlusion pattern (blue color) without anterior contact. The red marks show the canine guidance in optimal function during dynamic occlusion.

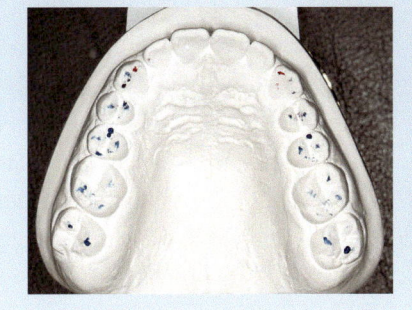

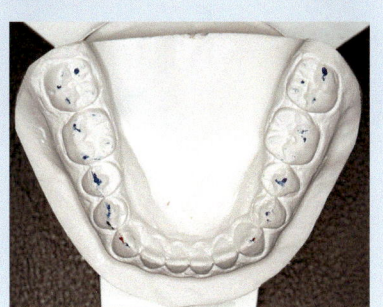

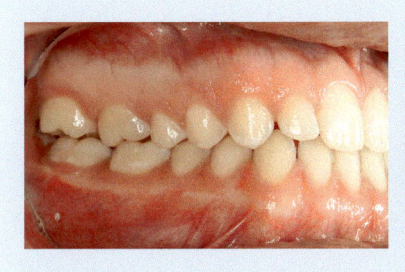

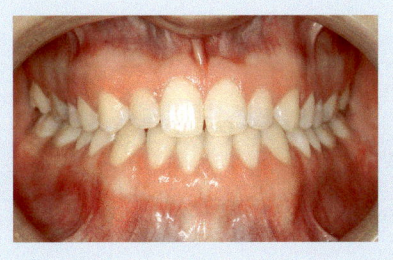

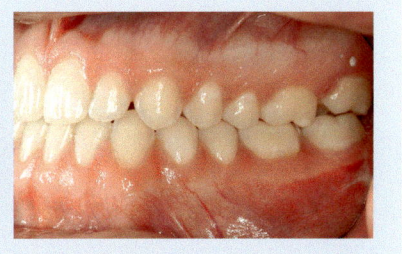

Fig 4-256 Intraoral pictures after 1 year of retention.

Topic 34
Class III relationship treated without surgery

Treatment:
- Invisalign treatment
- distalization in the lower arch
- non-surgical procedure

When considerable distalization of mandibular molars and premolars is required to correct a class III relationship with anterior crossbite, class III elastics are required in addition to the Invisalign system. In patients with TMJ dysfunction, anchorage with class III elastics can be critical, particularly if the condyle is already in a retral position. In some patients, the combination of Invisalign treatment with class III elastics worn intramaxillary to a skeletal anchorage such as a mini-implant represents a valuable approach (Yamaguchi et al, 2012).

This adult male showed a class III relationship, anterior crossbite, and mild crowding in both arches but no signs of CMD (Figs 4-257 and 4-258).

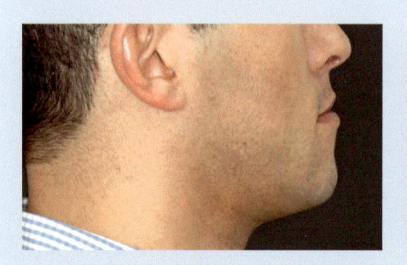

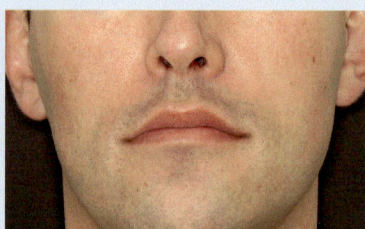

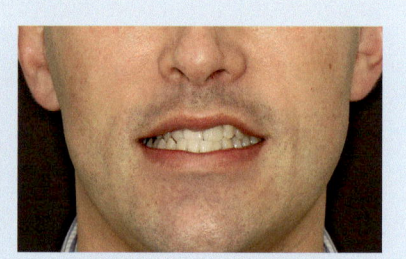

Fig 4-257 Initial presentation.

Diagnosis:
- class III relationship
- anterior crossbite
- transversally constricted maxillary arch
- mild crowding in both arches.

Therapy:
- Invisalign treatment
- class III elastics for anchorage during distalization in the mandibular arch.

Fig 4-258 Initial intraoral views.

Fig 4-259 Start of Invisalign treatment.

Treatment

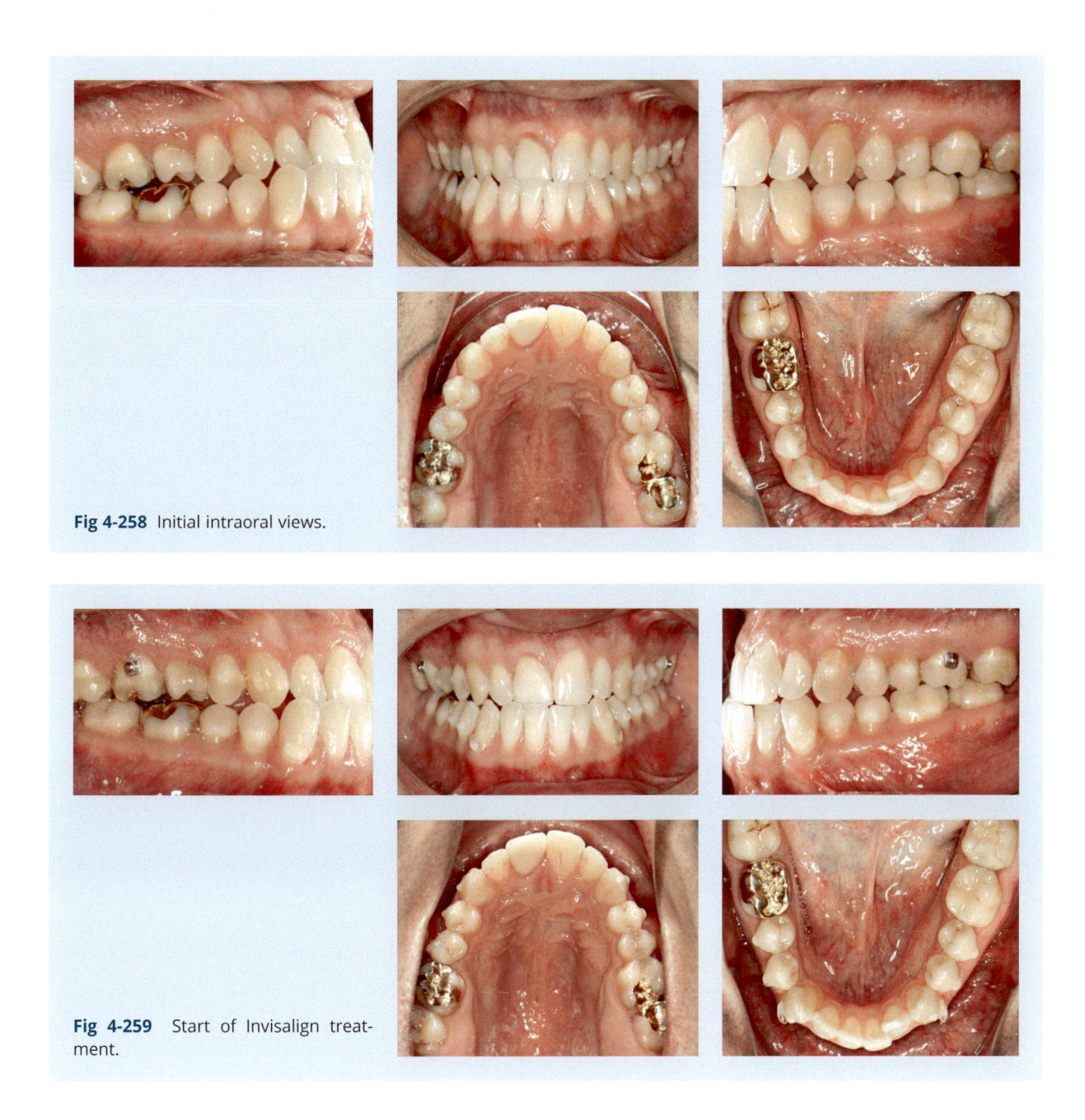

Invisalign treatment was commenced with ellipsoid attachments on premolars and canines, plus hooks on teeth 33 and 43 and buttons on teeth 16 and 26 for class III elastics for anchorage (Fig 4-259). The ClinCheck software with superimposition shows the planned movements (Fig 4-260). Distalization of 3 mm in the molar region with additional IPR was needed to obtain the desired class I relationship.

Figure 4-261 shows aligner 13 and distalization of mandibular molars as intraoral views and in the ClinCheck simulation.

The intraoral view and ClinCheck simulation show a perfect match in the mandibular arch at the end of distalization of the molars and beginning of distalization of the first premolars (Fig 4-262).

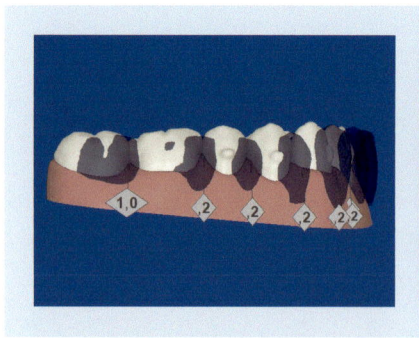

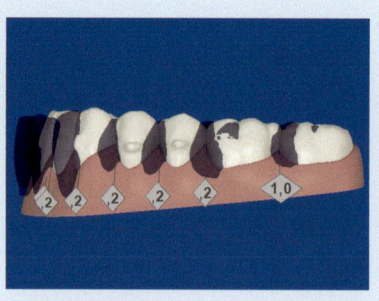

Fig 4-260 ClinCheck software showing superimposition of the planned movements (blue, initial tooth position; white, final tooth position).

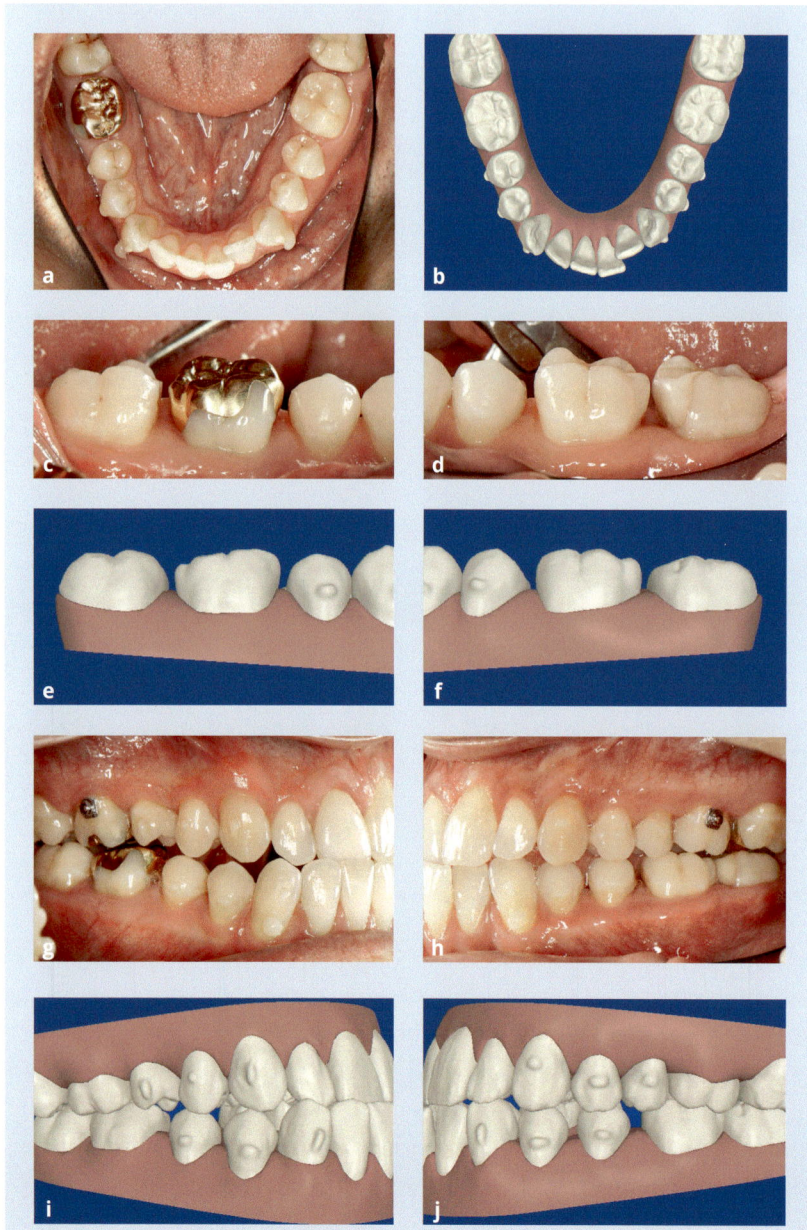

Fig 4-261 Aligner 13 and distalization of mandibular molars as intraoral views **(a,c,d,g,h)** and in the ClinCheck simulation **(b,e,f,i,j)**.

TREATMENT OF DIFFERENT MALOCCLUSIONS WITH ALIGNERS 4

Fig 4-262 The ClinCheck simulation and the intraoral situation show a perfect match at the end of distalization of the molars and beginning of distalization of the first premolars.

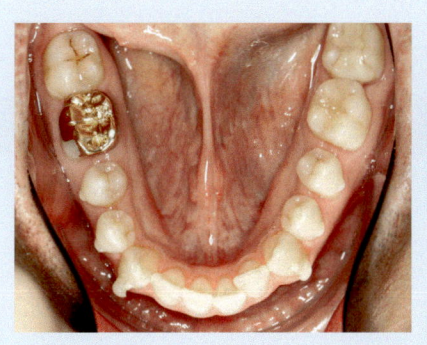

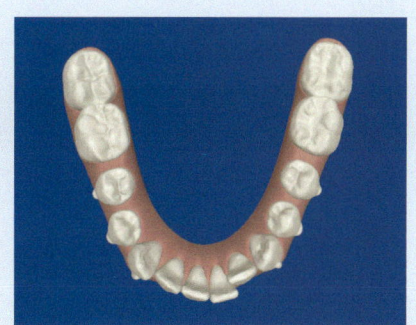

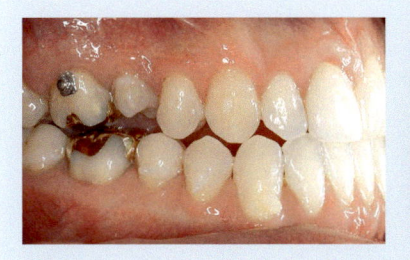

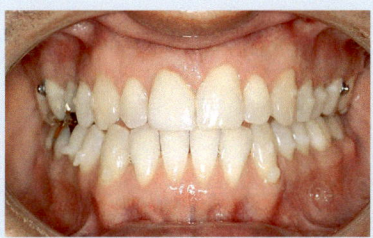

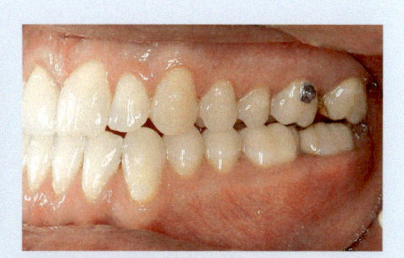

Fig 4-263 The intraoral pictures show the situation with stage at aligner number 14 of the refinement **(a-c)**. Tooth 15 was not planned to move with the aligners, but will be extruded with up and down elastics later on. **(d)** Situation with aligner number 14 and criss cross elastics on palatinal hooks on teeth 13, 14 and buccal hooks on teeth 43, 44, 45 in situ to solve crossbite tendency of the right side and fasten treatment course.

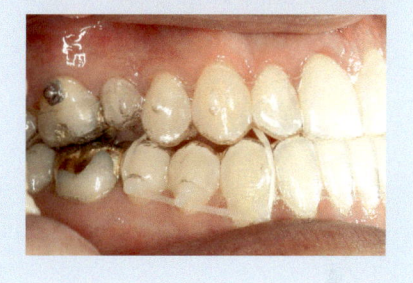

Figure 4-263 shows the result after further 14 aligners of refinement prior to additional up and down elastics on tooth 15 for better occlusion.

The patient is currently still in treatment with the final aligners. Retention is planned with a bonded lingual retainer and a removable aligner in the upper arch.

Topic 35
Intrusion of a maxillary molar with aligner therapy and miniscrews

Treatment:
- Invisalign system
- miniscrew anchorage (temporary anchorage device, TAD)

Mini-implants, so-called miniscrews, are well known in orthodontics for providing stong additional anchorage for tooth movements. Yamaguchi et al. (2012) commented, "Paradigms have started to shift in the orthodontic world since the introduction of mini-implants in the anchorage armamentarium." Lin et al. (2014) have described the issues of treating challenging malocclusions with Invisalign and miniscrew anchorage.

This patient had a missing mandibular first molar and an extruded maxillary first molar (Fig 4-264).

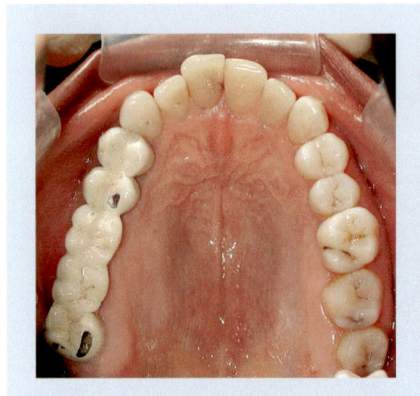

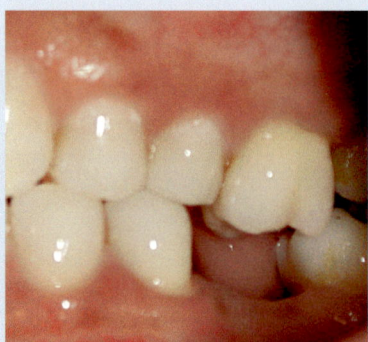

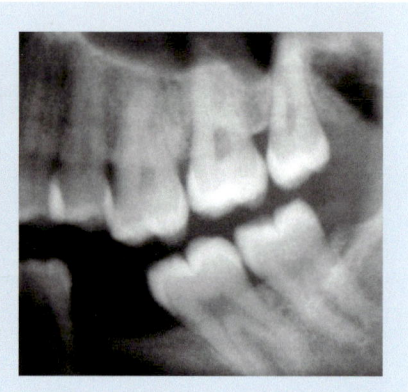

Fig 4-264 Initial presentation.

Diagnosis:
- missing tooth 36
- extruded tooth 26
- crowding
- anterior crossbite of tooth 12.

Therapy:
- aligner therapy
- miniscrews for anchorage.

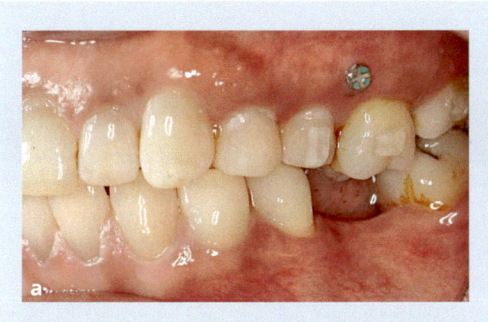

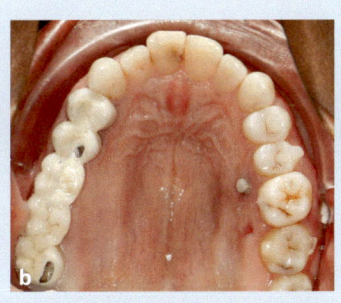

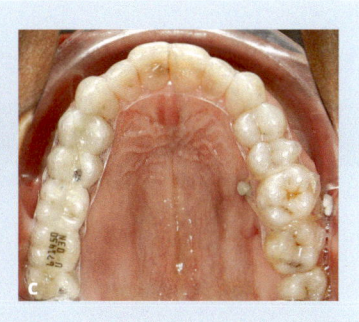

Fig 4-265 Intraoral views. **(a,b)** Miniscrews and attachments. **(c)** The aligner and an elastic from screw to screw over the aligner.

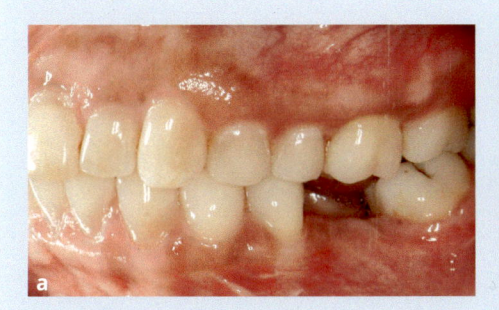

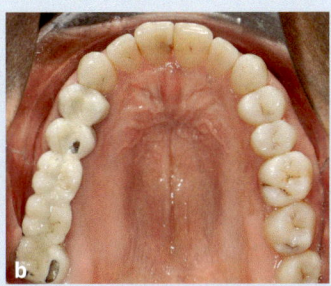

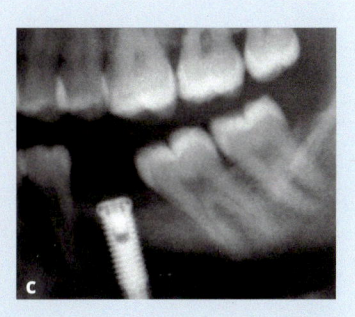

Fig 4-266 The intraoral pictures show the completed intrusion of tooth 26 at the end of the Invisalign treatment **(a,b)**. The X-ray shows the insertion of the implant area 36 **(c)**.

Treatment

Miniscrews were inserted buccally and lingually of tooth 26 (Fig 4-265). Attachments were bonded on teeth 25, 26, and 27 for major grip of the aligner. The patient wore the aligner and an elastic from screw to screw over the aligner.

At completion of treatment, tooth 26 had been completely intruded. The patient wore retention aligners in both arches until the prosthodontic treatment started (Fig 4-266).

Topic 36
Intrusion of a maxillary molar with aligner therapy

Treatment:
- Invisalign system without TAD's

Topic 35 demonstrated the intrusion of an extruded maxillary molar with aligner therapy combined with mini-screw anchorage. This topic is an example of intrusion using only the Invisalign system.

This patient had an extruded maxillary molar (Fig 4-267). Teeth 16 and 35 showed endodontic fillings (Fig 4-268).

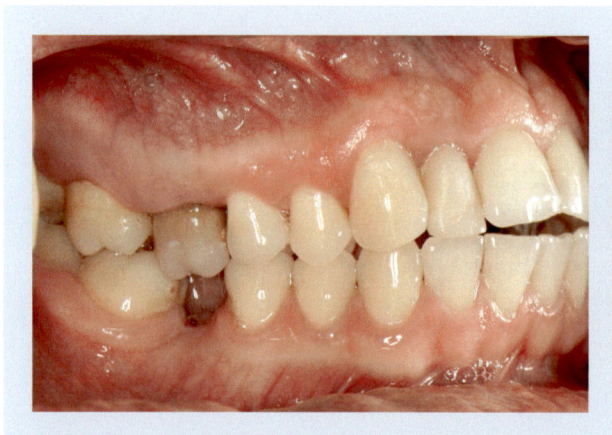

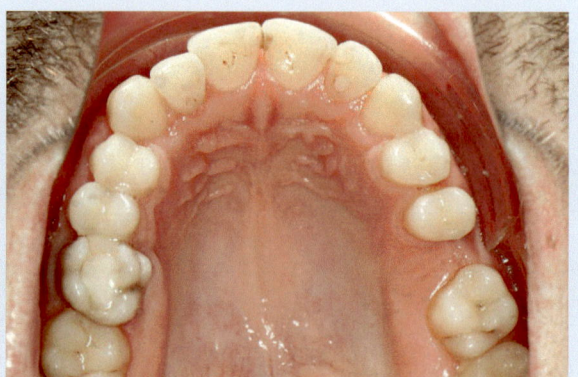

Fig 4-267 Initial presentation.

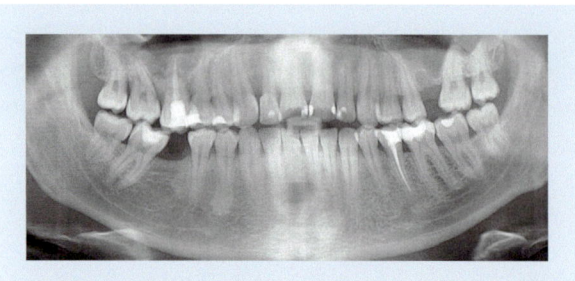

Fig 4-268 Initial orthopantomography.

Diagnosis:
- extruded tooth 16.

Therapy:
- alignment of maxilla and mandible
- intrusion of tooth 16
- space opening for later implants at positions 26 and 46.

Treatment

Eight months of aligner treatment with 17 aligners achieved completed intrusion of tooth 16 (Fig 4-269). The endodontically treated tooth 16 showed apical inflammation during the aligner treatment and was advised for endodontic revision.

Figure 4-270 compares the intraoral views and the ClinCheck planning image. A second phase of refinement (10 + 3 aligners in the maxillary arch, 10 aligners in the mandibular arch) and interdisciplinary treatment achieved correct position for tooth 16 and healthy gingival and periodontal situation (Fig 4-271).

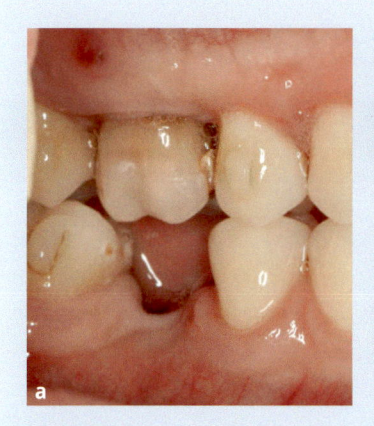

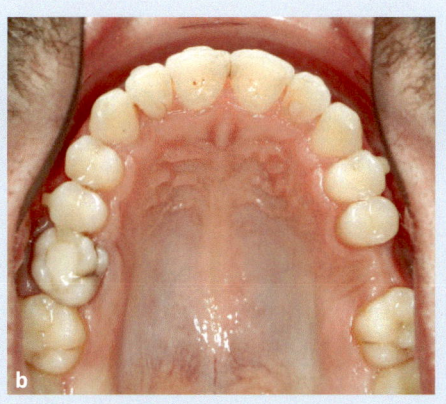

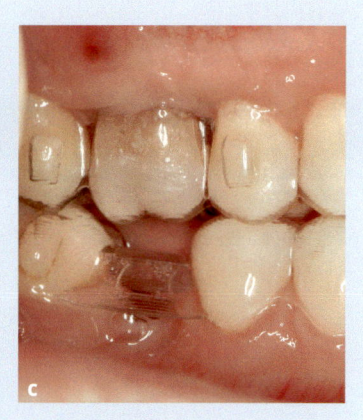

TREATMENT OF DIFFERENT MALOCCLUSIONS WITH ALIGNERS 4

Fig 4-269 Intraoral situation after the first phase. (a,b) Completed intrusion of tooth 16. (c) Aligner 17 in situ, demonstrating perfect fit after 8 months of treatment.

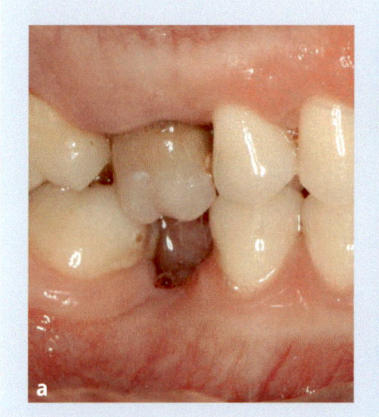

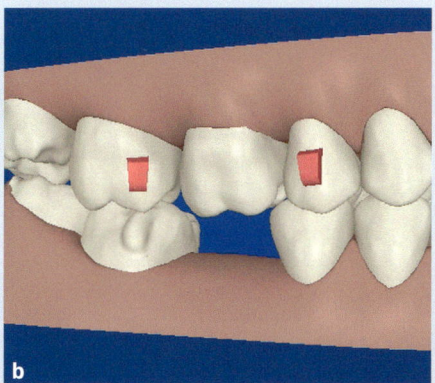

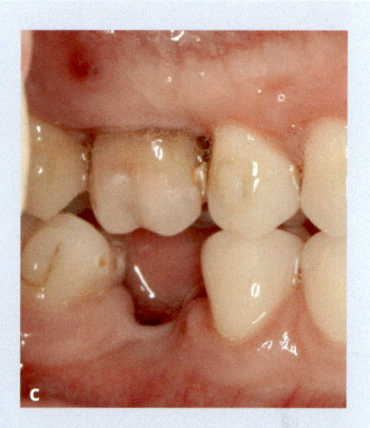

Fig 4-270 Intraoral initial (a) and final (b) views and the planned ClinCheck image (c).

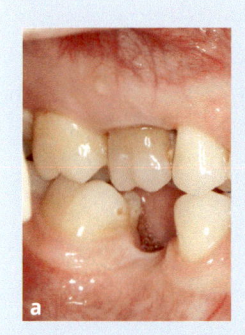

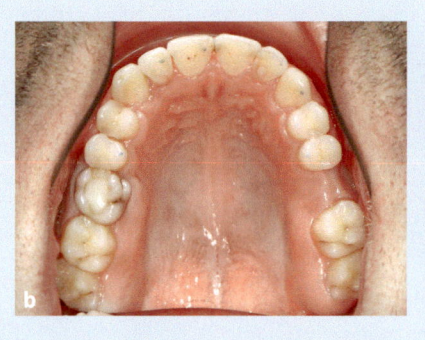

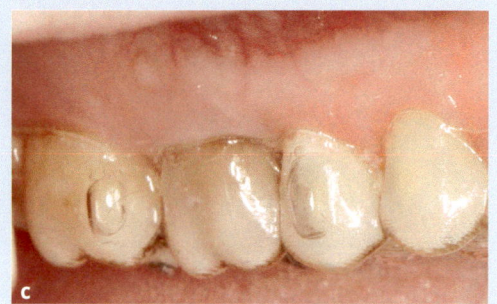

Fig 4-271 Final intraoral situation (a,b) Tooth 16 was endodontically revised and there was healthy gingiva and periodontium. (c) perfect fitting of the last aligner of treatment.

4 TREATMENT OF DIFFERENT MALOCCLUSIONS WITH ALIGNERS

Topic 37
Tipped molars

Treatment:
- uprighting of molars

Molars tipped into an extraction space can be uprighted and distalized with the Invisalign system to create space for a later implant or prosthetics. However, it appears to be impossible to obtain a mesial movement of the tipped tooth with the necessary root torque to close the dental space with an aligner technique alone.

This patient had lost several teeth and implants were chosen as the pathway for replacement (Fig 4-272). Orthopantomography showed the amount of space available before treatment (Fig 4-273).

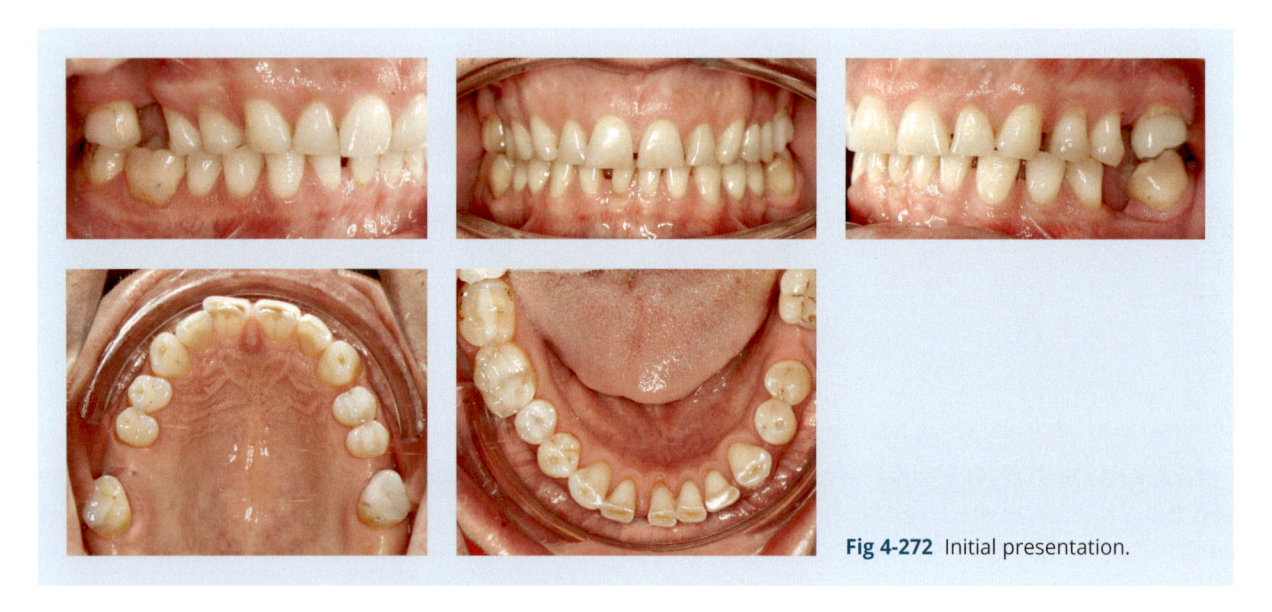

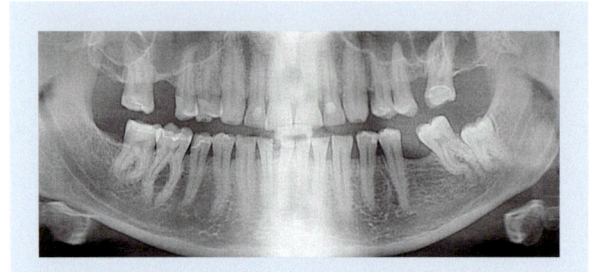

Fig 4-272 Initial presentation.

Fig 4-273 Orthopantomography showed the amount of space available before treatment.

Diagnosis:
- class I
- spaces in both arches with missing teeth 16, 26, and 36
- abrasions.

Therapy:
- alignment of maxilla and mandible with uprighting and distalization of teeth 17, 27, and 37
- space opening for later implants.

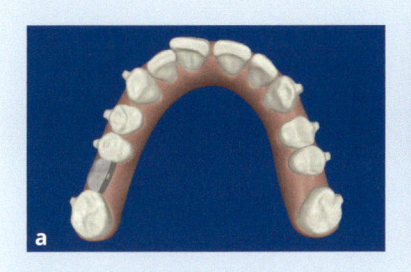

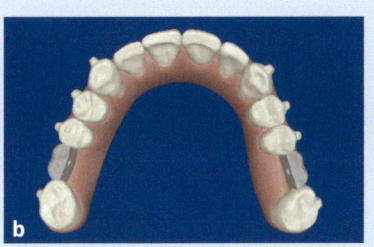

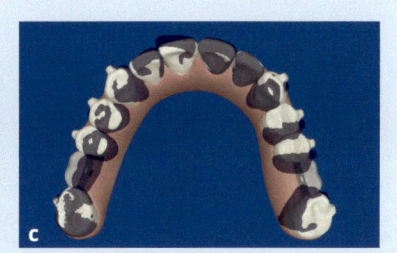

Fig 4-274 ClinCheck software results for the maxilla. **(a)** Initial situation with spaces in arch. **(b)** Final planned situation with opened spaces in regions 16 and 26 and virtual pontics. **(c)** Superimposition showing the planned teeth movement (blue, initial tooth position; white, final tooth position).

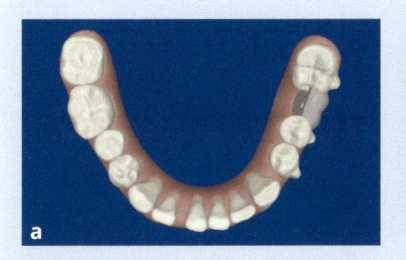

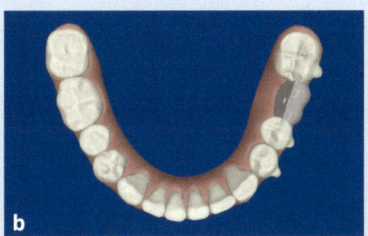

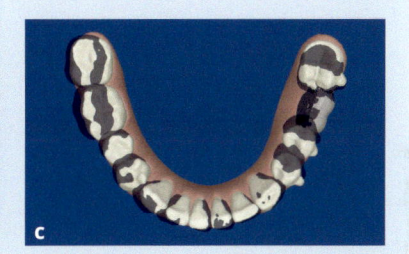

Fig 4-275 ClinCheck software results for the mandible. **(a)** Initial situation with spaces in the arch and a pontic in region 36. **(b)** Final planned situation with opened space in region 36. **(c)** Superimposition showing the planned teeth movement (blue, initial tooth position; white, final tooth position).

Treatment

The patient was advised to have tooth 38 extracted but declined. The spaces in regions 16, 26, and 36 did not offer sufficient space for an adequate implant insertion as the neighboring teeth had migrated into the spaces. The planned teeth movements in the maxilla included mesialization of premolars and distalization/uprighting of the second molars, with 25 aligners in the first phase (Fig 4-274). In the mandible, the planned movements included the mesialization of premolars and distalization/uprighting of tooth 37, with 25 aligners in the first phase (Fig 4-275). Studies performed by Align Technology have shown that there is no significant difference in uprighting force by using a pontic in the extraction area, or by using an aligner base without a pontic.

At the end of the first phase of the Invisalign treatment, all spaces for later implants have been opened sufficiently and a stable posterior occlusion with contact on all premolars and molars as well as canine guidance was achieved (Fig 4-276). The incisors are in a physiologic position just out of contact, leaving space for the Shimstock foil. A refinement was performed to align the midlines based on the patient's wishes. An additional eight aligners were used to obtain aligned midlines and create spaces for later implants in areas 16, 26, and 36 (Fig 4-277). Tooth reshaping with composite resin was planned on maxillary lateral incisors due to the convex tooth shape and black triangles.

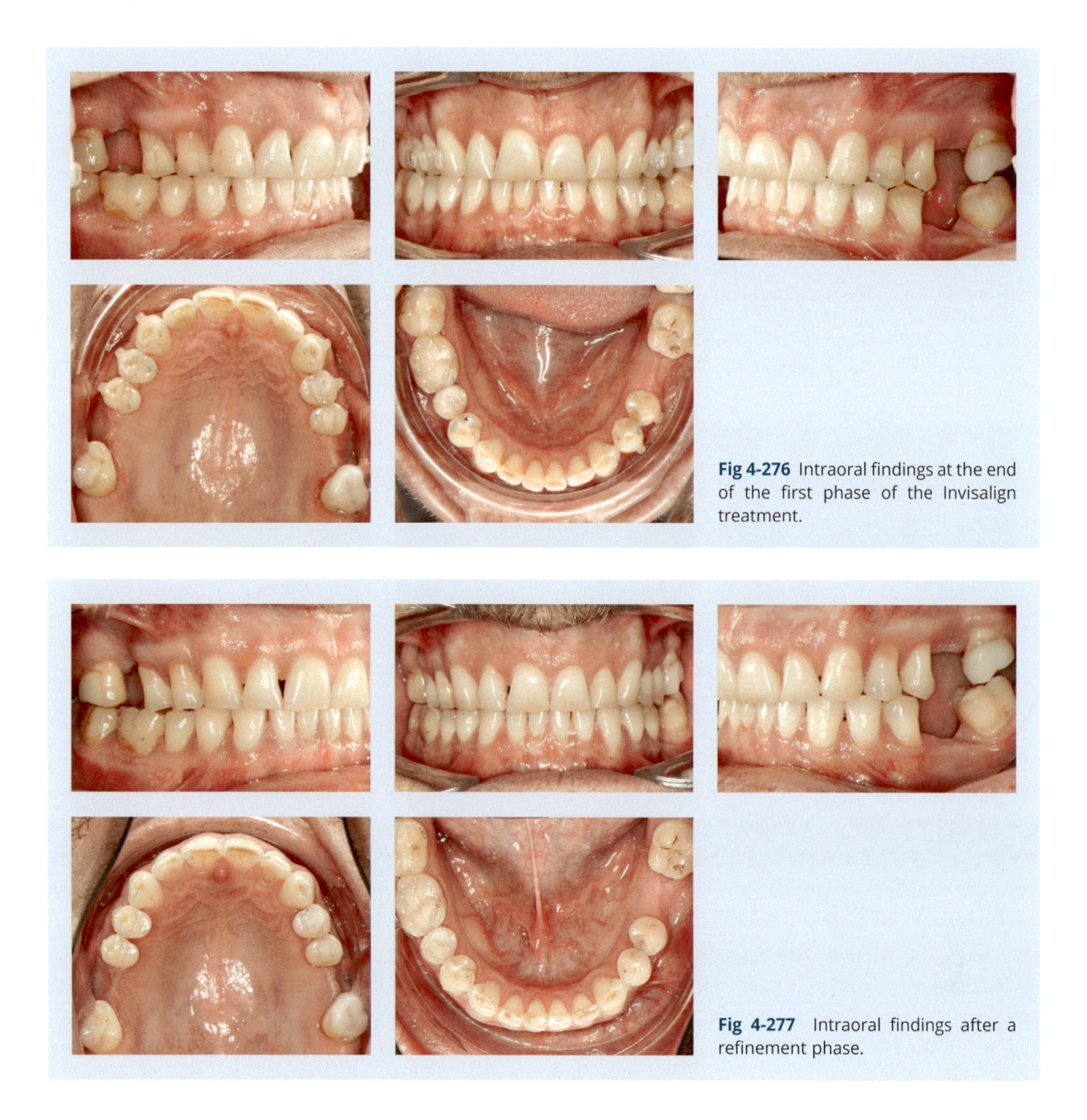

Fig 4-276 Intraoral findings at the end of the first phase of the Invisalign treatment.

Fig 4-277 Intraoral findings after a refinement phase.

Views before and after treatment show the changes achieved. Spaces for implants in region 16, 26, and 36 have been opened, with closure of all spaces from premolar to premolar and uprighting of tooth 37 (Figs 4-278 and 4-279). Tooth 38 was not removed as the patient was worried abut potential damage to the mandibular nerve during extraction. Removal of this tooth might have guaranteed even further uprighting of tooth 37.

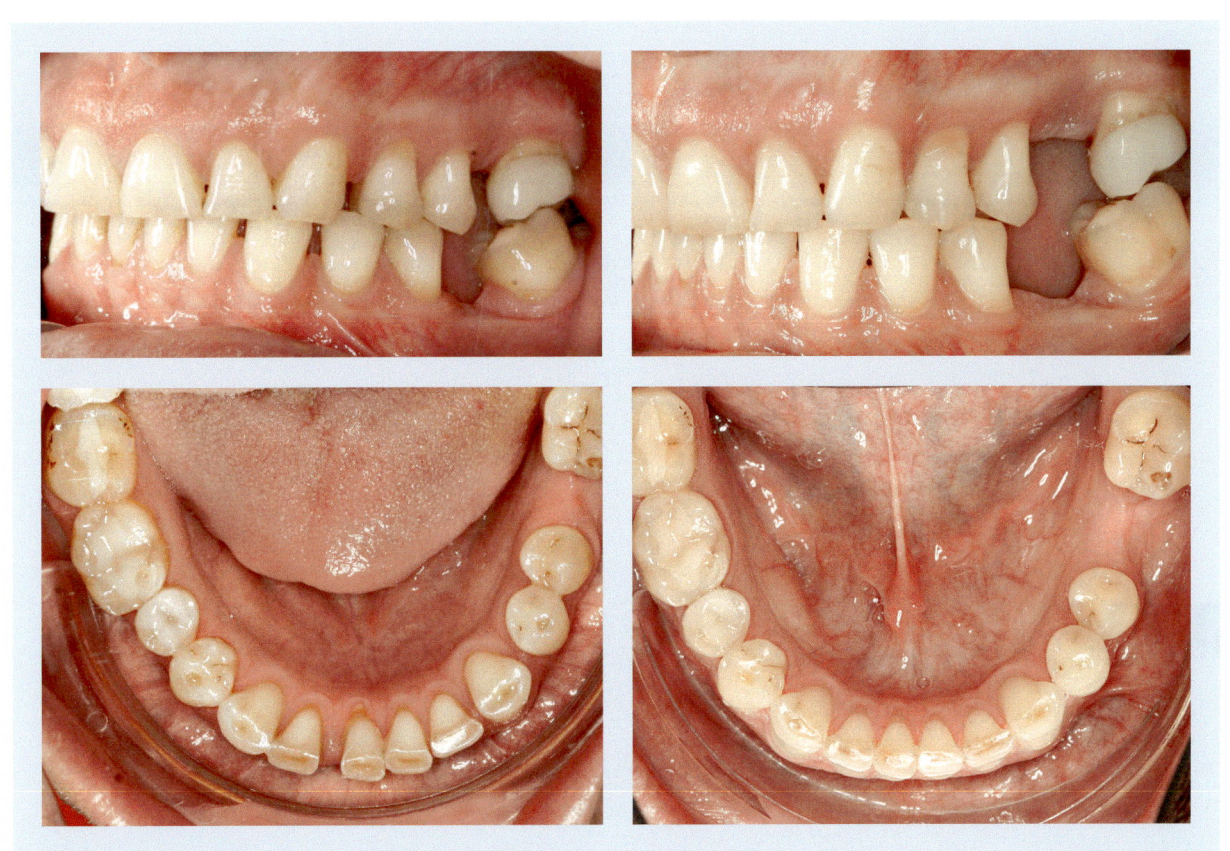

Fig 4-278 Initial **(left)** and final **(right)** left lateral and mandibular views.

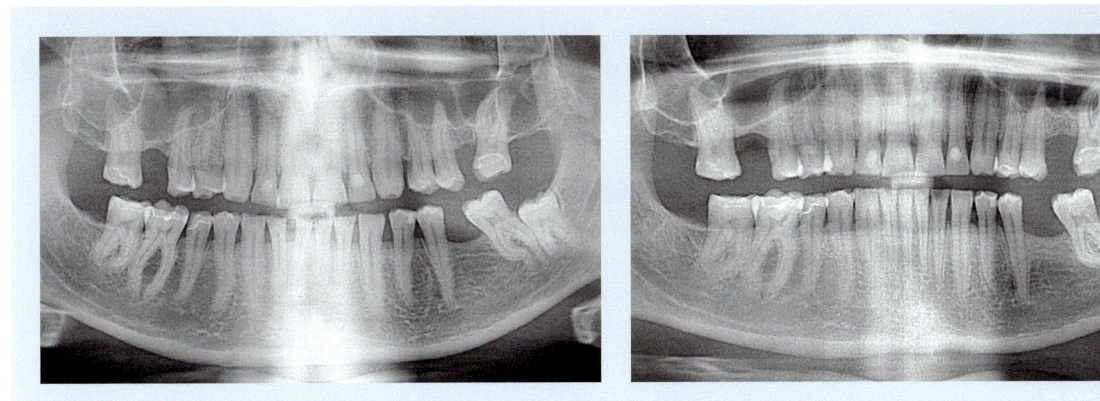

Fig 4-279 Orthopantomograms before **(left)** and after **(right)** Invisalign treatment.

Topic 38
Child with early loss of baby teeth

Treatment:
- distalization and space opening in the mixed dentition

Initially the Invisalign system was only licensed for adults with fully erupted teeth. With an extraordinary FDI license in 2003, we were able to treat the first child with Invisalign at the age of 7 years and 10 months. This topic demonstrates that distalization with aligners is perfectly realizable and highly predictable at every age and is one of the best ways to distalize teeth without any side effects.

The boy was nearly 8 years old and had early extraction of both maxillary second primary molars. Failure to use a retention appliance resulted in the spaces closing by undesired mesial movements of maxillary molars into the extraction spaces (Fig 4-280).

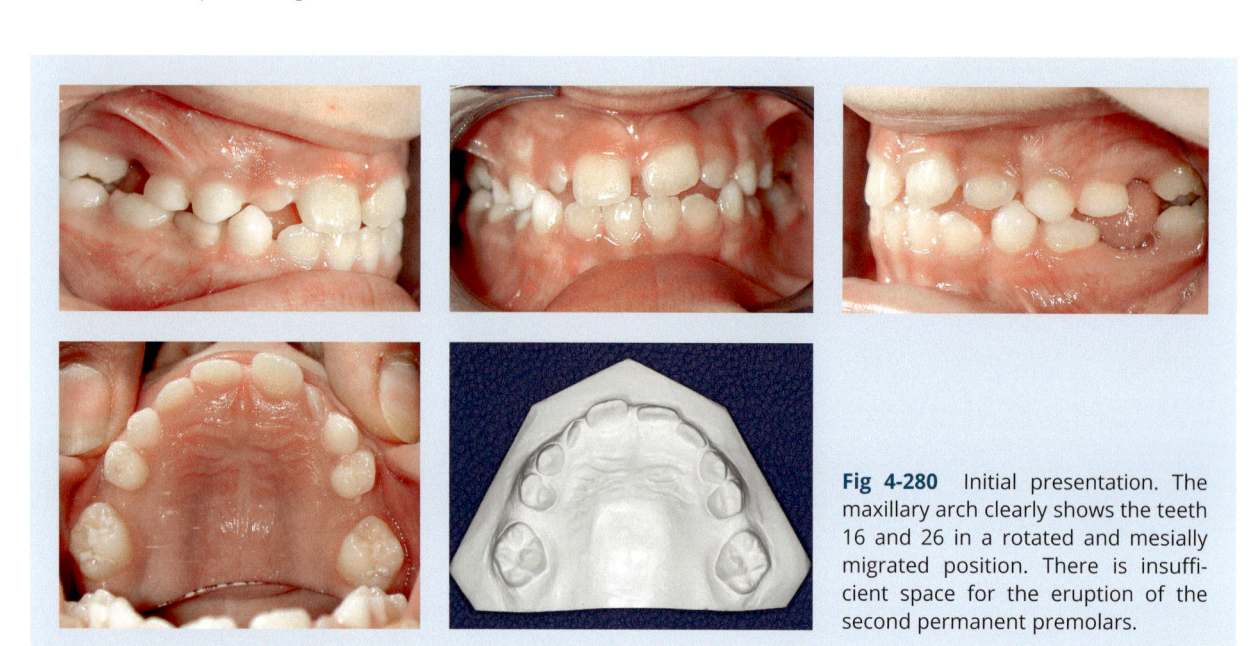

Fig 4-280 Initial presentation. The maxillary arch clearly shows the teeth 16 and 26 in a rotated and mesially migrated position. There is insufficient space for the eruption of the second permanent premolars.

Diagnosis:
- mesial migration of maxillary molars after early extraction of primary teeth 55 and 65.

Therapy:
- distalization of maxillary molars
- space opening for the eruption of permanent teeth 15 and 25.

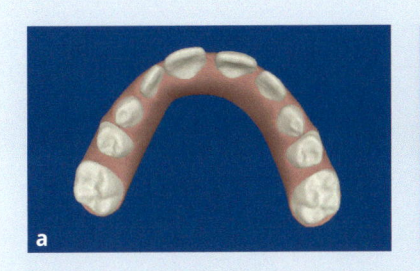

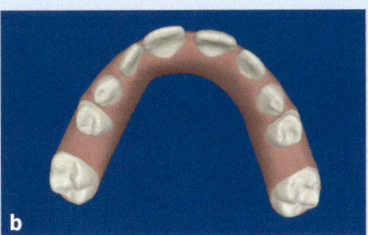

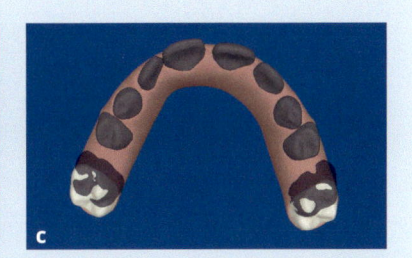

Fig 4-281 ClinCheck software results. The ClinCheck pictures show **(a)** Initial situation. **(b)** Final situation. **(c)** Superimposition to show the planned movement of the maxillary first molars (blue, initial tooth position; white, final tooth position).

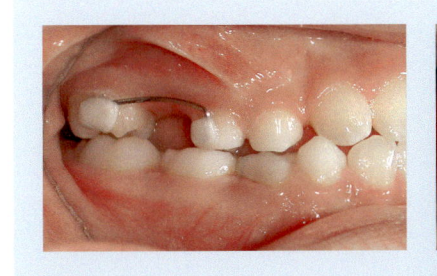

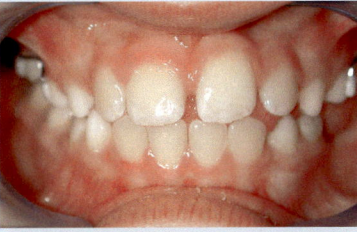

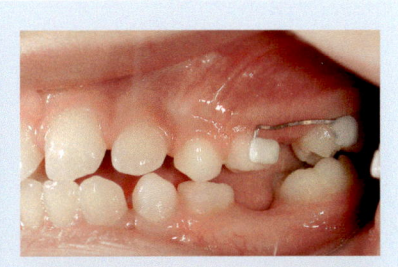

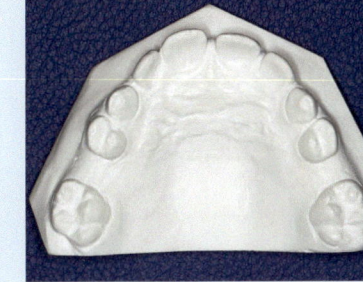

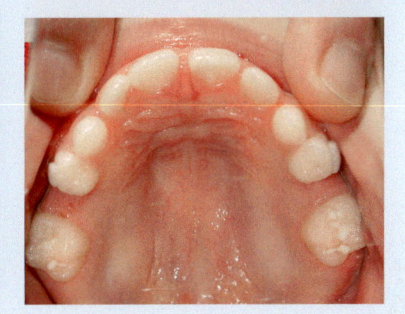

Fig 4-282 Intraoral situation after the Invisalign treatment with fixed sectional wires on teeth 54 to 16 and 64 to 26.

Treatment

A dentist had extracted primary teeth 55 and 65 without holding the spaces open with an intraoral appliance. As a consequence, permanent teeth 16 and 26 had migrated mesially and reduced the space for the eruption of the permanent teeth 15 and 25.

Based on the ClinCheck results (Fig 4-281), treatment used 14 aligners and, to obtain fast results, the wearing time of each aligner was reduced exceptionally to 9 instead of 14 days. The reduction from the usual 14 days is possible but should be performed with great care and requires substantial experience with the Invisalign system. In children and teenagers, this reduction can sometimes be an option when a high number of aligners are used. Should the patient not feel comfortable with the increased pressure on the teeth with the aligner change, the wearing time can be expanded again to 14 days.

After Invisalign treatment, the molars have been distalized and derotated; spaces have been opened with sufficient space for the eruption of teeth 15 and 25 (Fig 4-282). Teeth 16 and 26 show a correct axial inclination (Fig 4-283). Stainless steel sectional wires were bonded to the maxillary first molars and primary teeth 54 and 64 for retention.

The patient returned to have pictures taken a few years later (Fig 4-284). Teeth 15 and 25 had erupted perfectly and he had harmonious arches in class I rela-

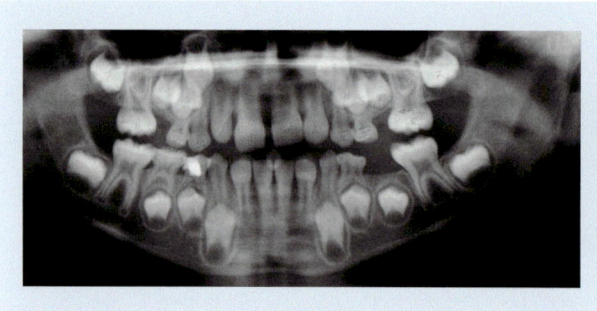

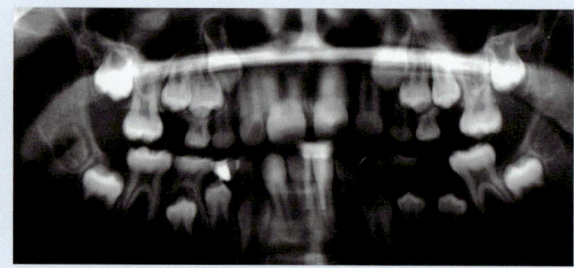

Fig 4-283 Orthopantomography before **(left)** and after **(right)** treatment.

Fig 4-284 Intraoral views several years after treatment and full eruption of all permanent teeth.

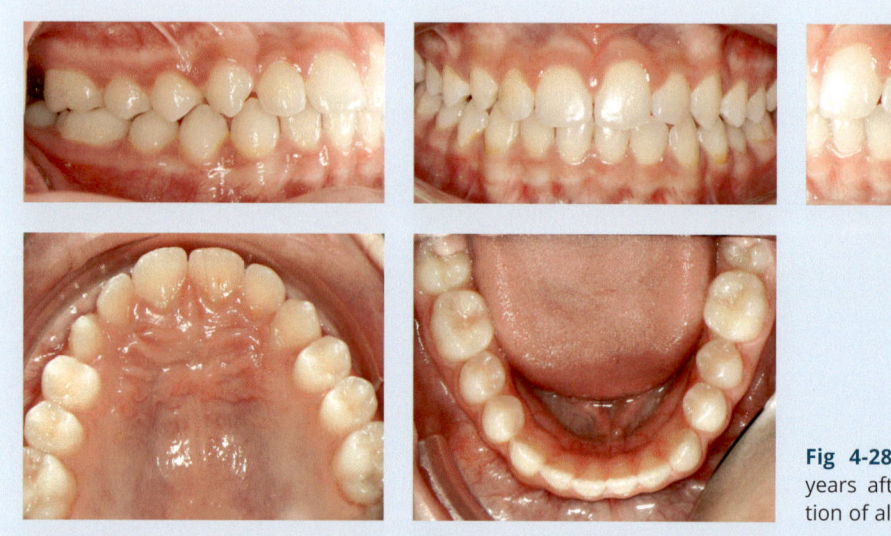

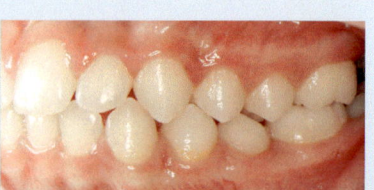

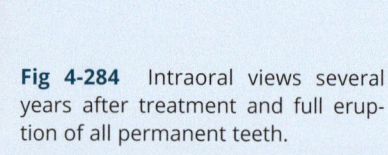

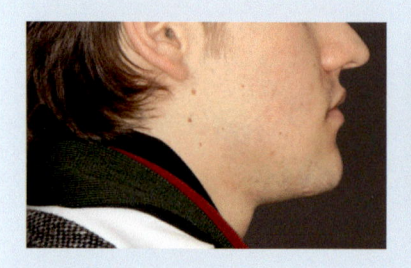

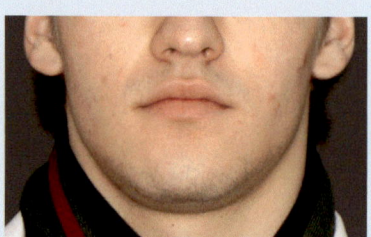

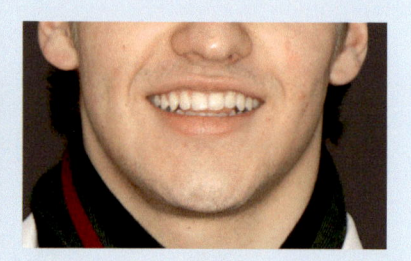

Fig 4-285 Extraoral views at age 17 after receiving a hit to the mandible.

tionship. Further orthodontic treatment was not needed. Without the distalization, performed with Invisalign system, extractions might have been inevitable.

Subsequent treatment
At age 17, the patient presented after receiving a hit to the left horizontal part of the mandible. The extraoral view showed swellings in the area (Fig 4-285). The patient reported pain in the right TMJ, which was his reason for returning, having already been examined at a hospital near his school abroad. He said that his bite had significantly changed after the accident.

Orthopantomography showed a slight fissure in the upper mandible (Fig 4-286) and intraoral views

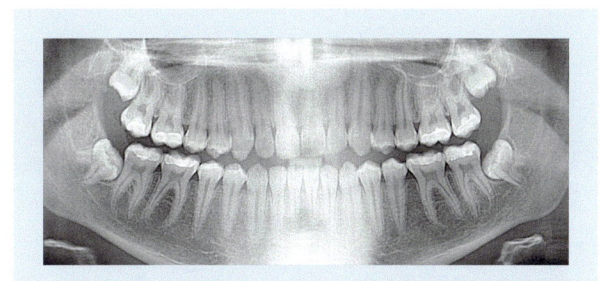

TREATMENT OF DIFFERENT MALOCCLUSIONS WITH ALIGNERS 4

Fig 4-286 Orthopantomography after the accident.

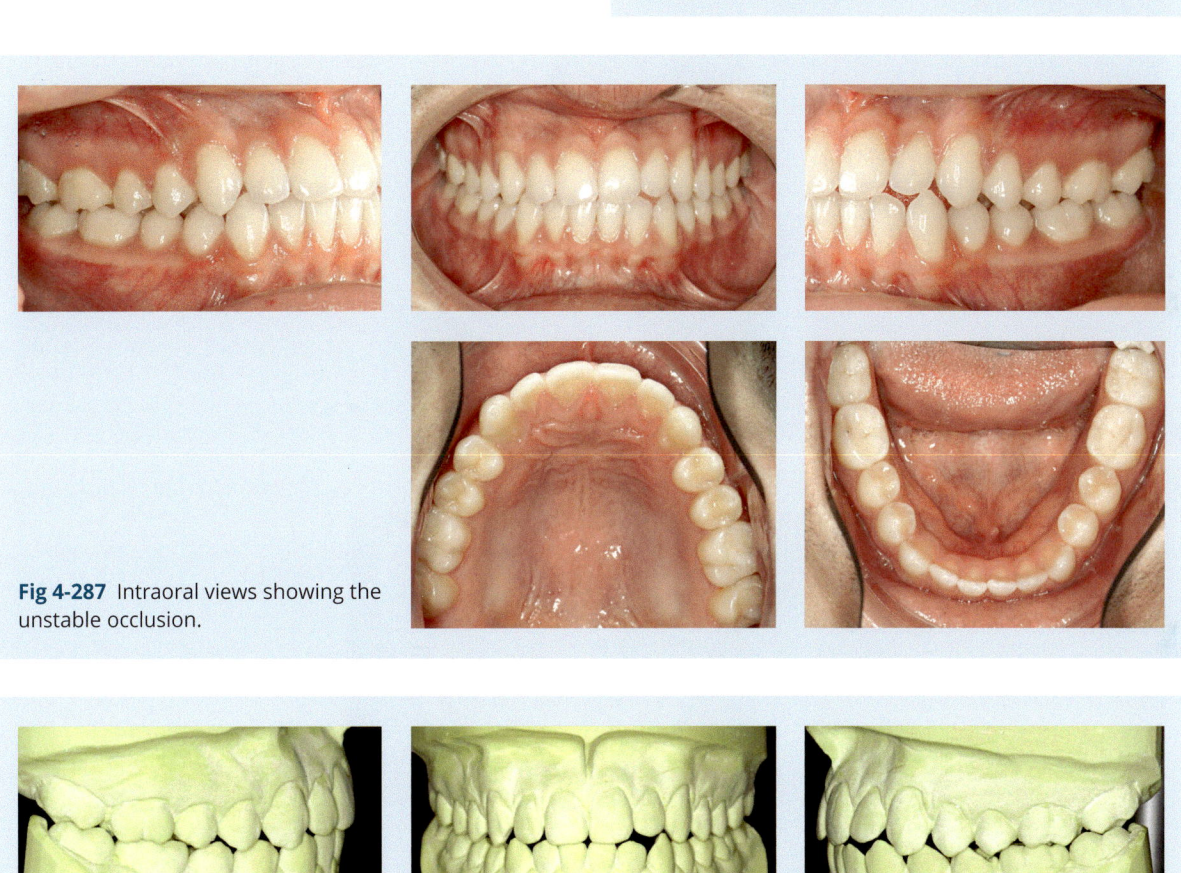

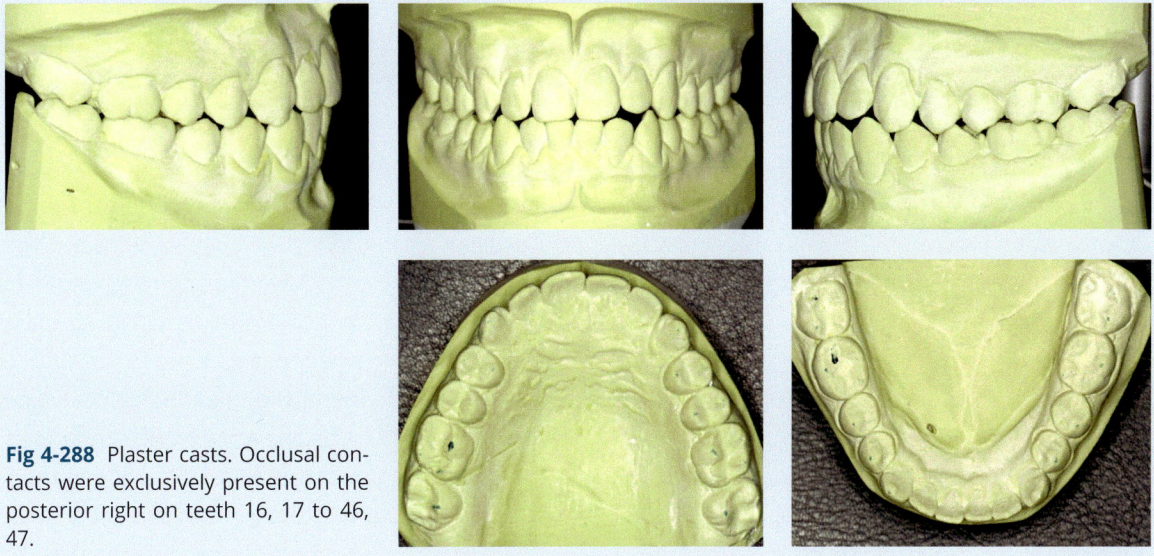

Fig 4-287 Intraoral views showing the unstable occlusion.

Fig 4-288 Plaster casts. Occlusal contacts were exclusively present on the posterior right on teeth 16, 17 to 46, 47.

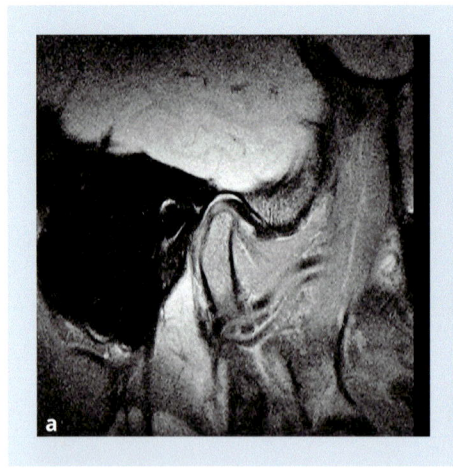

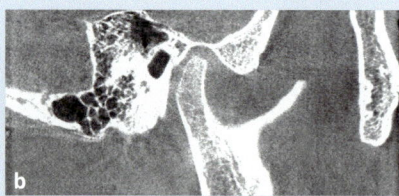

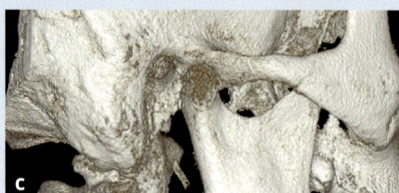

Fig 4-289 Imaging results. **(a)** MRT of the right mandible shows a disruption of the discus articularis. The bilaminar zone is ruptured in the posterior area and the disc dislocated anteriorly. **(b,c)** CBCT does not show any fractures in the area of the descending mandible or the condyle. The retral displacement of the condyle from traumatic anterior disc displacement is visible. (a, courtesy of Media-Park Clinic, Cologne; b, Picasso, Orange Dental.)

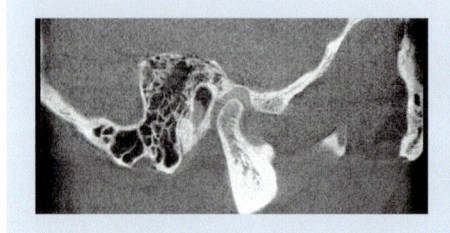

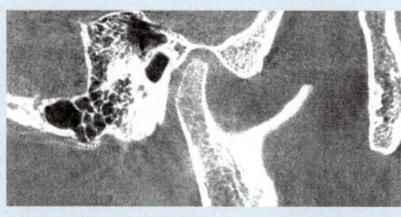

Fig 4-290 TMJ space. **(left)** Normal TMJ average joint space is 2.5 mm anterior, 3 mm superior, and 2.3 mm posterior. **(right)** CBCT indicated a reduced joint space of 1.2 mm.

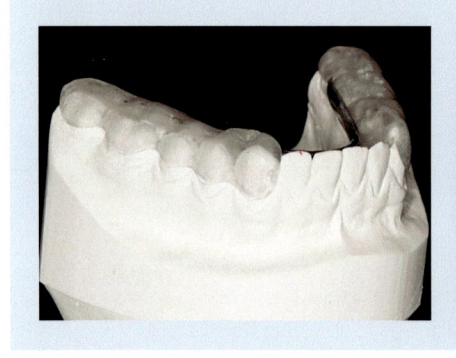

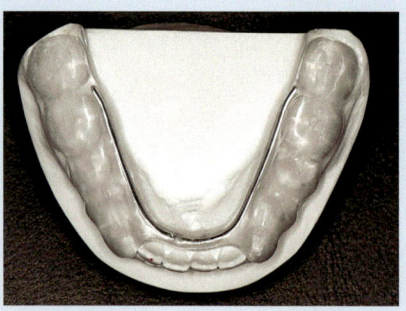

Fig 4-291 Plaster cast showing COPA fabrication.

and plaster casts showed unstable occlusion with non-occlusion of several teeth (Figs 4-287 and 4-288).

As orthopantomography is not suitable for condyle diagnostics, magnetic resonance tomography (MRT) and CBCT were performed (Fig 4-289). The CBCT image was used to assess the posterior joint space compared to average space (Dizidienda, 2011). He was advised to have his wisdom extracted after convalescence.

As a first step, a removable occlusal splint (craniomandibular orthopedic positioning appliance (COPA)) for the mandibular arch was fabricated to provide the patient with posterior height and, therefore, a less painful position for the condyle (Fig 4-291). Additionally, the patient was advised to have manual mobilization by a physiotherapist. The COPA was modified after every appointment for occlusal changes.

An alternative therapeutic option might have been the arthroscopic recapturing of the disc according to Yang. Once the patient was pain free, there was still unstable occlusion resulting from the traumatically

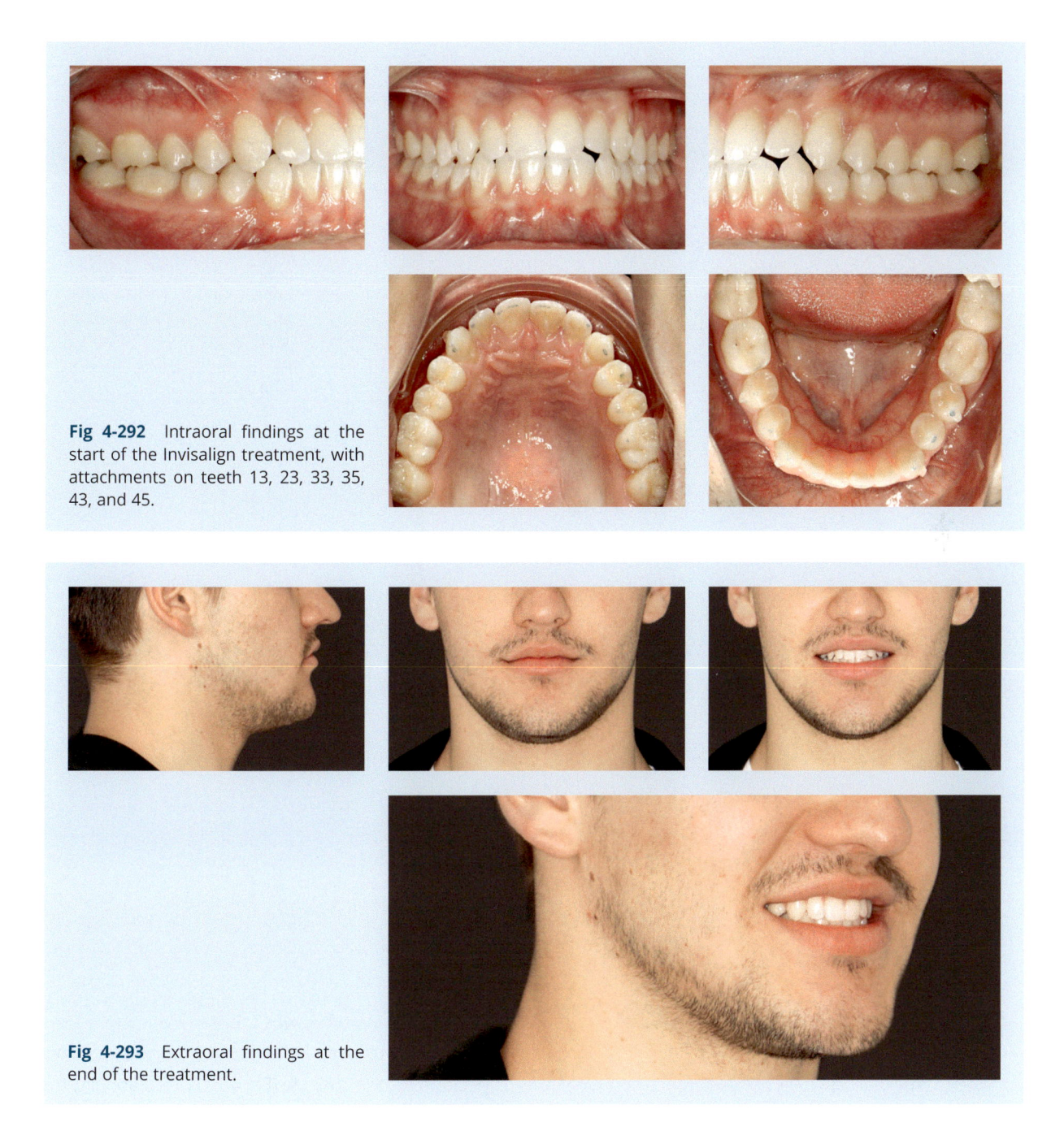

Fig 4-292 Intraoral findings at the start of the Invisalign treatment, with attachments on teeth 13, 23, 33, 35, 43, and 45.

Fig 4-293 Extraoral findings at the end of the treatment.

injured joint, which was planned to be treated with the Invisalign system (Fig 4-292).

After Invisalign treatment, there is harmonious facial symmetry (Fig 4-293); the arches are aligned in stable occlusion (Fig 4-294), and casts show equal contact points on all posteriors with canine guidance (Fig 4-295).

The patient was pain free, but arthrosis of the right joint was still a potential risk. This was assessed with CBCT at a later date (Fig 4-296).

4 TREATMENT OF DIFFERENT MALOCCLUSIONS WITH ALIGNERS

Fig 4-294 Intraoral findings at the end of the treatment.

Fig 4-295 Casts after the Invisalign treatment.

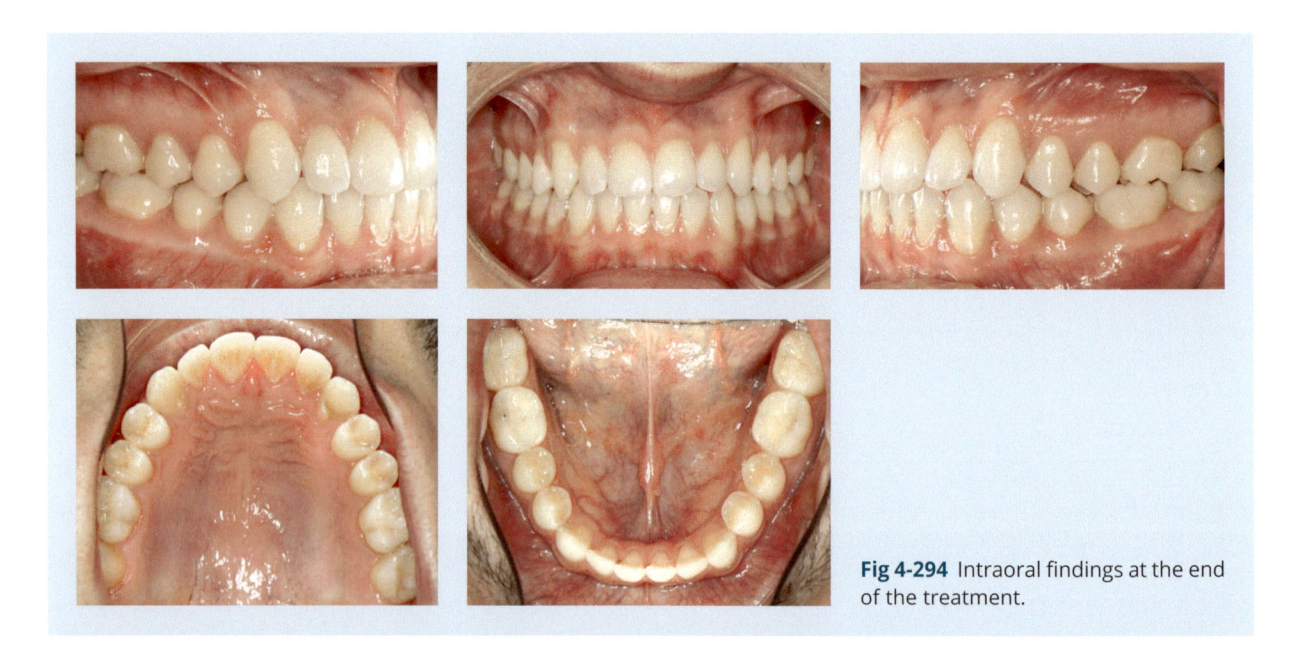

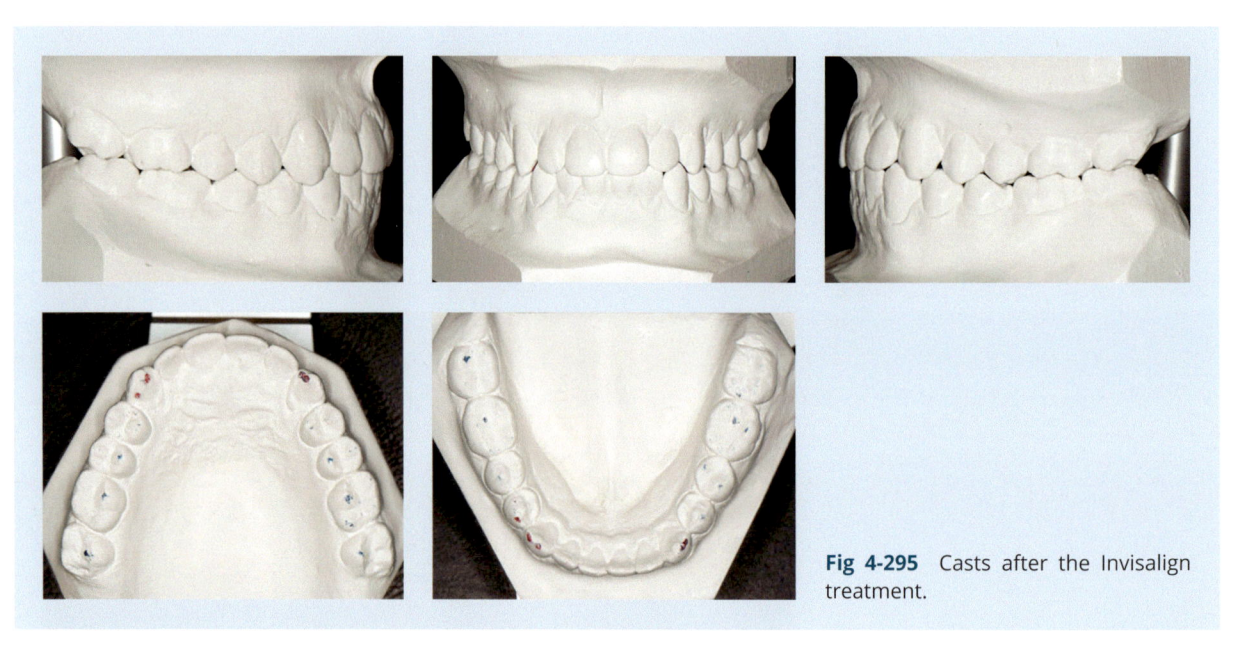

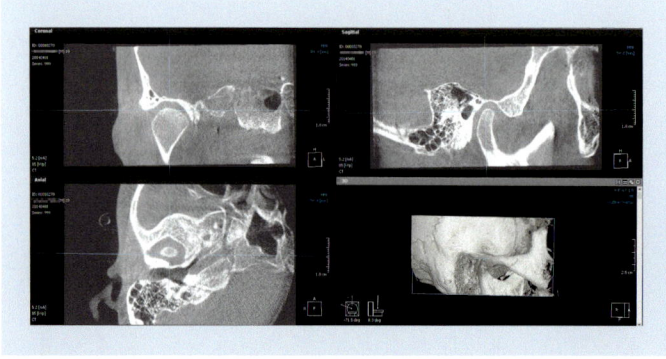

Fig 4-296 CBCT of the condyle 2 years and 9 months after the accident. There are no arthrosis alterations in the cortical bone. The condyle in the right joint is positioned slightly distally and the medial joint space has a minor reduction in size.

Topic 39
Creation of space for the eruption of a tooth in a young patient

Treatment:
- space opening

This topic shows the treatment of a young patient to create space for eruption of a mandibular canine without using extractions. Opening of spaces in teenagers is highly predictable with the Invisalign system.

This child had insufficient space for eruption of permanent tooth 43 due to mesially drifted molars and lower incisal shift to the right (Fig 4-297). Invisalign treatment started at the age of 8.5 years.

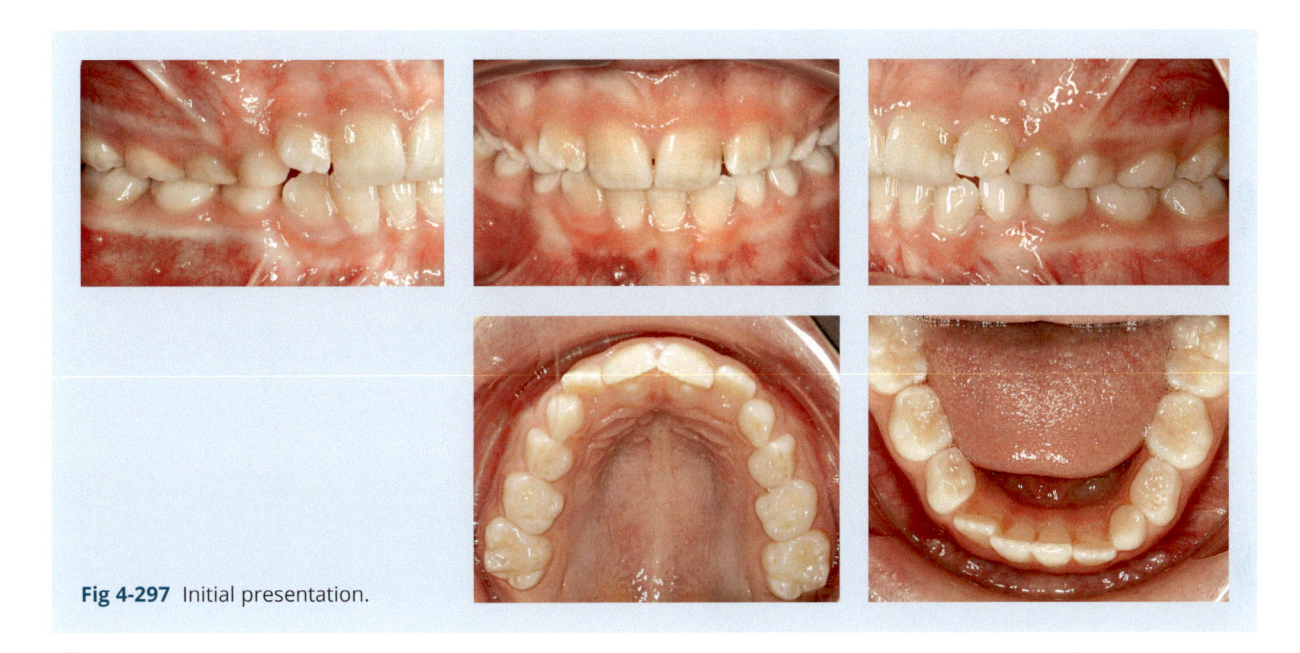

Fig 4-297 Initial presentation.

Diagnosis:
- insufficient space for eruption of tooth 43
- mesially drifted tooth 84 to almost approximal contact of tooth 42.

Therapy:
- distalization of tooth 46 and movement of lower incisors to the left
- space opening for the eruption of permanent tooth 43.

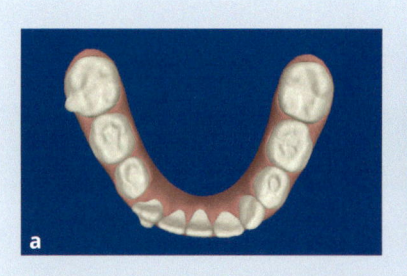

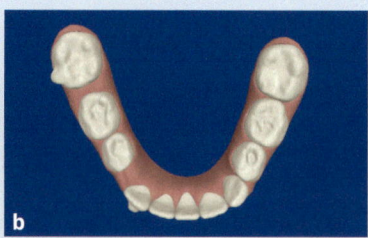

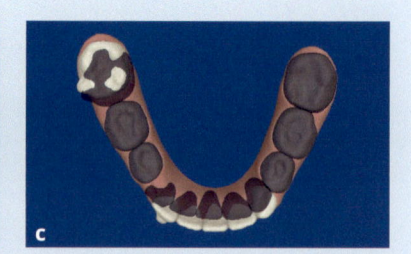

Fig 4-298 ClinCheck software results. **(a)** Initial situation with almost complete space closure regio 43. **(b)** Planned final situation. **(c)** Superimposition to show planned teeth movements in the mandibular arch (blue, initial tooth position; white, final tooth position).

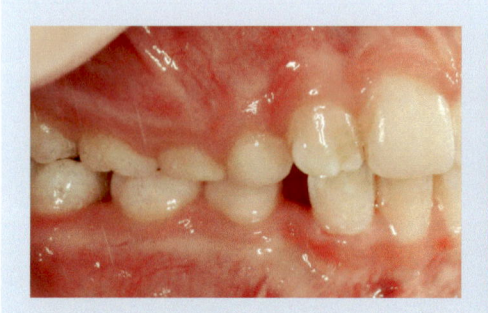

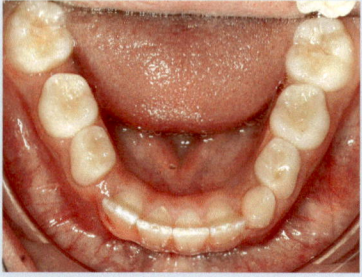

Fig 4-299 Final intraoral situation.

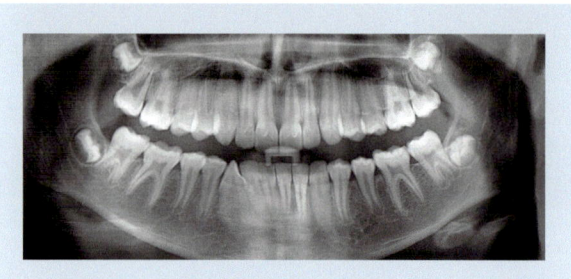

Fig 4-300 Orthopantomography 3 years after the Invisalign treatment start and full eruption of all permanent teeth. Tooth 43 has erupted in a rotated position.

Treatment

Invisalign treatment started when the child was 8.5 years of age. The ClinCheck images were used to plan treament (Fig 4-298). Tooth 46 was distalized 2 mm; tooth 42 was mesialized 2.5 mm. All mandibular anterior teeth were to be proclined for further space opening. The treatment consisted of 21 aligners, which the young patient changed every 10 days.

The final intraoral situation showed opening of space mesial of tooth 46 and distal of tooth 42 (Fig 4-299). By distalizing tooth 46 and protruding the mandibular incisors with bodily movement, space for the eruption of tooth 43 was created without needing extractions. The gingiva in the incisor and canine area is in healthy and stable conditions. A three year follow up Orthopantomography showed the eruption of the permanent dentition with rotation of tooth 43 (Fig 4-300).

After the complete eruption of all permanent teeth at age 11.5 years, a second phase of the Invisalign treatment was started, this time to treat the occlusion

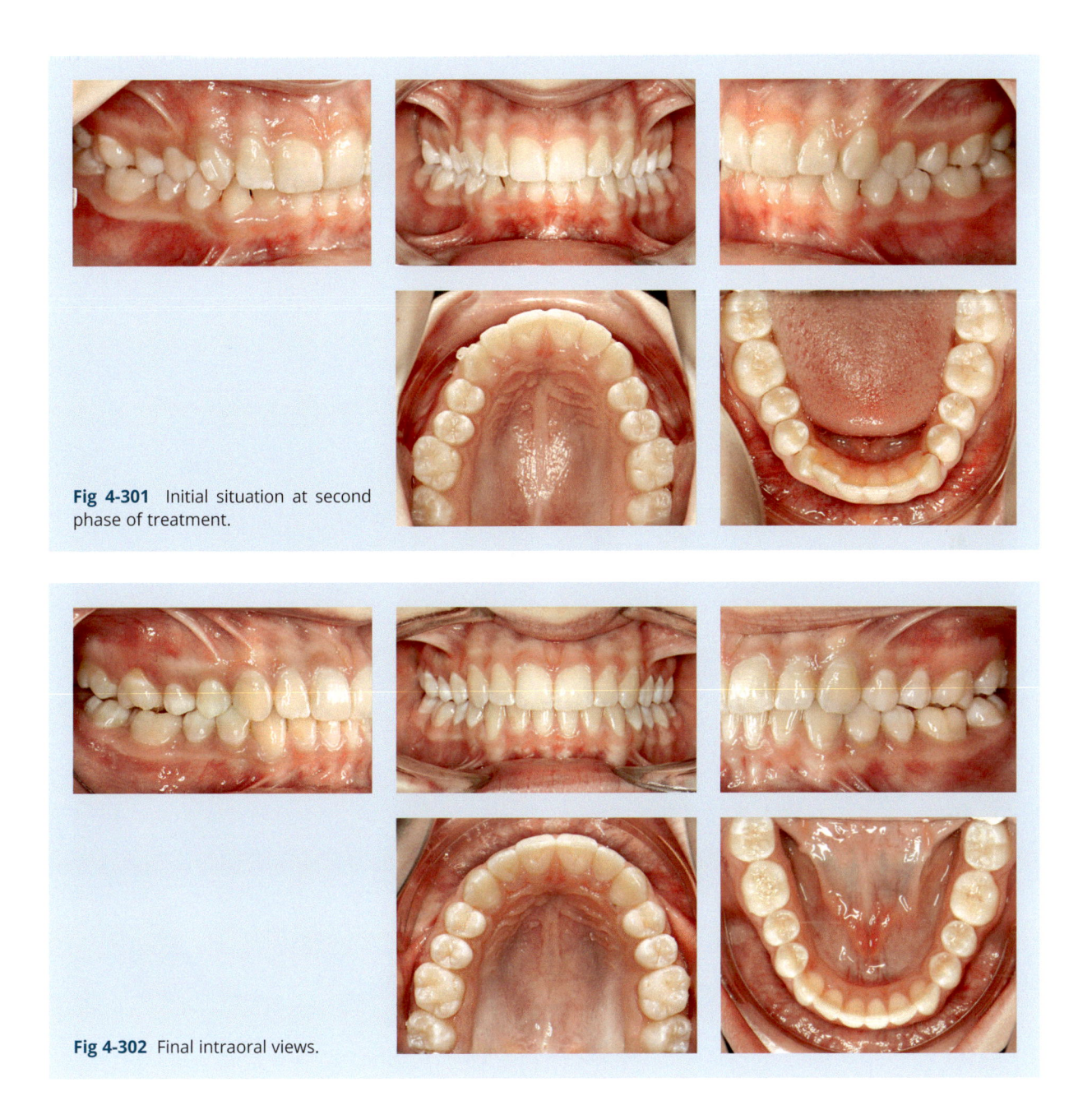

Fig 4-301 Initial situation at second phase of treatment.

Fig 4-302 Final intraoral views.

in detail. Tooth 43 had erupted rotated and needed derotation with overcorrection of the mesial aspect to lingual. To obtain space for alignment, 0.2 mm IPR was performed from mesial tooth 32 to distal 43, 30 aligners were used in the mandibular arch plus 20 aligners in the maxilla (Fig 4-301).

At the end of this phase, the mandibular arch has been well aligned and tooth 43 completely rotated. The lateral views (Fig 4-302) show a slightly posterior open bite on the first and second molars but full contact on premolars. The patient refused a refinement for posterior extrusion into hard collision. Therefore, a lingual retainer from mandibular first premolar to first premolar was bonded for retention, allowing the posterior teeth to settle into a stable occlusion. Orthopantomography shows no pathology (Fig 4-303). Wisdom teeth 18, 28, 38, 48 were advised for extraction.

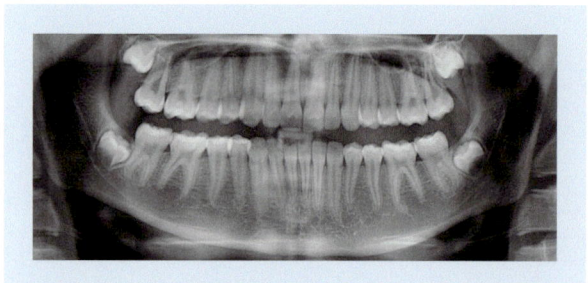

Fig 4-303 Orthopantomography.

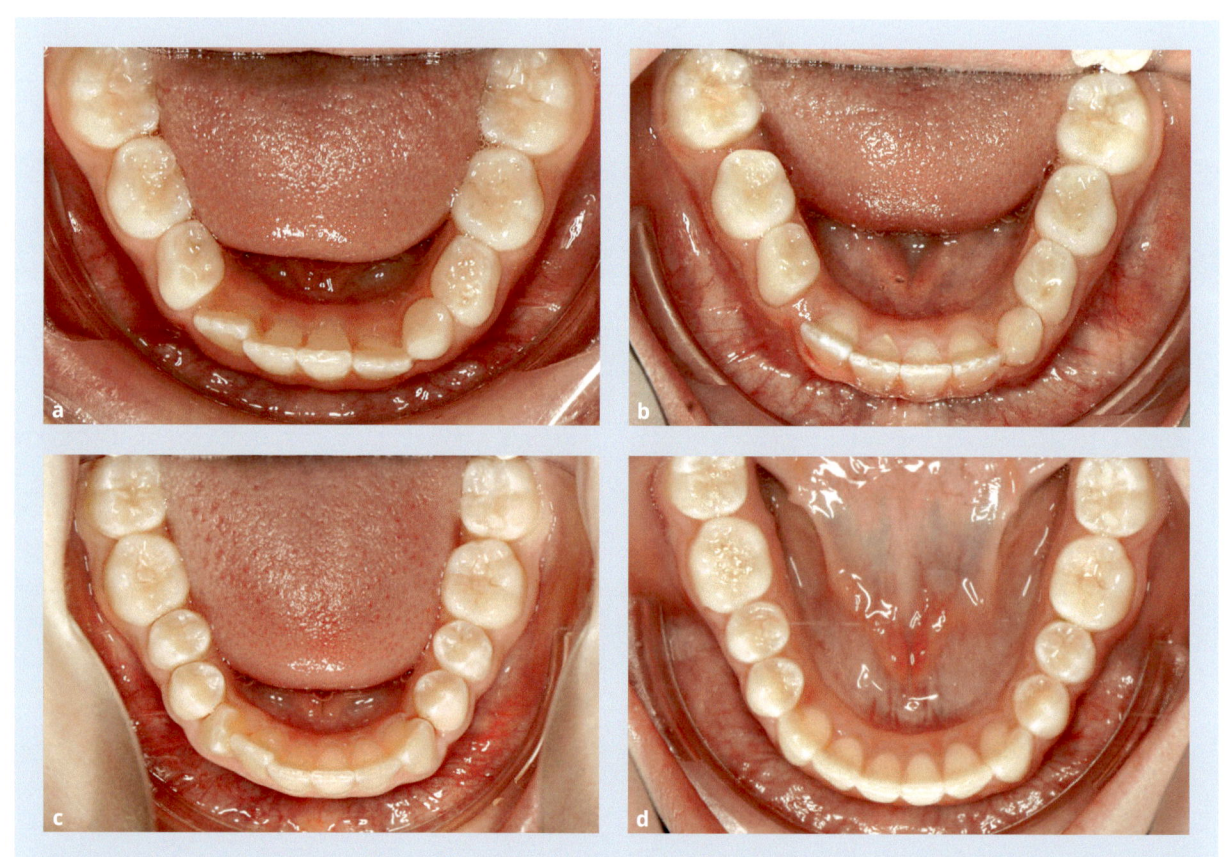

Fig 4-304 Intraoral views. **(a)** Initial situation before treatment. **(b)** End of the first phase with space for eruption of tooth 43 and protrusion of mandibular incisors and distalization of tooth 46. **(c)** Start of the second phase after the eruption of all permanent teeth with tooth 43 in a rotated position. **(d)** End of the second phase with harmonically aligned mandibular arch and derotated tooth 43.

Figure 4-304 shows the treatment pathway and Figure 4-305 the situation 2 years after completion of treatment. The patient wears additionally a removable aligner (Lamitec, Hinz Dental) at night in the maxilla. Both arches show equal occlusal contacts on all posteriors and canines.

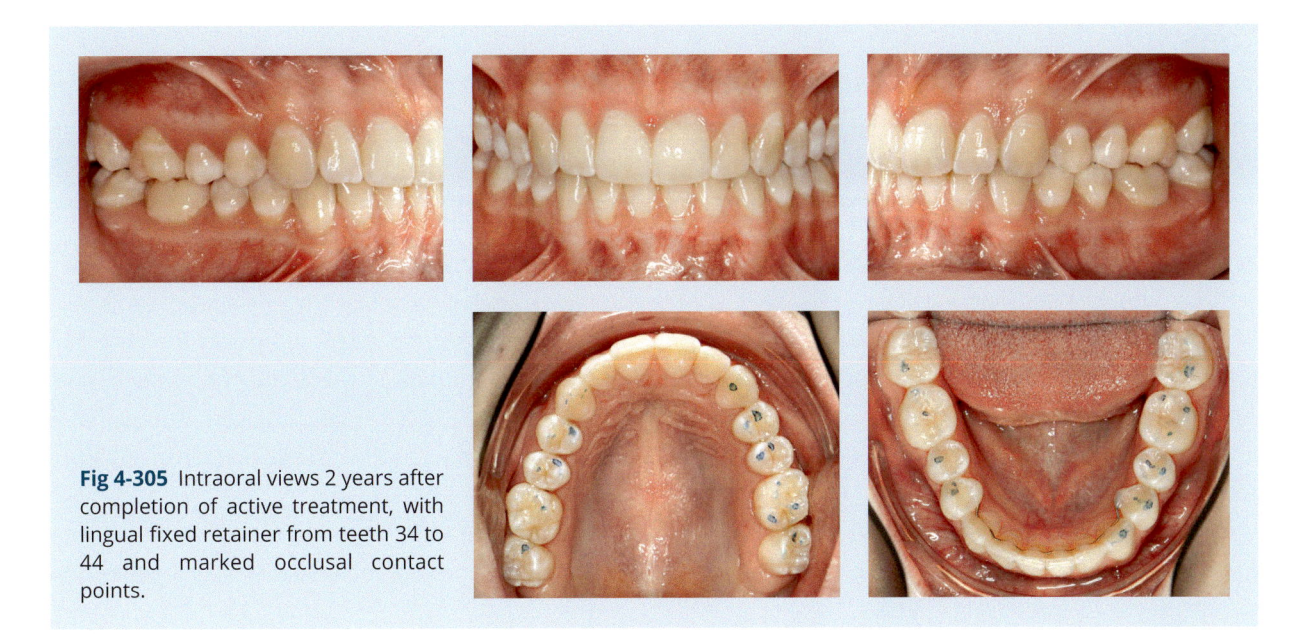

Fig 4-305 Intraoral views 2 years after completion of active treatment, with lingual fixed retainer from teeth 34 to 44 and marked occlusal contact points.

Topic 40
Teenager with spaces and agenesis of two teeth

Treatment:
- space opening for implants

In patients with agenesis, it is necessary to discuss different therapeutic possibilities, such as opening of spaces for later implants and restoratives or closing of spaces completely. Independent of the chosen option, space opening or space closure, the decision should be based on the advantages and disadvantages of the potential functional and esthetic results. For space closure, it is important to point out also the eventual necessity to deal with arch asymmetries with additional anchorage using temporary anchorage devices. Implants in regions of adequate bone seem to be a good option but the final decision must be taken by the patient, and parents/carers too for children.

This patient has the chin in optimal position in relation to the midline of the philtrum and the face has a harmonious skeletal midline (Fig 4-306). Orthopantomography shows agenesis of teeth 35 and 45 with persisting primary teeth 75 and 85 (Fig 4-307).

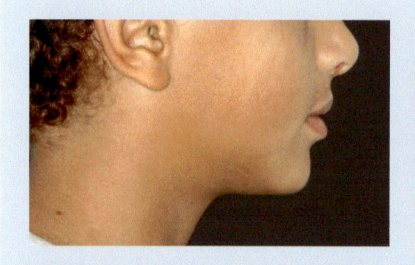

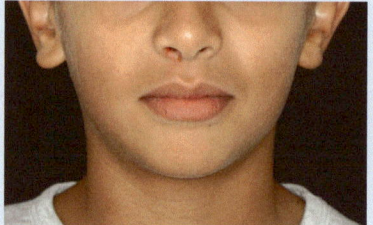

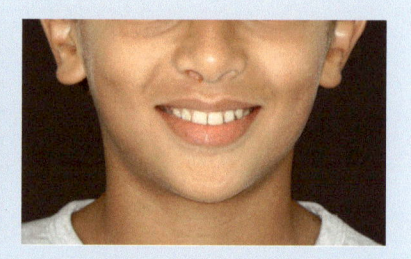

Fig 4-306 Initial presentation.

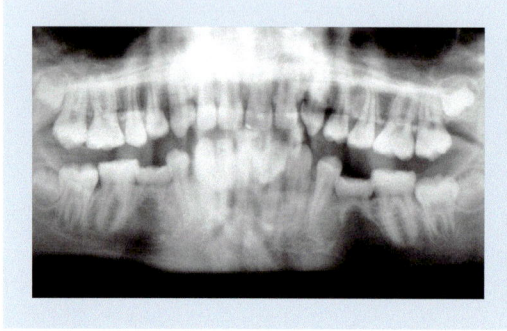

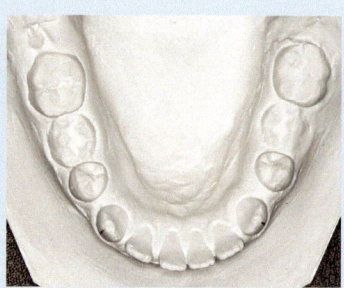

Fig 4-307 Agenesis of teeth 35 and 45 with persisting primary teeth 75 and 85. **(left)** Orthopantomography (performed alio loco). **(right)** Plaster cast of the mandibular arch at the beginning of the treatment.

Diagnosis:
- class I relationship on the right
- class II relationship on the left
- mandibular dental midline shift to the left
- slight enamel alteration and abrasion of first mandibular molars.

Therapy:
- Invisalign treatment
- implants for restoratives.

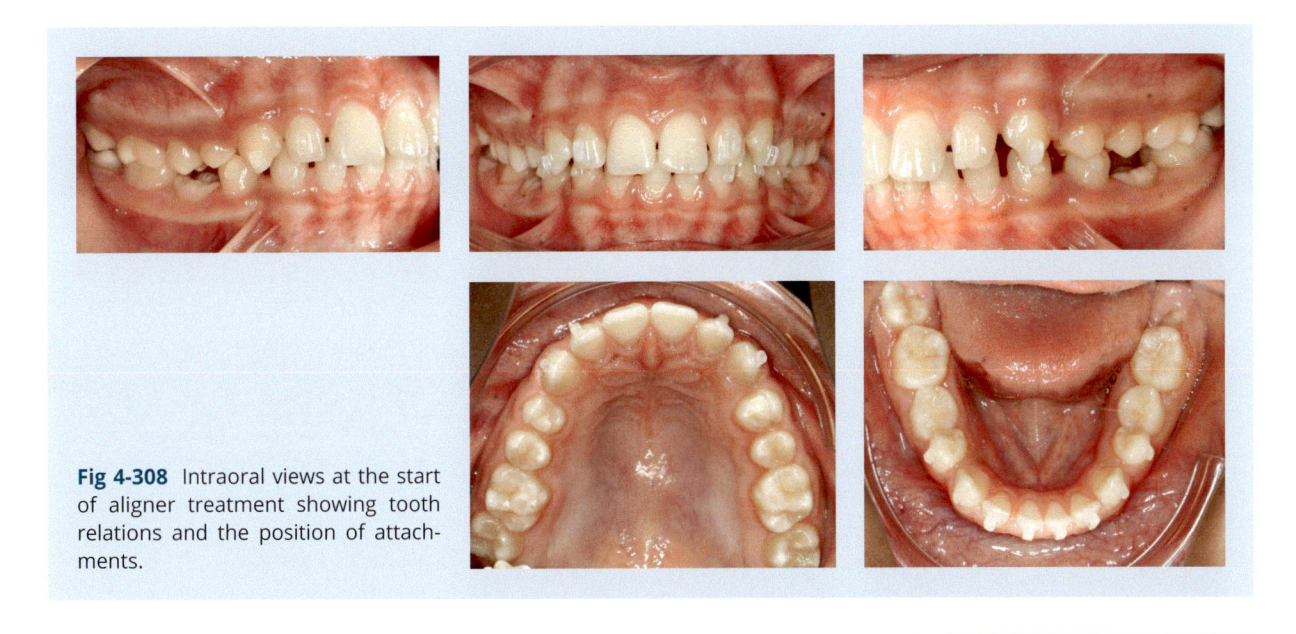

Fig 4-308 Intraoral views at the start of aligner treatment showing tooth relations and the position of attachments.

Fig 4-309 ClinCheck software results showing the planned changes.

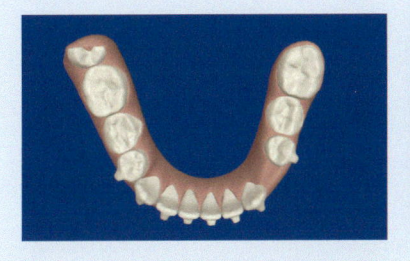

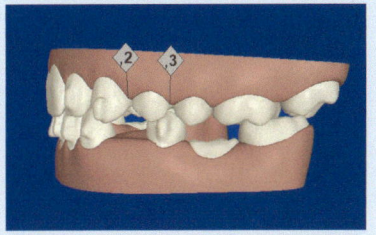

Treatment

The occlusion at the start of Invisalign treatment shows a class I relationship on the right side, a class II relationship on the left side, and a mandibular dental midline shift to the left of 3 mm. The first molars in the mandibular arch show slight enamel alteration and abrasion. Vertical rectangular attachments were bonded to teeth 13, 12, 22, 23, 34, 33, 32, 31, 41, 42, 43, and 44 (Fig 4-308).

The virtual images from the ClinCheck software show the treatment plan (Fig 4-309). Because of the existing mandibular midline deviation to the left, it was necessary to correct the mandibular midline to the right. As correction of the lower midline to the right while mesializing lower molars 36, 37 to reduce the spaces is a movement requiring high anchorage, we decided an alternative pathway with mesializing the lower left front teeth while remaining in the class II molar relationship. Consequently, two implants would be necessary on the mandibular left side, mesial of tooth 34 and after the extraction of tooth 75 also in region 35. Phase one used 28 aligners (Figs 4-310 to 4-314).

The occlusion after orthodontic treatment shows an optimal physiologic situation (Fig 4-315). At this point, the patient was transferred to the implantologist (Dr M Bäumer, Cologne).

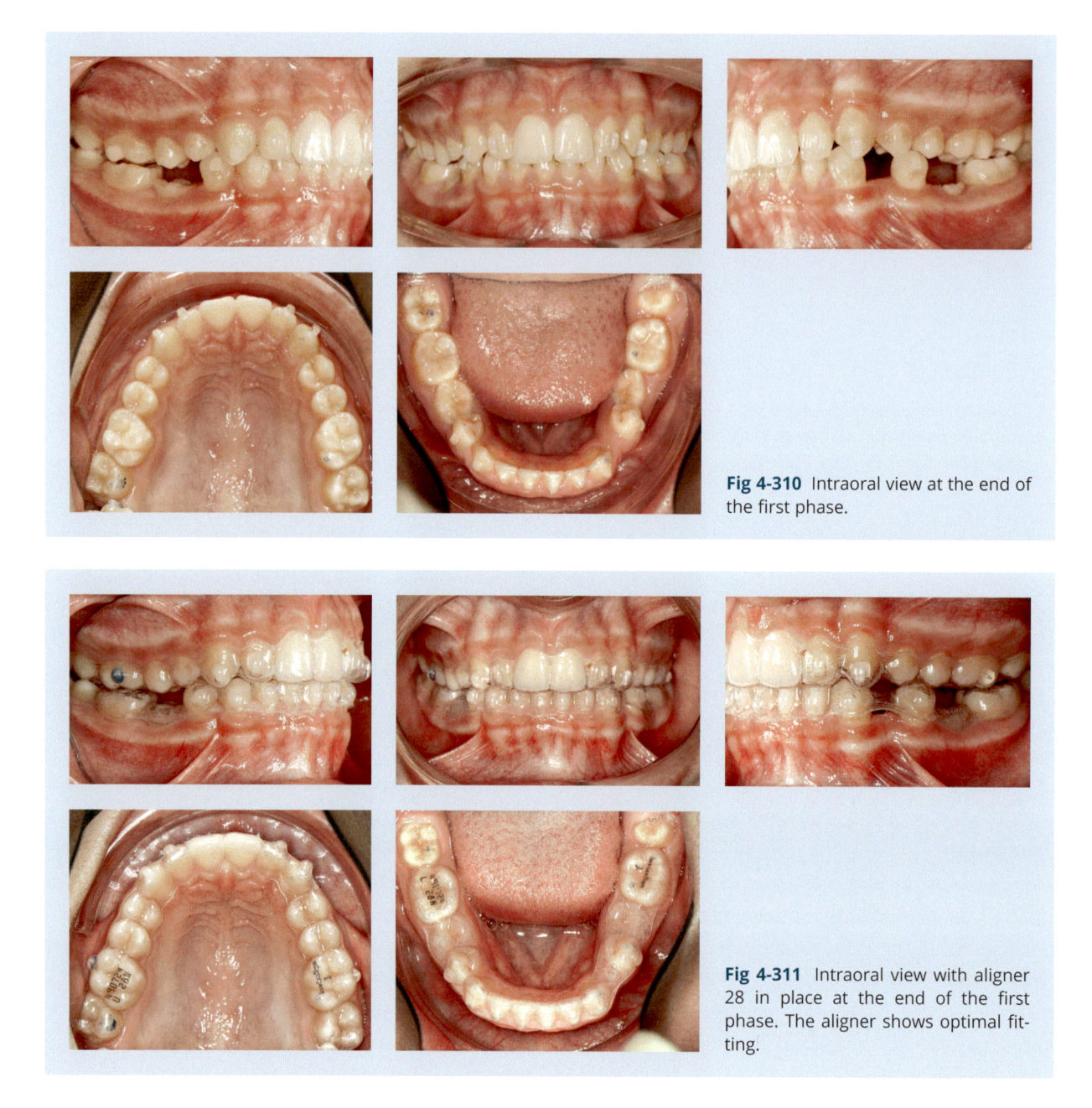

4 TREATMENT OF DIFFERENT MALOCCLUSIONS WITH ALIGNERS

Fig 4-310 Intraoral view at the end of the first phase.

Fig 4-311 Intraoral view with aligner 28 in place at the end of the first phase. The aligner shows optimal fitting.

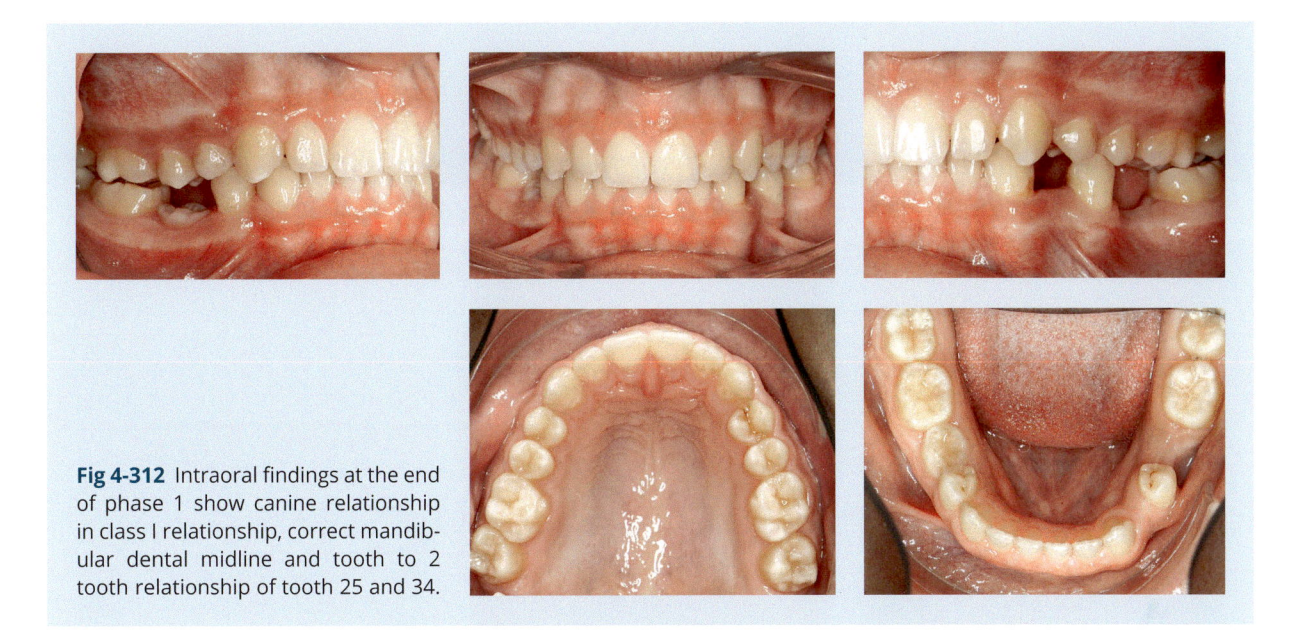

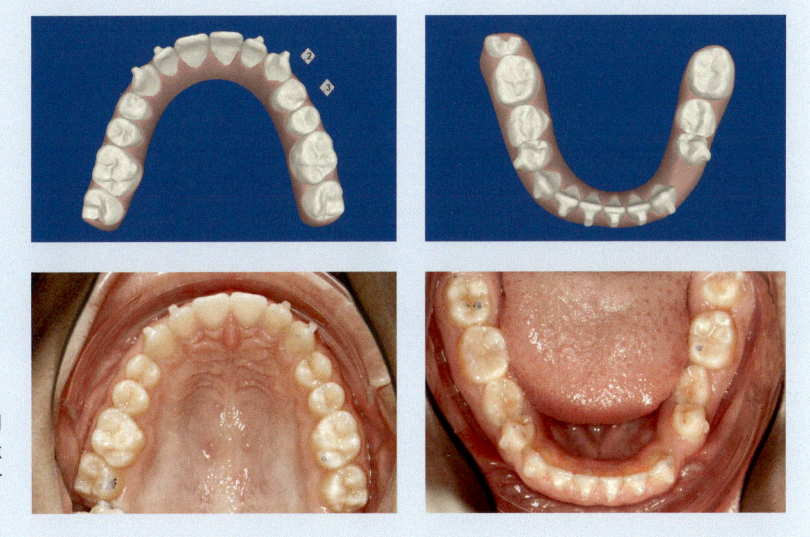

Fig 4-312 Intraoral findings at the end of phase 1 show canine relationship in class I relationship, correct mandibular dental midline and tooth to 2 tooth relationship of tooth 25 and 34.

Fig 4-313 Comparison of planned treatment outcome in the ClinCheck software and intraoral situation after phase 1.

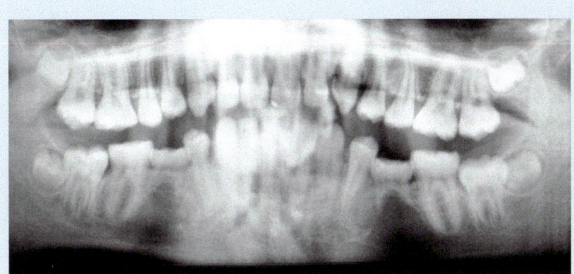

Fig 4-314 Orthopantomography before and after phase 1.

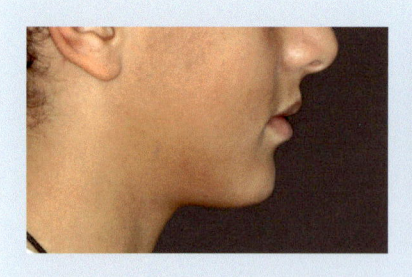

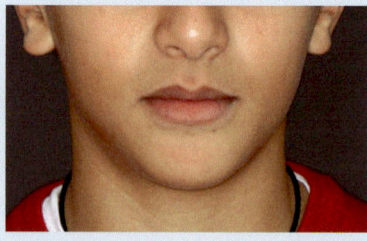

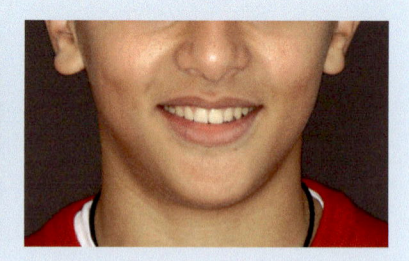

Fig 4-315 Facial views at the end of orthodontic treatment with maintained correct midline and symmetry.

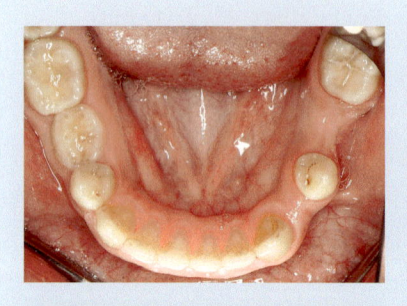

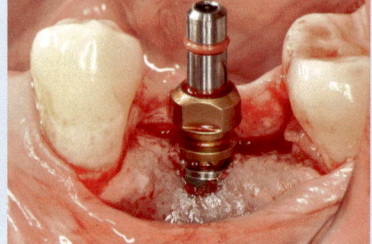

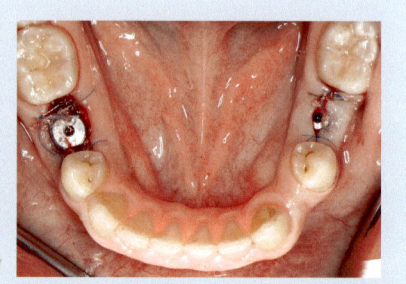

Fig 4-316 Implant insertion.

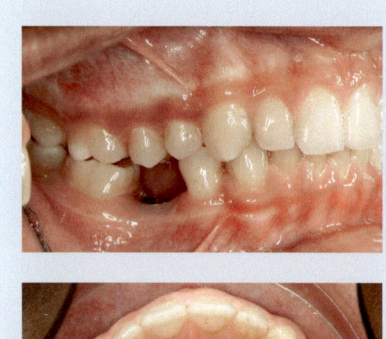

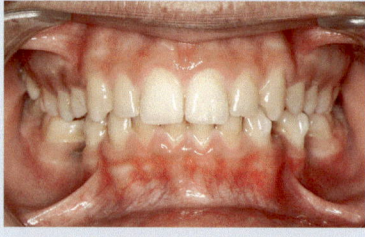

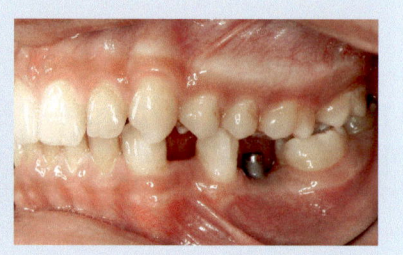

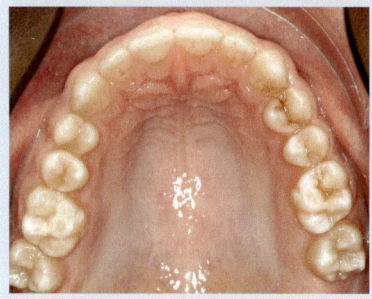

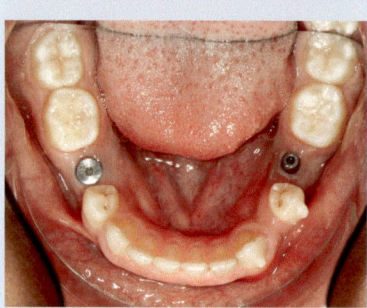

Fig 4-317 Intraoral situation with implants.

Primary tooth 85 was extracted and replaced with an implant (Fig 4-316).

Implants were placed in the sites of teeth 35 and 45. Roots of teeth 33 and 34 were still tipped and space for the planned implant was insufficient (Figs 4-317 and 4-318). Vertical rectangular attachments were added on teeth 33 and 34 and a refinement for root movement of tooth 33 to mesial, and of 34 to distal for space opening was planned (Fig 4-319). This refinement used IPR mesial on tooth 33 and 14 aligners for uprighting of the roots of teeth 33 and 34 to provide sufficient bone for the placement of the implant in this area.

Fig 4-318 Radiography. **(left)** Insufficient space for implant distal of tooth 33 because of tipped roots of 33 and 34. **(right)** Situation after insertion of implant distal of 34 and relation indicator mesial of 34.

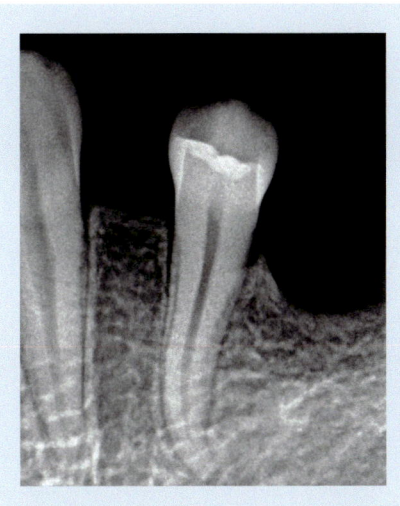

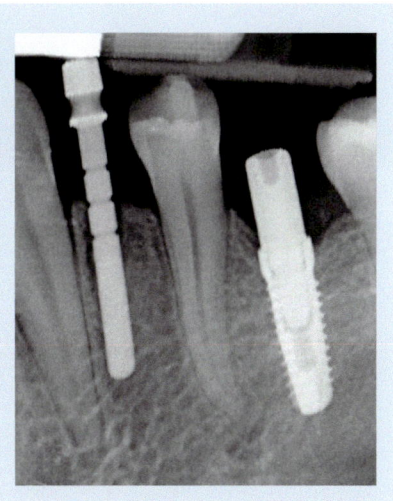

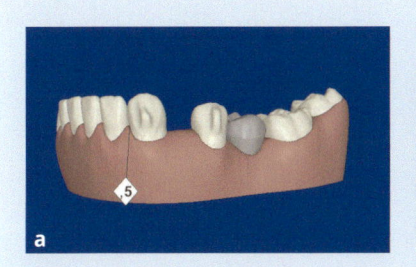

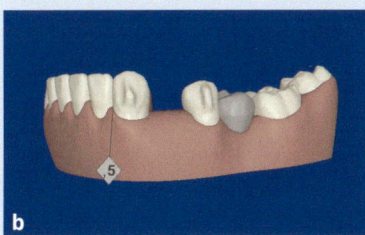

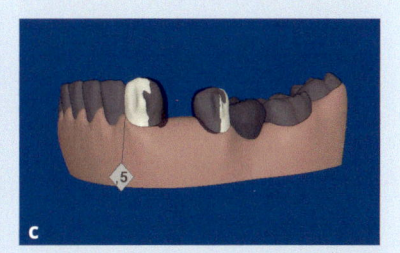

Fig 4-319 ClinCheck software results. **(a)** Before the additional deangulation of teeth 33 and 34 and IPR. **(b)** Planned outcome. **(c)** Superimposition showing the planned movement (blue, initial tooth position; white, final tooth position).

The implant in the region distal of tooth 33 was inserted following after the refinement (Fig 4-320).

Figure 4-321 shows the implants in regions 35, 34+, and 45.

The final result with implants and prosthetics is shown in Figures 4-322 and 4-323.

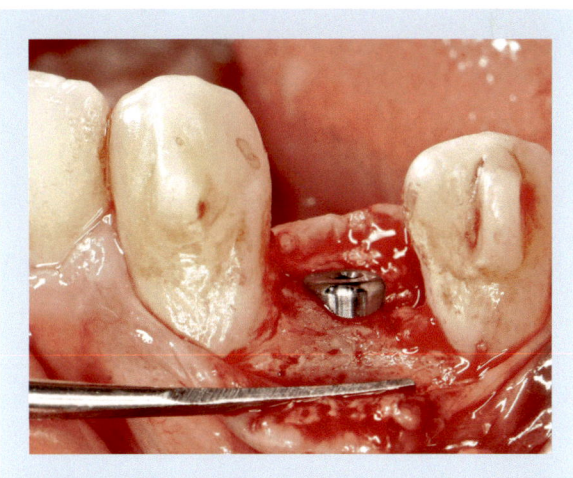

Fig 4-320 Insertion of implant in the region distal of tooth 33.

4 TREATMENT OF DIFFERENT MALOCCLUSIONS WITH ALIGNERS

Fig 4-321 Implants in regions 35, 34+, and 45.

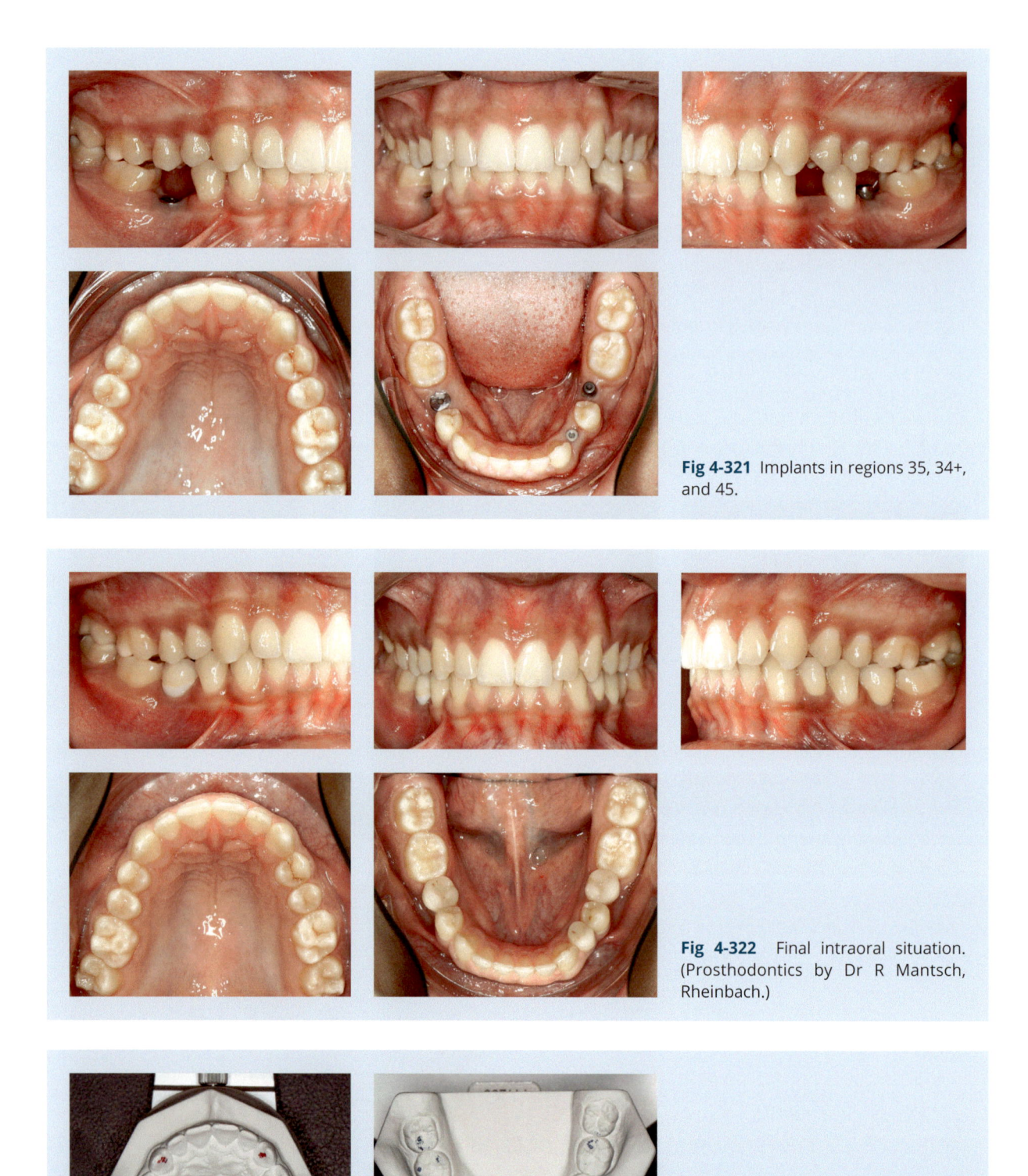

Fig 4-322 Final intraoral situation. (Prosthodontics by Dr R Mantsch, Rheinbach.)

Fig 4-323 Final plaster models in articulator with marked occlusal contact points.

Topic 41
Teenager with agenesis of four teeth and an impacted tooth

Treatment:
- space closure with space kept for later implant

Missing germs of permanent teeth can make orthodontic treatment difficult, with decisions needed about whether to close the space of the missing teeth or preserve it for later implants or prosthetics. Implantology is becoming more an more percise, but certain issues should be kept in mind treating young patients with missing permanent teeth. One important consideration is bone, and potential bone reduction resulting from the missing load where there are missing primary teeth. The second aspect is the esthetic aspects during puberty, as implant insertion is usually preferred after the age of 18 years.

This patient has several missing permanent teeth and a translocated tooth germ (Fig 4-324). She has primary teeth 54, 55, 65, 75, and 85 in situ and is missing teeth 34 and 44 (Fig 4-325).

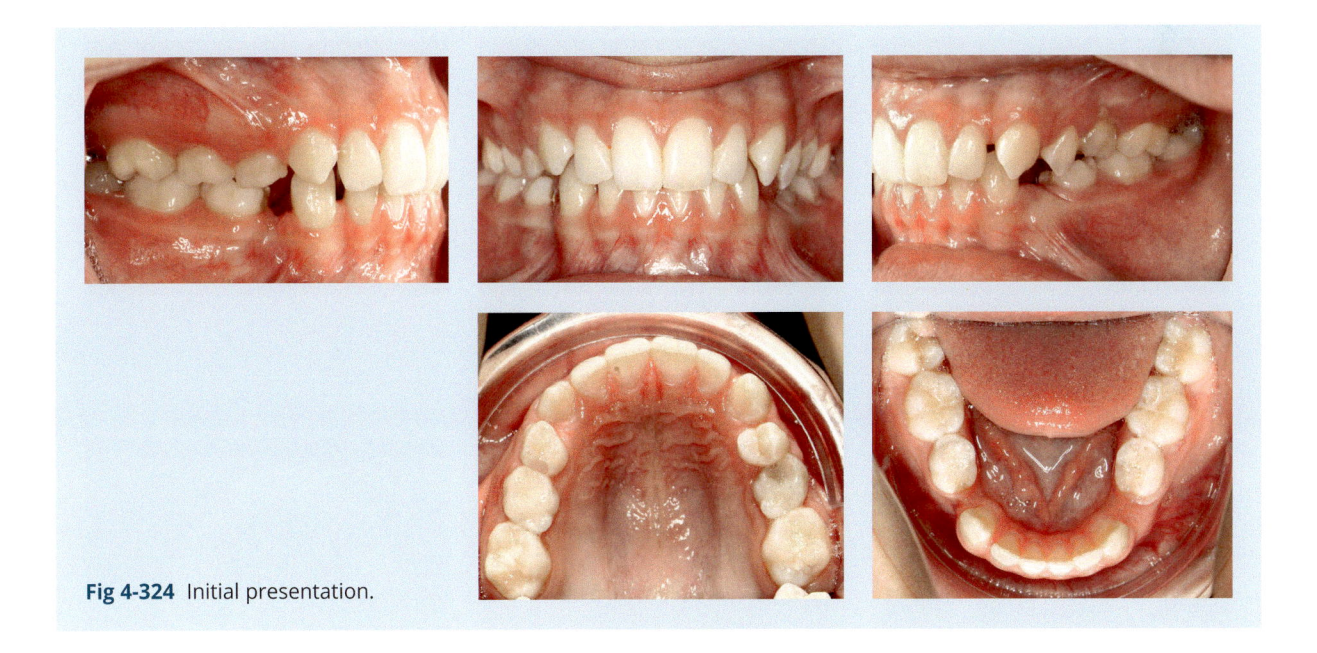

Fig 4-324 Initial presentation.

Diagnosis:
- missing teeth 15, 35, 44, 45
- translocated tooth germ 25
- germ of teeth 18 and 28 not visible.

Therapy:
- surgical removal of tooth germ 25
- Invisalign Teen treatment with mesialization for space closure of all missing teeth except implant site 44, which was planned for adulthood.

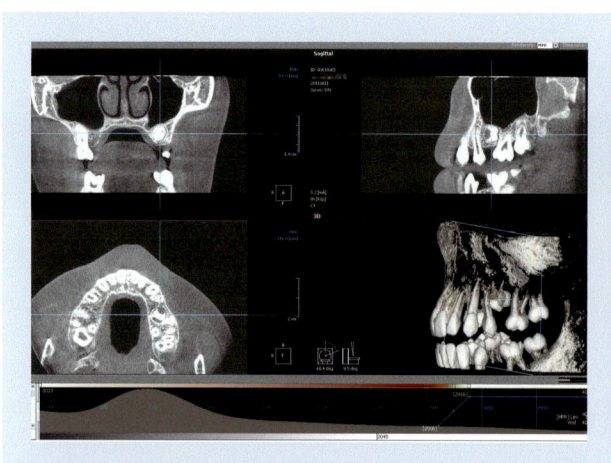

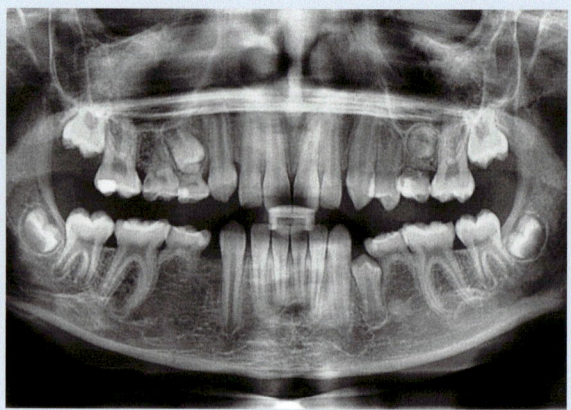

Fig 4-325 Initial orthopantomography and CBCT show the missing germs of 15, 35, 44, and 45 and the translocated germ of tooth 25.

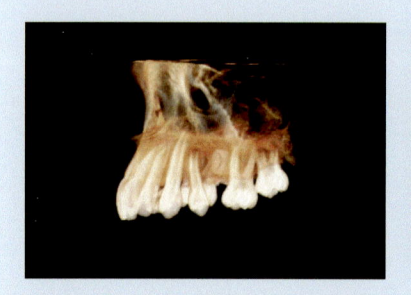

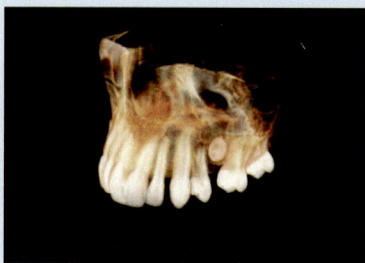

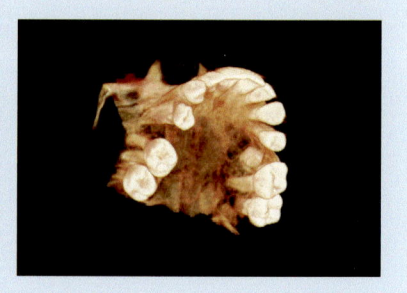

Fig 4-326 Invivo Software (Anatomage) images showing the translocated position of the permanent germ 25.

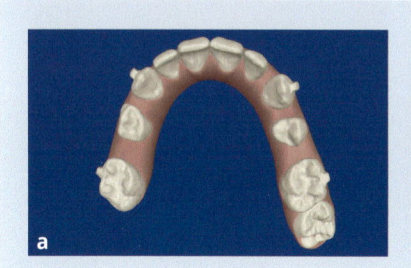

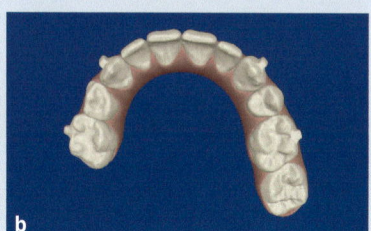

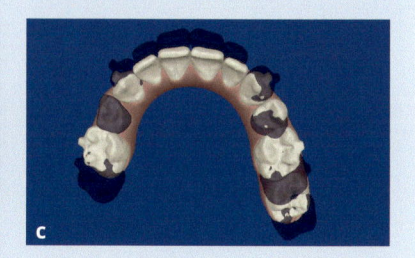

Fig 4-327 ClinCheck software results for the maxilla. **(a)** Initial situation. **(b)** Planned final result. **(c)** Superimposition to show planned tooth movement (blue, initial tooth position; white, final tooth position).

Treatment

Because of the missing permanent teeth 15, 35, 44, and 45 and the translocated germ 25, it was decided to start treatment when the patient was 12 years to obtain maximum mesialization of the first and second molars to close the space and to avoid a need for five implants. As both tooth 44 and tooth 45 were missing in the mandibular right arch, complete space closure here was not possible and space closure of 44 was planned with an implant. The CBCT images were transferred into three-dimensional software (Invivo Software, Anatomage) to outline the translocated position

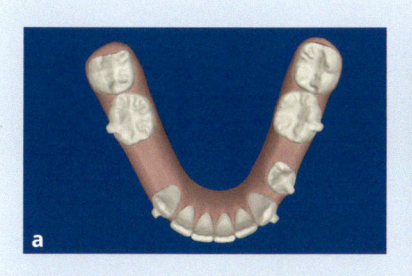

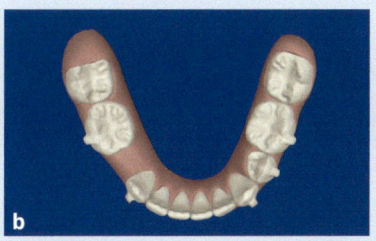

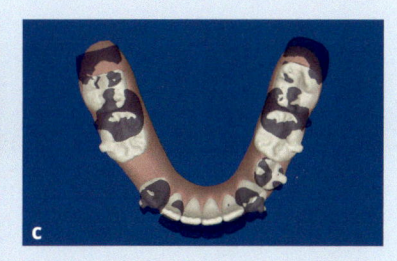

Fig 4-328 ClinCheck software results for the mandible. **(a)** Initial situation. **(b)** Planned final result. **(c)** Superimposition to show planned tooth movement (blue, initial tooth position; white, final tooth position).

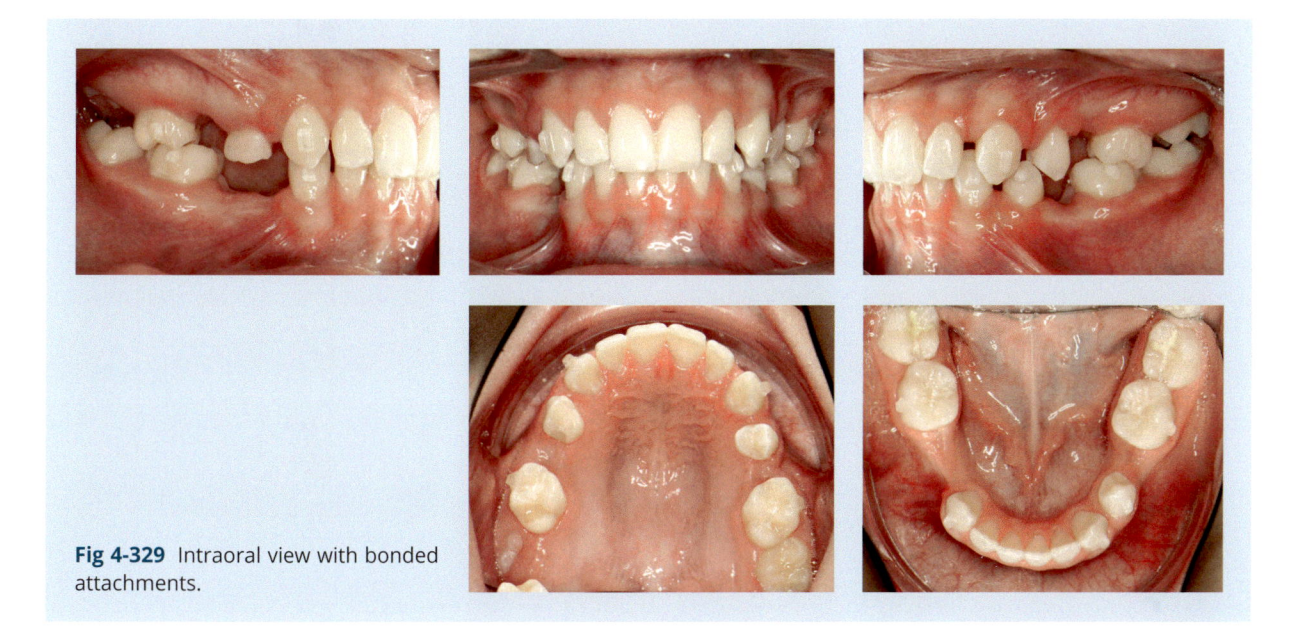

Fig 4-329 Intraoral view with bonded attachments.

of the permanent germ 25 in detail. Because of its rather complicated position, extraction with symmetric space closure to that on the other side of the arch was planned. ClinCheck software was used to create the treatment plan, which used 40 aligners in both arches (Figs 4-327 and 4-328). Tooth 54 was not moved as it is a primary tooth. The maxillary incisors were retracted and the maxillary molars mesialized to close all spaces. The planned mesialization was at least 5 mm, which is possible in young patients. The decision for distalization in the maxillary arch is highly depending on the patient's profile. In patients with flat facial profiles, a massive distalization in the maxillary arch with potential increase of the flattening should be avoided. The planned movements for the mandibular arch included the mesialization of the molars with retraction of the incisors, leaving space for a later implant in area 44.

After the extraction of the primary teeth excepting tooth 54 (14 was not yet erupted), Invisalign treatment was started with bonding of vertical rectangular attachments (Fig 4-329). After 14 aligners were placed, mesial movement of maxillary and mandibular molars occurred according to the treatment plan (Fig 4-330). With aligner 25, tooth 14 was erupting and the first molars were in their planned and correct position (Fig 4-331). Aligner 31 showed still optimal aligner fitting in both arches. Tooth 14 was erupting into the former position of primary tooth 54 via an eruption tab (Fig 4-332). Figures 4-333 and 4-334 show the situation at the end of the first phase. Tooth 14 was erupt-

Fig 4-330 Intraoral view after use of aligner 14.

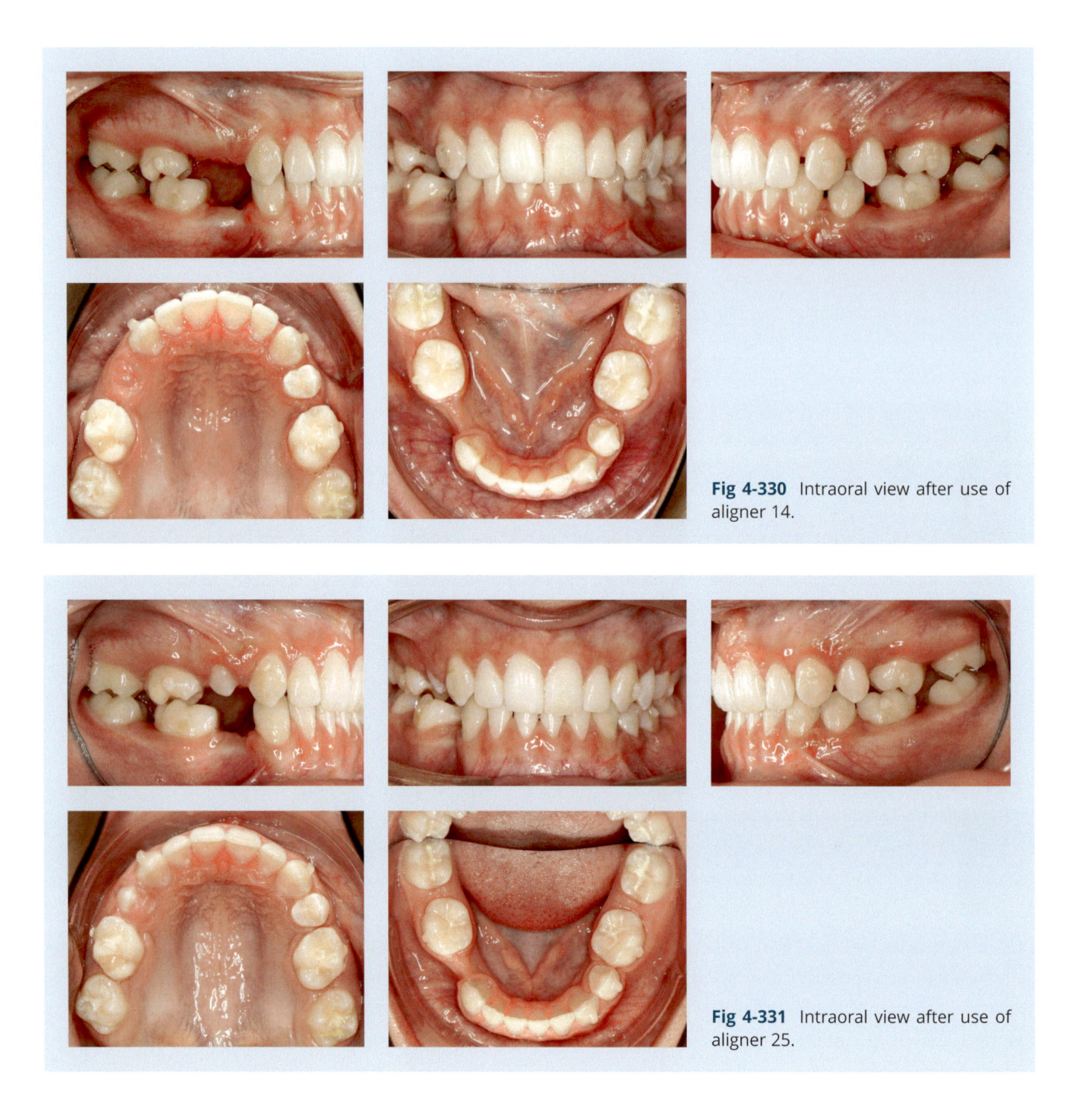

Fig 4-331 Intraoral view after use of aligner 25.

ing into the former aligner shape of primary tooth 54, according to an eruption tab. All movements planned in the ClinCheck software in the first phase of treatment had been completely accomplished.

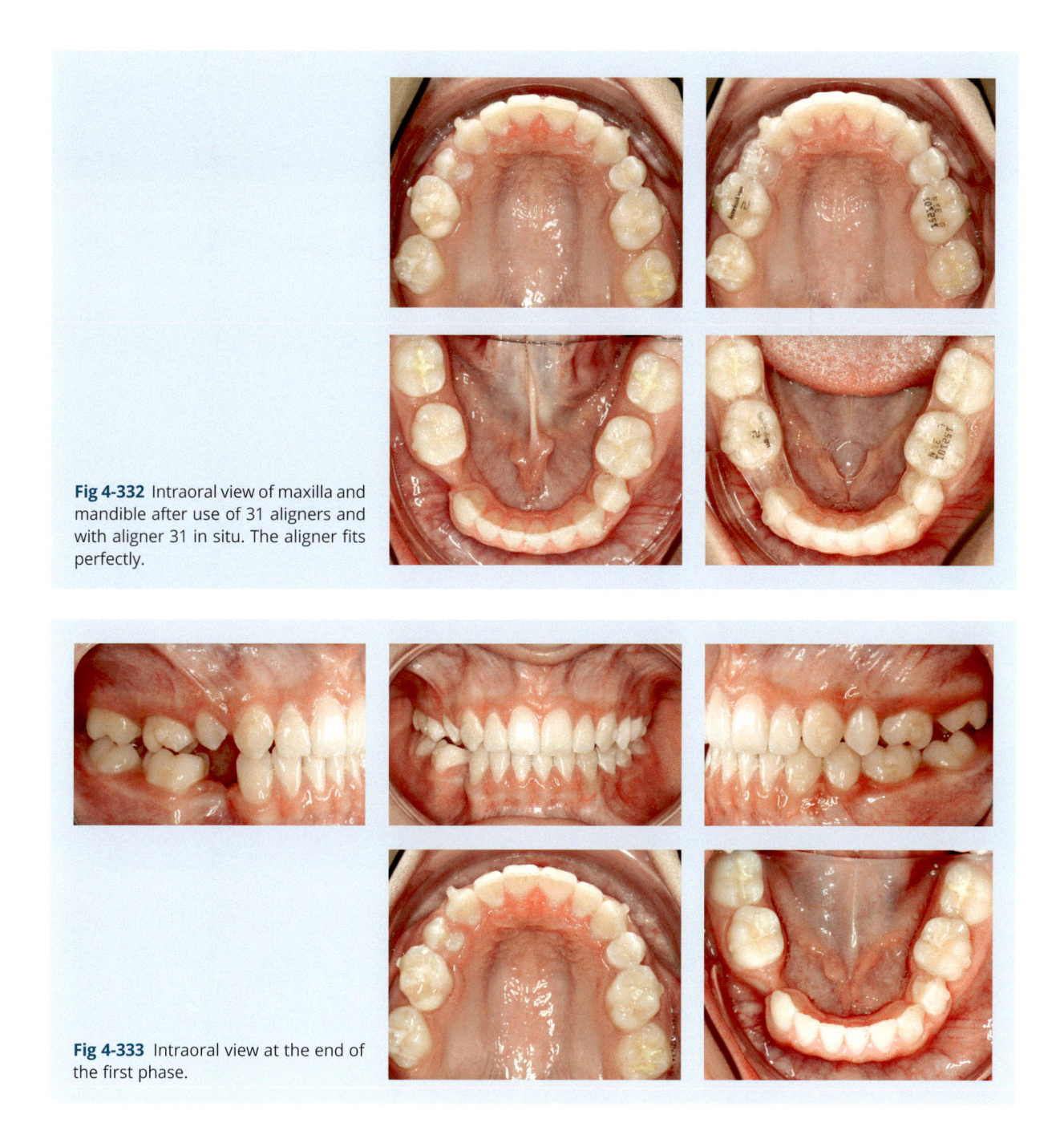

Fig 4-332 Intraoral view of maxilla and mandible after use of 31 aligners and with aligner 31 in situ. The aligner fits perfectly.

Fig 4-333 Intraoral view at the end of the first phase.

A further ClinCheck analysis allowed planning of the refinement (Fig 4-335). The refinement planned additional IPR on teeth 12, 13, and 14, and 32, 31, 41, and 42, to align maxillary and mandibular midlines and obtain better canine guidance on the right side. A beveled attachment was added on tooth 14 with planned extrusion. The refinement used 24 aligners in the maxillary arch and 10 in the mandibular arch.

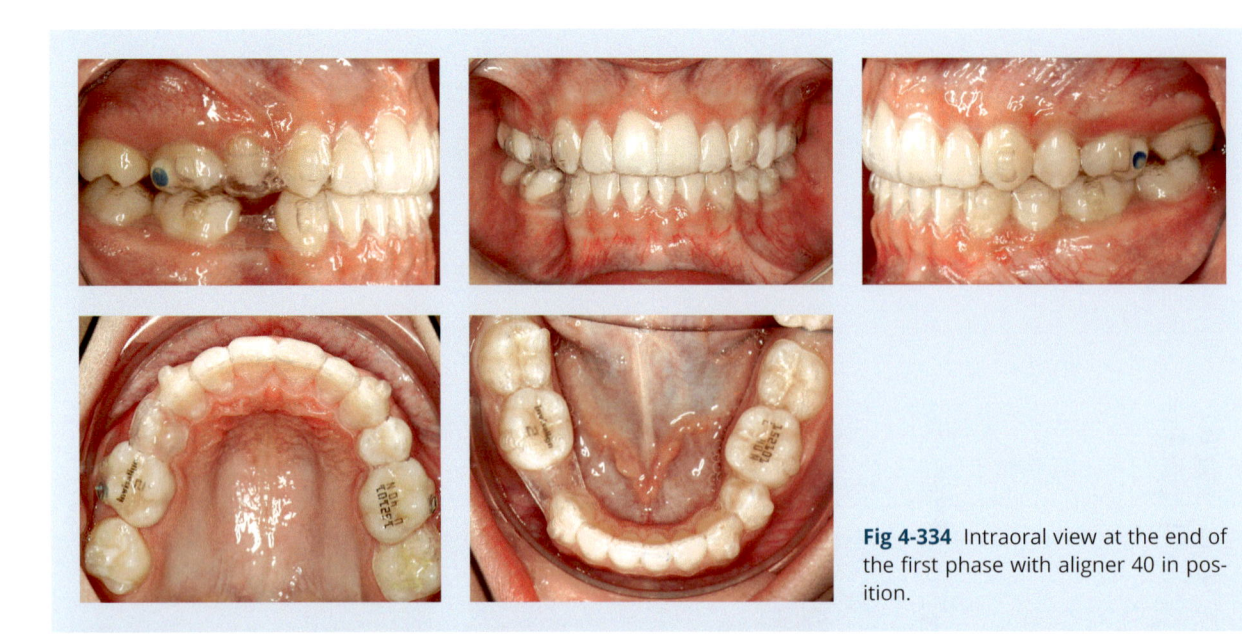

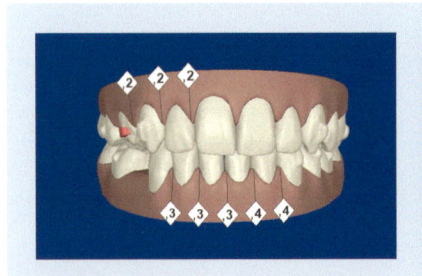

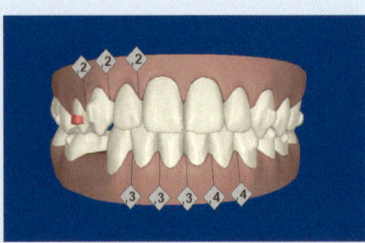

4 TREATMENT OF DIFFERENT MALOCCLUSIONS WITH ALIGNERS

Fig 4-334 Intraoral view at the end of the first phase with aligner 40 in position.

Fig 4-335 ClinCheck images at the end of the first phase **(left)** after refinement **(right)**.

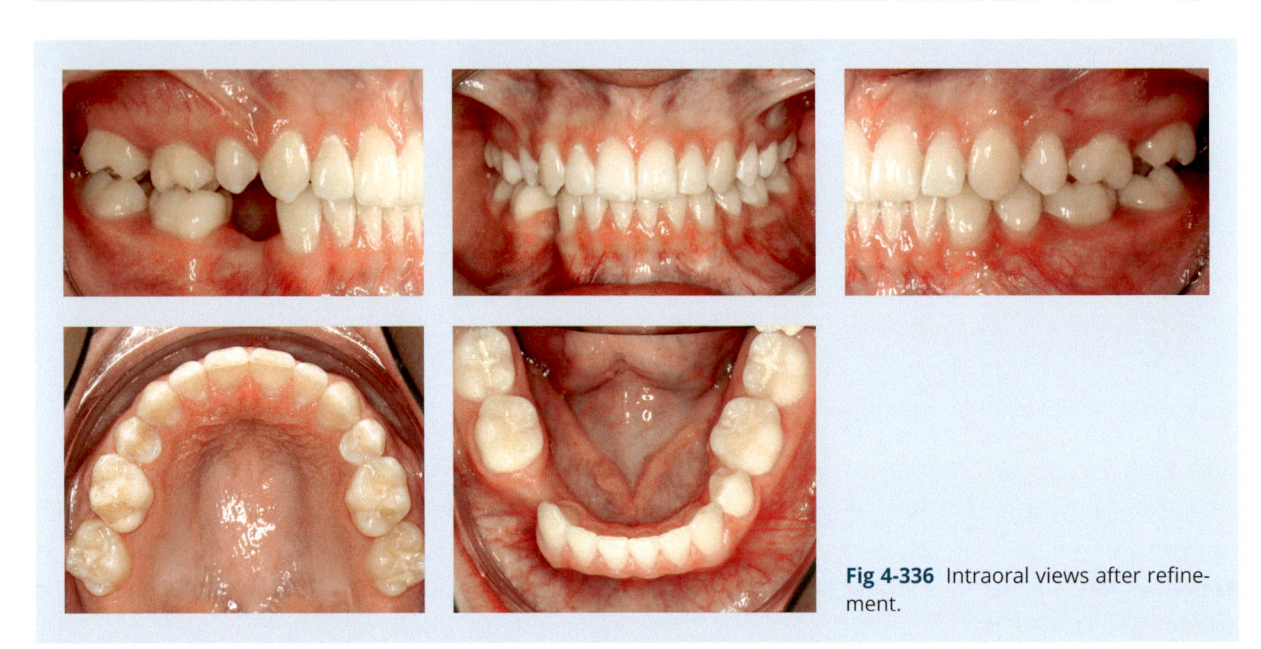

Fig 4-336 Intraoral views after refinement.

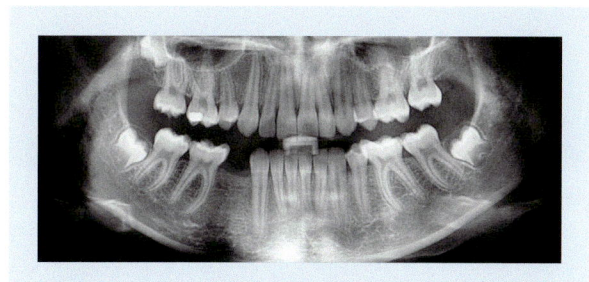

TREATMENT OF DIFFERENT MALOCCLUSIONS WITH ALIGNERS 4

Fig 4-337 Orthopantomography after refinement.

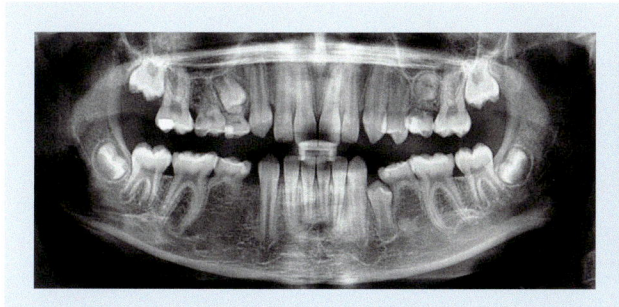

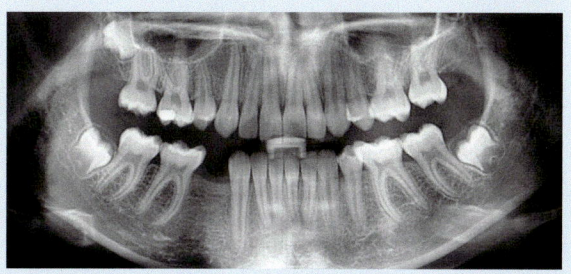

Fig 4-338 The initial (left) and final (right) orthopantomograms.

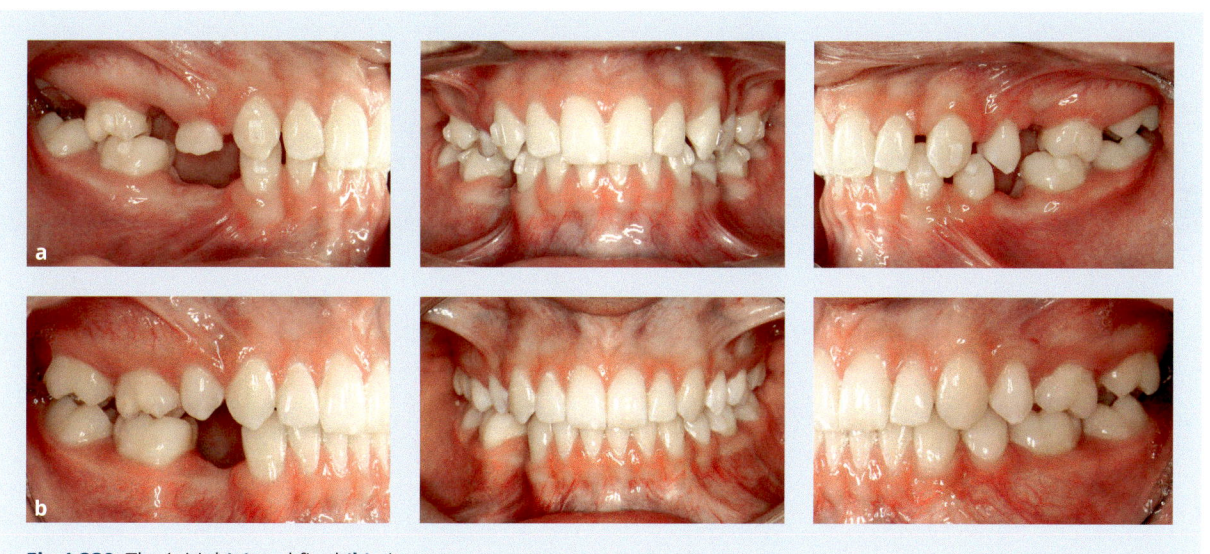

Fig 4-339 The initial (a) and final (b) views.

At the end of the refinement, there was complete space closure of teeth 14, 24, 34, and 44; a space in region 45 was maintained for later implant insertion (Figs 4-336 and 4-337).

The decision whether to extract teeth 18, 38, and 48 was postponed.

Figures 4-338 to 4-342 show the changes achieved with treatment.

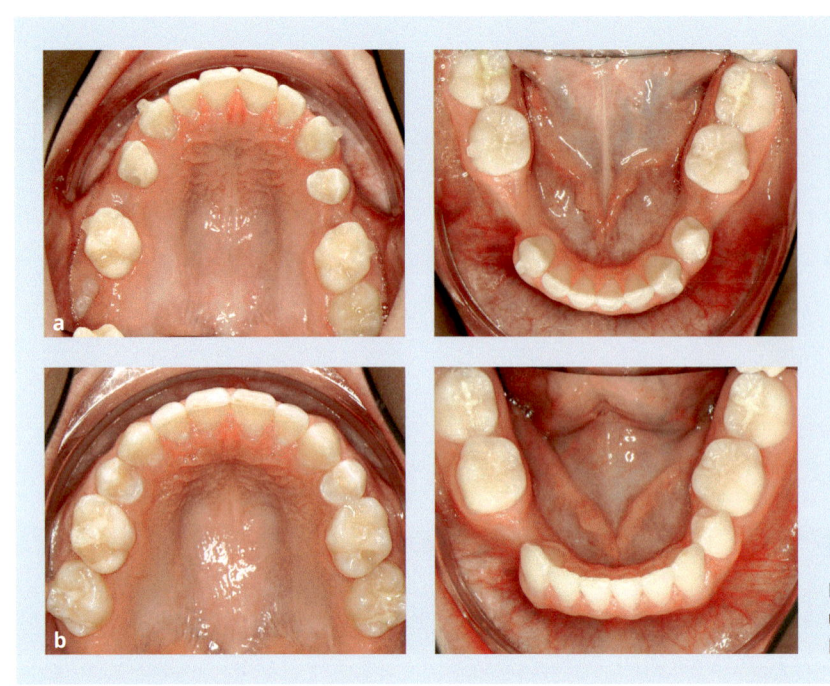

4 TREATMENT OF DIFFERENT MALOCCLUSIONS WITH ALIGNERS

Fig 4-340 The maxillary and mandibular arches before **(a)** and after **(b)** Invisalign treatment.

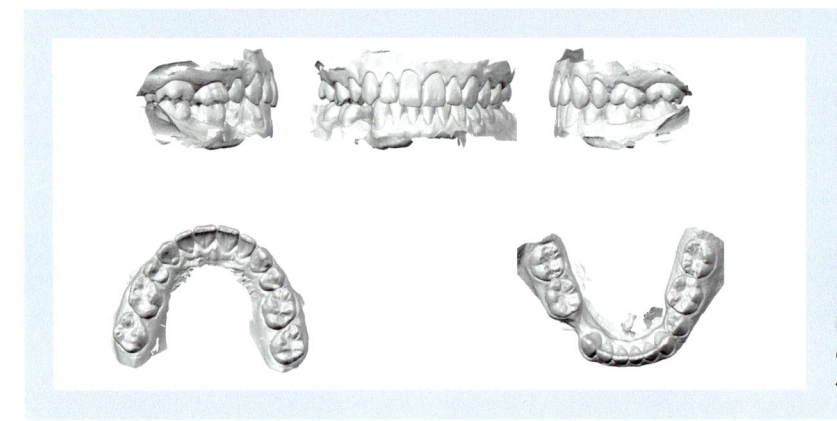

Fig 4-341 Final scans, showing space closure and bone situation in region 45.

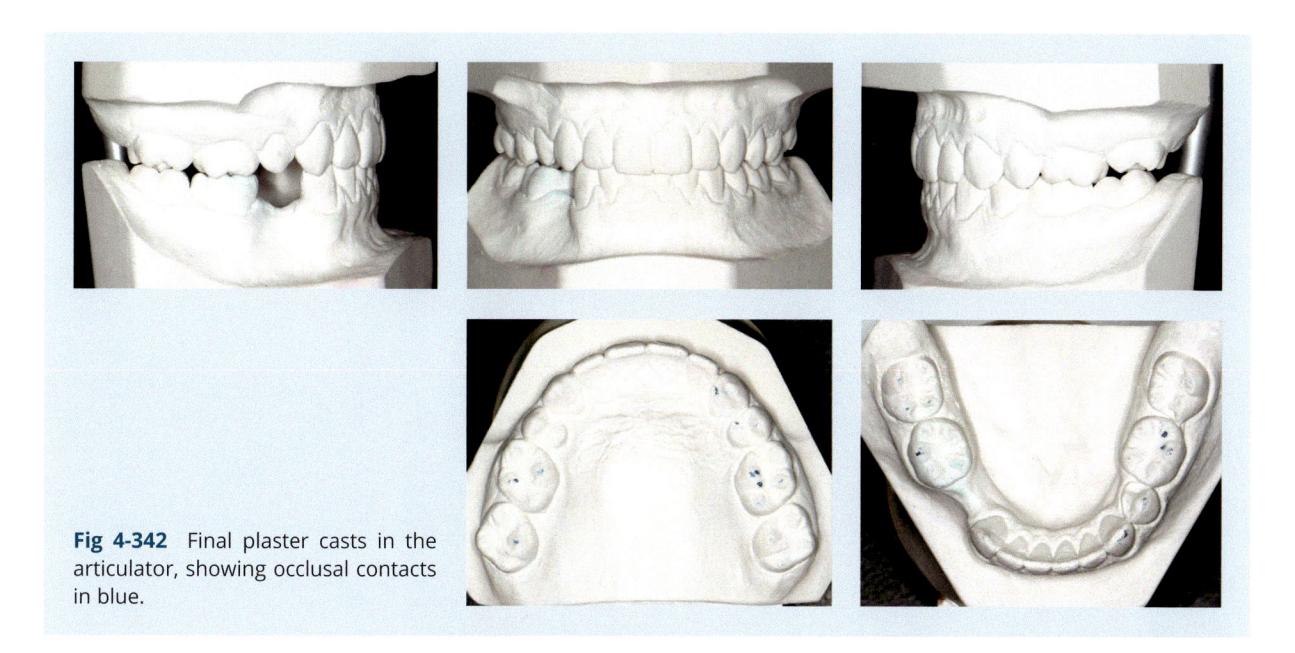

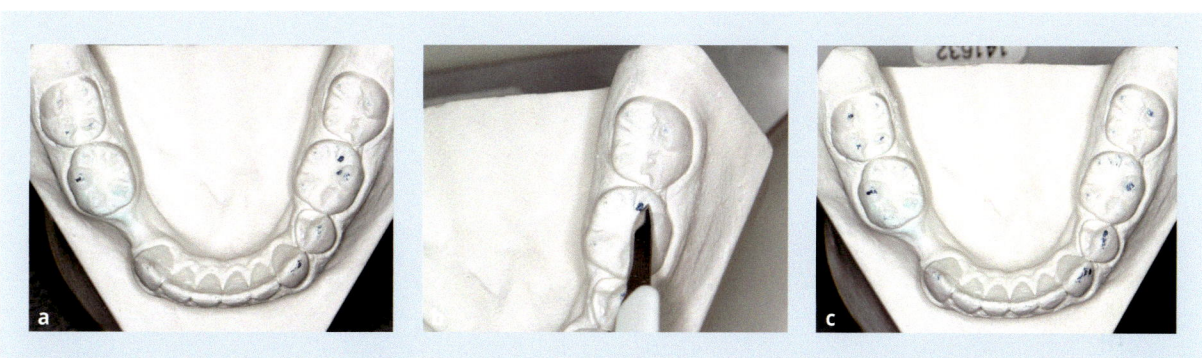

TREATMENT OF DIFFERENT MALOCCLUSIONS WITH ALIGNERS 4

Fig 4-342 Final plaster casts in the articulator, showing occlusal contacts in blue.

Fig 4-343 Simulation of intraoral grinding with removal of the first occlusal contact on tooth 36 **(a,b)** to obtain an equal occlusal contact pattern **(c)**.

Figure 4-343 shows a simulation of intraoral grinding to remove the first occlusal contact to obtain an equal occlusal contact pattern. After the correction of the occlusal contacts on the articulated plaster casts, slight grinding on the patient's teeth achieved the required occlusion (see also Topic 60).

Tooth 44 was planned to be replaced with an implant as soon as the patient reached 19 years and her growth was mainly completed. Until then, an adhesive fixed partial denture was bonded on teeth 43 and 46 to maintain the space for the later implant (Figs 4-344 and 4-345).

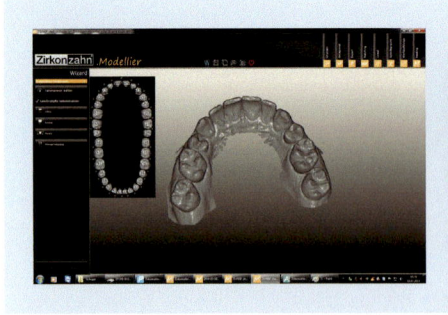

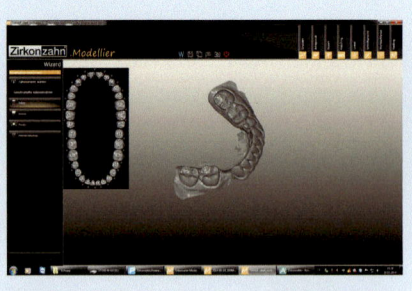

Fig 4-344 Fixed partial denture planned virtually with the Zirkonzahn software. The maxillary and mandibular arch forms were recorded with the iTero scanner and transferred into the software (matching).

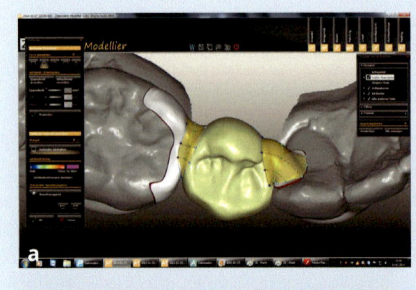

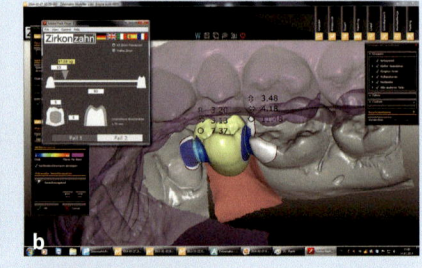

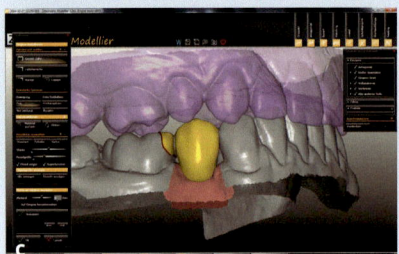

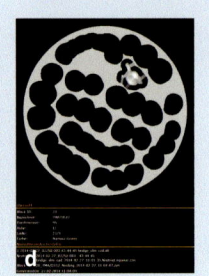

Fig 4-345 Virtual modeling of tooth 44, which was shaped without occlusal contact to avoid excessive overload. **(a,b)** The calculation and modeling of the occlusal base on the neighboring teeth can be very precise, making it possible to include potential occlusal load into the calculation for the dimension of the occlusal base. **(c)** The design of the fixed partial denture. **(d)** The actual appliance is milled out of green plastic (Burnout Green, Zirkonzahn), embedded, and transferred into ceramics (emax; Ivoclar) before characterization firing for coloring. (Fabrication planned and executed by M Läkamp with Zirkonzahn software.)

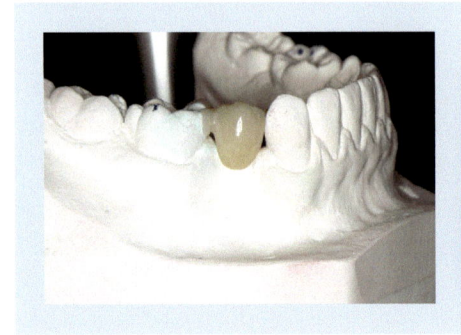

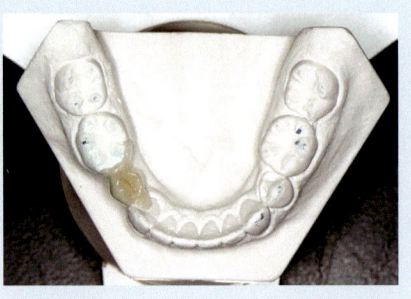

Fig 4-346 Completed denture for tooth 44 in lateral and occlusal view on an articulated plaster cast.

Figures 4-346 and 4-347 show the completed denture. Extraoral view and detail of the adhesive fixed partial denture of tooth 44 in situ show esthetic space closure (Fig 4-348). Intraoral views show the effect of slight tooth shaping for enamel defects in maxillary teeth 12, 11, 21, and 22. The curvature of the distal aspects were maintained and the mesial aspect shaped slightly more square according to standards of harmonious anterior tooth shape (Fig 4-349).

TREATMENT OF DIFFERENT MALOCCLUSIONS WITH ALIGNERS 4

Fig 4-347 Fixed partial denture in situ. Occlusal views show equal occlusal contacts on all posteriors except 44, which was taken completely out of contact.

Fig 4-348 Extraoral views showing esthetic space closure.

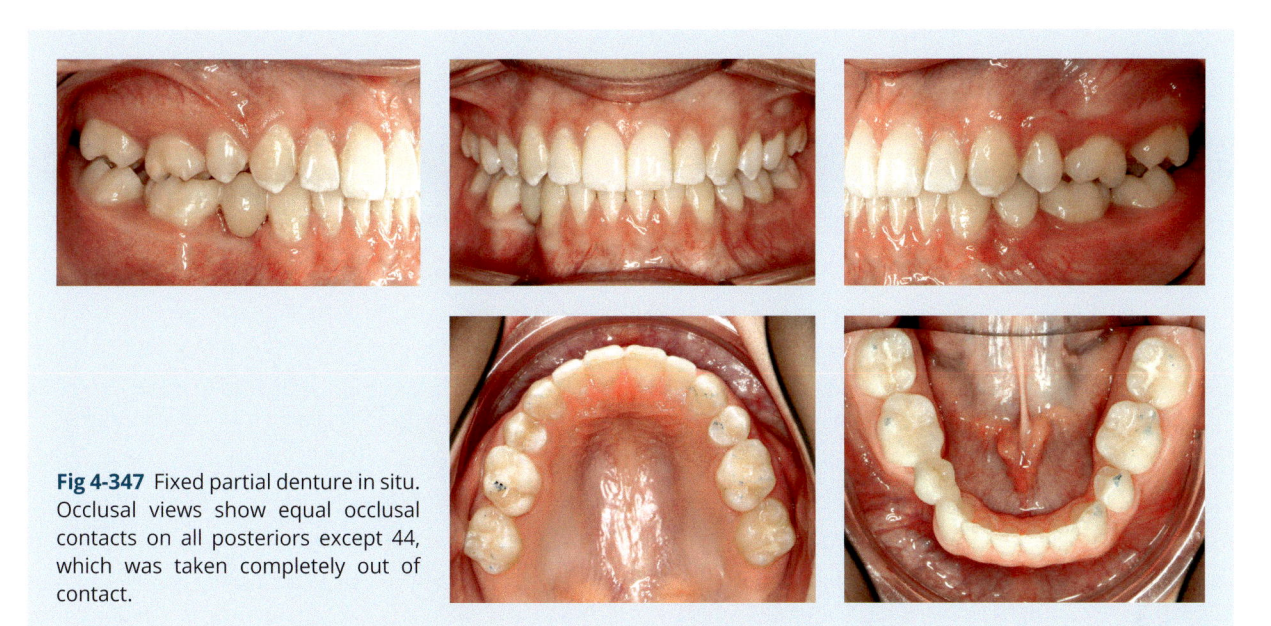

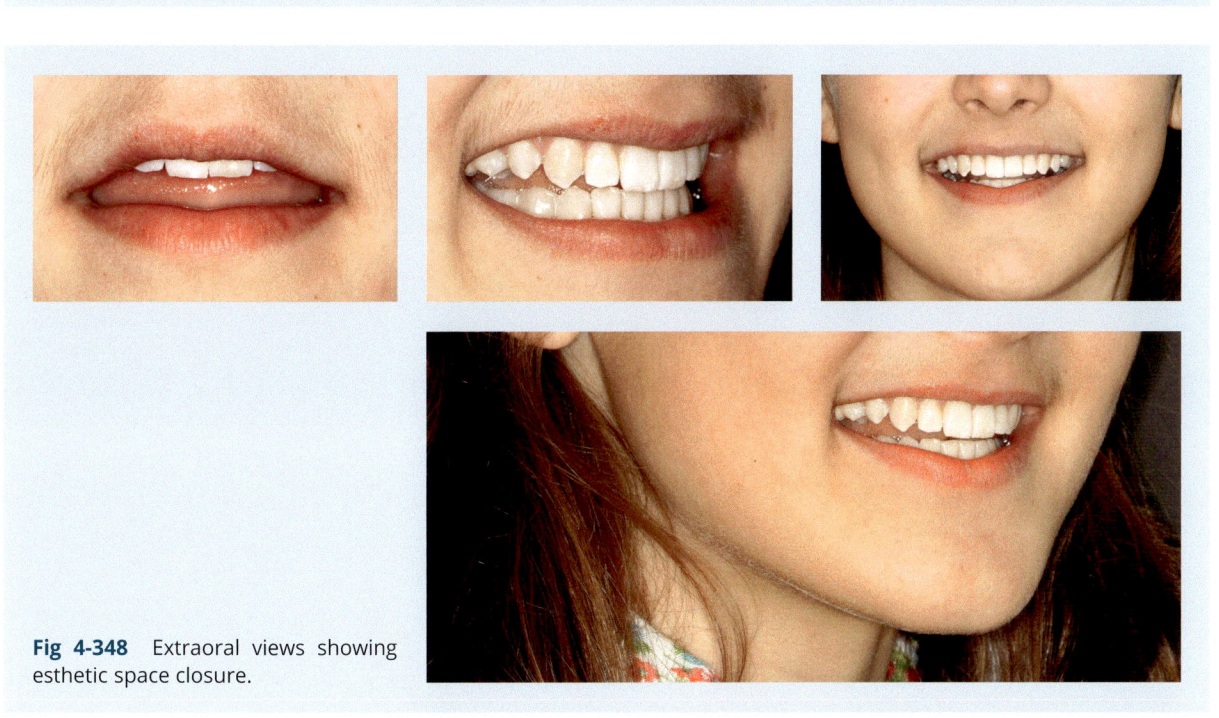

Fig 4-349 Intraoral final views before **(left)** and after **(right)** slight tooth shaping of enamel defects on anterior front teeth.

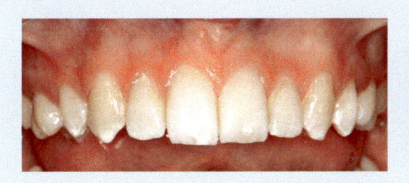

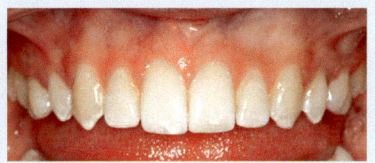

223

Topic 42
Skeletal class II relationship in a teenager

Treatment:
- functional appliance
- Invisalign system

In growing patients with a skeletal class II or class III relationship, it is usual in the author's practice to start treatment with a functional appliance. In class II without severe reclination of maxillary incisors, we use a Bionator or a Frankel appliance. Frankel appliance types 1 and 2 are our gold standard approach, particularly if the maxillary and mandibular arches are transversally restricted. The pelottes of the Frankel appliance eliminate the muscle force and pull on the periosteum to induce bone growth. In patients with severe reclination of maxillary incisors, we start with a torque and/or proclination of the reclined incisors using the Ricketts utility technique. As soon as the overjet is sufficient, a functional appliance is used. Some patients can start with the Invisalign system in combination with power ridges. The use of power ridges on the anterior teeth, with attachments added to teeth adjacent to the reclined teeth, can supply the additional anchorage control needed for the torque movement. A growing patient with a class III relationship can start wearing a Frankel appliance type 3 directly after the eruption of the mandibular permanent incisors.

In most patients who have been treated with a functional appliance, the arches and the occlusion have to be treated in detail after the eruption of all permanent teeth. This is now possible with the multibracket technique and with the Invisalign system.

Figure 4-350 shows production of the Frankel appliance. It is important to control the appliance carefully in the mouth, particularly the fitting of the pelottes. If the pelottes apply too much pull or lead to uncomfortable cutting of the cheek or tongue, reshaping and repolishing is necessary.

This patient had a class II relationship with crowding, an enlarged overjet, and deep bite. The circulating muscles of the mouth are in tension (Figs 4-351 and 4-352).

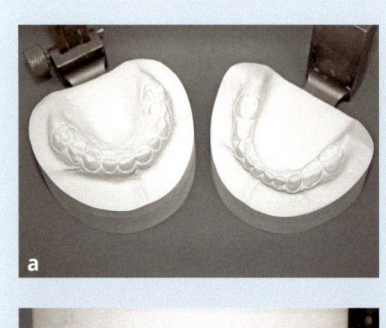

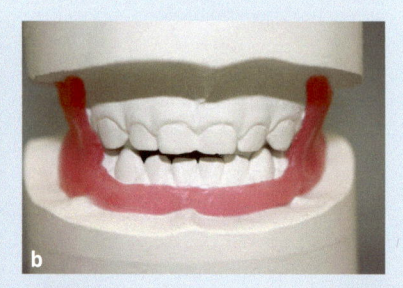

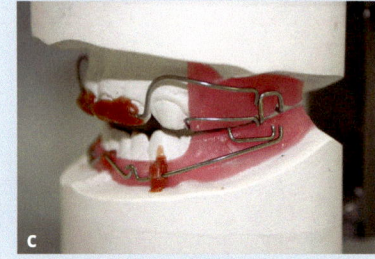

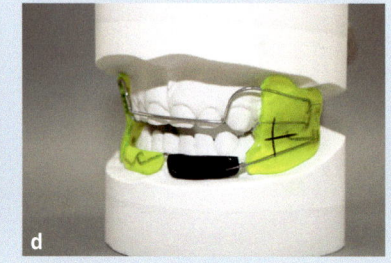

Fig 4-350 Production of the Frankel appliance. **(a)** Casts are ground in the buccal and lingual dimension for the extension of the pelottes. **(b)** Wax padding is needed where the pelottes have to eliminate the pressure of the muscles and thus pull on the periosteum. **(c)** The wire is bent in detail and fixed with wax. **(d)** Frankel appliance is fabricated and polished.

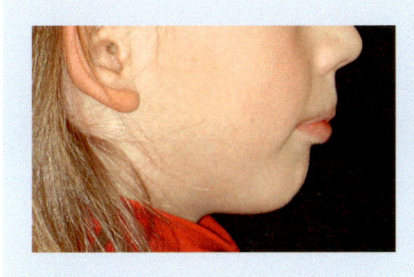

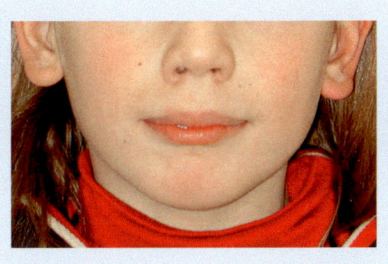

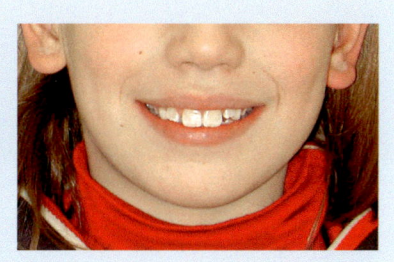

TREATMENT OF DIFFERENT MALOCCLUSIONS WITH ALIGNERS 4

Fig 4-351 Initial presentation shows orofacial muscle tension especially of m mentalis.

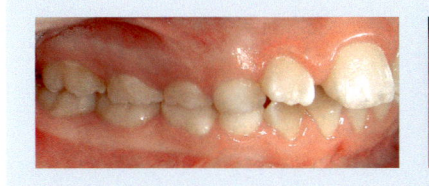

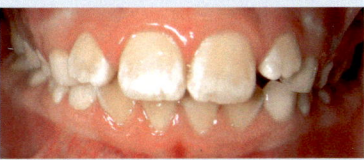

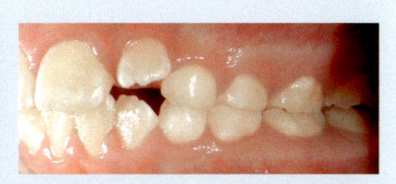

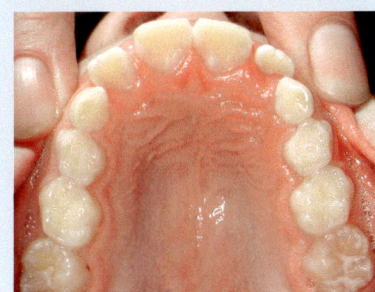

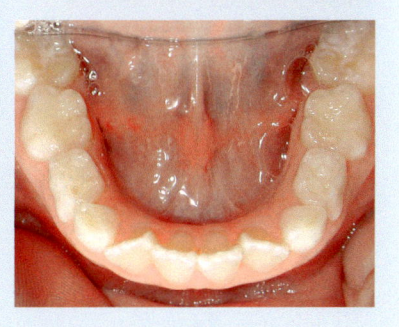

Fig 4-352 Intraoral views showing a full class II relationship, crowding, restricted arch forms and increased overjet.

Diagnosis:
- class II with crowding
- enlarged overjet
- deep bite
- severe tensing of orofacial muscles.

Therapy:
- orthopedic treatment with the Frankel appliance
- functional exercises for lip closure
- Invisalign Teen treatment.

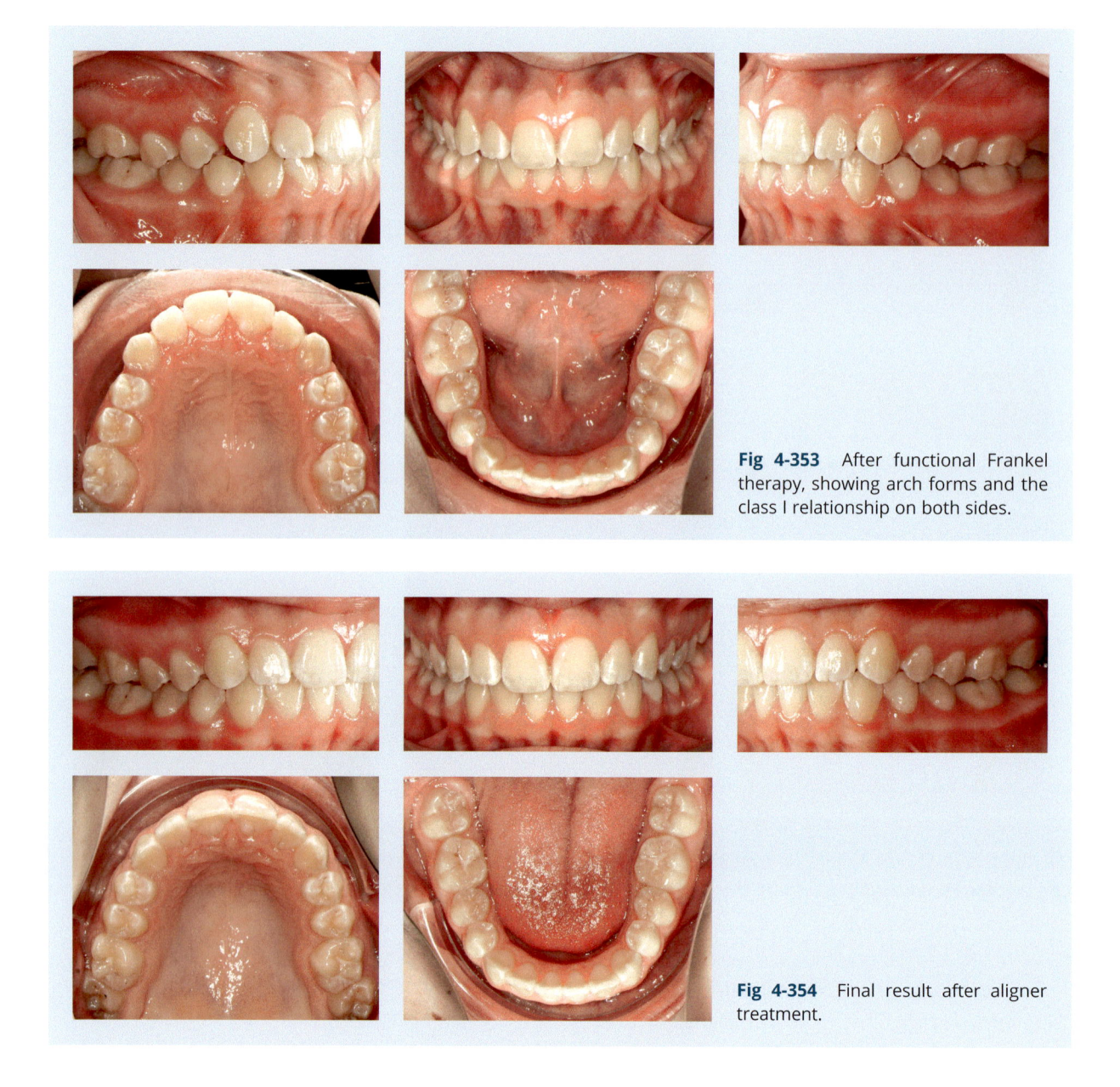

Fig 4-353 After functional Frankel therapy, showing arch forms and the class I relationship on both sides.

Fig 4-354 Final result after aligner treatment.

Treatment

The circulating muscles of the mouth (orbicularis oris; buccinator; depressor anguli oris; depressor labii inferioris; mentalis; levator anguli oris; risorius; and zygomaticus) have an important role in the growth of the maxilla and mandible. This patient showed severe hyperactivity of these muscles. The pressure of the tensed muscles has led to growth obstruction and, therefore, to the retruded mandibular position. The Frankel appliance needs to be worn ideally 16 hours a day at the beginning. Once the patient has reached a skeletal class I and the arch form has improved, the patient wears the Frankel appliance only at night for retention. After full eruption of the permanent teeth, function and esthetics are the main aspects to decide if a detailed treatment is still necessary.

After Frankel therapy, there was a physiologic upper and mandibular arch form, still with mild crowding, and a full class I relationship on both sides (Fig 4-353).

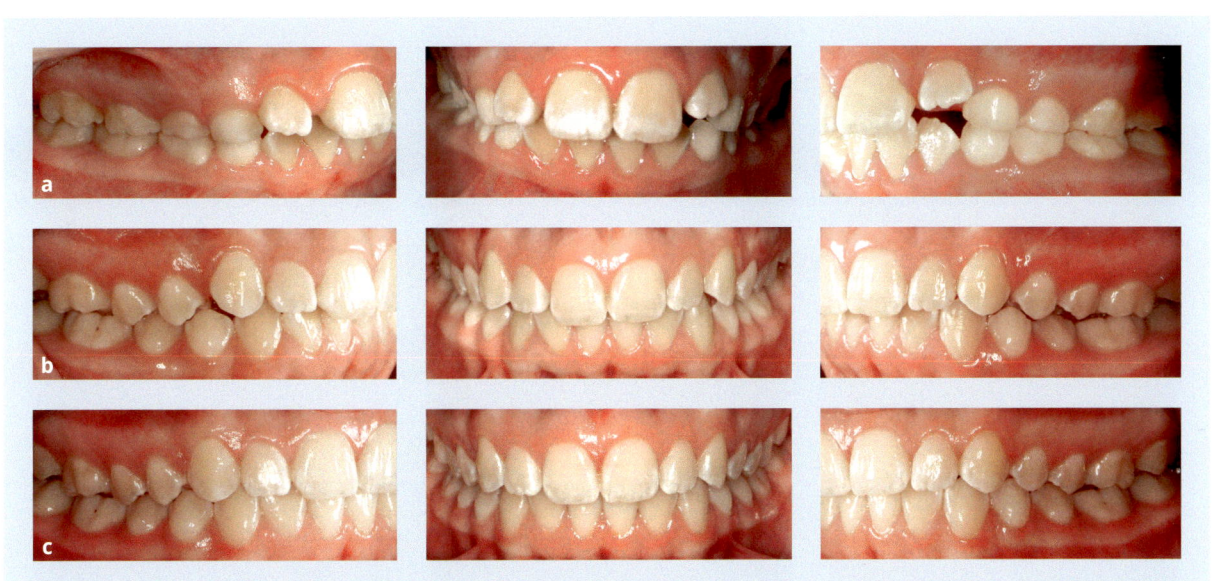

Fig 4-355 Course of the treatment. **(a)** Before the start of Frankel therapy, at age 9.5 years. **(b)** After Frankel therapy and before Invisalign treatment at age 13.5 years. **(c)** Final views.

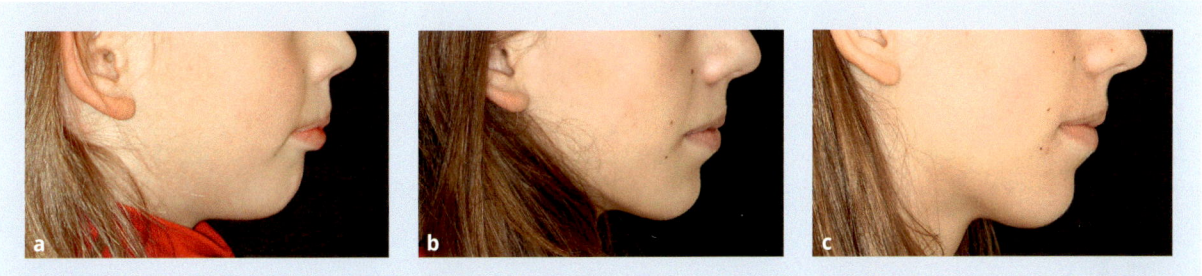

Fig 4-356 Facial views during treatment. **(a)** Before Frankel therapy, with severe tension of orofacial muscles. **(b)** After Frankel therapy and before Invisalign treatment. **(c)** Final view. The circulating muscles of the mouth are relaxed and the muscular pressure is eliminated. The lip closure is competent and the orofacial esthetics are improved.

Details of occlusion and esthetics were solved using the Invisalign system, with 21 aligners over 10.5 months (Fig 4-354). Changes over the course of treatment are shown in Figures 4-355 and 4-356.

Topic 43
Skeletal class II relationship in a teenager

Treatment:
- Functional appliance in combination with the Invisalign system

Topic 42 discussed the sequential use of the Frankel appliance and Invisalign treatment in a growing patient with a skeletal class II relationship. However, these approaches can be undertaken simultaneously with success (Aquilio, 2013). The fabrication process for the Frankel appliance is undertaken with the aligner in situ.

This 11-year old girl had a a class II relationship, mild crowding in the maxilla and mandible, a slight midline deviation, and dental deep bite. Her maxillary canines and premolars were still in eruption phase (Fig 4-357).

Fig 4-357 Initial presentation.

Diagnosis:
- class II with mild crowding
- slight midline deviation
- deep bite.

Therapy:
- Frankel appliance
- simultaneous alignment using Invisalign Teen system.

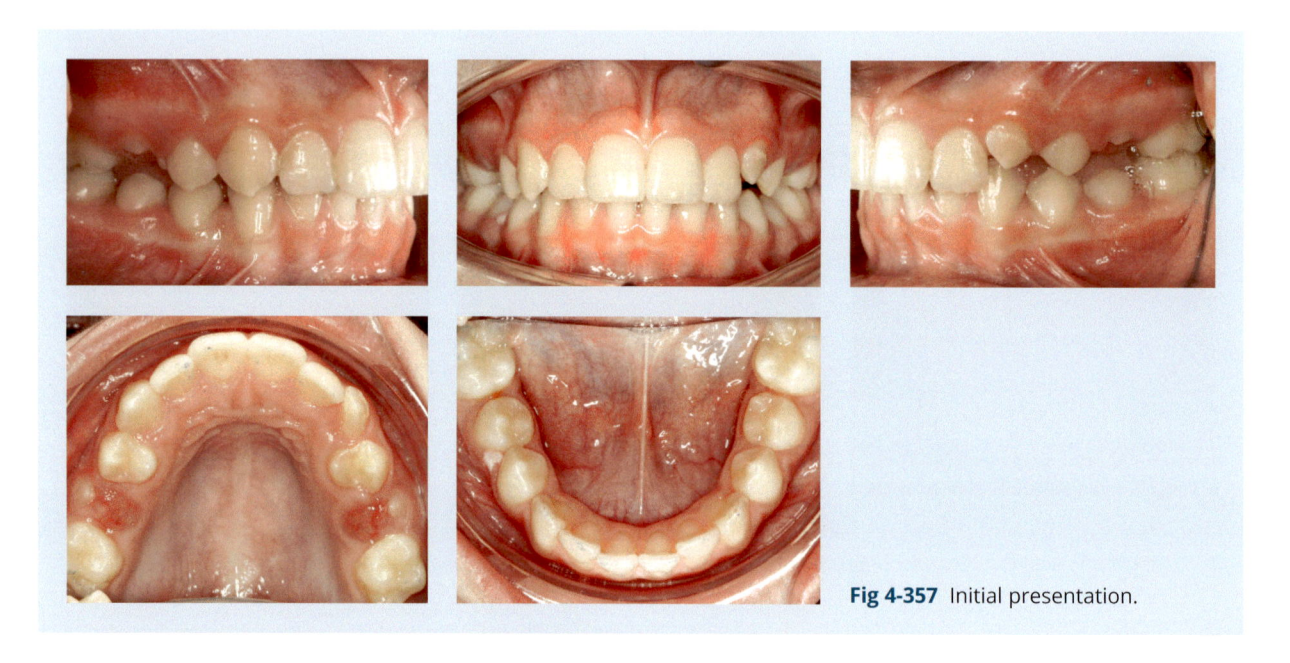

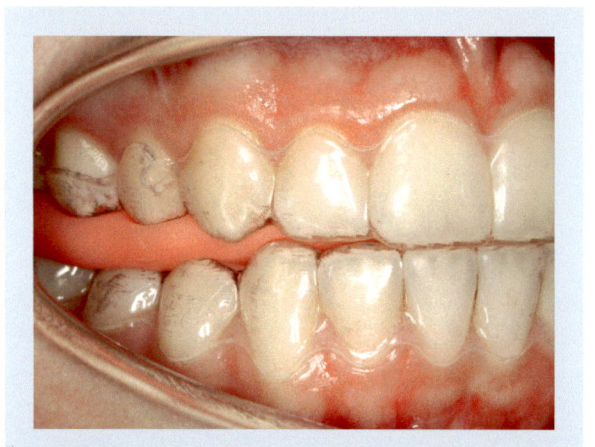

Fig 4-358 Therapeutic wax construction bite in place with the aligner.

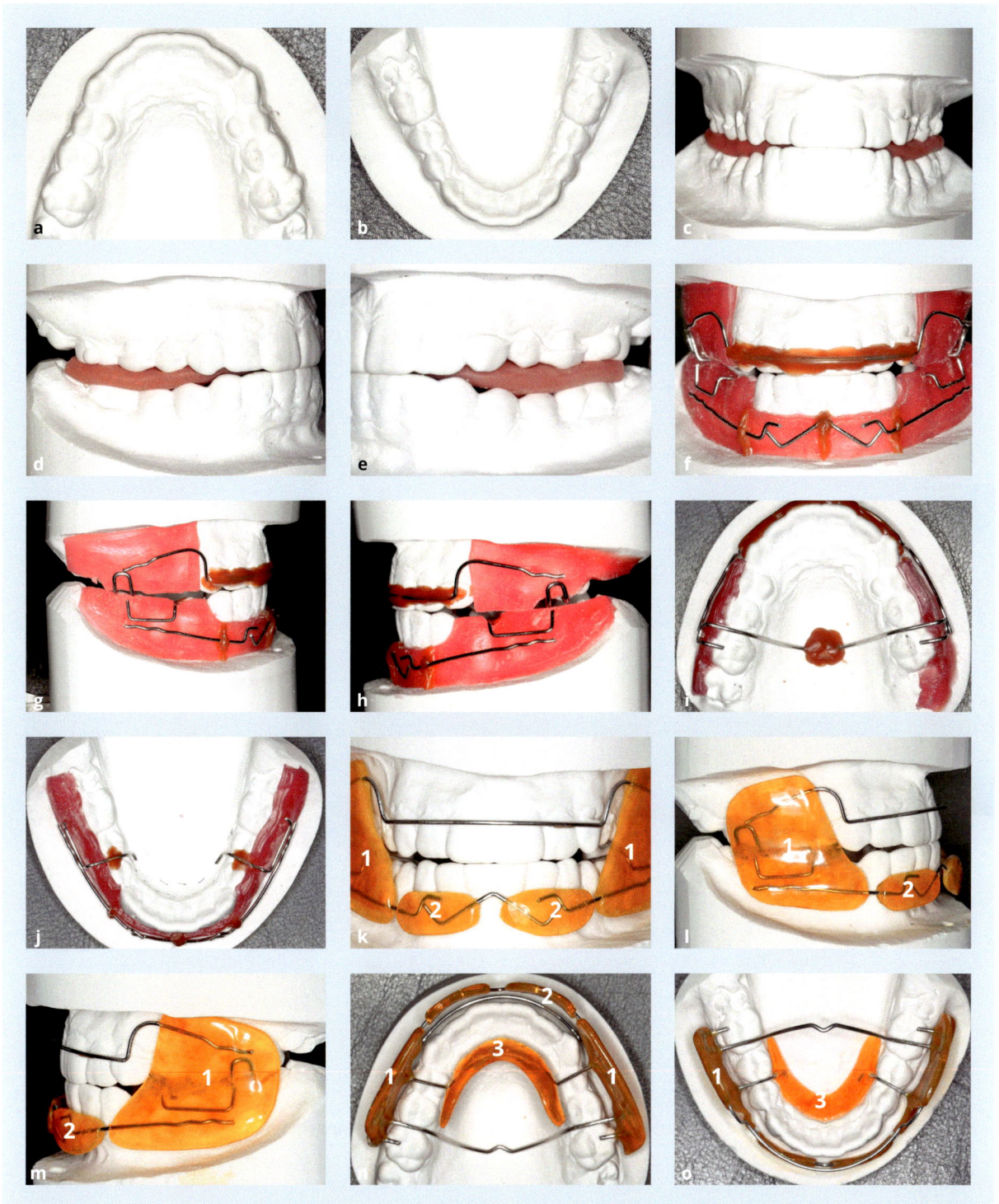

TREATMENT OF DIFFERENT MALOCCLUSIONS WITH ALIGNERS 4

Fig 4-359 Production of the Frankel appliance. **(a,b)** Preparation of the plaster casts with the aligners in situ and plaster reduction in the buccal and lingual dimension for the extension of the pelottes. **(c–e)** The plaster casts with the therapeutic bite in situ. **(f–j)** The wax padding is necessary in all areas where the pelottes need to eliminate pressure from muscles. The wire is bent in detail and fixed with wax. **(k–o)** The finished appliance on the plaster cast. 1, buccal shield; 2, labial shield; 3, lingual shield.

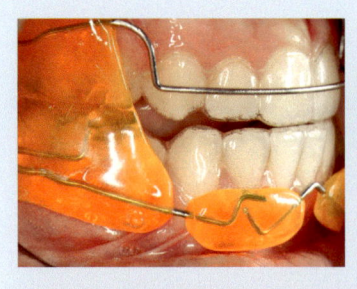

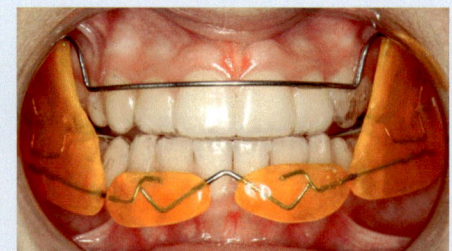

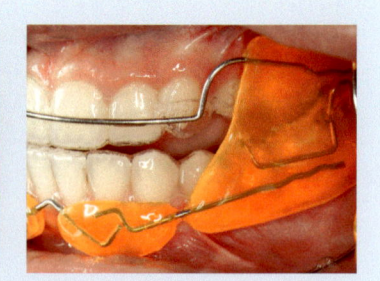

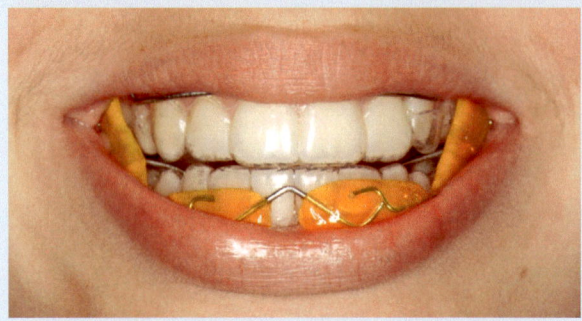

Fig 4-360 The Frankel appliance combined with the aligner in situ.

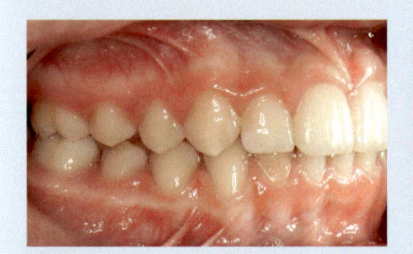

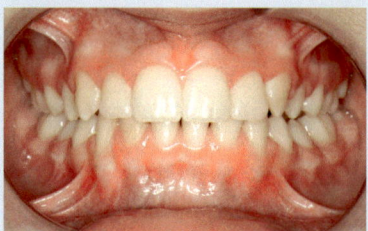

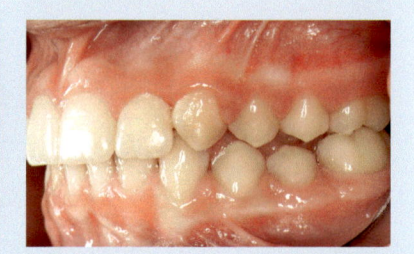

Fig 4-361 Intraoral views after 8 weeks of combined treatment.

Treatment

Invisalign therapy was planned with simultaneous wearing of a Frankel type 1 functional appliance (Fig 4-358). The buccal and lingual shields work in the same way as without aligners. The lingual shield is below the aligner and keeps the mandible forward in a more anterior position to let it grow forward into a class I. The lip shield keeps the force of the orofacial muscles off the mandible and contributes to the advancement of mandibular growth. The Frankel appliance was manufactured as described in Topic 42 but the therapeutic construction bite was taken with the mouth in class I canine relationship with the aligners in situ (Fig 4-359).

The appliance with the aligners in the mouth needs to be checked carefully to ensure that the pelottes are fitted correctly (Fig 4-360). If they apply too much pull or lead to uncomfortable cutting of the cheek or tongue, reshaping and repolishing is needed.

After 8 weeks of combined Invisalign and Frankel treatment, the mandible had slightly advanced and there was improvement of the class II relationship (Fig 4-361). At 6 months, there is a class I molar relationship on both sides (Fig 4-362).

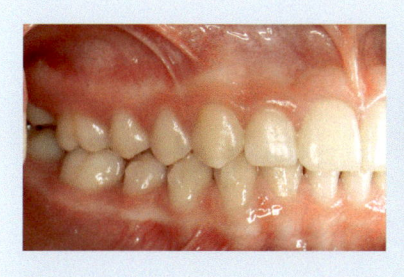

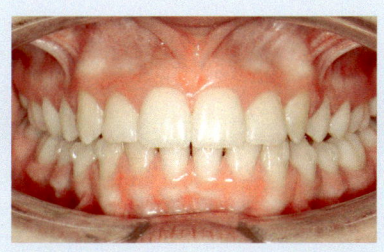

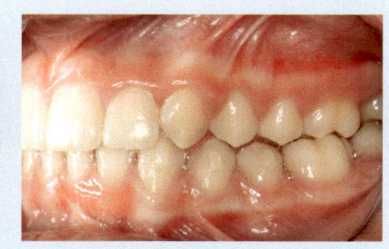

Fig 4-362 Intraoral situation after 6 months of combined Invisalign and Frankel treatment. The patient shows a class I molar relationship on both sides.

Fig 4-363 Intraoral situation after 12 months of combined Invisalign and Frankel treatment, and 4 weeks of class II elastics used on the right side.

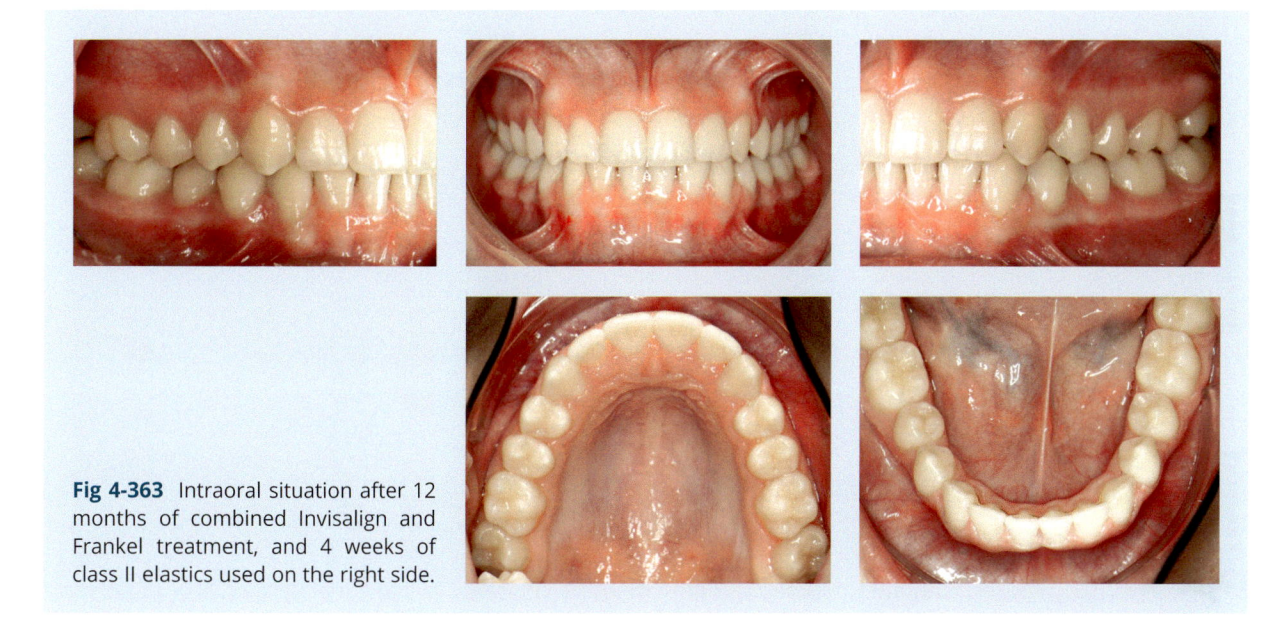

Figure 4-363 shows the situation after 12 months of combined Invisalign and Frankel treatment with 4 weeks of class II elastic wearing on the right side. A lingual retainer was bonded in the lower arch from teeth 33 to 43 and the patient wore in the upper arch the last aligner for 3 hours during daytime and the Frankel at night-time for retention for the next 4 months. After this period, retention was performed with the lingual retainer in the lower arch and a removable aligner in the upper arch at night-time.

Topic 44
Periodontitis with bone loss, extruded teeth, and spaces

Treatment:
- periodontal treatment
- Invisalign treatment
- implantology
- prosthodontics

Sometimes treatment is required in a patient with severe bone loss. We consider that small and intermittent forces are the best way to treat these patients, which is why the Invisalign system is highly suitable. Forces can be reduced by increasing the number of aligners and slowing the staging. As patients take aligners out for eating and tooth cleaning, the Invisalign system is always an intermittent force system. During the aligner-free period, blood flow continues without restriction in the periodontal ligament and so risks of resorptions are minimized.

One big advantage of the Invisalign system is the opportunity to perform oral hygiene at the dental office without any requirement to remove archwires or ligatures, which is time consuming and uncomfortable for the patient. Patients can visit the periodontist whenever needed for treatment with no additional appointments with the orthodontist to reposition wires after professional oral hygiene has been performed.

This adult male had a periodontally reduced bone situation with extruded teeth and spaces in both arches (Fig 4-364). He showed signs of CMD with anterior disc displacement without repositioning and headache.

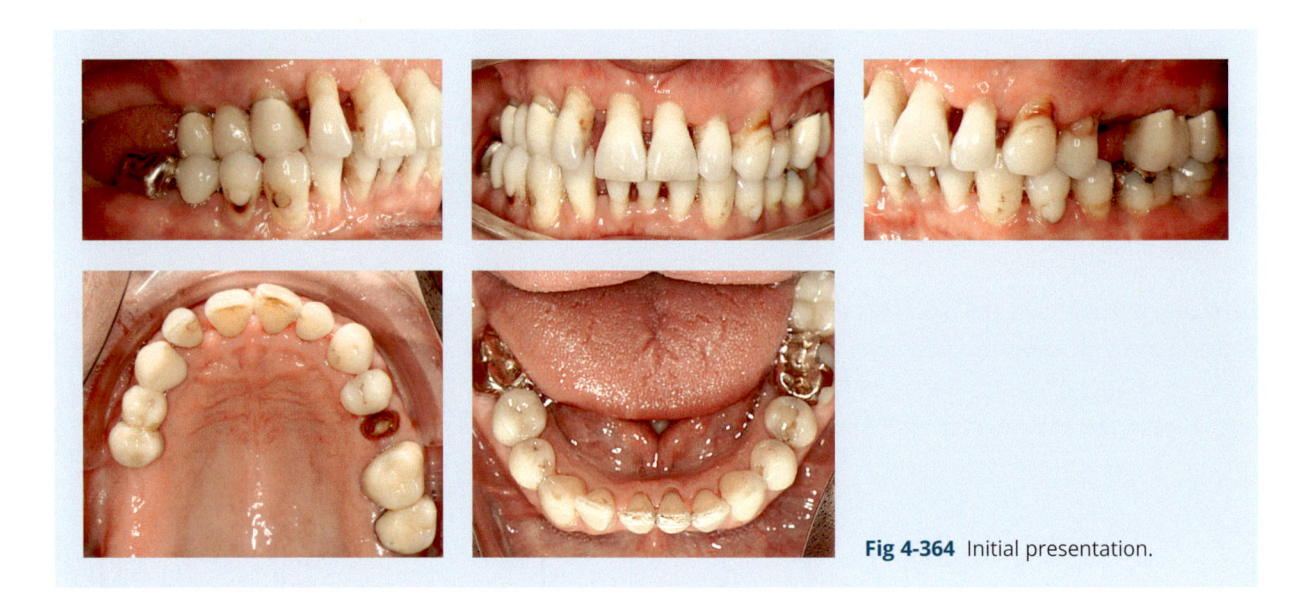

Fig 4-364 Initial presentation.

Diagnosis:
- CMD with anterior disc displacement without repositioning
- headache
- periodontitis
- deep bite and loss of posterior support in centric relation
- crowding.

Therapy:
- Invisalign treatment
- implantology
- prosthodontics.

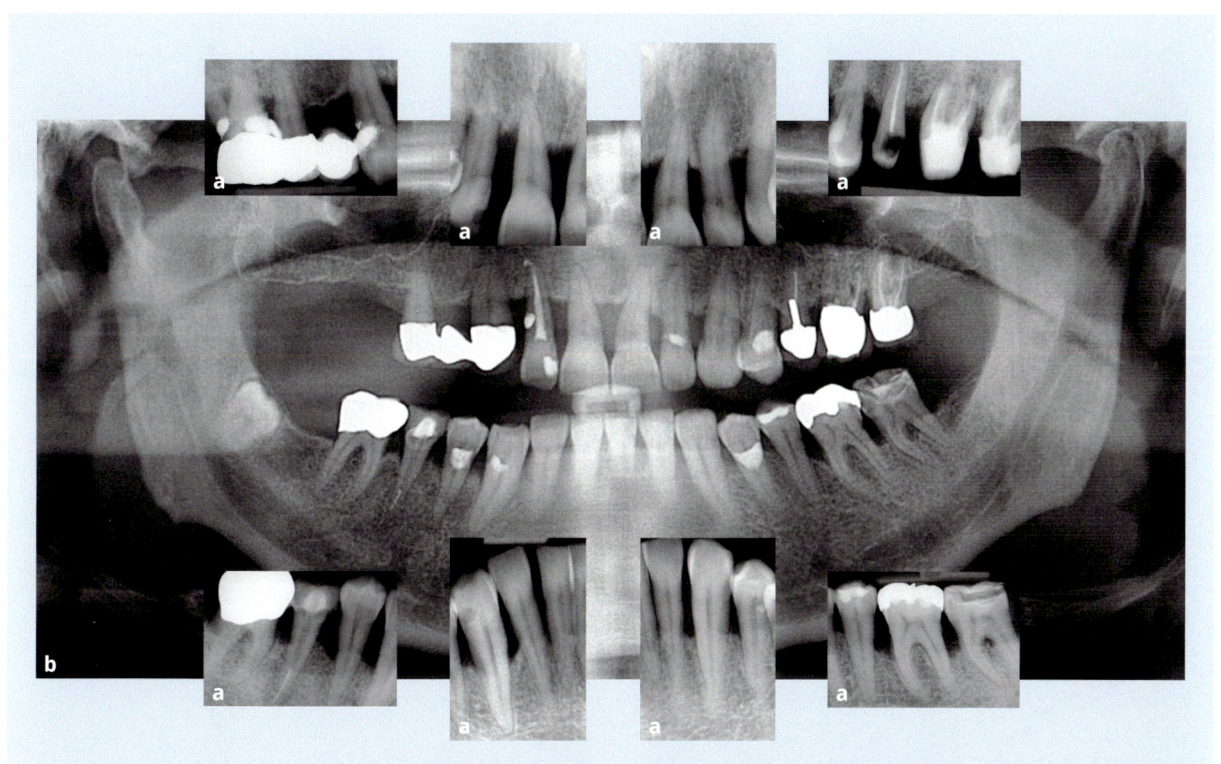

Fig 4-365 Orthopantomography. **(a)** There is severe bone loss in a clinically stable situation at the beginning of orthodontic treatment. **(b)** At the end of the Invisalign treatment, the bone situation seems improved.

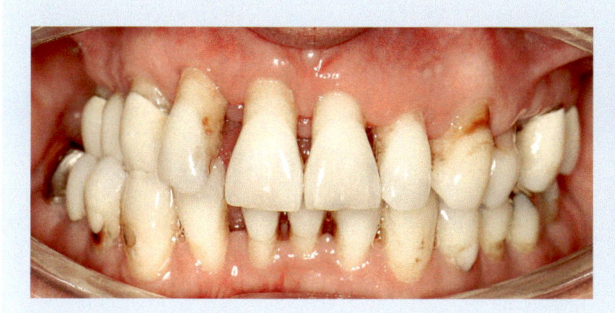

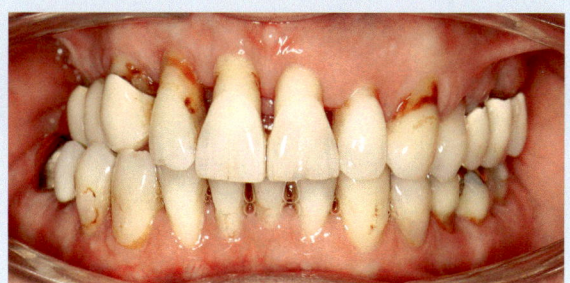

Fig 4-366 The periodont was stable before **(left)** and after **(right)** Invisalign treatment.

Treatment

Radiology at the end of periodontal treatment showed severe bone loss, but a clinically stable situation (Fig 4-365). Periodontal recall was performed every 3 months during orthodontic treatment.

The periodontal tissues were stable both before and after Invisalign treatment (Fig 4-366). Orthodontic treatment included intrusion in the maxillary and mandibular incisor area with space closure. The crossbite on the right posterior side was planned to be maintained.

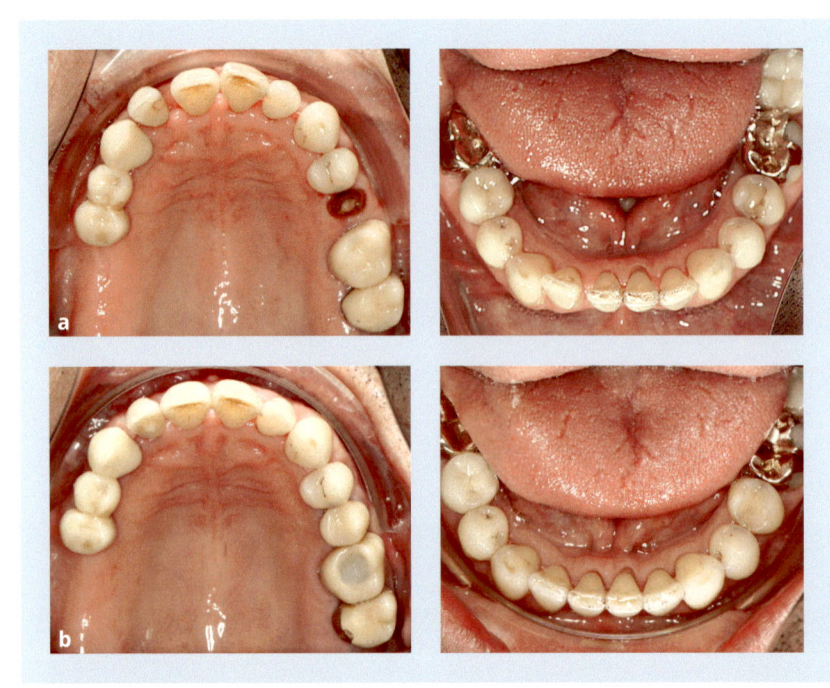

4 TREATMENT OF DIFFERENT MALOCCLUSIONS WITH ALIGNERS

Fig 4-367 Intraoral views before **(a)** and after **(b)** treatment, with a provisional crown on tooth 25.

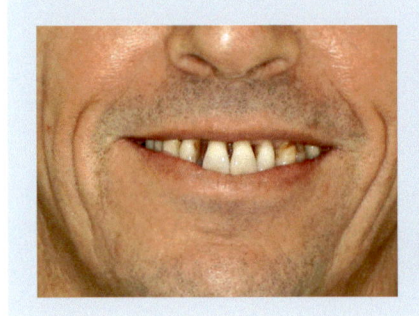

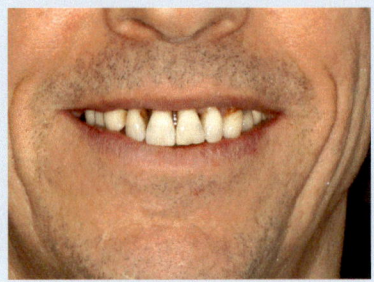

Fig 4-368 Facial view before **(left)** and after treatment **(right)**.

The patient was treated in an interdisciplinary approach (implants and prosthodontics by Dr F Bröseler, Aachen). Comparison of views before and after treatment show that space closure is highly predictable in patients with bone loss (Fig 4-367). The facial esthetics have been enhanced, with improved functional relationship of the anterior teeth (Fig 4-368).

Topic 45
CMD and bone loss in a patient with class II/2 relationship

Treatment:
- invisalign system
- implantology
- prosthodontics

One of the most important benefits of the Invisalign system is the possibility it offers of discussing the virtual end-result of treatment, as shown by the ClinCheck software, with an interdisciplinary team and the patient.

This patient presented with CMD with anterior disc displacement and headache. In addition to crowding and a deep bite, there was loss of posterior support in centric relation and the patient showed periodontitis (Figs 4-369 and 4-370).

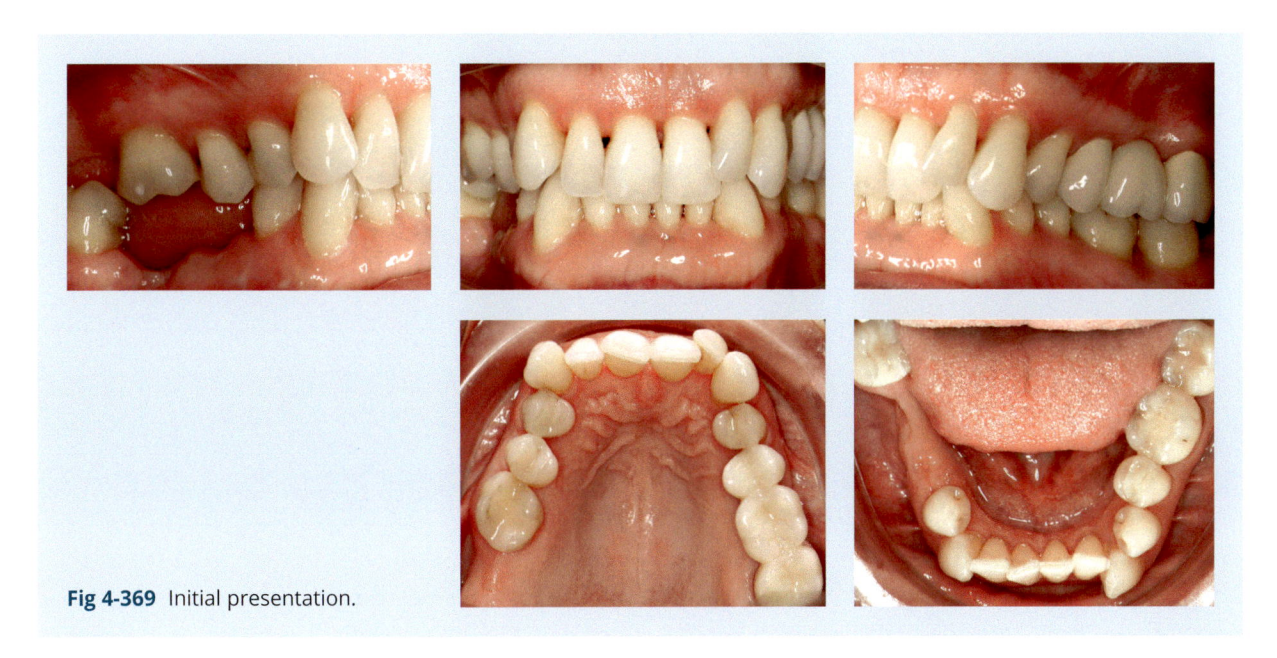

Fig 4-369 Initial presentation.

Diagnosis:
- CMD with anterior disc displacement
- headache
- periodontitis
- class II/ 2 relationship
- deep bite and loss of posterior support in centric relation
- crowding.

Therapy:
- periodontal pretreatment
- Invisalign system
- implantology
- prosthodontics.

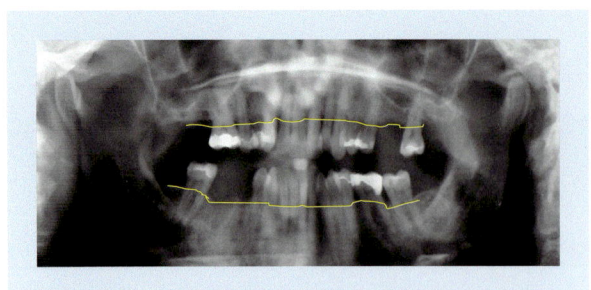

4 TREATMENT OF DIFFERENT MALOCCLUSIONS WITH ALIGNERS

Fig 4-370 Initial conventional orthopantomogram showing severe bone loss and spaces from periodontal tooth loss in both arches.

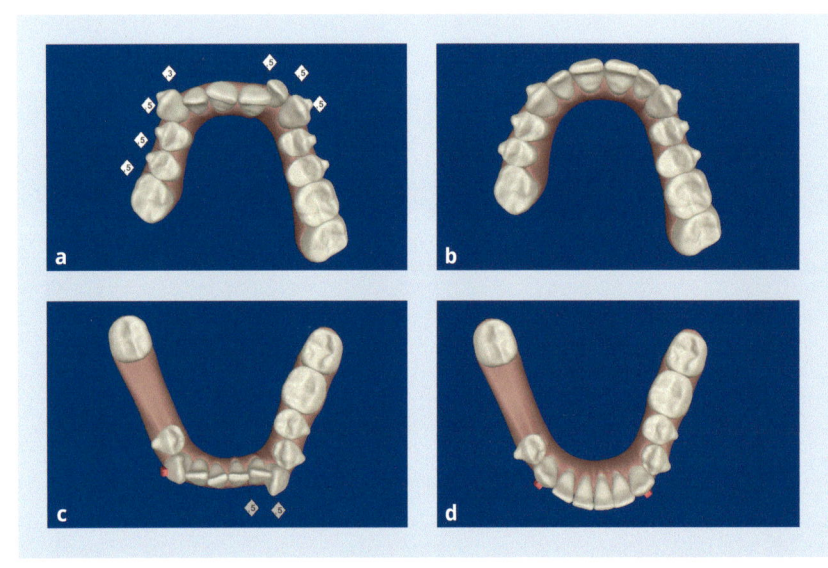

Fig 4-371 ClinCheck software results. **(a,c)** Initial situation with the IPR required. **(b,d)** Planned final result.

Treatment

After the periodontist had finished the periodontal pretreatment, and after bone augmentation in regions 45 and 46, Invisalign treatment was started. The patient remained in periodontal recall during the whole orthodontic treatment period. The ClinCheck images of the maxilla and mandible show the proposed treatment plan (Fig 4-371) using 41 aligners in the maxilla and 45 aligners in the mandible. IPR was planned for reduction on the maxillary right canine, right premolars, lateral left incisor, and left canine, as well as in the mandibular arch on teeth 32 and 33.

The maxillary incisors were torqued and the maxillary right posterior teeth were distalized into the spaces created with IPR. The mandibular incisors were proclined and moved with very little force during slow staging. The mandibular canines were planned to derotate with overcorrective movement of the mesial aspect to the lingual aspect. Expansion was performed in the maxillary arch over the whole treatment time. The overjet was set as 0.5 mm.

After Invisalign treatment, there was still a class II relationship on the right side. As the correction of the class II into a class I relationship here required a substantial amount of distalization, with an additional risk for the periodontal situation, distalization was not carried out and the uncorrected occlusal relationship was retained (Fig 4-372). Implants were inserted (Dr Meier, Cologne) with provisional crowns.

Figures 4-373 and 4-374 show the treatment pathway. The class I on the left and class II on the right was maintained but the arches were aligned and the

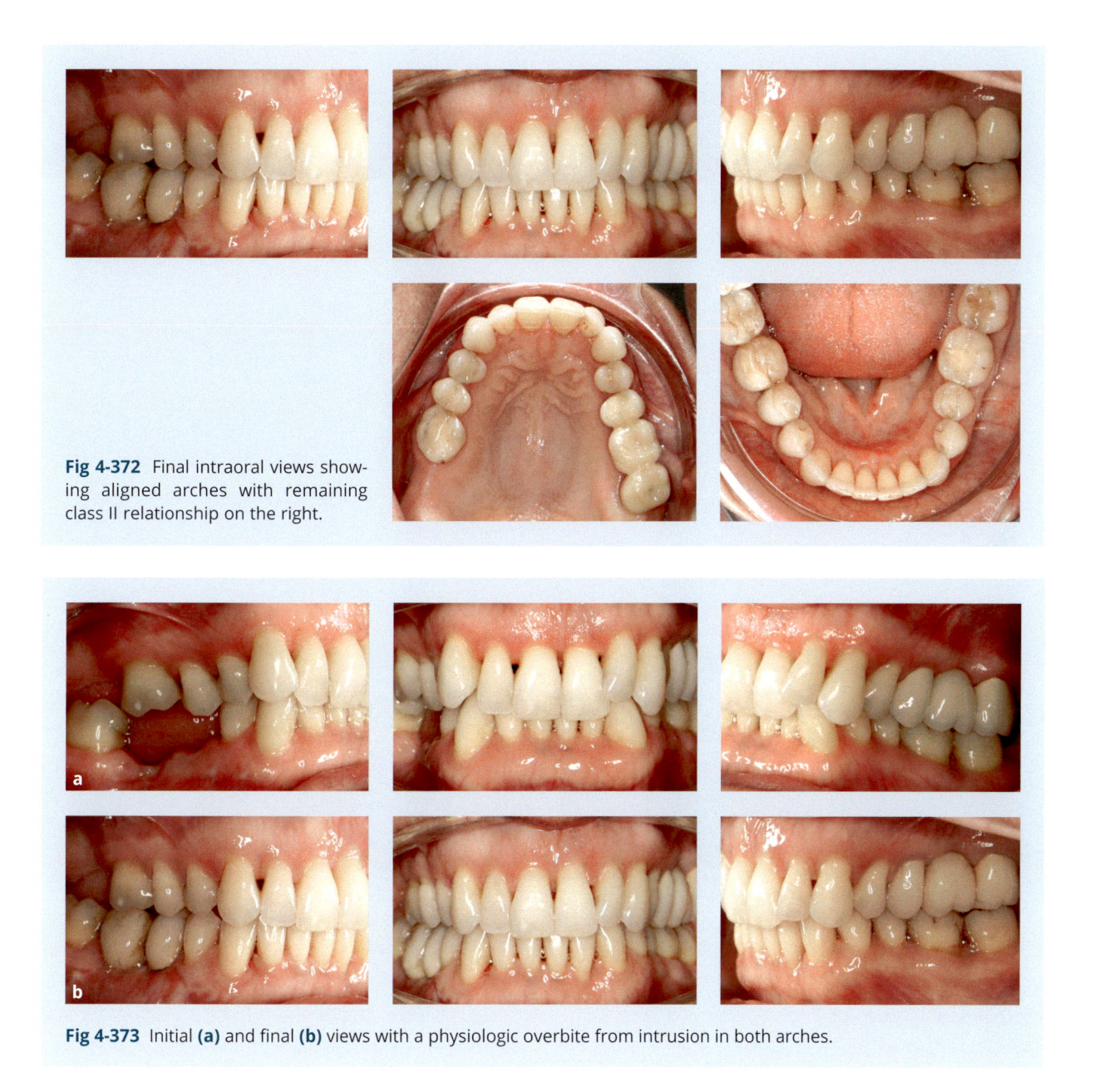

Fig 4-372 Final intraoral views showing aligned arches with remaining class II relationship on the right.

Fig 4-373 Initial (a) and final (b) views with a physiologic overbite from intrusion in both arches.

crowding resolved. The alignment of arches with solving of crowding and arch form development was achieved exclusively with aligners. A slight gingival recession has occurred in the anterior region on teeth 32 and 31. The availability of power ridges now would enable more torque to be generated. Implants were inserted in regions 45 and 46 and provided with provisional crowns.

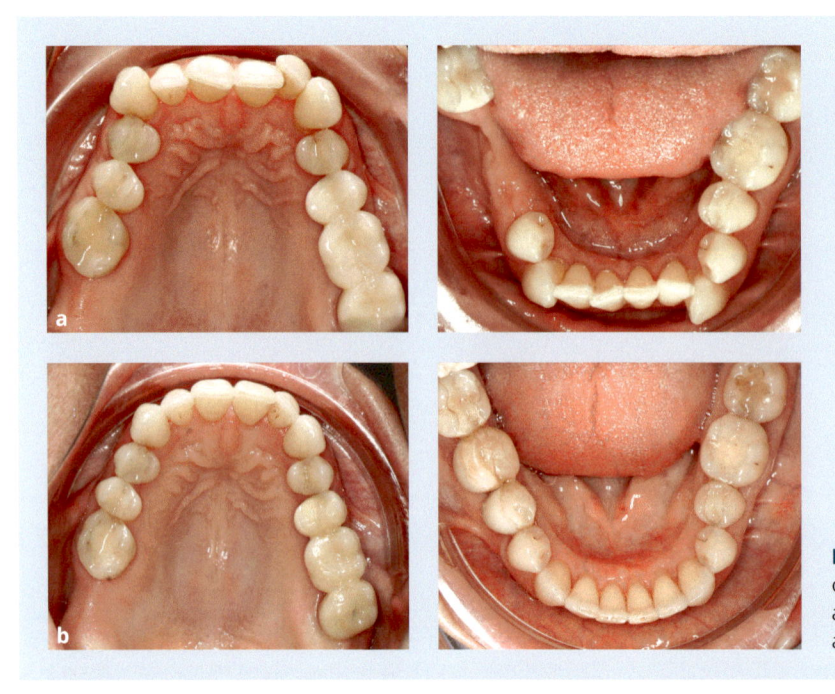

Fig 4-374 Initial **(a)** and final **(b)** views of the arches, demonstrating their alignment with resolution of crowding and arch form.

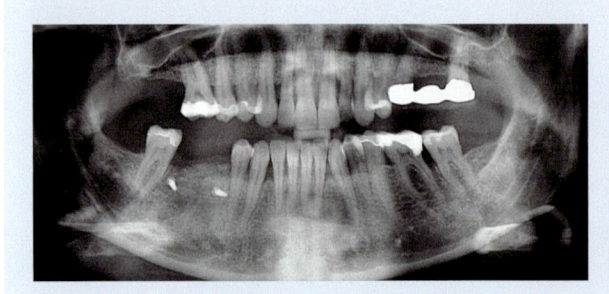

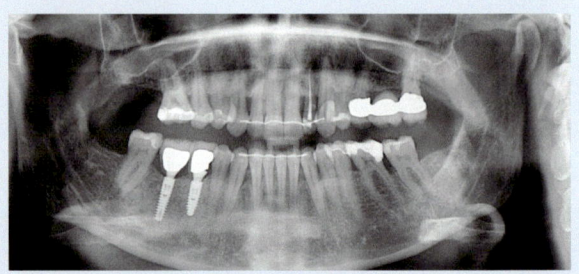

Fig 4-375 Orthopantomography. **(left)** At the start of the Invisalign treatment and after bone augmentation in regions 45 and 46. After the orthodontic treatment **(right)** showing a stable bone situation with implants inserted.

Orthopantomography shows the changing bone status during therapy (Fig 4-375).

The initial orthodontic treatment plan included the removal of the existing restoratives and prosthodontics after orthodontic pretreatment. However, because of the numerous insufficient restoratives at the beginning of orthodontic treatment, development of adequate posterior support was not included in the orthodontic treatment, but was planned for the following prosthodontic treatment (Dr W Boisserée, Cologne).

Figure 4-376 shows the intraoral findings at the beginning of the prosthodontic and restorative supply. This started with fixed splints on mandibular canines, premolars, and molars to create posterior support.

After restorative dentistry with lingual bonded retainers in both arches from canine to canine for retention, the class II relationship was maintained on the right side (Fig 4-377). Premolars and molars have been supplied with new restoratives (e.max, Ivoclar) and sufficient posterior support in a physiologic man-

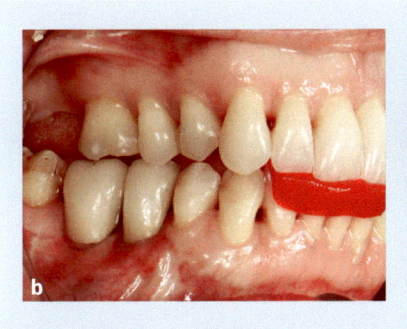

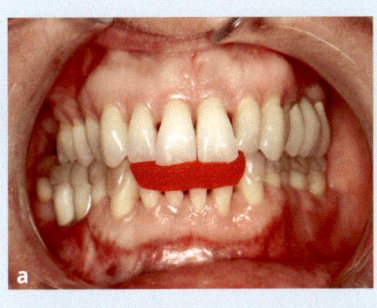

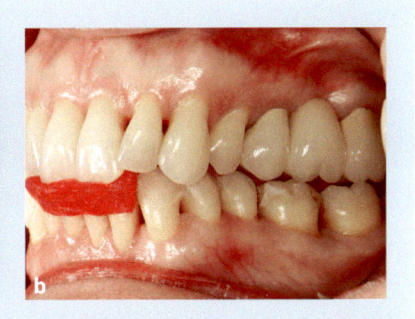

Fig 4-376 Intraoral findings at the beginning of prosthodontic and restorative treatment. **(a)** The anterior reference bite (red) represents the three-dimensional orthopedic position of the mandible in a physiologic condyle position. **(b)** After removal of the fixed posterior splints with the anterior reference bite, demonstrating the lack of posterior support.

Fig 4-377 After restorative dentistry with lingual bonded retainers in both arches from canine to canine.

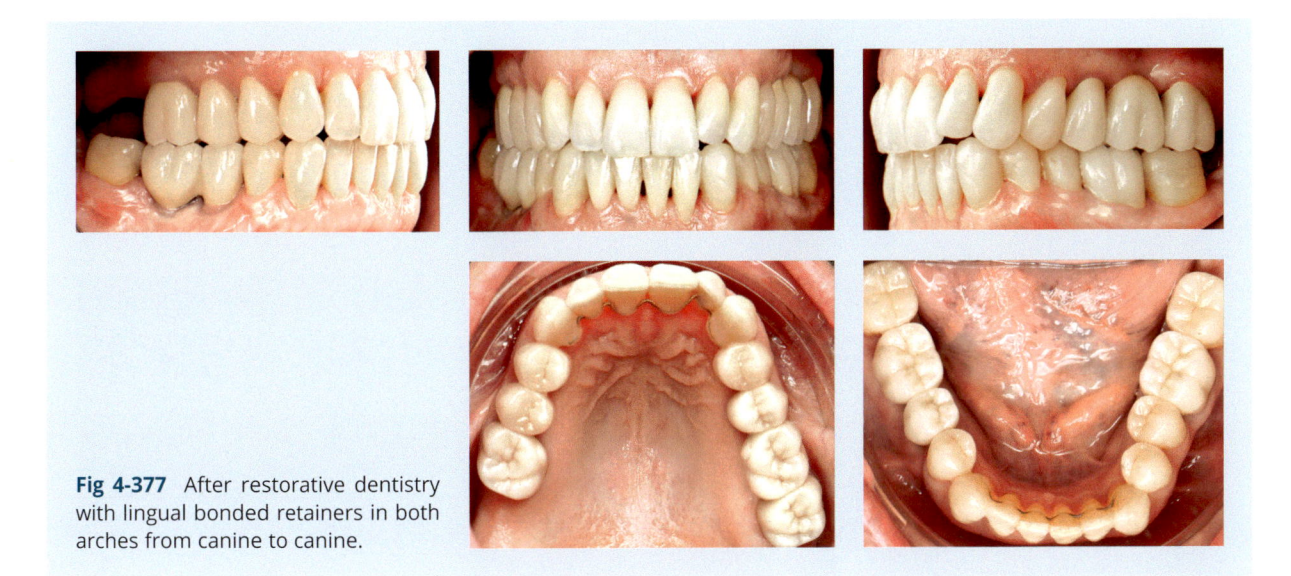

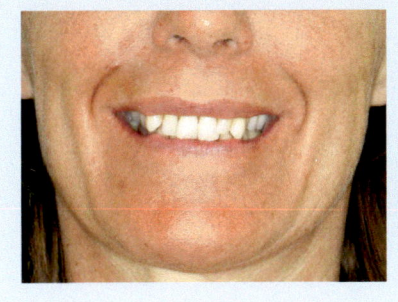

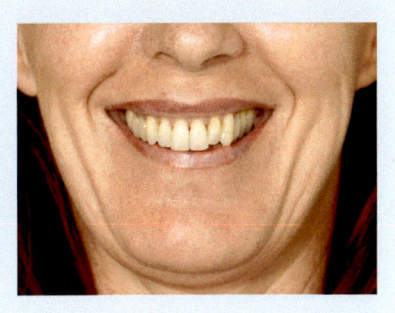

Fig 4-378 Initial **(left)** and final **(right)** extraoral views.

dibular position. Fixed partial dentures and crowns (Prettau Zirkon) were fabricated by M Läkamp (Ostbevern). Black triangles have been reduced with composite resin in the anterior area (Enamel plus HFO, Vanini).

There was a significant improvement in the esthetic appearance (Fig 4-378) and the patient no longer had pain and headache associated with the CMD.

Topic 46
Class II relationship treated with alignment before surgery

Treatment:
- Invisalign treatment
- orthognathic surgery

Preparing the arches for an orthognathic surgery is possible with the Invisalign system, using the ClinCheck software to plan for arch alignment and preparation for surgery. The software has a "bite jump" to allow simulation of surgery for changes in sagittal relationship. After surgery, an orthodontic refinement might be necessary for finishing in detail.

This patient had an asymmetric class II relationship with a midline shift in the mandibular arch to the left, deep bite, and crowding in both arches (Fig 4-379). The patient was advised for periodontics due to several gingival inflammations. Lateral cephalography gave the following results (Fig 4-380):

- convexity of A: 11.4 mm
- facial depth: 86.4 degrees
- lower facial height: 38.2 degrees.

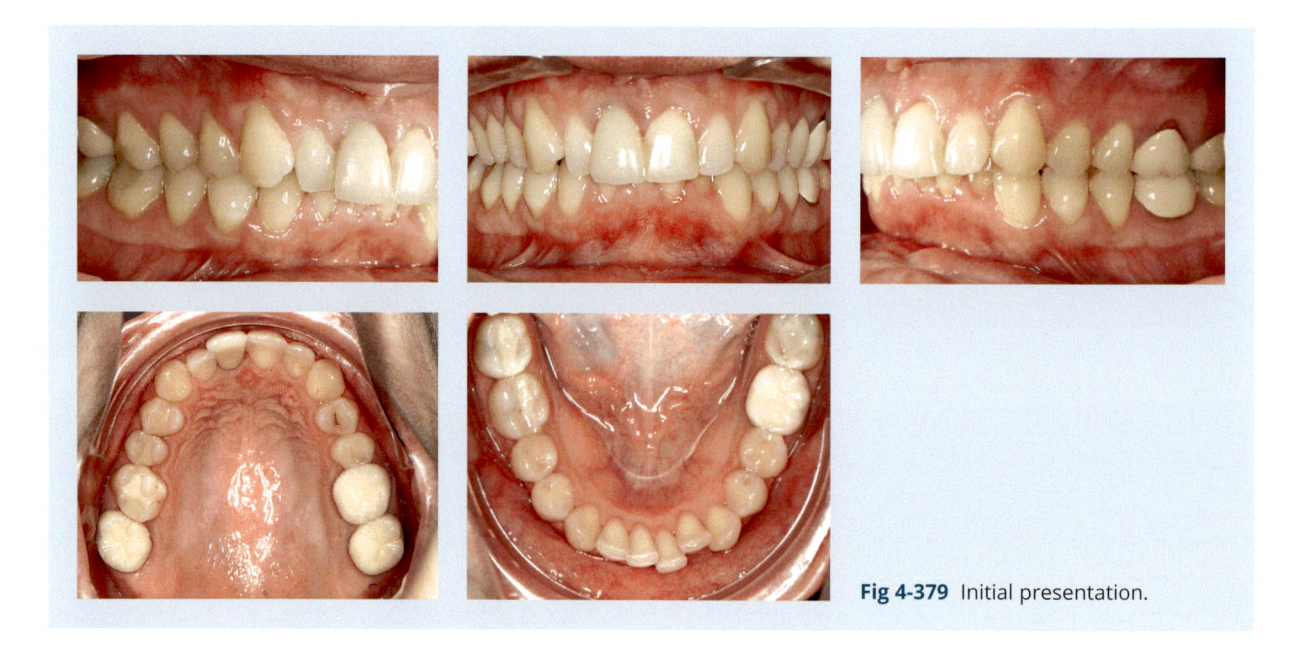

Fig 4-379 Initial presentation.

Diagnosis:
- skeletal class II
- crowding
- deep bite
- gingival inflammations.

Therapy:
- Invisalign treatment
- orthognathic surgery (Prof Dr Dr U Meyer, Münster).

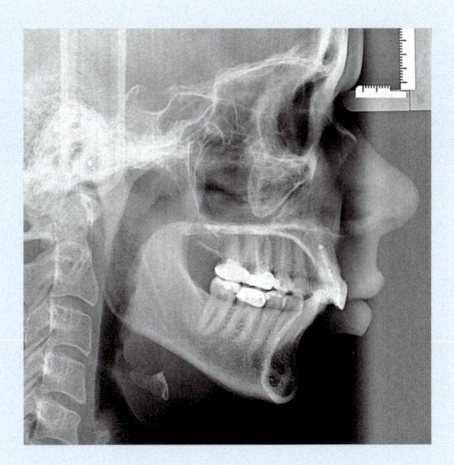

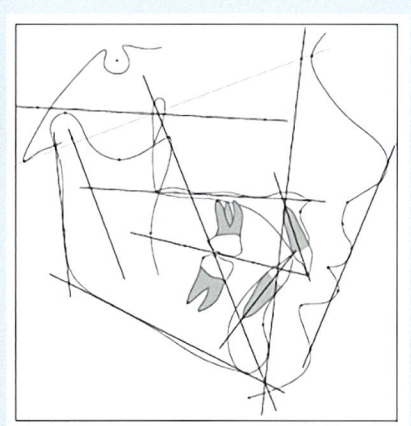

TREATMENT OF DIFFERENT MALOCCLUSIONS WITH ALIGNERS 4

Fig 4-380 Lateral cephalography for skeletal parameters.

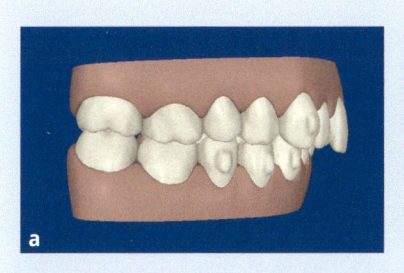

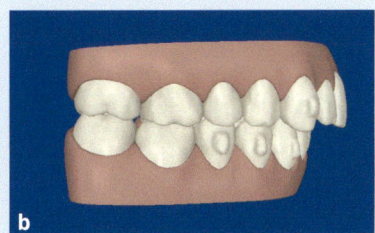

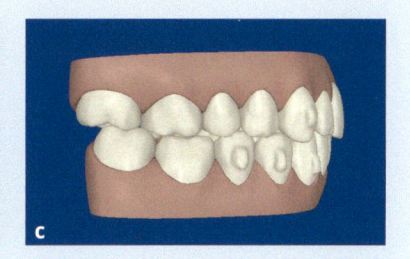

Fig 4-381 ClinCheck software results in lateral views. **(a)** Initial situation. **(b)** Planned treatment result; the overjet was slightly increased to create space for mandibular surgery with intrusion of lower anteriors 3-4 mm and an overjet of 5 mm. **(c)** Final situation after use of the "bite jump" and mandible movement.

Treatment

The patient was advised to have professional dental hygiene and periodontal therapy because of severe gingival inflammation, particularly of the maxillary anterior teeth. The patient wished to have correction of the retrognathic mandibular position, which was apparent in external views. An alternative treatment with dental correction and distalization in the maxillary arch was proposed but was rejected by the patient.

ClinCheck software shows the class II relationship with a deep bite and increased overjet with crowding (Fig 4-381). Planned treatment used 16 aligners and increased the overjet up to 5 mm to obtain the optimal situation for surgery and sufficient space for the mandible to be set forward. Use of the "bite jump" allowed virtual planning of that stage, too (Fig 4-381c).

The surgical stage was carried out by Prof Dr Dr U Meyer (Münster). The adjusted skeletal relation achieved with surgery requires fixation after setting of the arches. In multibracket therapy, this fixation can be obtained with elastics on wires, brackets, or bands. This is not an option if Invisalign therapy is used. Consequently, the surgically adjusted skeletal relation in this patient was fixed and maintained with elastics worn from miniscrews inserted in the maxilla and mandible.

Fig 4-382 Intraoral views showing the final outcome of Invisalign pretreatment and surgery.

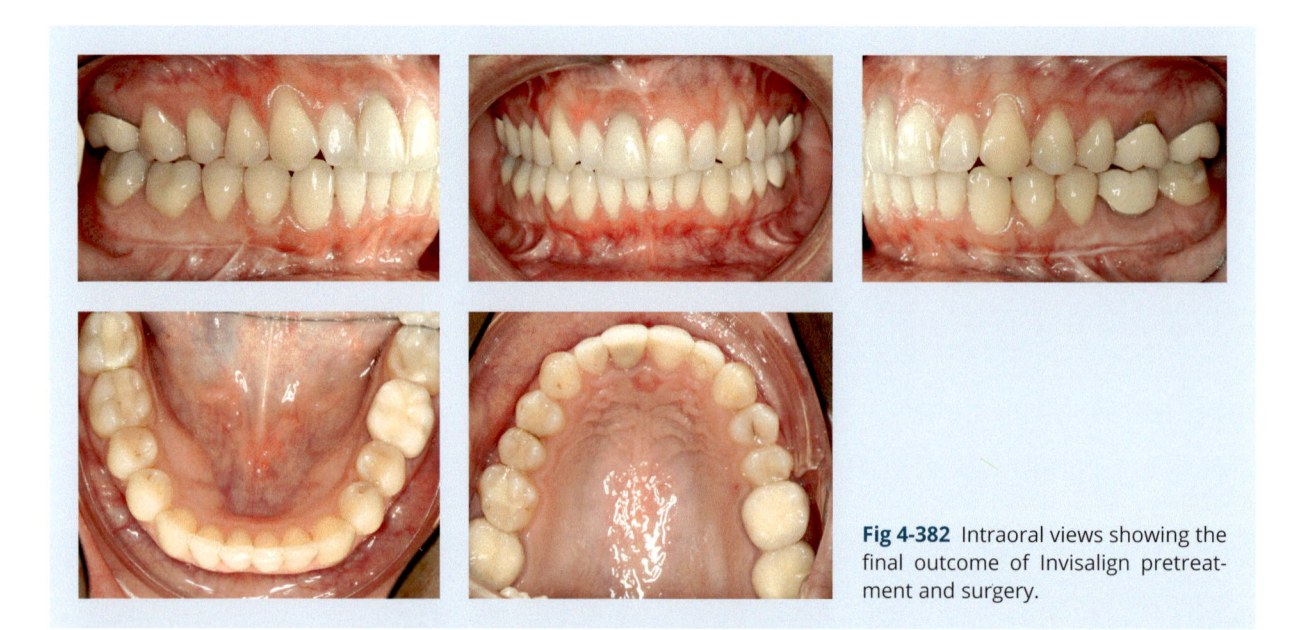

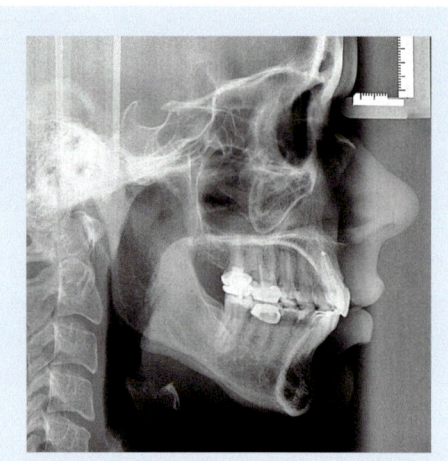

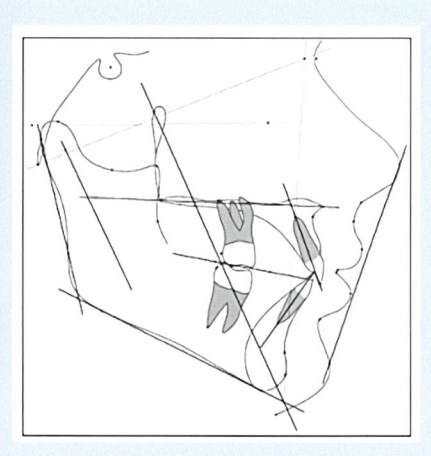

Fig 4-383 Lateral cephalography showing final skeletal parameters.

After Invisalign pretreatment and surgery, the mandible had been advanced into a class I relationship; there was midline correction and a physiologic overbite (Figs 4-382 and 4-383). Final skeletal parameters were:

- convexity of A: 12.3 mm
- facial depth: 85.8 degrees
- lower facial height: 40.8 degrees.

Figures 4-384 to 4-386 shows the changes achieved with this treatment path. There is a class I relationship, aligned midlines, and physiologic overjet and overbite. Visually, there is an improved final smile and lateral profile. The disproportionate lower facial height has been adjusted to give improved harmonious esthetics, an additional chin plastic might have even improved the esthetic result but was declined by the patient.

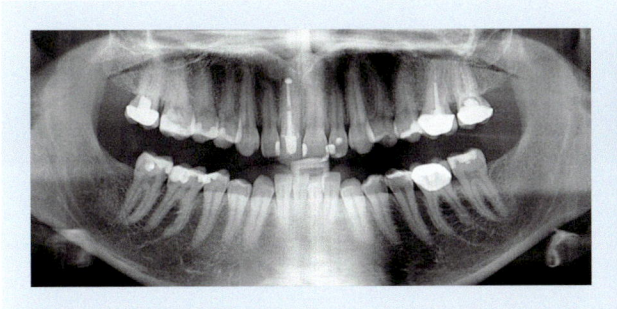

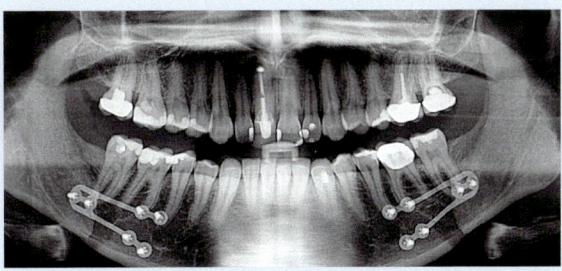

Fig 4-384 Orthopantomography initial view **(left)** and after surgery **(right)**. Osteosynthesis plates and screws can be seen. (Craniofacial Orthognathic Mandibular Fixation Plate, Medartis.)

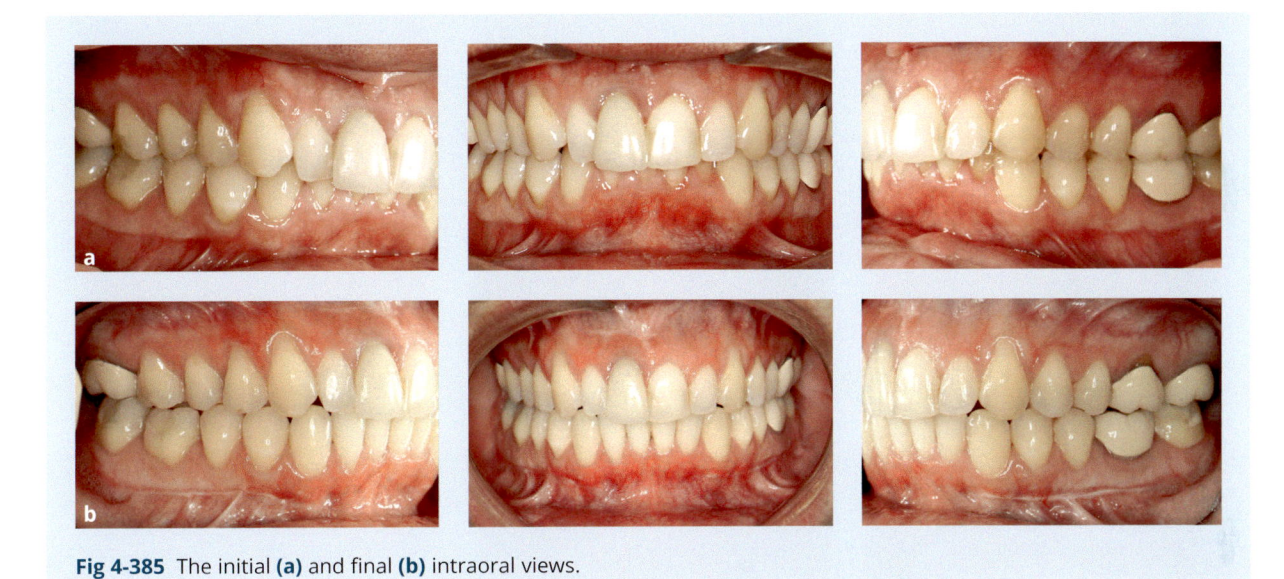

Fig 4-385 The initial **(a)** and final **(b)** intraoral views.

Fig 4-386 Initial **(a,c)** and final **(b,d)** views showing the changed esthetics in profile and frontal views.

4 TREATMENT OF DIFFERENT MALOCCLUSIONS WITH ALIGNERS

Topic 47
Class III relationship treated with alignment before surgery

Treatment:
- Invisalign treatment
- orthognathic surgery

A skeletal class III relationship is more likely to require orthognathic surgery than class II. In both groups, it is necessary to first check the condyle position as it is not advisable to plan a surgical intervention until the physiologic mandibular position is defined.

This patient had an anterior crossbite from tooth 13 to tooth 22 in a class III relationship, midline deviation, crowding in the maxillary arch, and spaces distal of teeth 33 and 43 in the mandibular arch (Fig 4-387). Lateral cephalography gave the following results (Fig 4-388):

- convexity of A: 16.2 mm
- facial depth: 100.0 degrees
- lower facial height: 36.9 degrees.

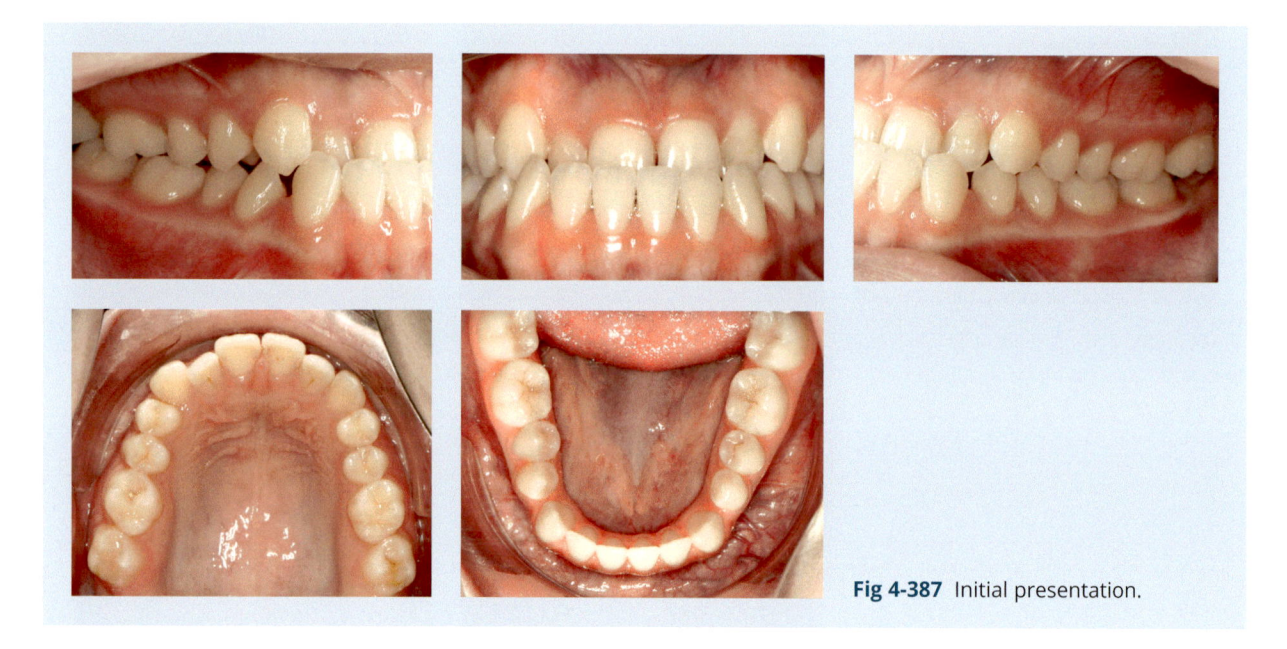

Fig 4-387 Initial presentation.

Diagnosis:
- skeletal class III with midline deviation
- anterior crossbite
- crowding in the maxilla, spaces in the mandible.

Therapy:
- Invisalign treatment
- orthognathic surgery (Prof Dr Dr hc mult U K Joos, Münster).

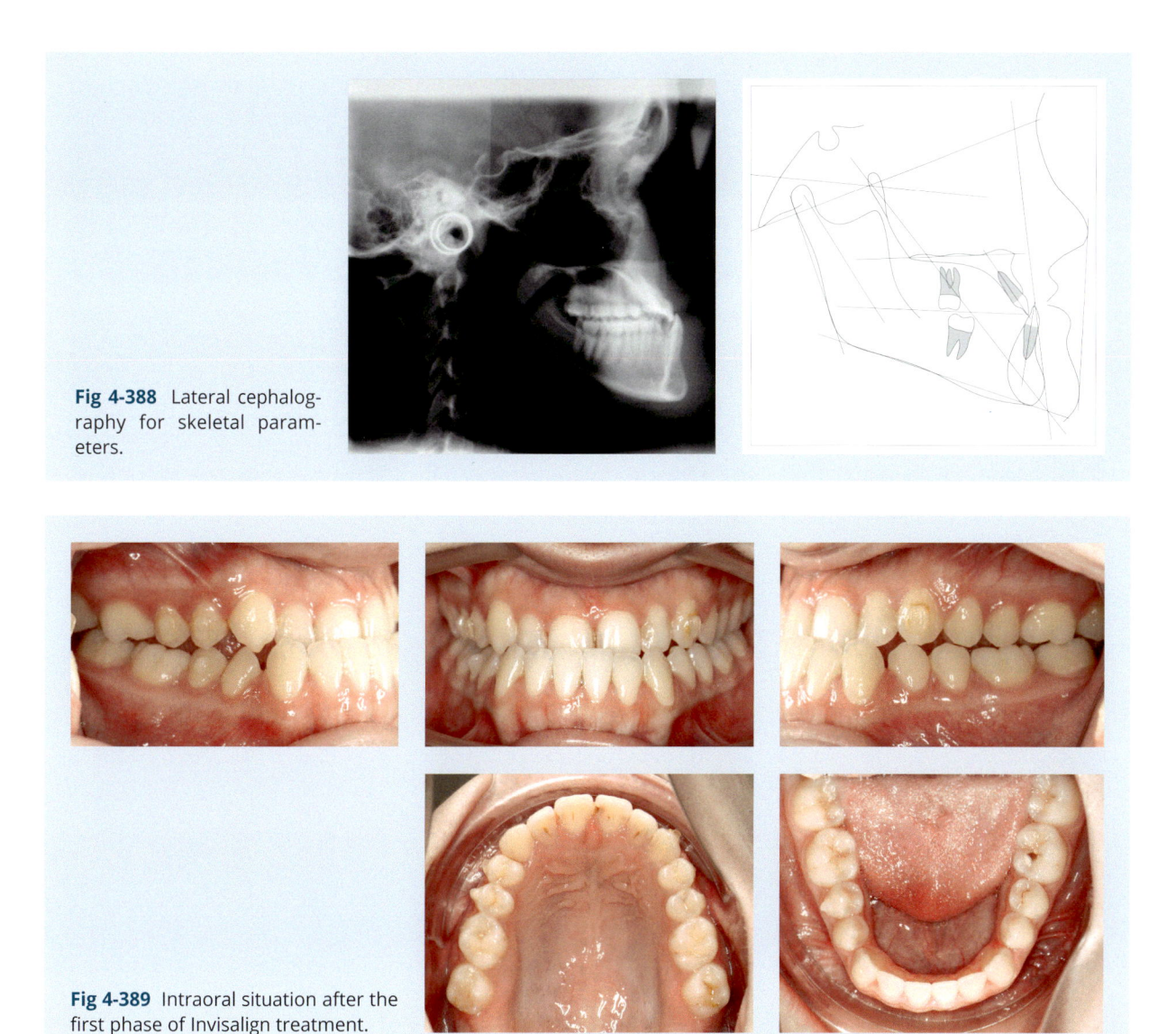

TREATMENT OF DIFFERENT MALOCCLUSIONS WITH ALIGNERS 4

Fig 4-388 Lateral cephalography for skeletal parameters.

Fig 4-389 Intraoral situation after the first phase of Invisalign treatment.

Treatment

The first phase of Invisalign treatment aligned the maxilla and mandible for the planned surgery using 23 aligners in the maxilla and 34 in the mandible (Fig 4-389).

ClinCheck software at the end of the first phase, with the aligned arches, allowed planning of the mandibular movement (Fig 4-390). Use of the "bite jump" in the software enables very precise planning of the treatment outcome from the very beginning through to after surgical intervention.

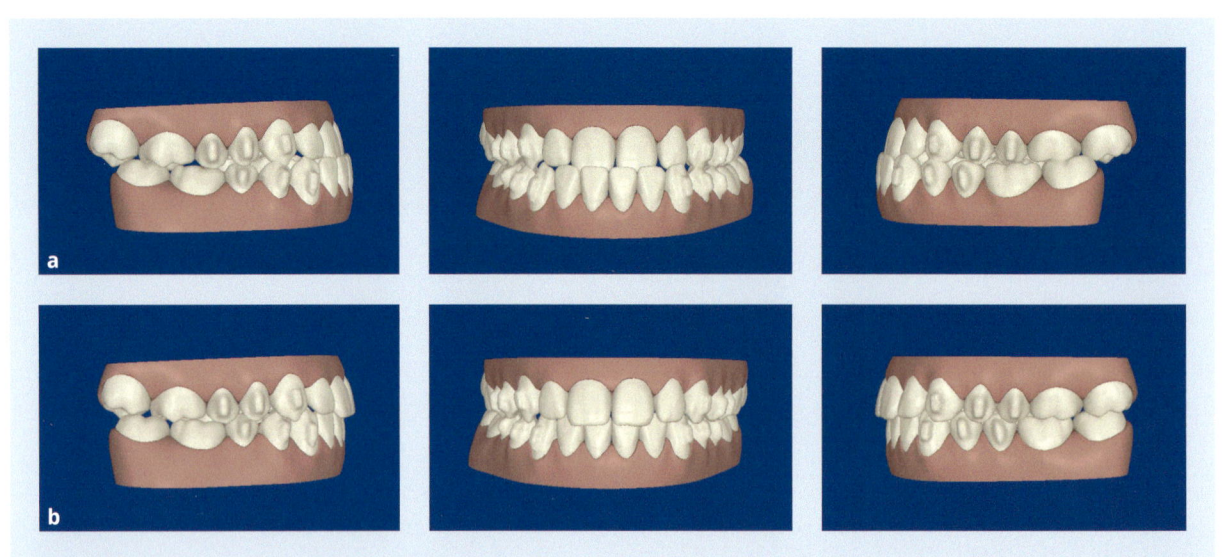

4 TREATMENT OF DIFFERENT MALOCCLUSIONS WITH ALIGNERS

Fig 4-390 ClinCheck images at the end of the first phase. **(a)** Aligned arches. **(b)** Final occlusion after the surgical simulation.

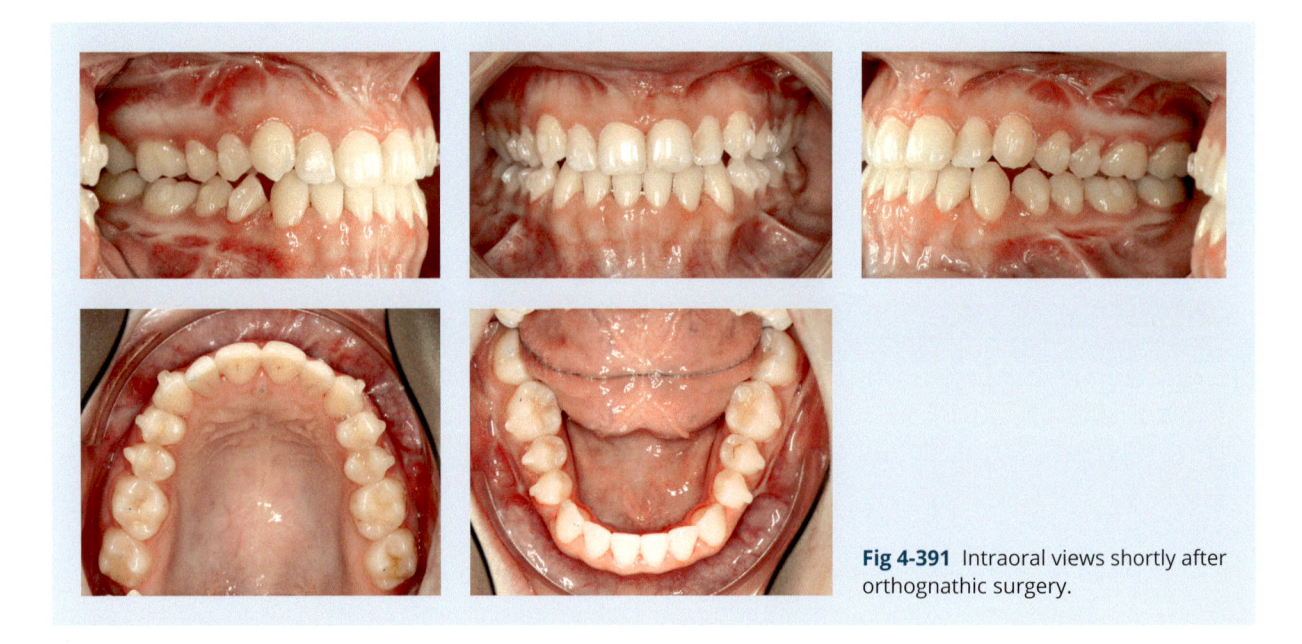

Fig 4-391 Intraoral views shortly after orthognathic surgery.

After surgery (Prof Dr Dr hc mult U K Joos, Münster), the new sagital position of the mandible was maintained with intermaxillary elastics worn from miniscrews in the maxilla and mandible for several weeks (Fig 4-391). A refinement was planned to align the arches in detail (Fig 4-392).

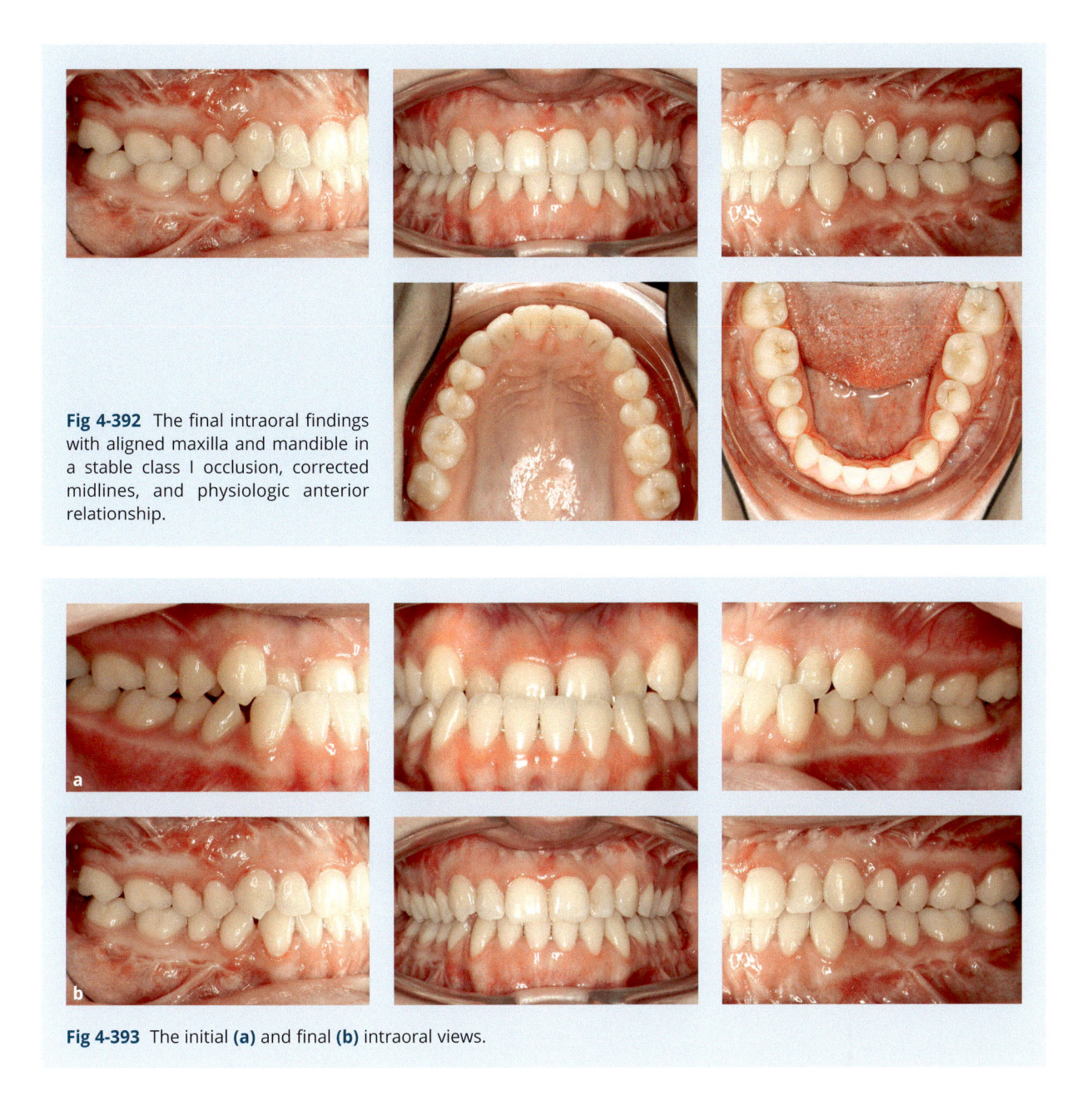

Fig 4-392 The final intraoral findings with aligned maxilla and mandible in a stable class I occlusion, corrected midlines, and physiologic anterior relationship.

Fig 4-393 The initial **(a)** and final **(b)** intraoral views.

After Invisalign pretreatment and surgery, the mandible has been advanced into a class I relationship; there is a corrected midline and a physiologic anterior relationship (Figs 4-393 and 4-394). The patient shows increased lower facial height and a significantly improved smile esthetic (Fig 4-394c, d) Skeletal changes performed with surgery were:

- maxilla: 4 mm advancement
- mandible right: 3 mm advancement
- mandible left: 2 mm set back.

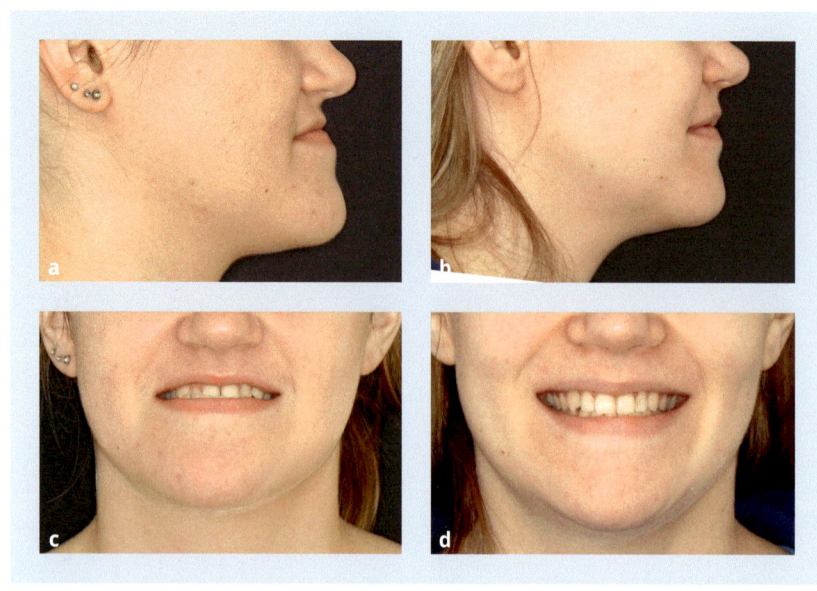

Fig 4-394 Extraoral initial **(a)** and final **(b)** lateral views. Initial **(c)** and final **(d)** frontal views show the improved smile esthetic.

Topic 48
Craniomandibular dysfunction: General considerations

In nearly all patients with craniomandibular dysfunction and musculoskeletal disorders, treatment starts with a removable occlusal splint (Boisserée and Schupp, 2012). If orthodontic treatment is subsequently necessary, this can be performed with the Invisalign system, which allows precise and highly predictable results.

Figure 4-395a shows a class I relationship with physiologic posterior support, physiologic position of the condyles, and physiologically positioned discus articularis. In most TMJ disorders, there is a lack of posterior support (Fig 4-395b). When the patient takes habitual occlusion position, contact will occur first on incisors followed by the molars but this will move the condyles posteriorly into a backward position and displace the disc anteriorly (Fig 4-395c). The TMJ is then positioned on the bilaminar zone, not on the disc. The bilaminar zone is one of the body areas with the most nociceptors, which transmit the pain to the lower nucleus of the trigeminal nerve and then on to the brain (Fig 4-396).

Fig 4-395 TMJ disorders. **(a)** Class I relationship with physiologic posterior support, physiologic position of the condyles, and physiologically positioned discus articularis. **(b)** Lack of posterior support with contact limited to the incisor area in physiologic condyle position, giving a posterior open bite. **(c)** Habitual contact on the molars then moves the condyles into a backward position, displacing the disc to anterior and positioning the joint on the bilaminar zone. **(d)** A removable splint stabilizes the condyle in its centric position. The area showing the disc (blue) and the alignment of the joint (red) is referred to as the "black box" in subsequent topics.

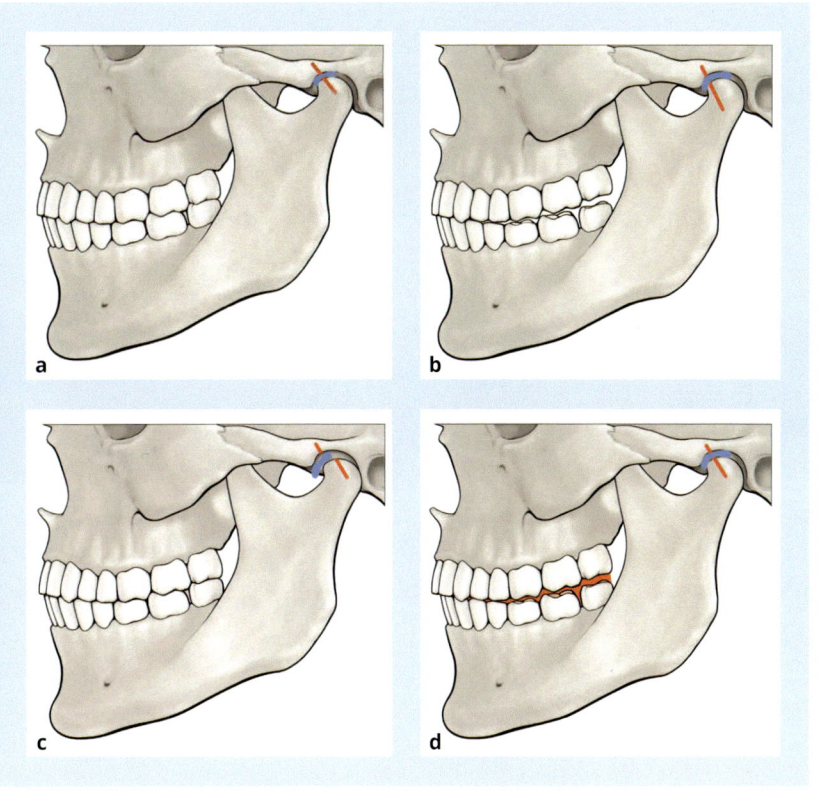

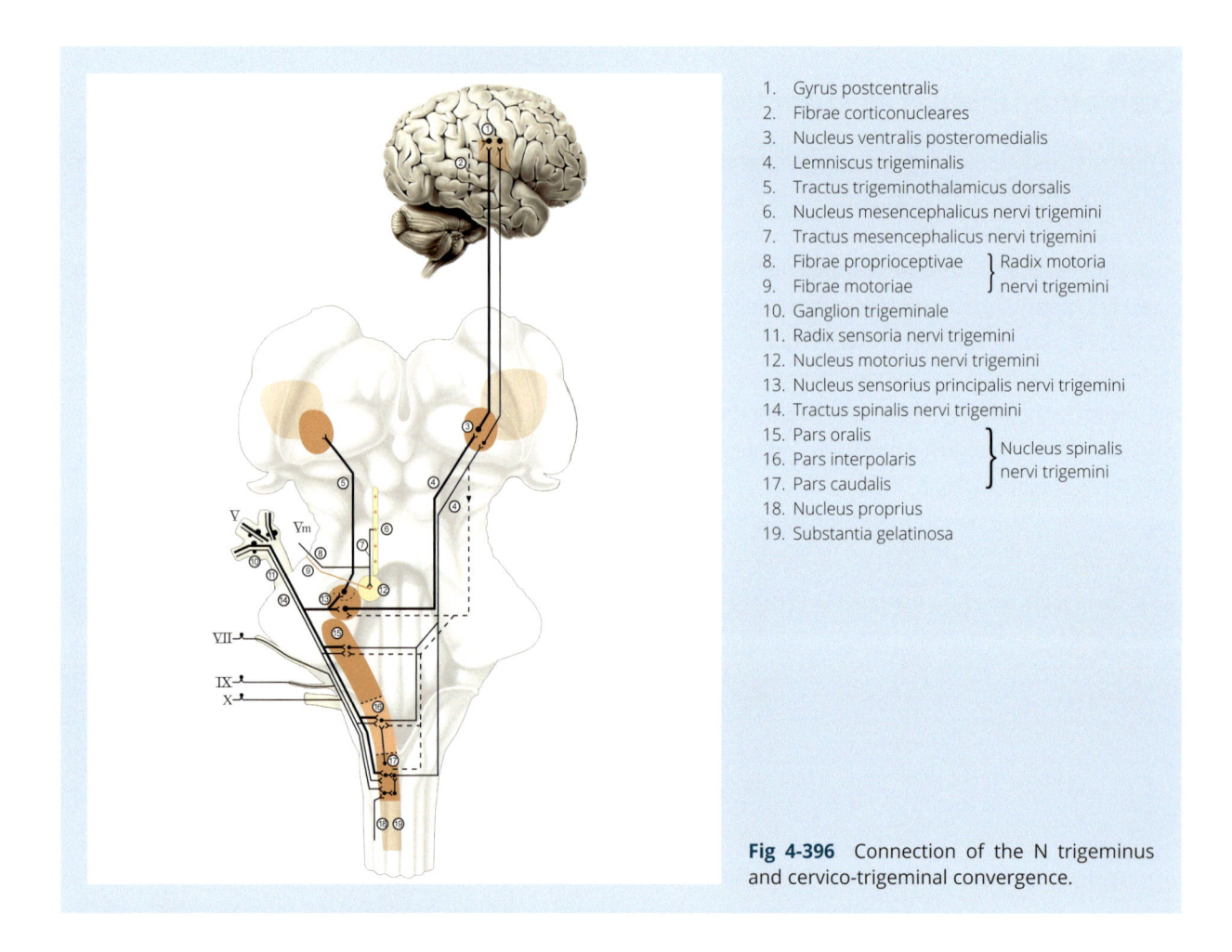

4 TREATMENT OF DIFFERENT MALOCCLUSIONS WITH ALIGNERS

1. Gyrus postcentralis
2. Fibrae corticonucleares
3. Nucleus ventralis posteromedialis
4. Lemniscus trigeminalis
5. Tractus trigeminothalamicus dorsalis
6. Nucleus mesencephalicus nervi trigemini
7. Tractus mesencephalicus nervi trigemini
8. Fibrae proprioceptivae } Radix motoria
9. Fibrae motoriae } nervi trigemini
10. Ganglion trigeminale
11. Radix sensoria nervi trigemini
12. Nucleus motorius nervi trigemini
13. Nucleus sensorius principalis nervi trigemini
14. Tractus spinalis nervi trigemini
15. Pars oralis } Nucleus spinalis
16. Pars interpolaris } nervi trigemini
17. Pars caudalis
18. Nucleus proprius
19. Substantia gelatinosa

Fig 4-396 Connection of the N trigeminus and cervico-trigeminal convergence.

In the lower nucleus of the trigeminus (nucleus spinalis nervi trigemini pars caudalis), which is positioned at the height of C3, a convergence of the N trigeminus with the N facialis, N accessorius, N glossopharyngeus, N vagus and the spinal nerves C2-C5 occurs. We call this the cervico-trigeminal convergence. In the lower receptor of the trigeminus nucleus, information from all the different above-mentioned nerves can arrive. The joining of the different information requires a differentiation in perception.

The lower trigeminal nucleus has input from a number of facial and cervical nerves (trigeminal, facial, glossopharyngeal, N trigeminal, N facialis, N glossopharyngeus, N vagus, N accessorius, and spinal nerves C2–C5) and TMJ dysfunction has always impact on these nerves (Fig 4-396). Often "referred pain" is seen, where the patient describes a pain that is located distant from its orgin. The origins for TMJ pain can be trigger points in the muscles. A frontal and parietal headache may also have its origin in dysfunction of the TMJ. Pain needs to be treated at its origin, not at the site of the pain; for example, pain can be experienced in the shoulder and arm with a mycardial infarction.

Insertion of a removable splint stabilizes the condyle in its centric position (Fig 4-395d). The patient is advised to wear the splint day and night except for eating and tooth cleaning, just like an aligner. Patients often undergo manual or physiotherapeutic treatment at the same time.

The removable occlusal splint we use is the COPA (craniomandibular orthopedic positioning appliance). The splint helps to center the condyle in a therapeutic and physiologic position and lead the muscles into a neutral, adapted neurologic balance.

Topic 49
Craniomandibular dysfunction: diagnosis and treatment planning

Treatment:
- assessment of the root cause (open the "black box")

This topic describes the essential diagnosis and treatment planning before embarking on treatment in patients with craniomandibular and musculoskeletal disorders. The vertical dimension is the most important dimension for the TMJ. The discussion centers around "black box," the components and alignment of the TMJ (see Fig 4-395 in Topic 48).

The diagnosis and treatment planning pathway is described for a patient who presented with severe back pain, who in fact had TMJ anterior disc displacement with a posterior positioned condyle (Fig 4-397).

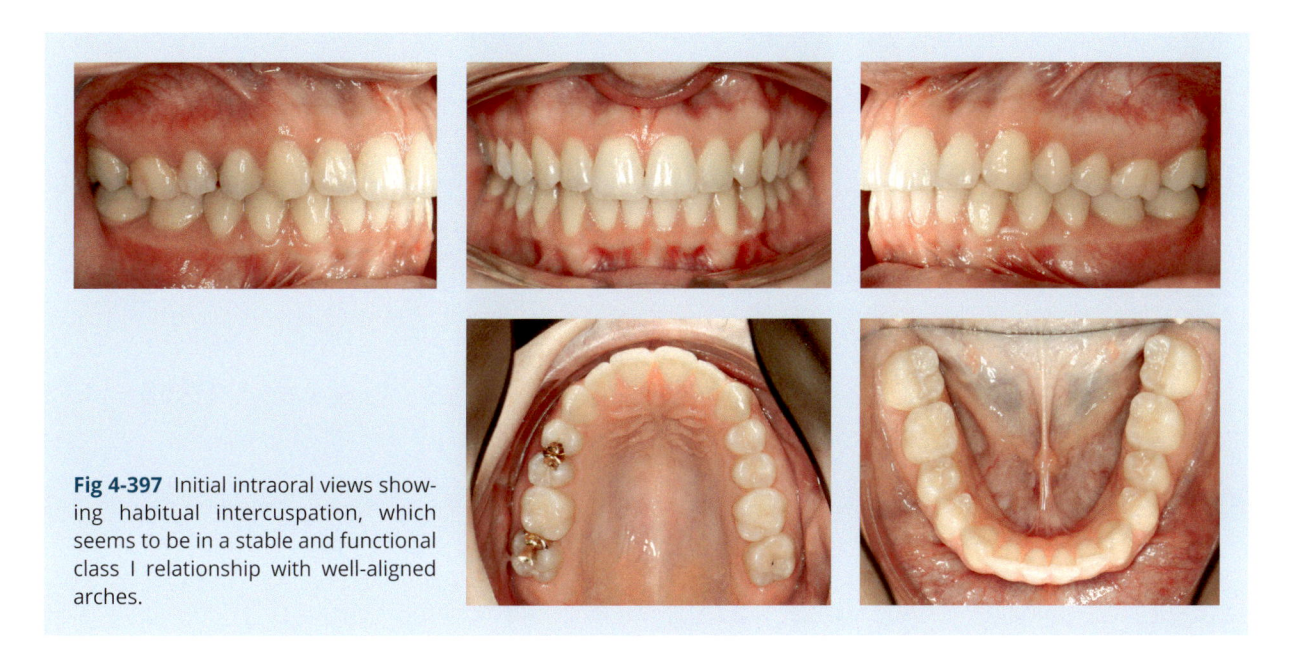

Fig 4-397 Initial intraoral views showing habitual intercuspation, which seems to be in a stable and functional class I relationship with well-aligned arches.

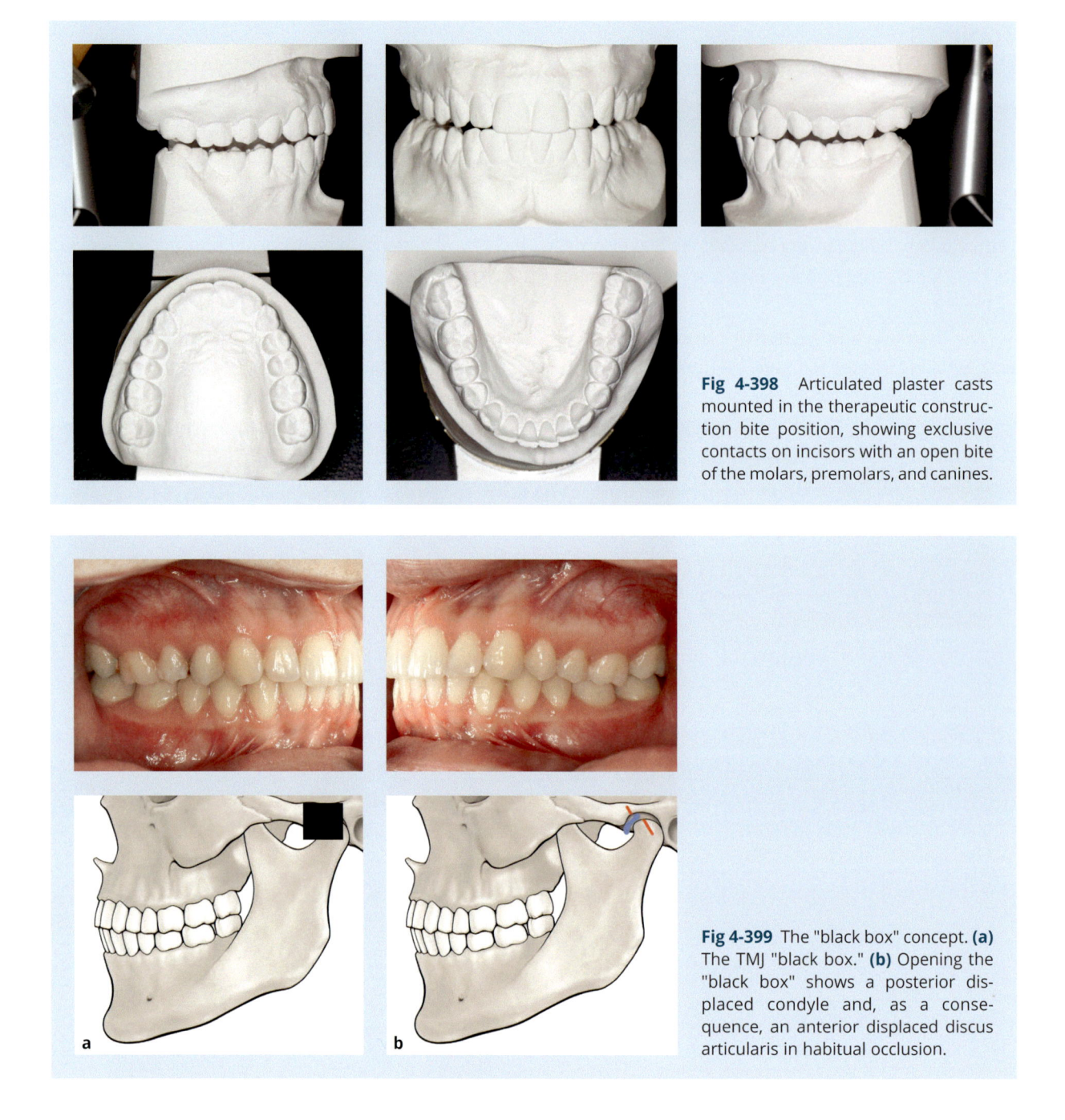

Fig 4-398 Articulated plaster casts mounted in the therapeutic construction bite position, showing exclusive contacts on incisors with an open bite of the molars, premolars, and canines.

Fig 4-399 The "black box" concept. **(a)** The TMJ "black box." **(b)** Opening the "black box" shows a posterior displaced condyle and, as a consequence, an anterior displaced discus articularis in habitual occlusion.

Articulated plaster mounted in therapeutic relation (see Chapter 1) clarifies the problems of occlusion (Fig 4-398) that had looked reasonable visually. There is exclusive contacts on incisors with an open bite at the molars and premolars. Under muscle forces, the TMJ condyle shifts posterior and upwards from the centric relation into the habitual intercuspation during jaw closure. Non-mounted, hand-held casts would not have been able to show more than the intraoral views in habitual occlusion did.

If the components of the TMJ is considered as a "black box," its opening is indispensable for the therapeutic approach (Fig 4-399). In this patient, if treatment, orthodontic or other, had been commenced

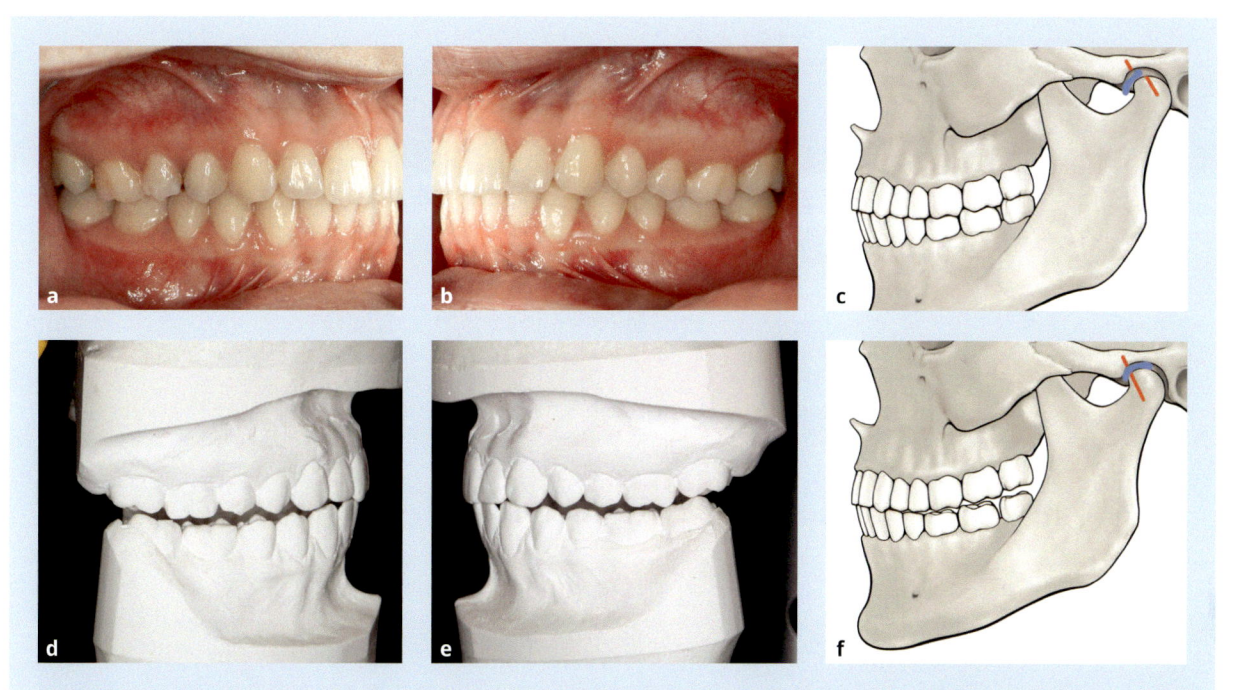

TREATMENT OF DIFFERENT MALOCCLUSIONS WITH ALIGNERS 4

Fig 4-400 Treatment planning. **(a,b)** Intraoral views in habitual intercuspation. **(c)** Representation of the habitual intercuspation, with the "black box" opened to show the posterior positioned condyle with the anterior displaced disc. **(d,e)** Mounted plaster casts showing the occlusion in therapeutic relation with the lack of posterior vertical support. **(f)** Occlusion in centric relation with a physiologic condyle, showing the disc position and lack of posterior support.

without consideration of the TMJ and the musculoskeletal system, the whole treatment would have failed. As Harold Gelb (1994) said: "Think orthopedic first – then teeth."

Figure 4-400 shows a treatment following these components.

To assess the TMJ, open the "black box":
- manual diagnosis (see Chapter 1)
- mounted plaster casts in centric relation (see Chapter 1).

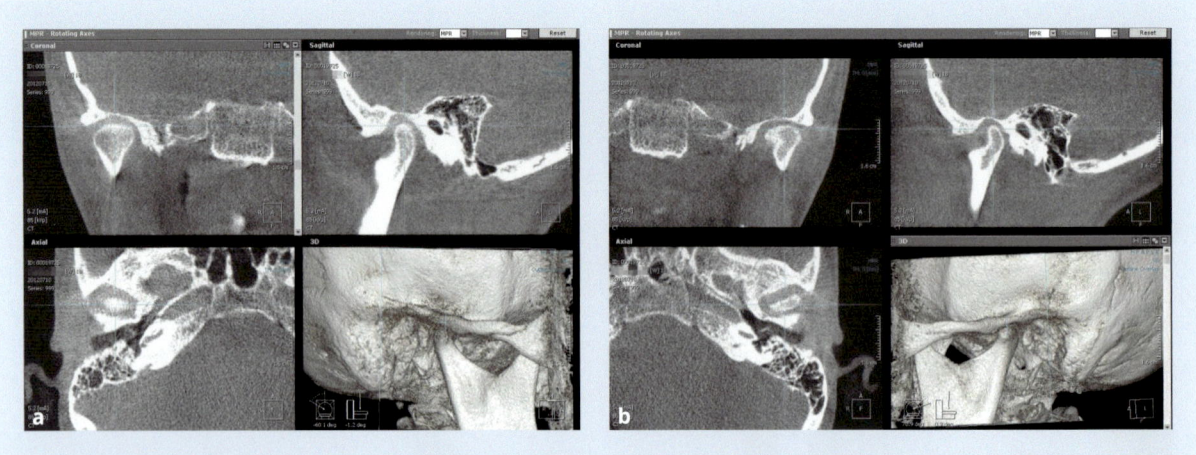

4 TREATMENT OF DIFFERENT MALOCCLUSIONS WITH ALIGNERS

Fig 4-401 CBCT of the TMJs (Picasso, Orange Dental). **(a)** Right side showing retruded condylar position. **(b)** Left side also with retruded condyle position but more dislocation. No cortical bone pathology on either side.

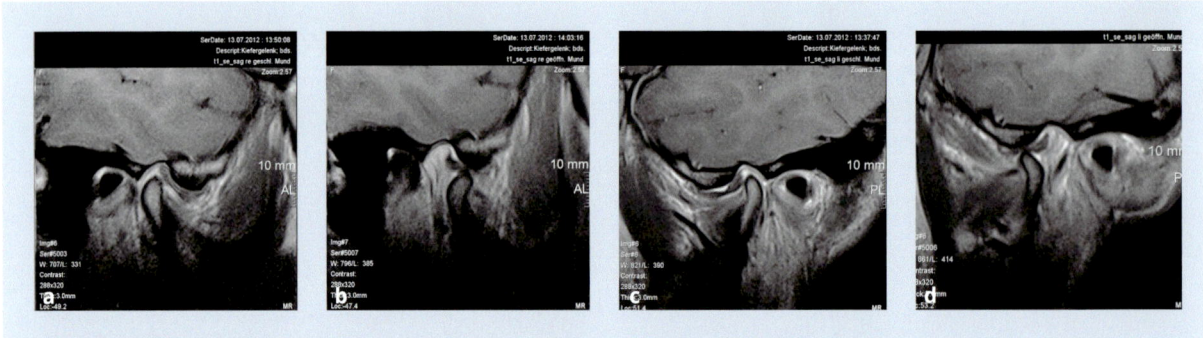

Fig 4-402 MRT (MediaPark Clinic, Drs Andersson and Steimel). **(a,b)** Right TMJ with anteriorly displaced disc **(a)** that repositions during mouth opening **(b)**. **(c,d)** Left TMJ with complete anterior displaced disc **(c)** with repositioning during mouth opening **(d)**. As with the CBCT findings, the condyle is more retral on the left than on the right.

Depending on the findings, CBCT (Fig 4-401) and MRT (Fig 4-402) may be needed.

Once the assessments had been completed, treatment of the patient commenced with a COPA in the mandibular arch (Fig 4-403). The patient was advised to wear the splint continually apart from eating and tooth cleaning. Parallel treatment by a manual therapist or physiotherapist is indispensable (M Becker, Much). Manual treatment takes place first and then the COPA is adjusted for the changed contact points. In the following weeks, the COPA is adjusted regularly according to the joint and neuromuscular changes.

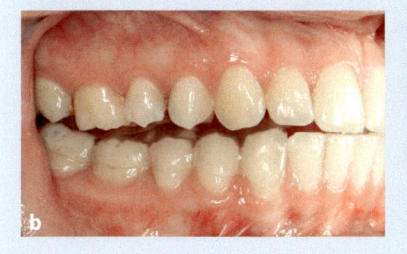

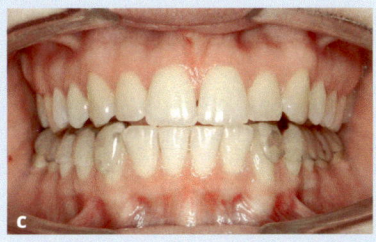

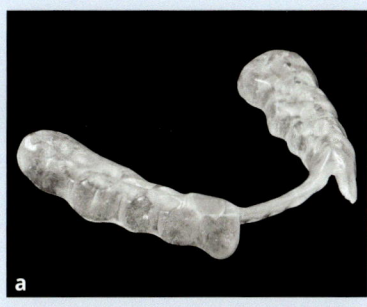

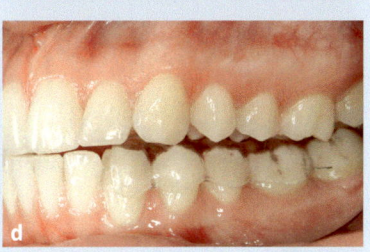

TREATMENT OF DIFFERENT MALOCCLUSIONS WITH ALIGNERS 4

Fig 4-403 Treatment pathway. **(a)** Removable COPA for the mandibular arch made of resin without metall arch, light hardened (Dreve). **(b–d)** Initial intraoral situation with a therapeutic mandible position.

Fig 4-404 CBCT (Picasso, Orange Dental) with the COPA in place, showing a physiologic condyle position.

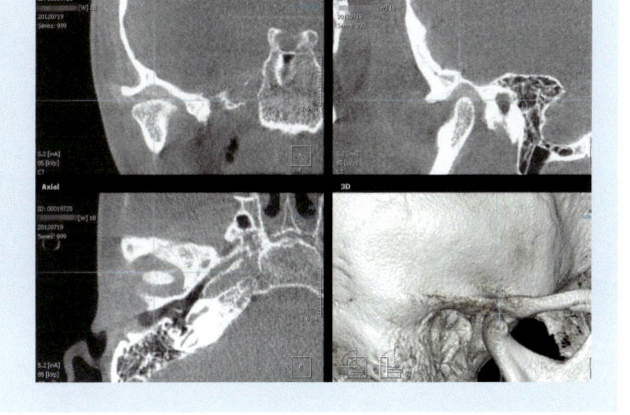

The final CBCT shows the physiologic condyle position achieved with the COPA in position (Fig 4-404).

This patient commenced treatment with:
- back pain
- scoliosis
- leg length discrepancy (left +1.5)
- difference in Prien abduction test (left hard)
- pain and clicking of the TMJ
- deviation of the mandible during opening and closing.

After 5 weeks of treatment with the COPA and accompanying physiotherapy, the patient had no more back or TMJ pain. Currently the patient wears the COPA only during the night and is pain free. The COPA should be assessed every 6 months. For night wearing only, we cover the incisors with the COPA, too.

Topic 50
Craniomandibular disorder in a teenager

Treatment:
- fixed splints
- Invisalign Teen treatment

While treatment of CMD is definitely possible with the Invisalign system, fixed splints are also required.

This patient had been treated previously with an activator in another orthodontic office. After 2 years of therapy, she presented with TMJ problems and the following extraoral findings in habitual intercuspation (Fig 4-405):
- convexity of the face to the left
- reduction of the facial height on the right
- skeletal mandibular midline shift 2 mm to the left.

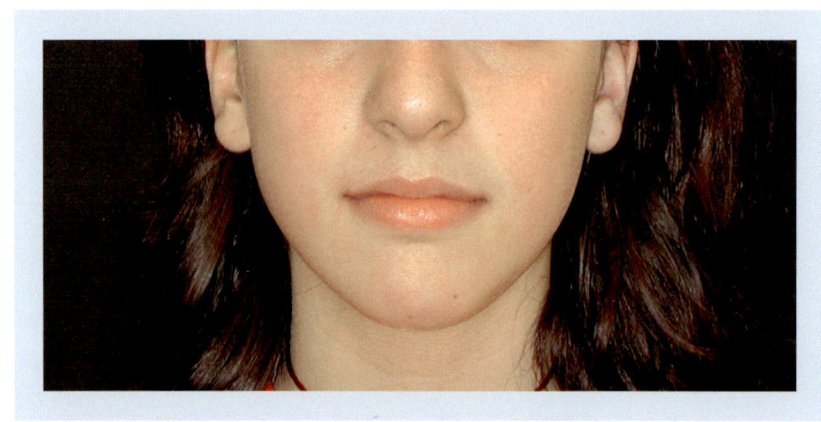

Fig 4-405 Initial facial view.

The intraoral findings at the start of the treatment in habitual intercuspation (Fig 4-406) provided the following diagnosis from intraoral and hand-held casts:
- lateral open bite
- dental class II on the left side
- midline deviation
- gingival recessions in the mandibular incisor area
- rotations and anterior crowding
- transversal constriction of the maxillary arch in the premolar region.

Fig 4-406 Initial intraoral views.

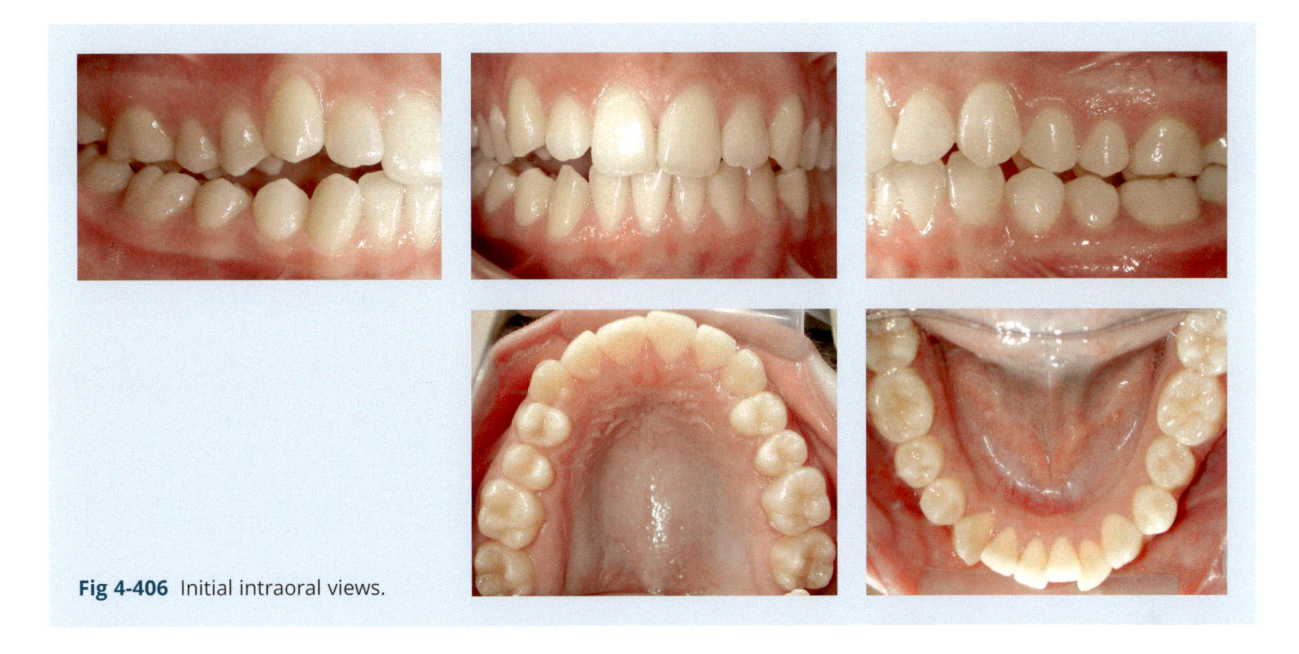

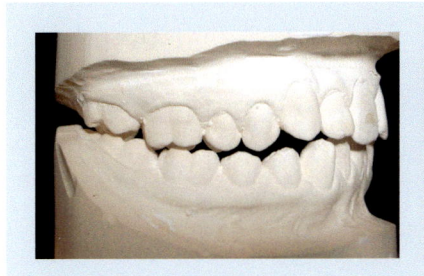

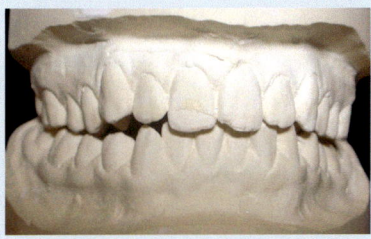

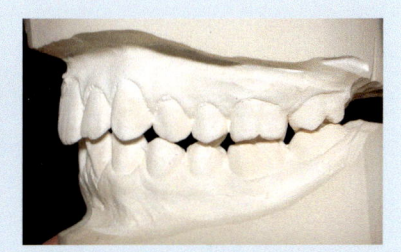

Fig 4-407 Hand-held plaster casts at the start of treatment.

Non-mounted, hand-held plaster casts at the start of treatment in habitual intercuspation showed:
- lateral open bite
- dental class II on the left side
- midline deviation.

Therapy based on the intraoral views and non-mounted casts (Fig 4-407) includes:
- distalizing in the maxillary arch on the left side to obtain a class I relationship and a correct maxillary midline
- potential extraction of maxillary premolar
- transversal expansion of maxillary arch
- posterior extrusion to close the lateral open bite and intrusion of the mandibular anterior teeth to level curve of Spee
- alignment and derotation of mandibular anterior teeth using IPR.

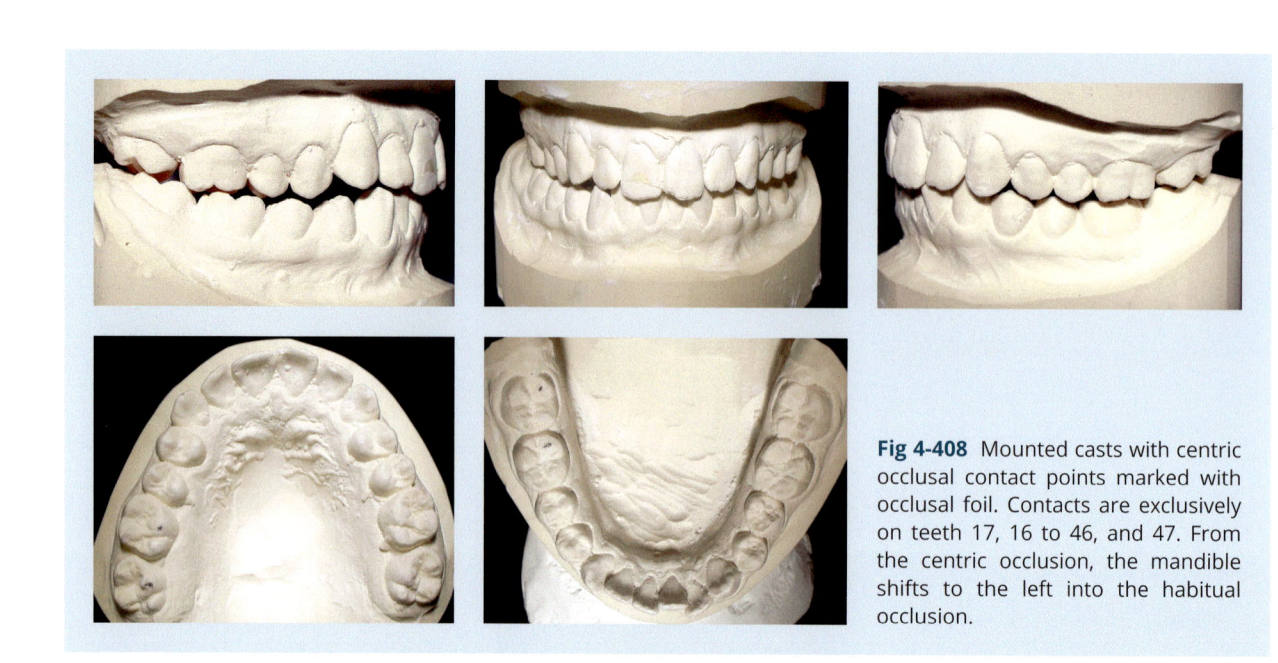

4 TREATMENT OF DIFFERENT MALOCCLUSIONS WITH ALIGNERS

Fig 4-408 Mounted casts with centric occlusal contact points marked with occlusal foil. Contacts are exclusively on teeth 17, 16 to 46, and 47. From the centric occlusion, the mandible shifts to the left into the habitual occlusion.

Using mounted casts in centric relation (Fig 4-408) gave a different diagnosis:
- lateral open bite
- dental class I on left and right
- no midline deviation.

Therapy based on mounted casts in physiologic centric relation provides:

- adjustment of the physiologic centric position with fixed splints
- no distalization needed
- transversal expansion in the maxillary arch
- posterior extrusion to close the lateral open bite and intrusion of the mandibular anterior teeth to level curve of Spee
- alignment of the arches with solving of crowding by IPR.

Treatment

Comparison of non-mounted and mounted casts in centric relation (Fig 4-409) shows the difference in findings and hence the completely different approaches that would be suggested for orthodontic treatment.

Treatment in centric relation is possible with the Invisalign system in combination with fixed splints. The splints are fabricated in the SAM articulator on the mounted casts in centric relation. The fixed splints are bonded on the mandibular molars, to keep the condyle in a physiologic position during the first phase of treatment (Figs 4-410 and 4-411).

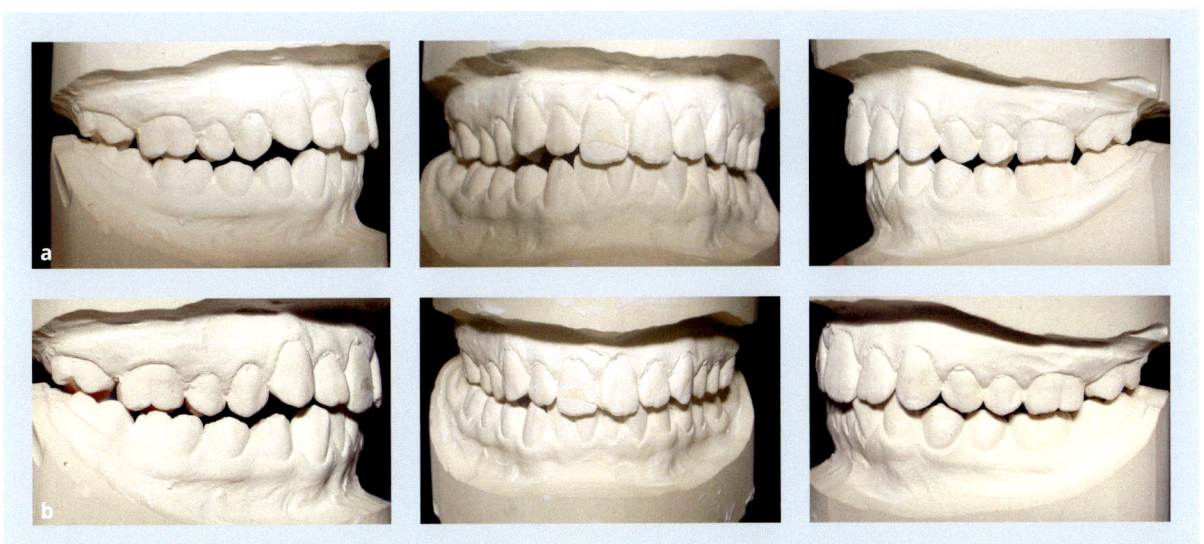

Fig 4-409 Comparison of non-mounted casts **(a)** and mounted casts in centric relation **(b)**.

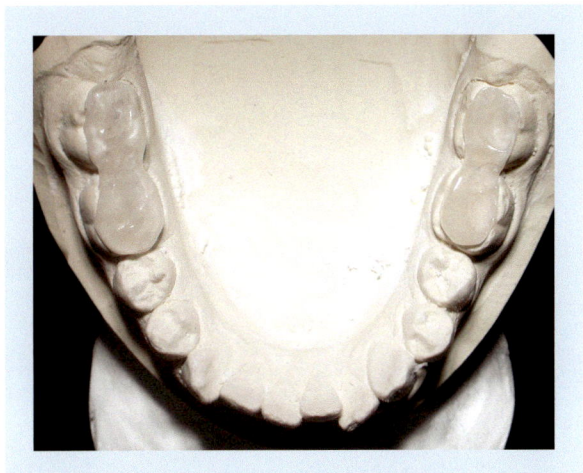

Fig 4-410 Splint fabrication on the cast.

Treatment with the Invisalign system started with the bonding of fixed splints on the mandibular molars (Fig 4-411). After obtaining the correct condyle position, the patient had a bilateral class I relationship and aligned midlines.

The online treatment plan asked for attachments on all teeth that were planned for extrusion (Fig 4-412). The first phase corrected the malposition of all premolars, canines, and incisors. The molars in the maxillary and mandibular arches were not moved as they keep the mandible and the condyles in the correct centric relation. Alignment of the arches and crowding was treated with 23 maxillary and 20 mandibular aligners.

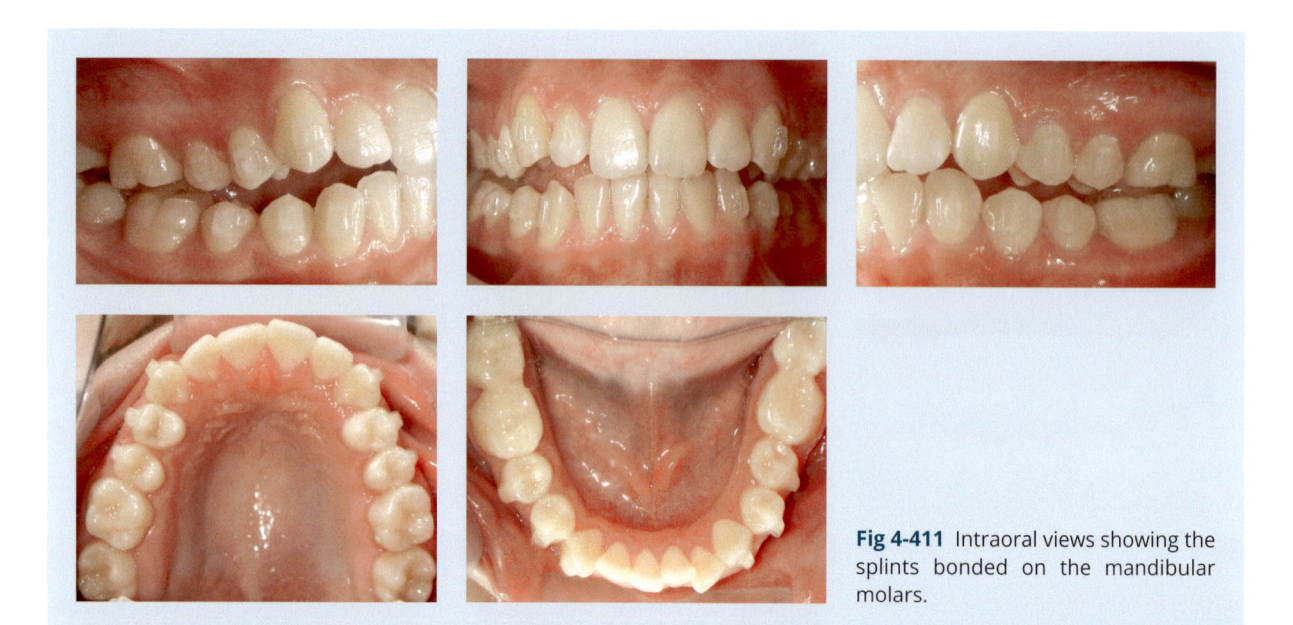

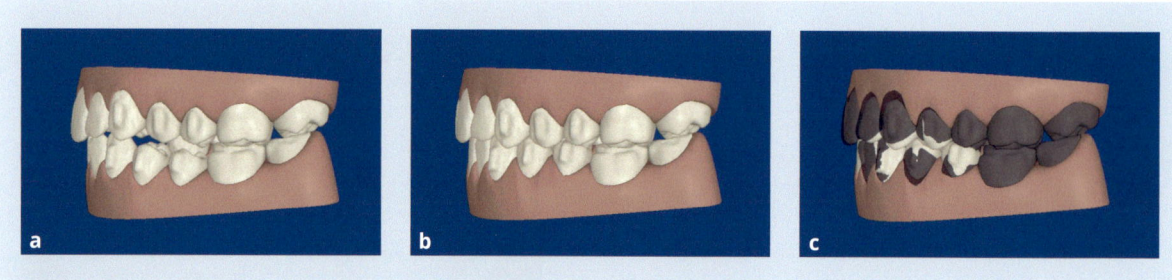

4 TREATMENT OF DIFFERENT MALOCCLUSIONS WITH ALIGNERS

Fig 4-411 Intraoral views showing the splints bonded on the mandibular molars.

Fig 4-412 ClinCheck software results. **(a)** Initial situation with fixed splints on mandibular first and second molars. **(b)** Planned result at the end of the first phase. **(c)** Superimposition showing extrusion planned for premolars, canines, and incisors (blue, initial tooth position; white, final tooth position).

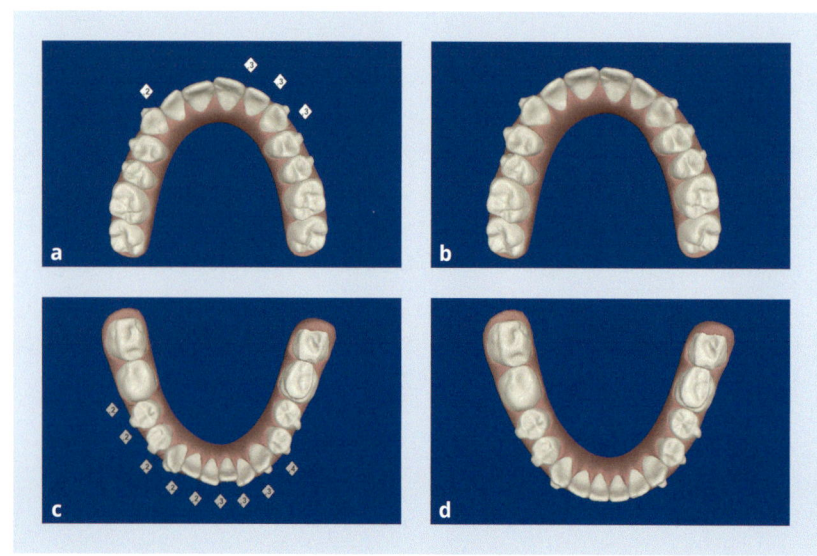

Fig 4-413 ClinCheck software results for both arches. **(a,c)** IPR required. **(b,d)** Planned result.

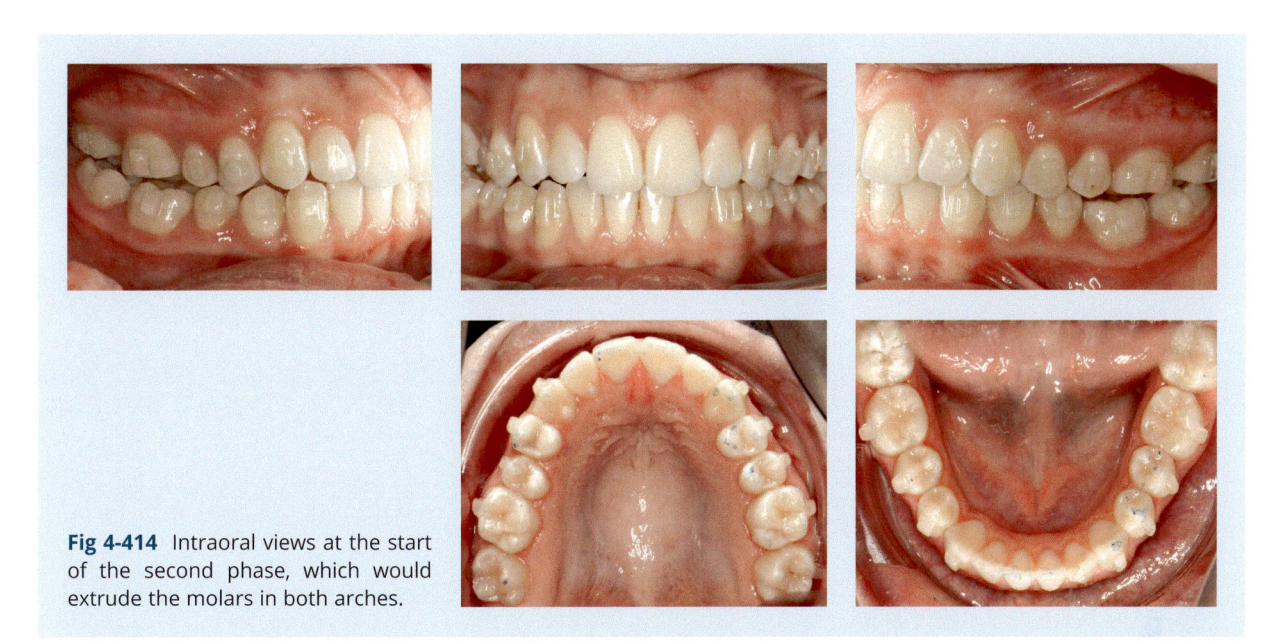

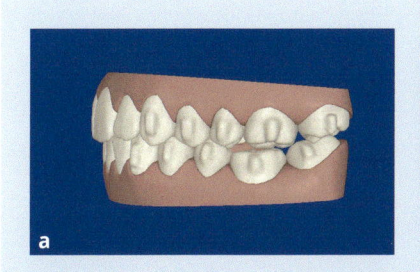

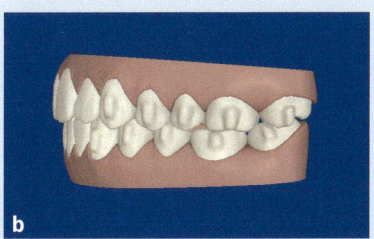

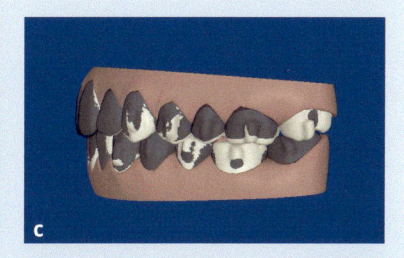

Fig 4-414 Intraoral views at the start of the second phase, which would extrude the molars in both arches.

Fig 4-415 ClinCheck software results in lateral view. **(a)** Initial situation after removal of the fixed splints. **(b)** Planned result at the end of the second phase. **(c)** Superimposition showing extrusion planned for molars but also a slight extrusion of premolars and canines to obtain even better occlusal contact (blue, initial tooth position; white, final tooth position).

ClinCheck images were also used to decide the amount of IPR needed (Fig 4-413).

After the first phase of treatment, the fixed splints were removed as the premolars and canines could keep the mandible in correct centric relation once they had achieved their new positions. At this point, attachments were also added on maxillary and mandibular molars to extrude them into the correct vertical height for hard collision and a stable occlusion (Figs 4-414 and 4-415). The second phase of treatment included 16 maxillary and 12 mandibular aligners.

4 TREATMENT OF DIFFERENT MALOCCLUSIONS WITH ALIGNERS

Fig 4-416 Intraoral situation at the end of the second phase with contact points on all premolars and molars (as marked with occlusal foil) and harmonically aligned arches.

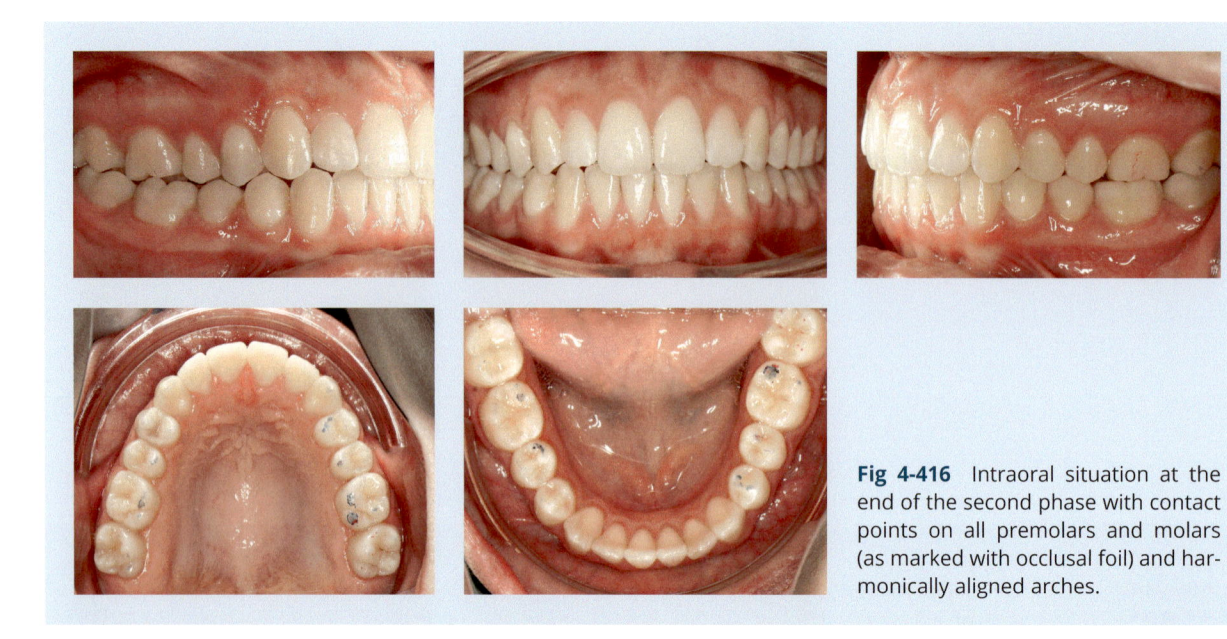

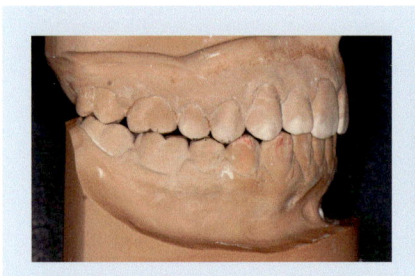

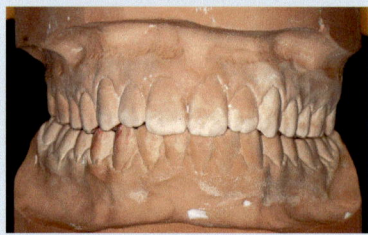

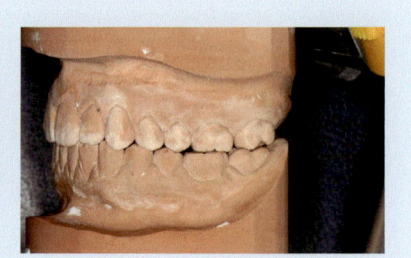

Fig 4-417 Mounted plaster casts showing good molar occlusion.

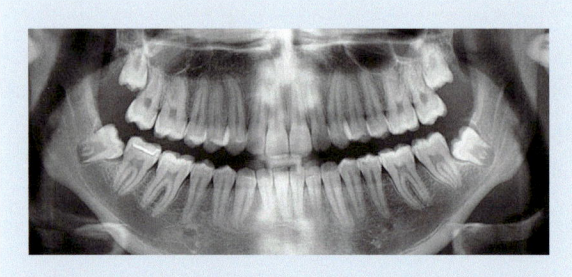

Fig 4-418 Orthopantomography at end of the second phase, showing no pathology.

At the end of the second phase, there were contact points on all premolars and molars (Figs 4-416 and 4-417). Orthopantomography showed no pathology but the removal of the wisdom teeth was advised (Fig 4-418).

Comparisons of initial and final views show the successfully treated teeth (Figs 4-119 to 4-421). There is stable occlusion with corrected midlines, physiologic anterior relation, and canine guidance. Smile esthetics have improved, with the curve of the upper dentition following the curve of the lower lip harmonically. Gingival levels are well aligned in the vertical dimension.

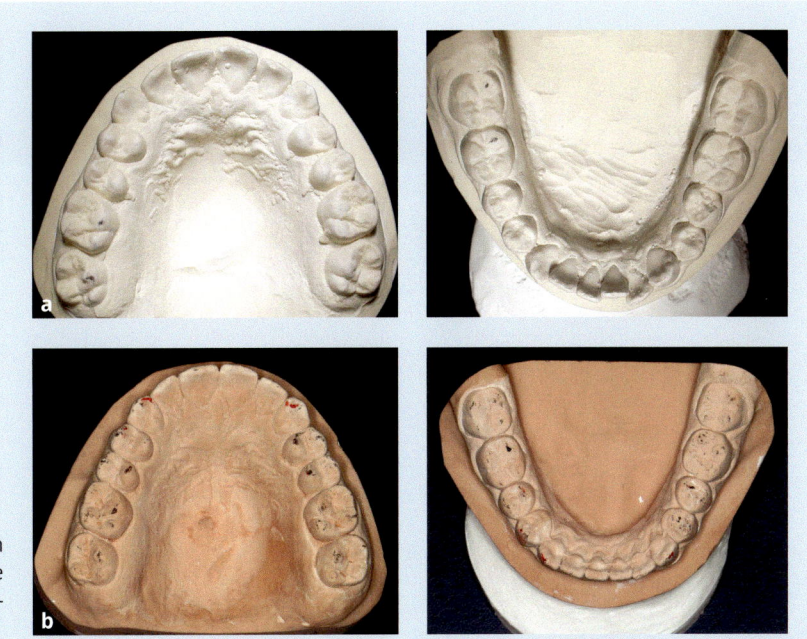

TREATMENT OF DIFFERENT MALOCCLUSIONS WITH ALIGNERS 4

Fig 4-419 Mounted plaster casts with marked occlusal contact points at the beginning **(a)** and end **(b)** of orthodontic treatment.

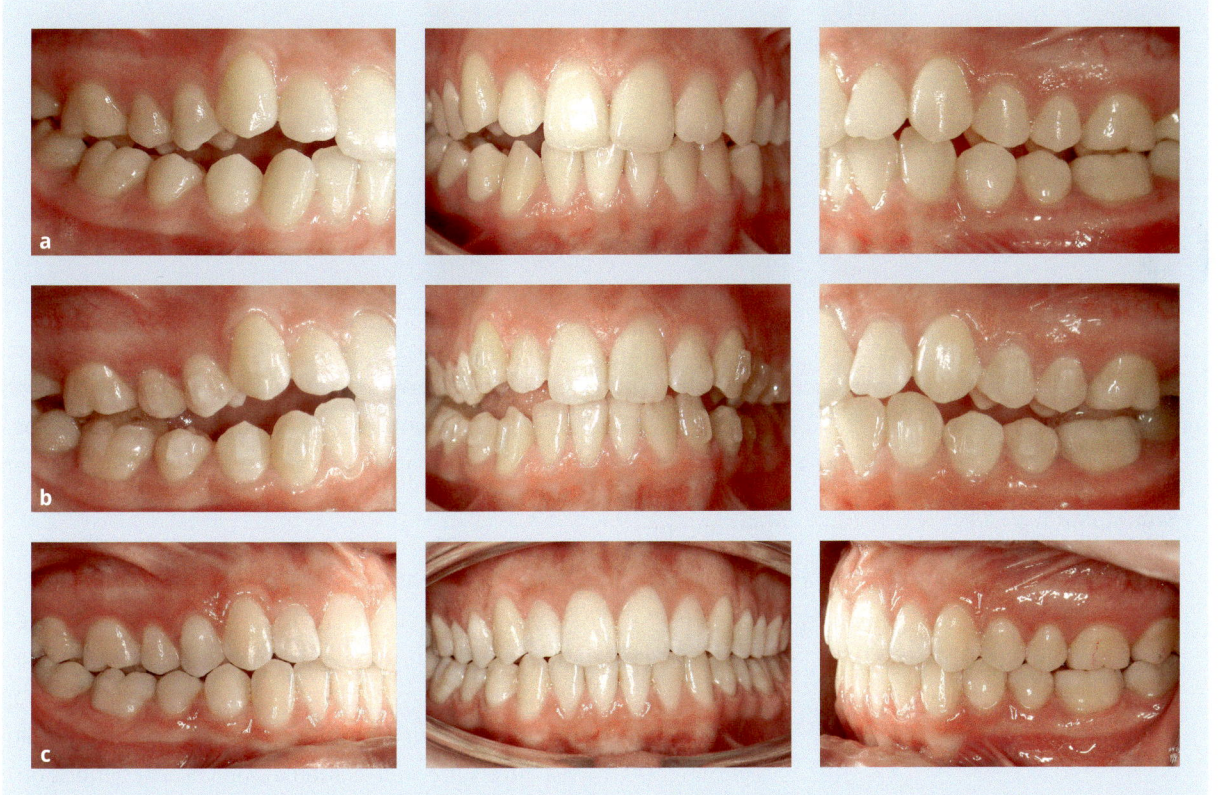

Fig 4-420 Intraoral views. **(a)** Initial views showing a side shift to the left and the lateral open bite. **(b)** The fixed splints maintaining centric relation. **(c)** Final views showing a stable occlusion with corrected midlines, physiologic anterior relation, and canine guidance.

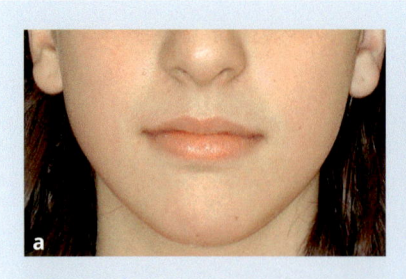

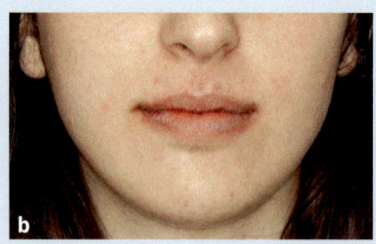

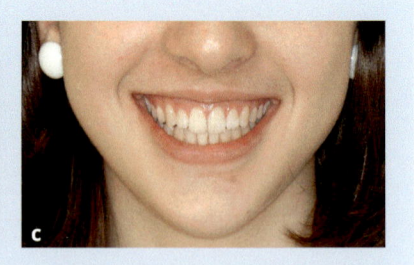

Fig 4-421 Extraoral views initially with face convexity to the left **(a)** and finally **(b)** with facial symmetry. **(c)** Final smile esthetics.

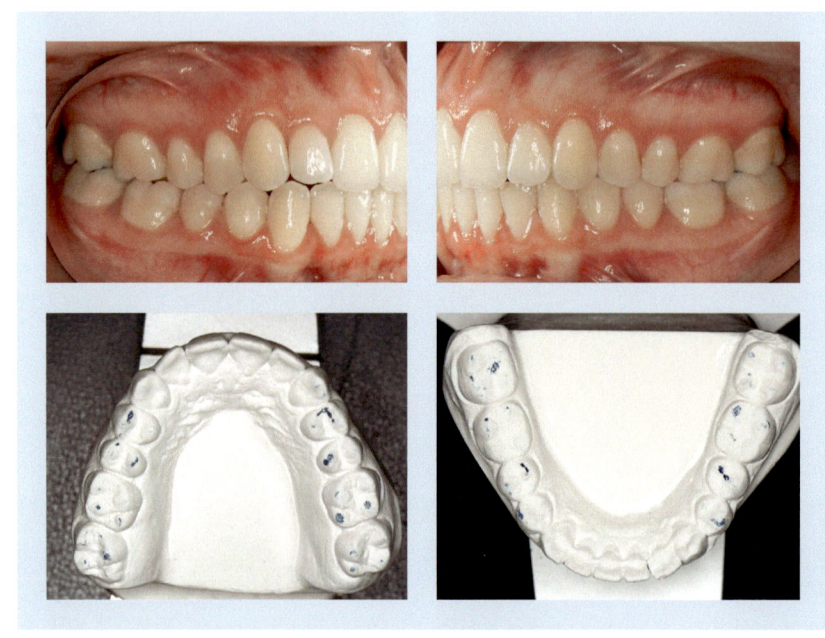

Fig 4-422 Intraoral lateral views 5 years after treatment **(top)** show class I relationship with equal occlusal contacts. Casts **(bottom)** confirm the posterior contact pattern (blue).

Examination at 5 years after orthodontic treatment, in the retention phase (still with a maxillary removable retainer and a mandibular fixed retainer on teeth 33 to 43), shows a class I relationship with equal occlusal posterior contact patterns (Fig 4-222).

Topic 51
Craniomandibular disorder with pain

Treatment:
- removable splint therapy
- Invisalign treatment plus fixed splints

This patient was referred from a pain clinic because of headache, migraine, and neck pain for which she was taking continuous medication. She had crowding and rotations in both arches, plus loss of posterior support (Fig 4-423).

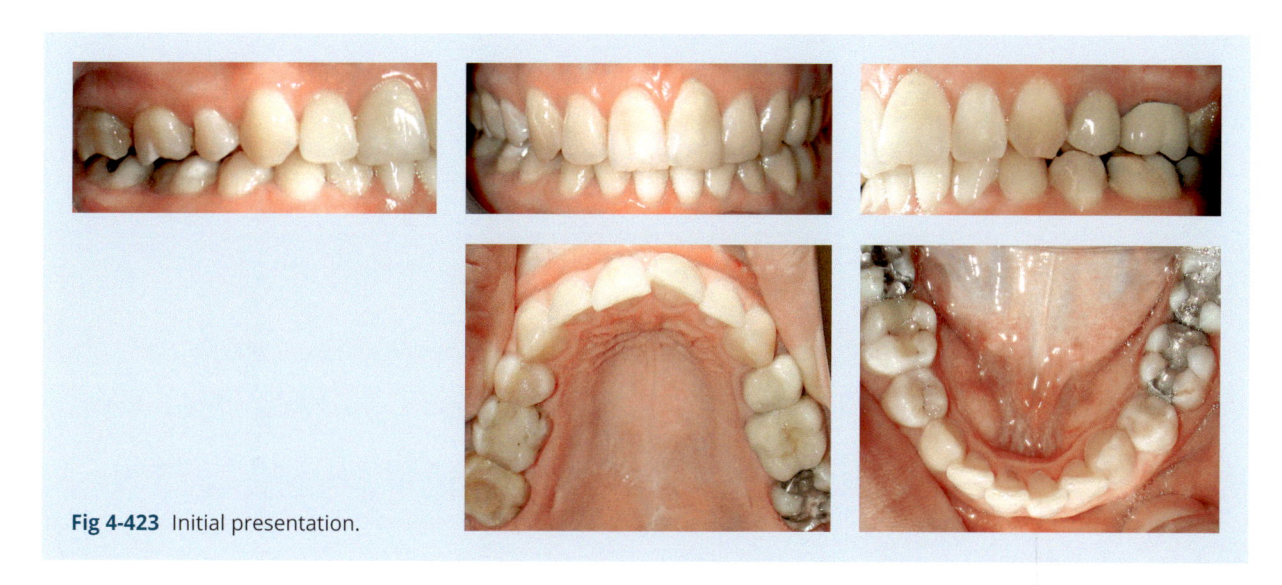

Fig 4-423 Initial presentation.

Diagnosis:
- headache, migraine, and neck pain
- crowding and rotations in both arches
- posterior missing support and infraocclusion.

Therapy:
- therapy with COPA
- Invisalign treatment with fixed splints.

Fig 4-424 Intraoral views with the removable occlusal splint on the mandibular arch.

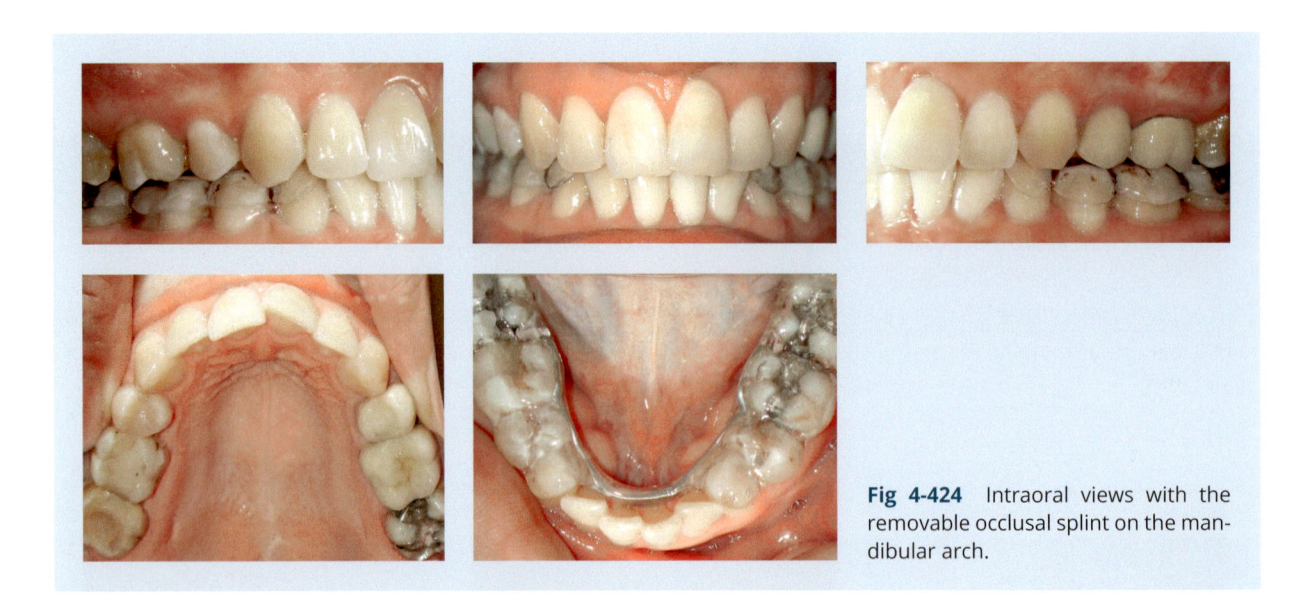

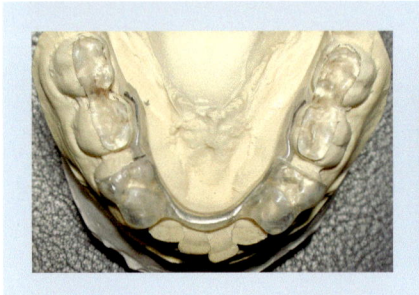

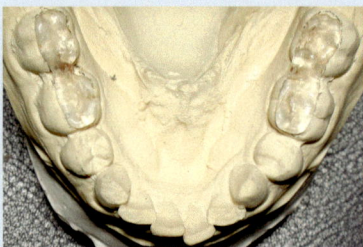

Fig 4-425 Plaster casts with the initial removable splint and the already cut out occlusal splints for molars (**left**) and the redesigned and reduced single splints on the molars (**right**).

Treatment

Treatment was started with a removable occlusal splint on the mandibular arch (Fig 4-424). A removable splint in this arch appears to be more comfortable for the patient and so helps with compliance. It also allows better articulation and avoids undesired blocking of the maxilla. The COPA contains a sublingual arch and does not cover the mandibular anterior teeth, which helps to reduce potential disturbance of articulation to a minimum and thus avoids upper incisor contact to the splint.

Alginate impressions were performed to produce a retention aligner (vacuum-formed splint) in the mandibular arch for retention until the inset of the first Invisalign aligner. Patients with infraocclusion usually cope well with the removable aligner retainer or the Invisalign aligner on the bonded splints. The additional height is mostly welcome, because it contributes to pain reduction. In supraocclusion (Topic 53), the additional vertical height from aligner thickness can sometimes lead to difficulties for the patient and rejection. If a patient has problems, additional manual therapy and acupuncture is advised.

The patient is advised to wear the COPA day and night, and therapy usually takes 3 to 4 months. In this particular patient, 8 months was needed. At the end of this period, there was a significant improvement in her pain and she had a stable centric relation, which allowed Invisalign treatment to start. The patient was advised to wear the retention splint at night only until the aligners were available. Impressions/scans were taken with the splints in place.

The orthodontic treatment plan included the transfer of the exact position of the splint into the dental occlusion. For this, the existing removable splint can be redesigned and reduced to two single splints

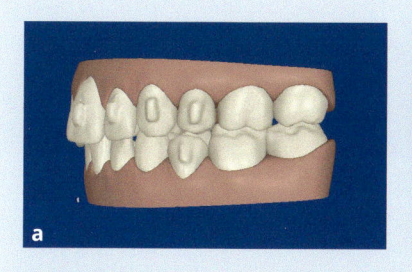

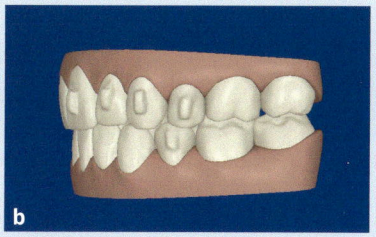

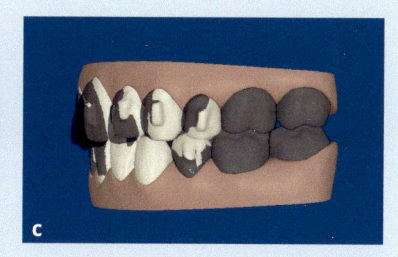

TREATMENT OF DIFFERENT MALOCCLUSIONS WITH ALIGNERS 4

Fig 4-426 ClinCheck software results for phase 1. **(a)** Initial view with the fixed splints on the mandibular molars to maintain the therapeutic mandibular position. **(b)** Planned result with extrusion of premolars and canines into hard collision and alignment of the arches. **(c)** Superimposition shows the amount of planned movement (blue, initial tooth position; white, final tooth position).

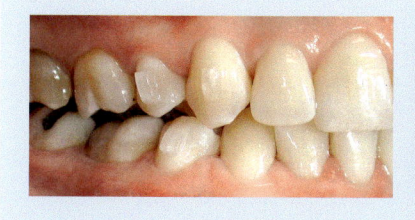

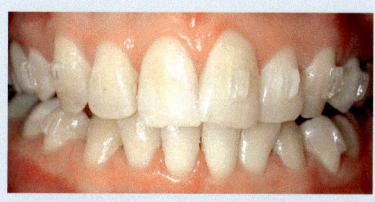

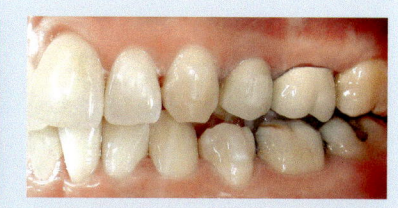

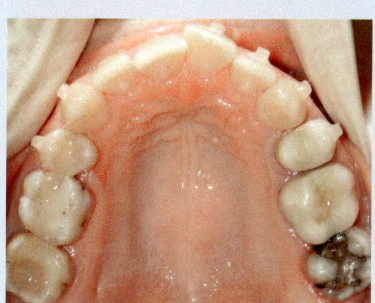

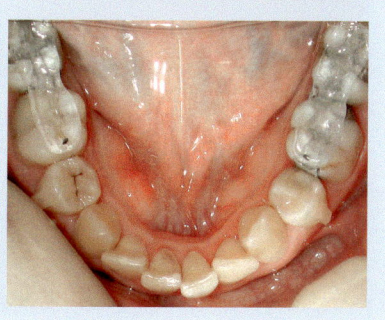

Fig 4-427 Intraoral views with bonded attachments and splints on mandibular molars.

(Fig 4-425). These splints can be bonded onto the teeth with thin fluid resin (e.g. Maximum Cure unfilled, Reliance Orthodontic Products). The advantage of a thin fluid resin is the reduced depth of the bonding layer, which avoids changes in height and thus maintains the exact therapeutic position of the splints.

Phase 1 of aligner treatment

For the first phase, the following requirements were entered into the online ClinCheck software:
- correct anterior malocclusion from 15 to 25 and 35 to 45
- real extrusion of premolars into hard collision (heavy occlusal contacts)
- attachments on every tooth with needed extrusion additionally to any other attachment required
- no movement of the maxillary and mandibular molars in this phase to maintain the therapeutic mandible position
- any other movement is possible.

The ClinCheck software shows the proposed pathway for the first phase (Fig 4-426). Movements would be restricted to teeth anterior to the first molars in both arches in order to maintain the therapeutic mandibular position with the first and second molars. The first phase used 27 aligners. Figure 4-427 shows the bonded attachments and the splints on mandibular molars.

267

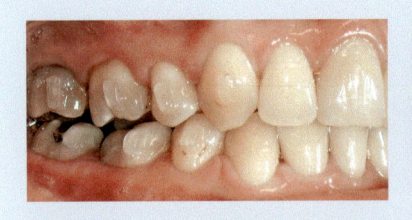

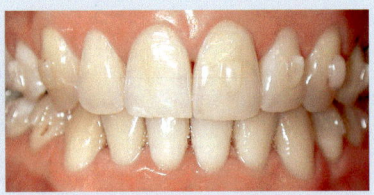

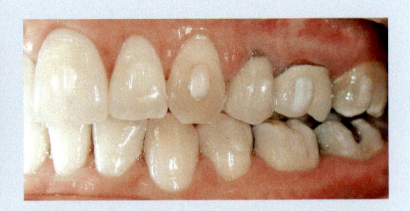

Fig 4-428 Intraoral situation at the end of the first treatment phase – splints are removed.

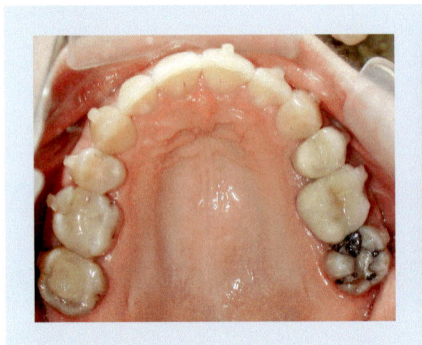

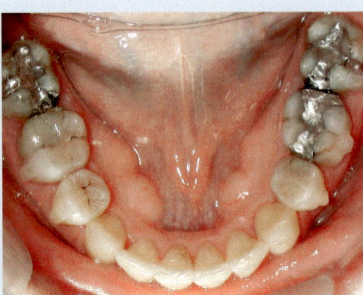

Fig 4-429 Intraoral view of the maxillary and mandibular arches at the end of the first phase with vertical rectangular attachments added on all maxillary and mandibular molars and without splints.

ClinCheck evaluation of the first phase included the following:
- the mounting of the maxilla to mandible
- the contact of maxillary molars to the fixed splint, thus maintaining the therapeutic mandibular position
- no movement of the molars should occur but there should be hard collision of the premolars at the end of phase 1
- all other tooth movements as intended.

At the end of the first treatment phase, the premolars and canines were in full occlusal contact, maintaining the vertical height of the therapeutic splint position (Fig 4-428).

Phase 2 of aligner treatment

The second phase of treatment (midcourse correction) included:
- removal of fixed splints
- patient wearing retention aligners 22 hours a day
- attachment planning for all molars that need extrusion
- new impressions/scans and intraoral views (Fig 4-429).

Crowding in both arches has been resolved by this point. The requirements entered into ClinCheck for the second phase were:
- correct malocclusion of the molars, with real extrusion of molars to hard collision
- attachments on molars for extrusion
- any additional attachments needed
- any other tooth movements needed.

The ClinCheck superimposition shows the planned extrusive movement of the molars into hard collision (Fig 4-430). The premolars were already in full occlusal contact and so could maintain the correct vertical dimension.

The final orthodontic result has improved posterior support (Fig 4-431). The vertical dimension, which was preset using the COPA, has been transferred completely into dental occlusion. The patient was pain free with the removable splint and stayed pain free at the end of the Invisalign treatment. The maxillary and mandibular arches are well aligned and retained with a lingual retainer bonded on teeth 35 to 45. Retention in the maxillary arch is with a removable retention aligner.

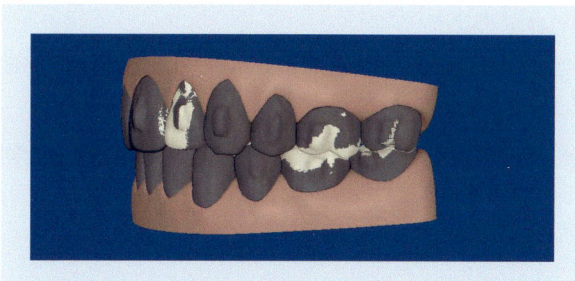

TREATMENT OF DIFFERENT MALOCCLUSIONS WITH ALIGNERS 4

Fig 4-430 Lateral view of the superimposition in ClinCheck to show the planned extrusive movement of the molars into hard collision.

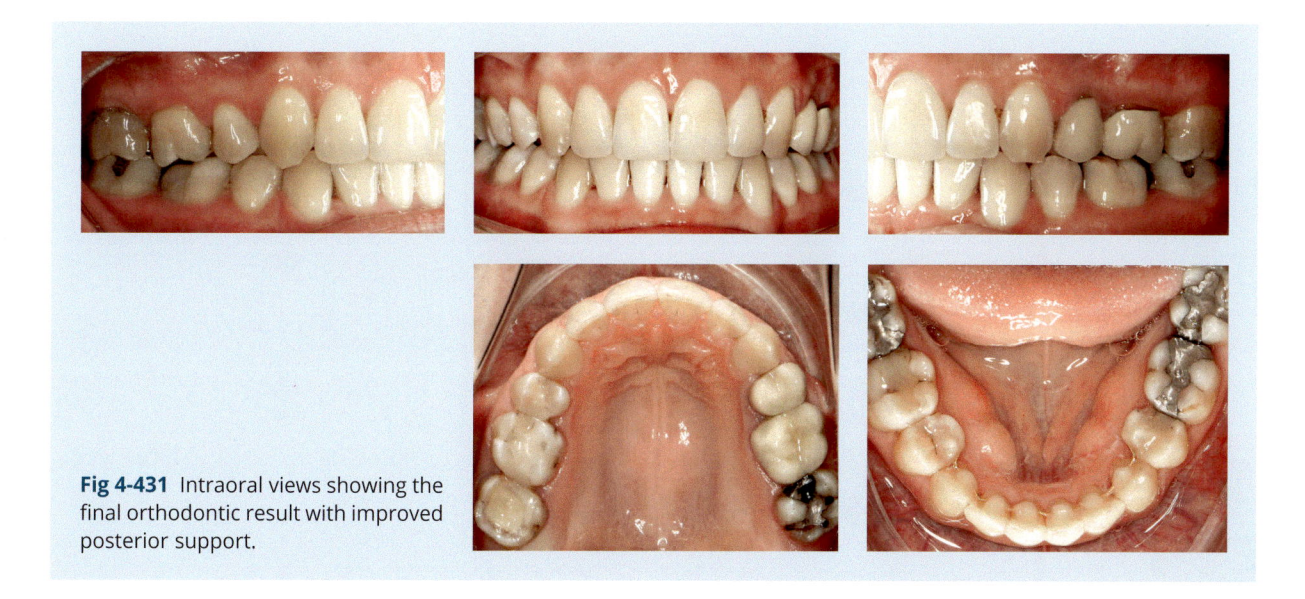

Fig 4-431 Intraoral views showing the final orthodontic result with improved posterior support.

The patient was sent to a dentist to replace inadequate restoratives. It is important that the three-dimensional position of the mandibular arch, and therefore the therapeutic condyle position, is not changed with the new dental supply.

Topic 52
Craniomandibular disorder with pain treated with the Invisalign system followed by prosthodontics

Treatment:
- removable splint
- Invisalign treatment plus fixed splints
- prosthodontics

Patients with CMD require a comprehensive range of treatments in an interdisciplinary team. Whenever we start treatment, we start with a functional analysis (Fig 4-432).

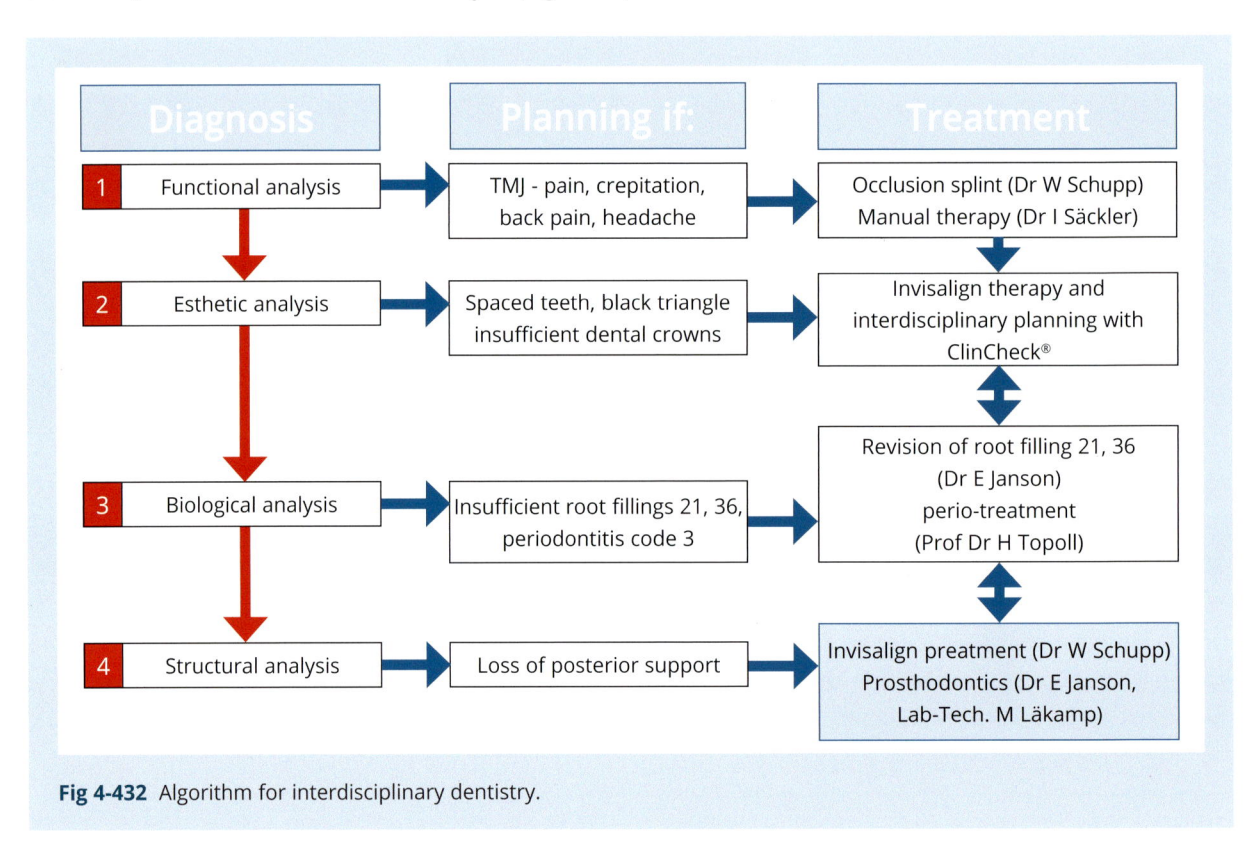

Fig 4-432 Algorithm for interdisciplinary dentistry.

This patient presented with the major problem of back pain and tension headache; there was TMJ pain on the left side and crepitation. A lingual retainer had been placed after a previous treatment with a fixed appliance in another office (Fig 4-433).

Diagnosis:
- TMJ pain on the left side and crepitation
- back pain and tension headache
- loss of posterior support (guiding symptom).

Therapy:
- removable splint accompanied with manual therapy
- periodontal therapy
- endodontics
- Invisalign treatment with fixed splints in phase 1
- prosthodontics.

Fig 4-433 Initial presentation.

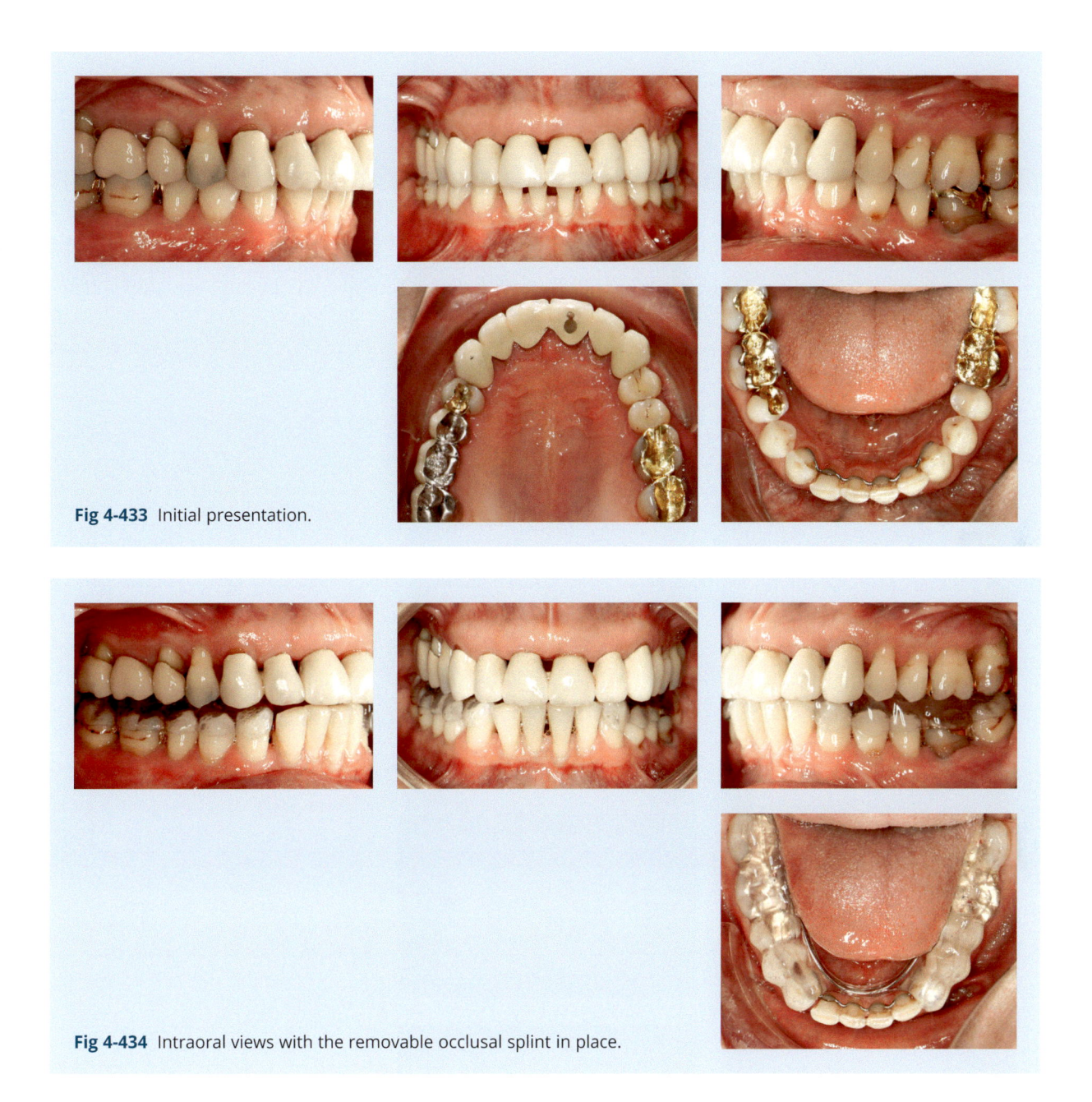

Fig 4-434 Intraoral views with the removable occlusal splint in place.

Treatment

Although the patient clearly needed new restoratives, the first step was removable splint therapy accompanied by manual therapy, because of the TMJ problems and back pain (Fig 4-434). This would be followed by Invisalign treatment in the mandibular arch. It was planned not to treat the maxillary arch because of the numerous partial dentures.

The patient was advised to wear the splint permanently except for eating and tooth cleaning. Control and modification of the occlusal splint pattern take place directly after manual therapy; initially within the first week and then every 2 weeks.

Once the patient was pain free and a stable occlusion pattern using the splint was achieved (Fig 4-435), Invisalign treatment was started.

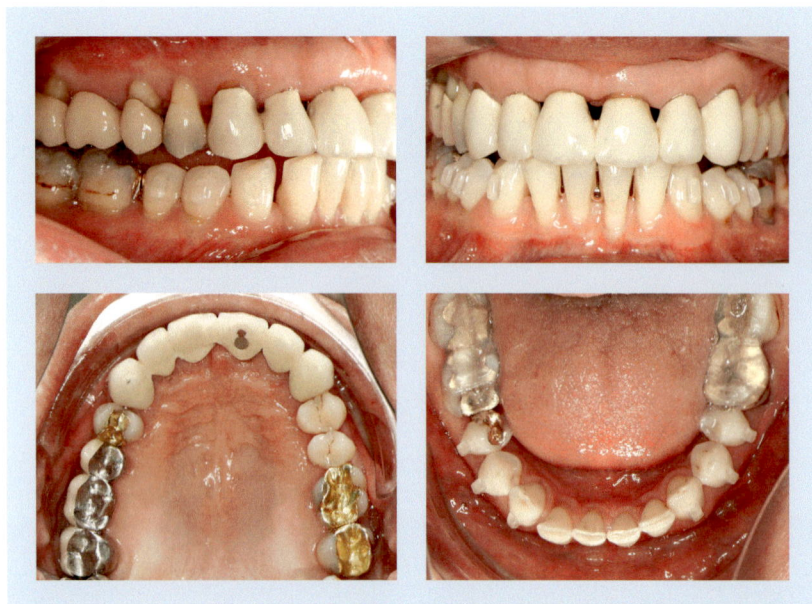

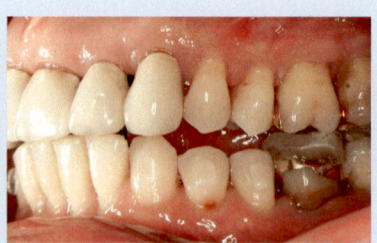

4 TREATMENT OF DIFFERENT MALOCCLUSIONS WITH ALIGNERS

Fig 4-435 Initial situation with fixed splints on lower molars, and attachments on lower canines and premolars at the start of the Invisalign treatment.

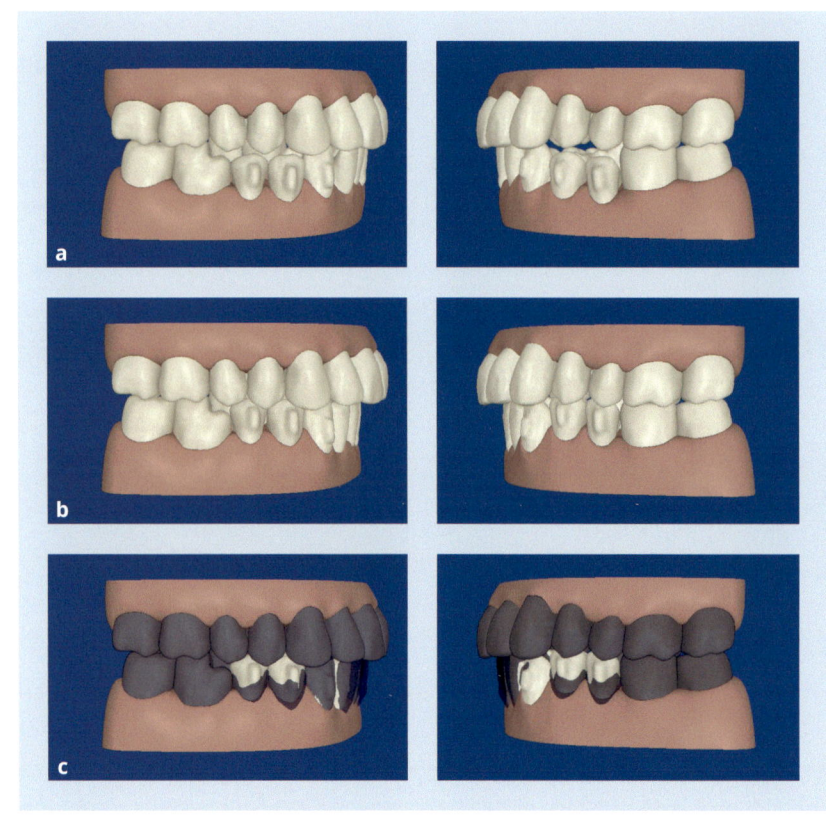

Fig 4-436 ClinCheck software results. **(a)** Initial situation with fixed splints on mandibular molars and vertical rectangular attachments on mandibular premolars and canines. **(b)** Planned outcome with extrusion of mandibular premolars and canines into hard collision. **(c)** Superimposition showing the planned extrusion in the mandibular premolar and canine region (blue, initial tooth position; white, final tooth position).

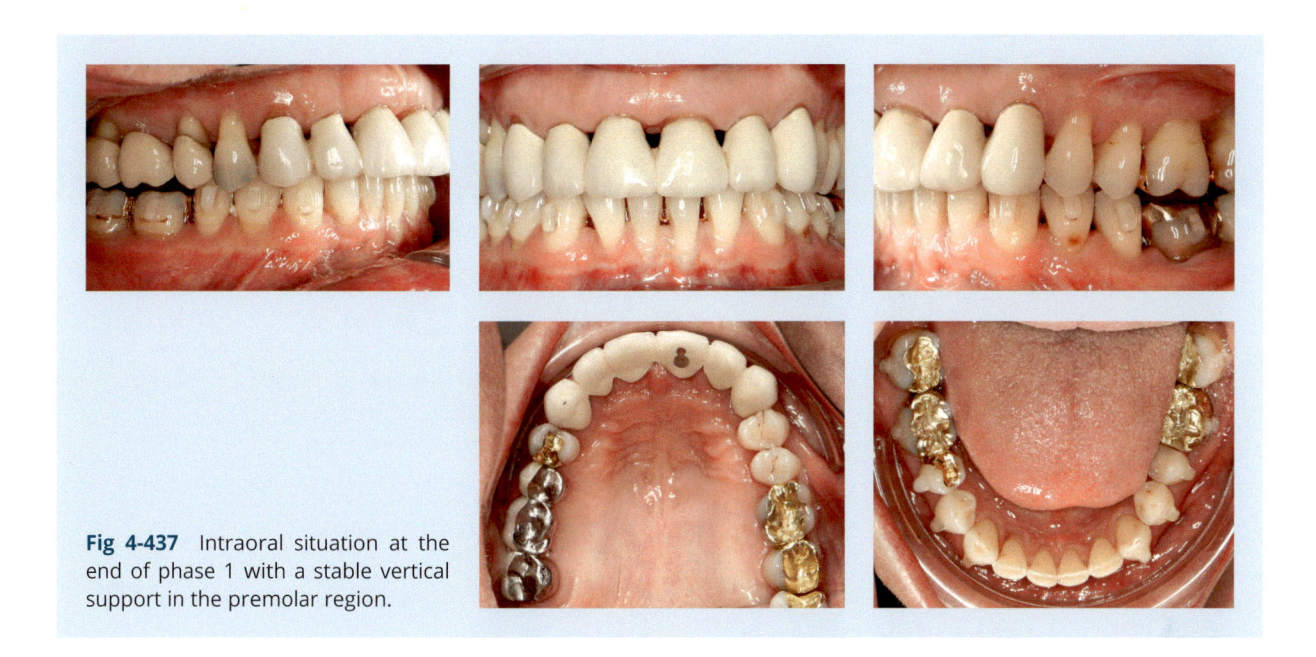

Fig 4-437 Intraoral situation at the end of phase 1 with a stable vertical support in the premolar region.

Phase 1 of aligner treatment

The therapeutic splint was transferred into bonded fixed splints on the mandibular molars. Vertical rectangular attachments were added to obtain anchorage for extrusive force on all premolars and canines.

The intraoral position was transferred into the ClinCheck software for treatment planning (Fig 4-436). Extrusion of mandibular premolars and canines into hard collision was carried out with 25 aligners in the mandibular arch. No treatment was planned in the maxillary arch.

At the end of the first phase, there was stable vertical support in the premolar region. Fixed splints were removed and attachments for extrusion were added to mandibular molars (Fig 4-437). Impressions/scans were taken to start the second phase of the Invisalign treatment, the midcourse correction.

Phase 2 of aligner treatment

The fixed splints in the mandible could be removed as the premolars were maintaining the occlusion. Extrusion of mandibular molars into hard collision was planned in the ClinCheck software with an additional 12 mandibular aligners (Fig 4-438).

The second phase achieved stable occlusion with physiologic vertical height (Fig 4-439). The patient remained pain free.

Figure 4-440 shows the course of treatment.

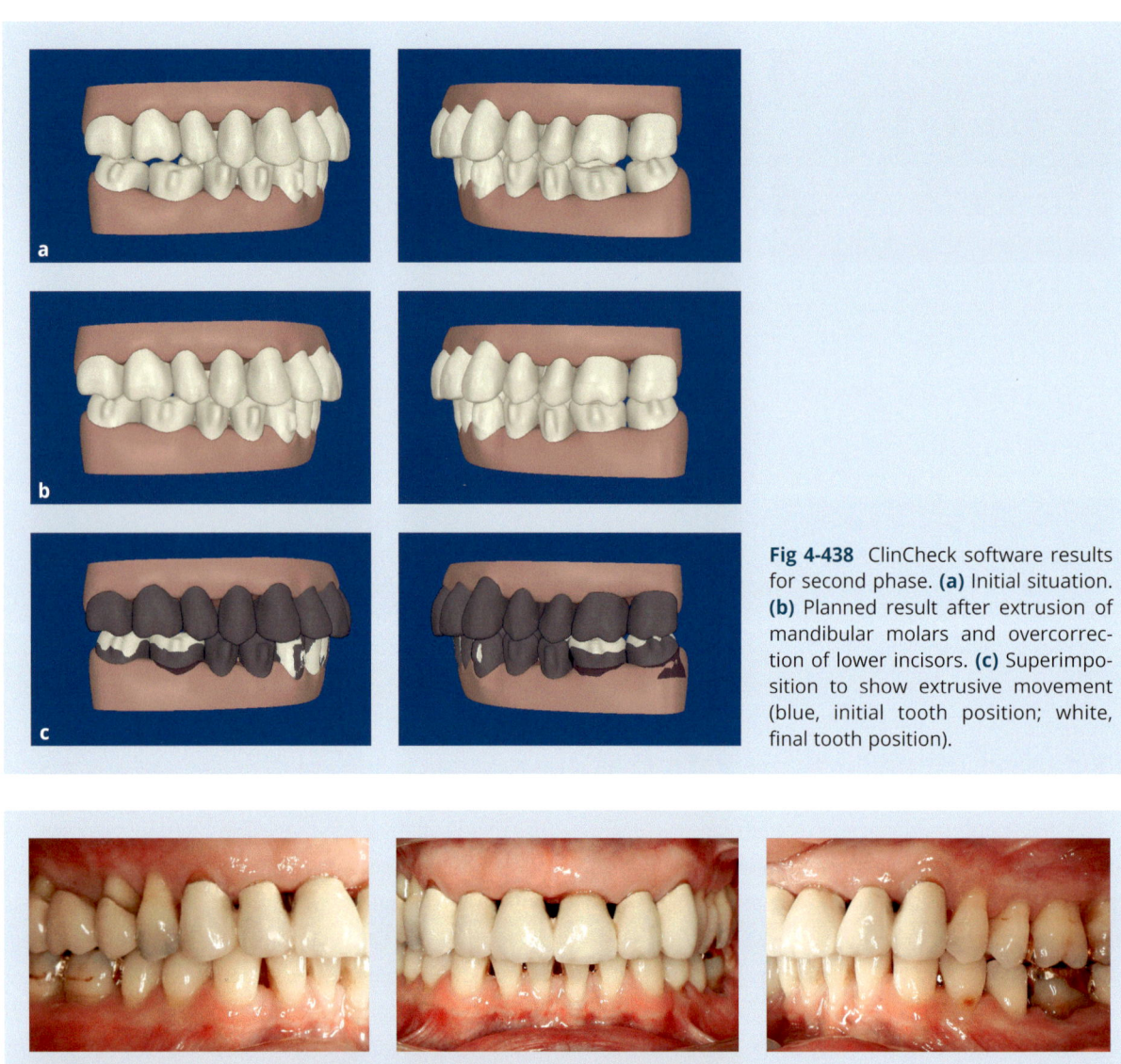

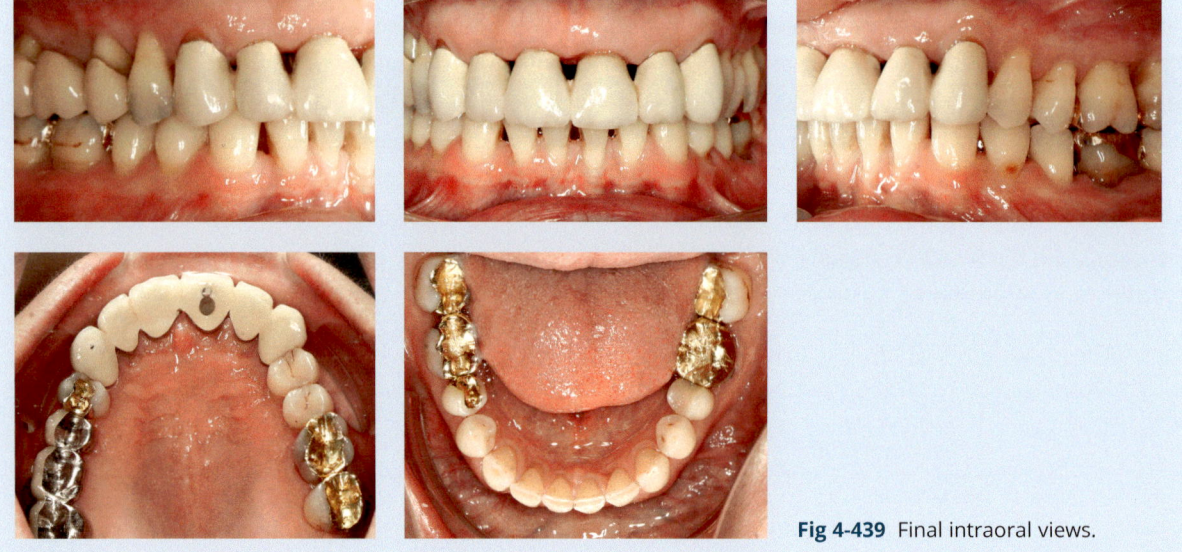

Fig 4-438 ClinCheck software results for second phase. **(a)** Initial situation. **(b)** Planned result after extrusion of mandibular molars and overcorrection of lower incisors. **(c)** Superimposition to show extrusive movement (blue, initial tooth position; white, final tooth position).

Fig 4-439 Final intraoral views.

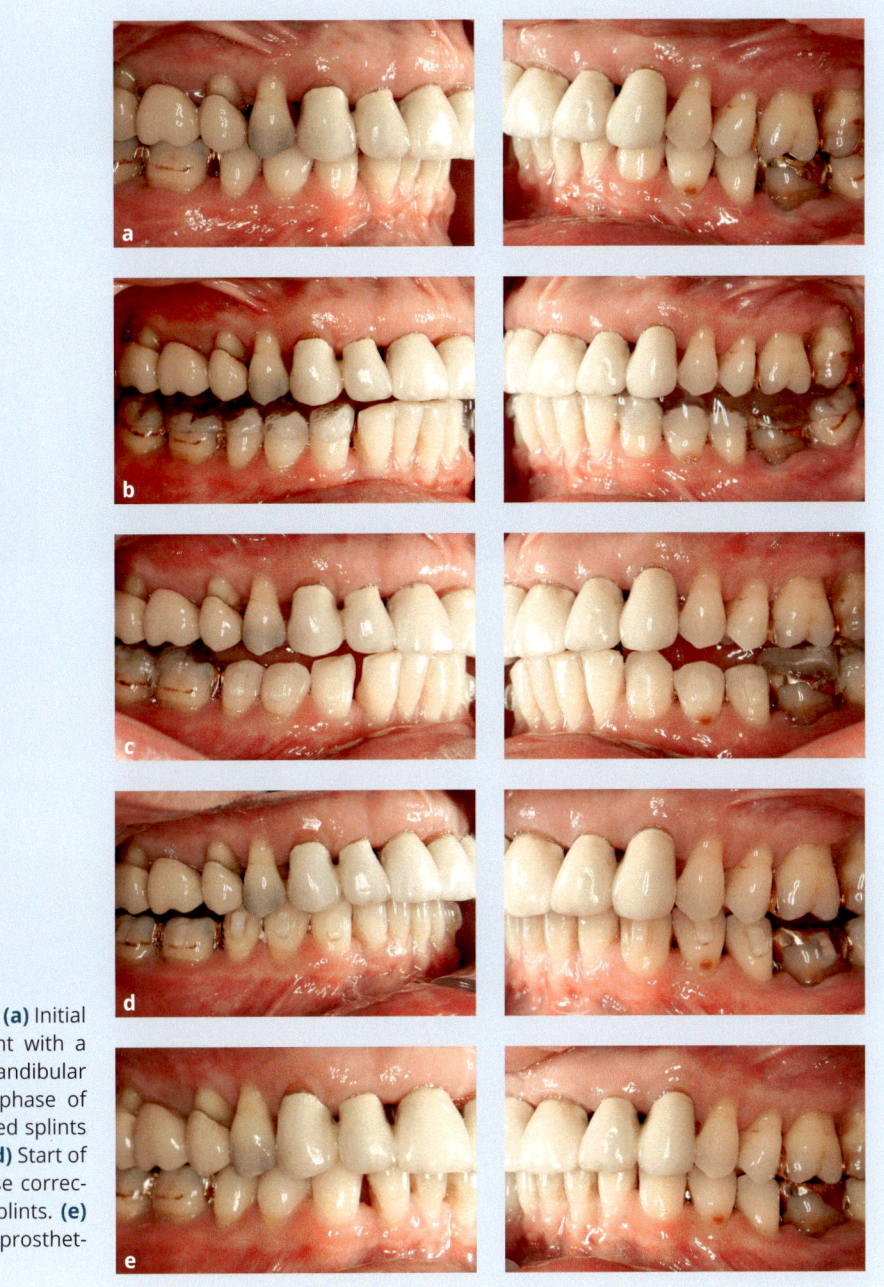

Fig 4-440 Treatment course. **(a)** Initial views. **(b)** Start of treatment with a removable splint in the mandibular arch. **(c)** Start of the first phase of Invisalign treatment with fixed splints on the mandibular molars. **(d)** Start of the second phase, midcourse correction and removal of fixed splints. **(e)** Final occlusion prior to new prosthetics.

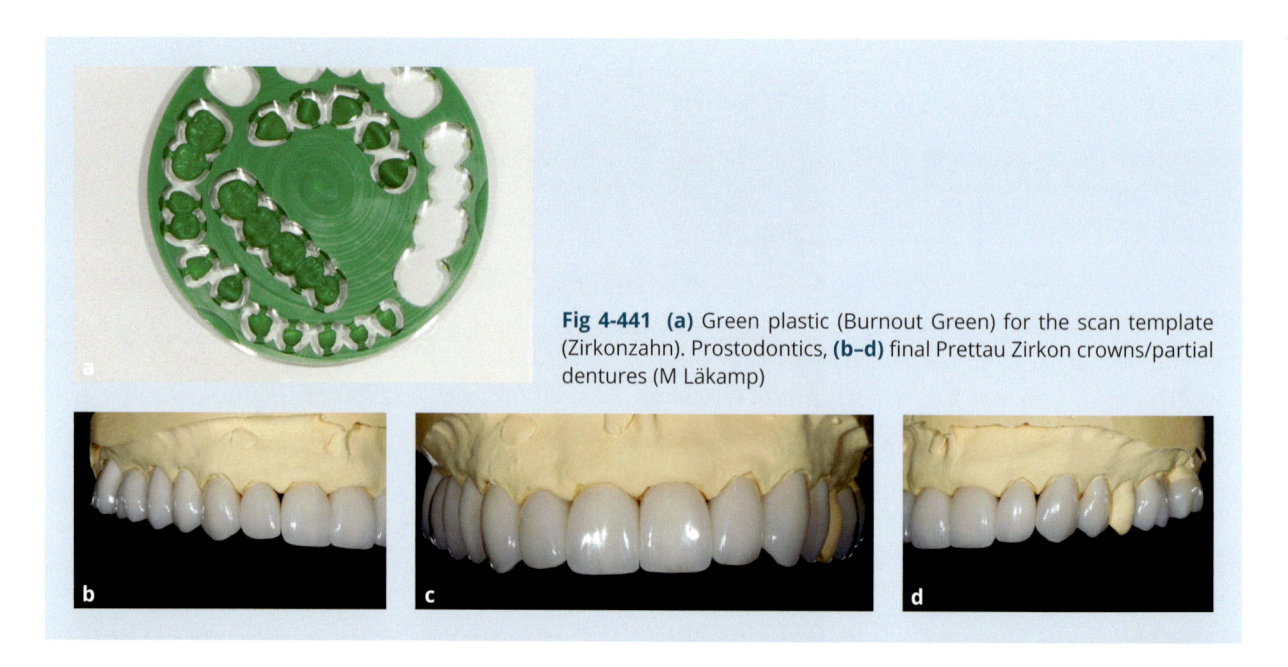

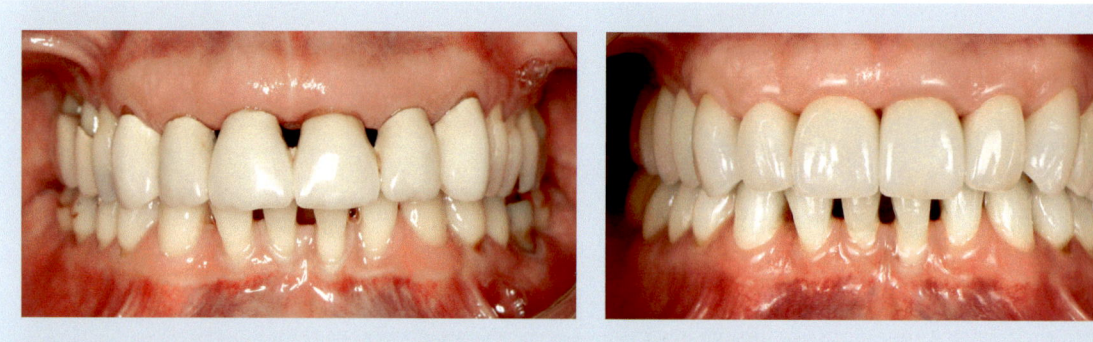

Fig 4-441 (a) Green plastic (Burnout Green) for the scan template (Zirkonzahn). Prostodontics, (b–d) final Prettau Zirkon crowns/partial dentures (M Läkamp)

Fig 4-442 Initial (**left**) prior to the orthodontic treatment and final (**right**) views after the restorative was given an improved esthetic and functional result.

Five months after Invisalign treatment, the final restoratives were inserted (prosthodontics, Dr E Janson, Wetter, laboratory, M Läkamp, Ostbevern) (Fig 4-441).

Treatment produced an improved esthetic result. The mandibular incisors do not show during smiling and speaking, which was the reason to avoid additional restoratives, with composite resin or veneers, on the mandibular anterior teeth (Fig 4-442).

Topic 53
Craniomandibular disorder with headache and cervical spine syndrome

Treatment:
- Invisalign treatment
- prosthodontics

In a few patients, supraocclusion and missing anterior guidance can be a factor for CMD. Often these patients are difficult to treat as any occlusal splint will increase vertical height while creating the needed anterior guidance. This can sometimes lead to problems of rejection and lack of compliance. If problems occur, the patient is advised to undergo additional manual therapy and acupuncture.

This patient had CMD with posterior supraocclusion, which needed interdisciplinary treatment (Fig 4-443).

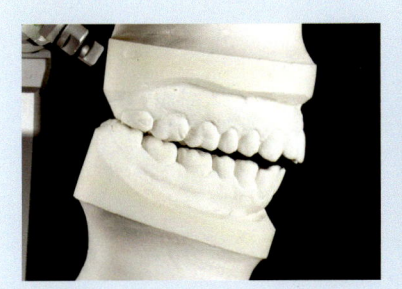

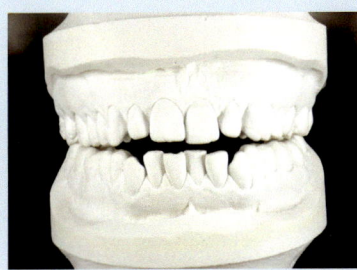

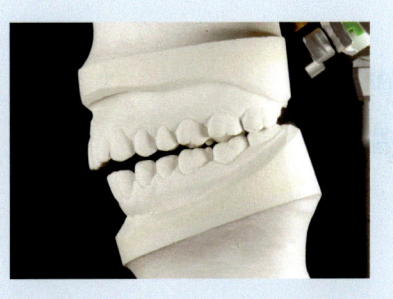

Fig 4-443 Plaster casts mounted in SAM articulator in centric relation showed contact exclusively on teeth 28 to 38.

Diagnosis:
- CMD
- headache
- cervical spine syndrome
- posterior supraocclusion.

Therapy:
- removable splint and osteopathy
- wisdom tooth extraction
- Invisalign treatment
- restorations.

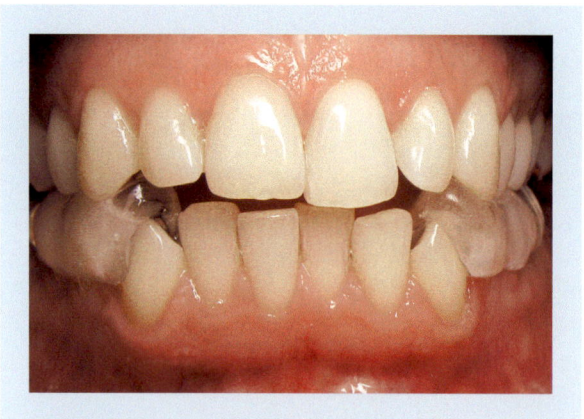

4 TREATMENT OF DIFFERENT MALOCCLUSIONS WITH ALIGNERS

Fig 4-444 Removable splint (COPA) in situ.

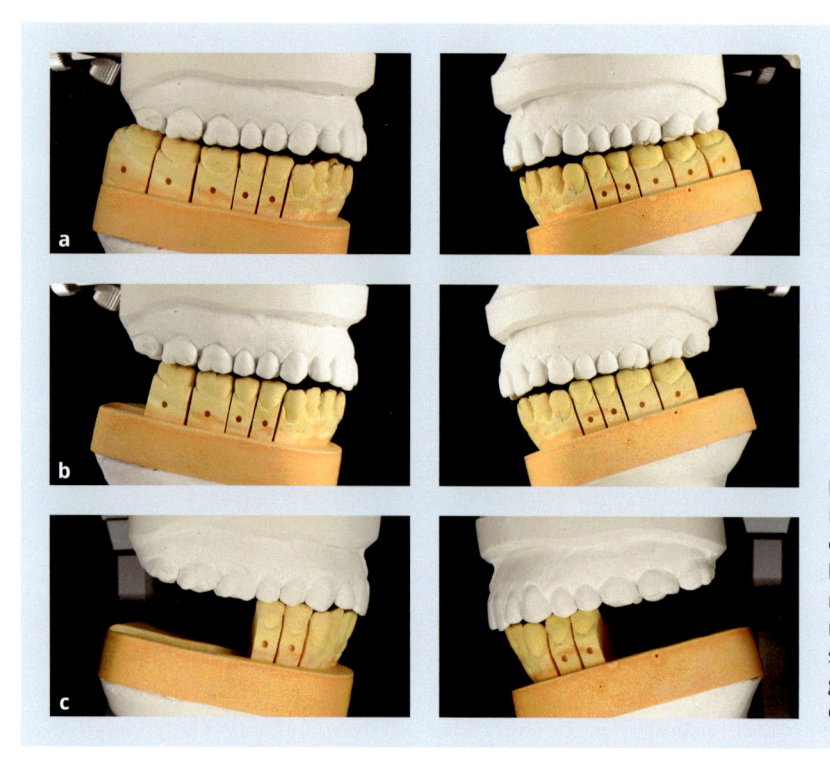

Fig 4-445 Mounted plaster casts **(a)** Initial situation mounted in centric occlusion. **(b)** Teeth 38 and 48 have been taken out, which leads to a slight reduction of the open bite. **(c)** After removal of the molars: the premolars shift into a class I relationship and good vertical support, the anterior open bite is even more reduced.

Treatment

Treatment was started with with a removable splint (Fig 4-444), which the patient wore 24 hours a day (Dr W Boisserée, Cologne). The patient also had osteopathic therapy.

Mounted plaster casts and with closing of the anterior open bite with the removal of posterior teeth showed the right strategy for treatment planning in this patient (Fig 4-445). The wisdom teeth needed to be removed, followed by reduction of the posterior vertical height.

An interdisciplinary treatment plan was intended from the beginning. The first step, removal of wisdom teeth and use of provisional crowns to give decreased vertical height, created a class I relationship with posterior contacts (Fig 4-446). However, the patient still does not have any physiologic anterior relation or canine guidance. As it would not be feasible to build

Fig 4-446 Provisional crowns with decreased vertical posterior height.

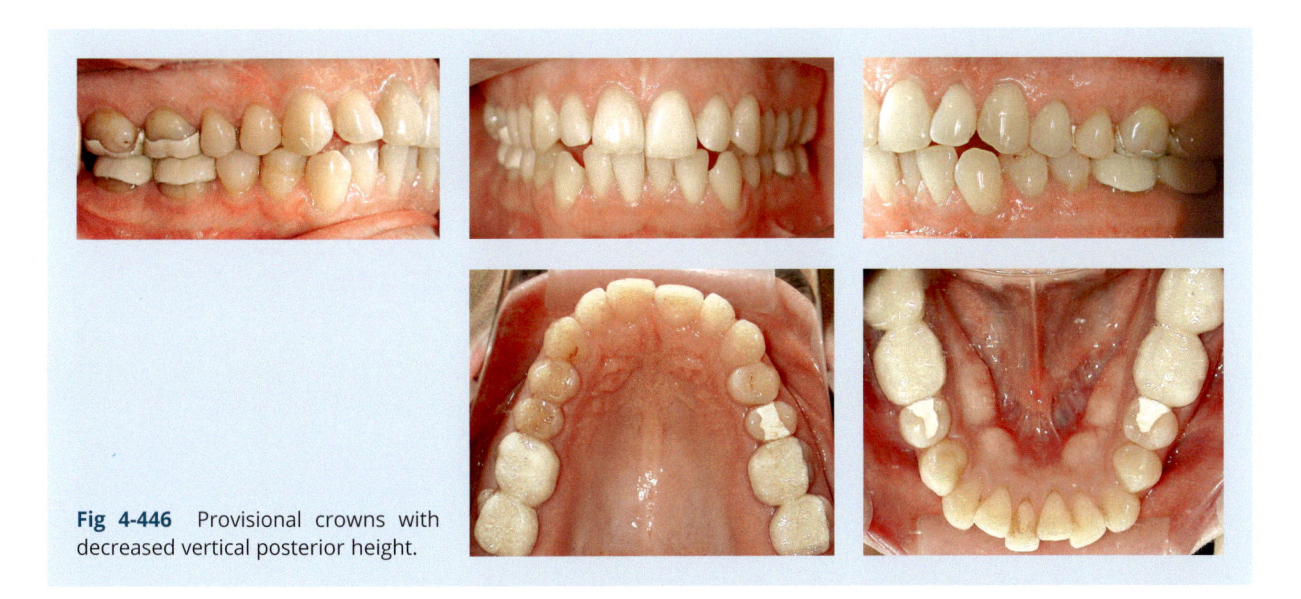

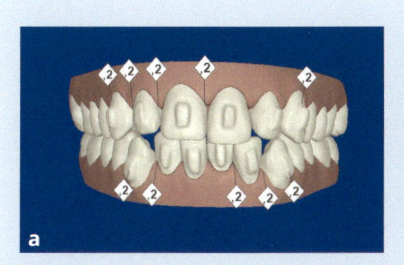

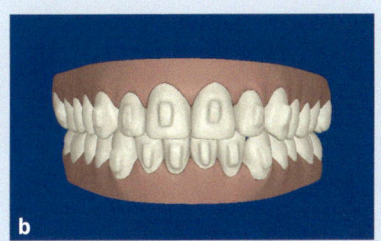

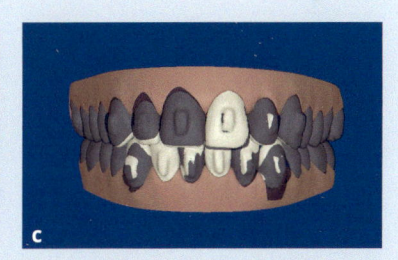

Fig 4-447 ClinCheck software results. **(a)** Initial situation with attachments and planned IPR. **(b)** Final planned result with closing of the anterior open bite and alignment of both arches. **(c)** Superimposition to show planned movement (blue, initial tooth position; white, final tooth position).

up all canines and incisors to achieve a physiologic overbite, overjet, and canine guidance, the next step proposed was orthodontic treatment with the Invisalign system.

ClinCheck software shows the initial intraoral situation with attachments on all maxillary and mandibular incisors and canines with planned IPR of 0.2 mm on maxillary teeth 11, 12, 13, and 23 as well as on mandibular canines and lateral incisors (Fig 4-447). The treatment with the Invisalign system here was a formerly available therapy option for "anterior treatment," with planned movements only in the incisors and canines. This was to use 9 maxillary and 12 mandibular aligners.

Comparison of the initial and final findings show that the overjet and overbite have been adjusted and the patient has a physiologic canine relation (Fig 4-448). The position of the premolars and molars was not changed during Invisalign treatment. The canines with insufficient restorations were to be renewed and the provisional crowns on maxillary and mandibular molars are showing signs of wear and attrition after 18 months of orthodontic treatment (Fig 4-449).

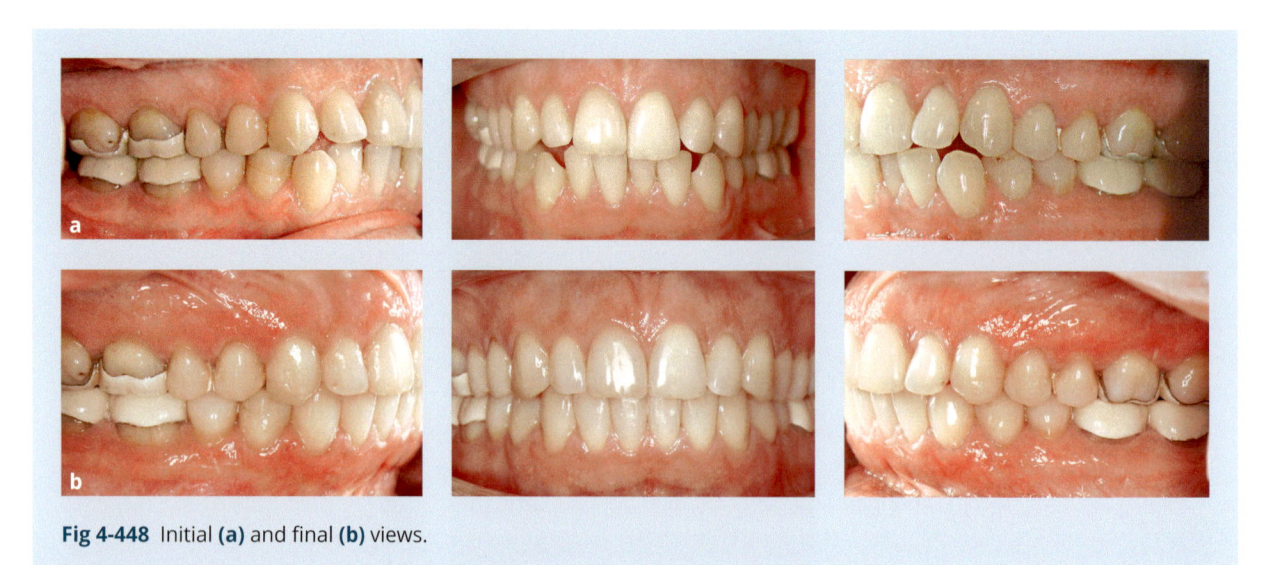

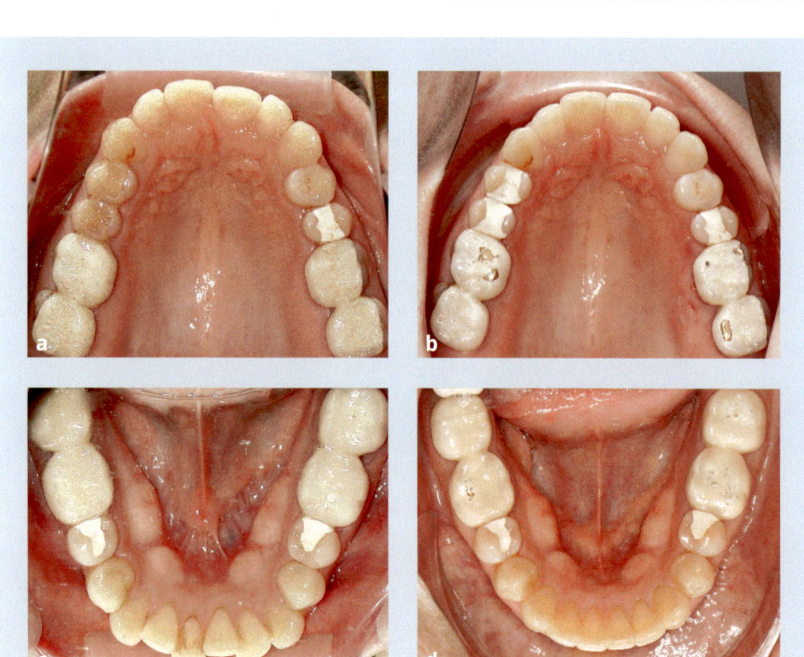

4 TREATMENT OF DIFFERENT MALOCCLUSIONS WITH ALIGNERS

Fig 4-448 Initial **(a)** and final **(b)** views.

Fig 4-449 Initial **(a,c)** and final **(b,d)** views of the maxillary and mandibular arches. The upper canines show insufficient restorations. The provisional crowns are also showing signs of wear.

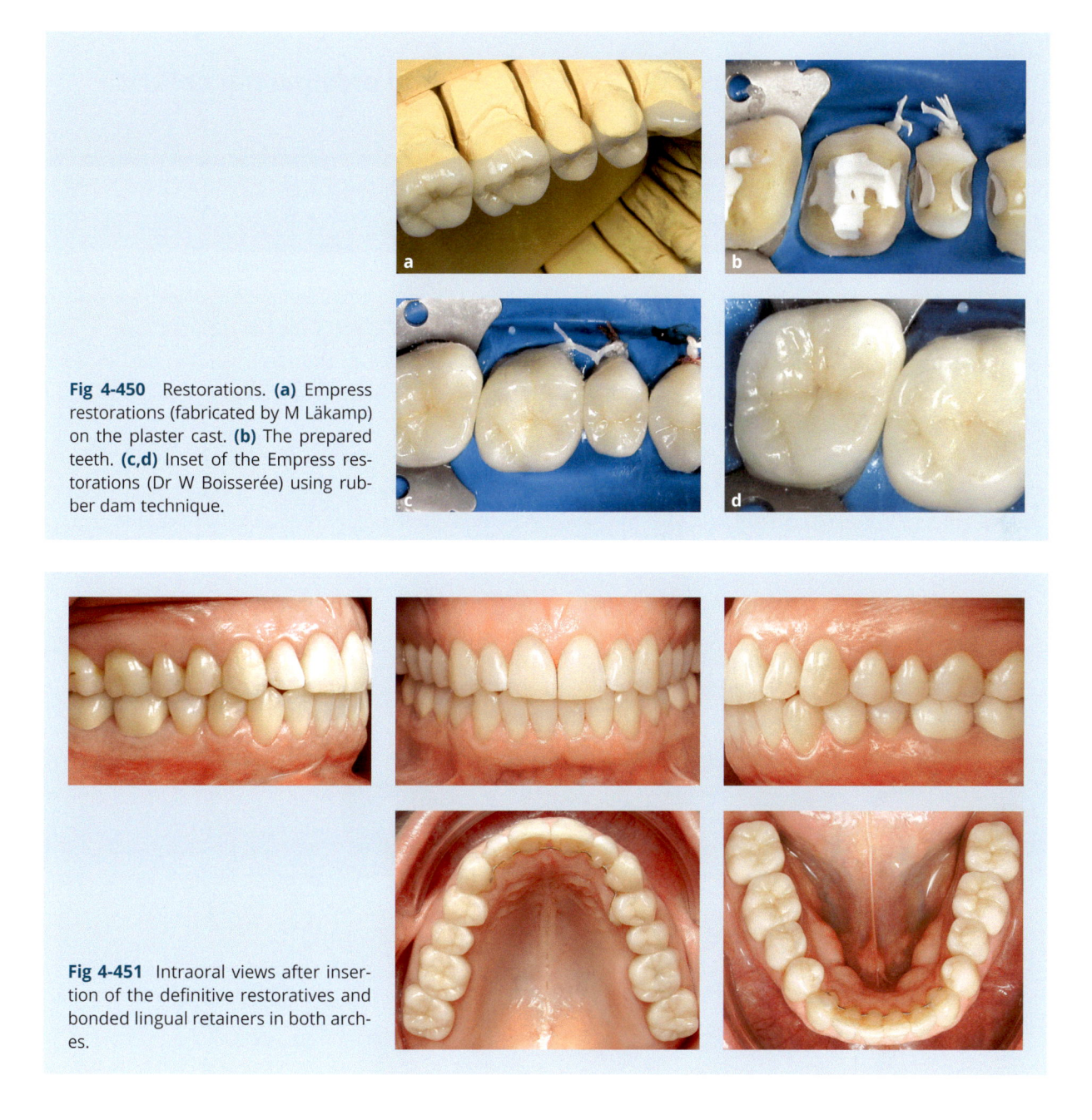

TREATMENT OF DIFFERENT MALOCCLUSIONS WITH ALIGNERS 4

Fig 4-450 Restorations. **(a)** Empress restorations (fabricated by M Läkamp) on the plaster cast. **(b)** The prepared teeth. **(c,d)** Inset of the Empress restorations (Dr W Boisserée) using rubber dam technique.

Fig 4-451 Intraoral views after insertion of the definitive restoratives and bonded lingual retainers in both arches.

Figure 4-450 shows the restoration process and Figure 4-451 the final intraoral views.

Topic 54
Craniomandibular disorder with a crossbite and only partial centric contact on two molars

Treatment:
- bonding a vertical hook
- Invisalign treatment with criss-cross elastics

A crossbite can be treated with the Invisalign system. If it is a single tooth crossbite and the neighboring teeth are not also in a crossbite position, the force of the aligners is mostly sufficient. If the last molars show a crossbite situation, the addition of a criss-cross elastics to the aligner is advisable. Criss-cross elastics require buttons on the teeth. Originally these were metal buttons or laboratory-prepared buttons, but also individual hooks can be made that are smaller and more esthetic.

The fabrication of an individual hook is shown in Figure 4-452. The aligner needs to be cut out at the hook site but the amount is very small and it does not affect the fit of the aligner.

This patient had a crossbite on the right side from the canine to the last molar on all teeth, with centric contact only on teeth 17/47 (Fig 4-453).

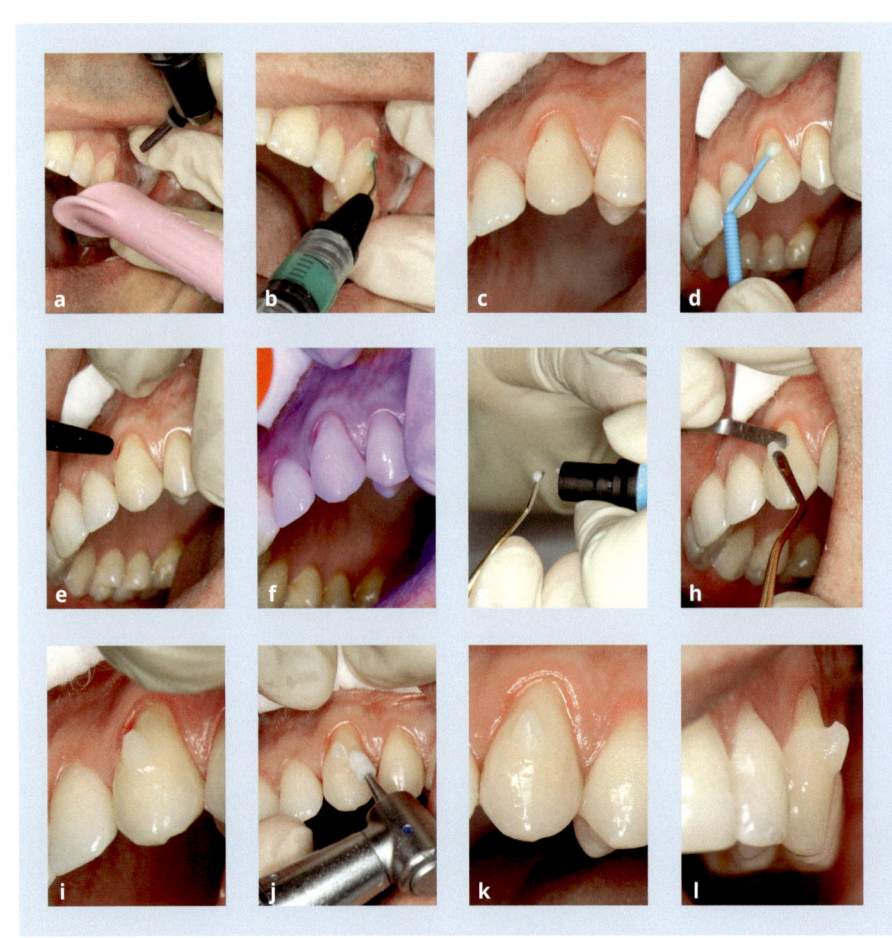

Fig 4-452 Fabrication and bonding of a vertical hook. (**a**) The enamel is sandblasted with aluminum oxide 50 μm. (**b**) The surface is etched with phosphoric acid for 5 seconds. (**c**) The prepared tooth has a slightly abraded buccal surface. (**d,e**) Primer (OptiBond FL primer) is applied (**d**) and coated with air syringe onto the tooth (**e**). (**f**) Primer is light cured. (**g,h**) The chosen composite resin (e.g. Enamel plus HFO, Vanini) is formed onto the tooth as a hook; this only takes a few minutes using two instruments. (**i**) A gingival cut is made for the elastic. (**j**) The hook is polished. (**k,l**). The final vertical hook, which is very small and comfortable for the patient.

Fig 4-453 Initial presentation.

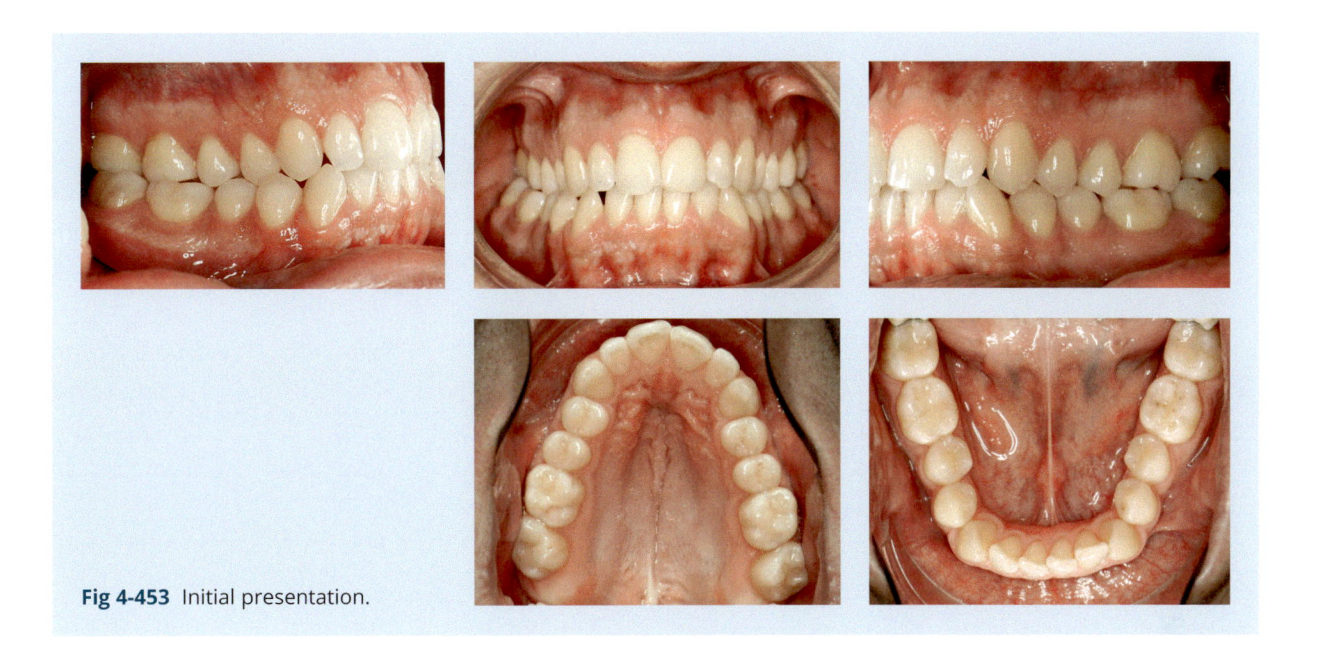

Diagnosis:
- CMD
- crossbite on the right side with sliding of the mandible from centric into habitual occlusion
- mild crowding
- excessive lower Curve of Spee.

Therapy:
- Invisalign treatment combined with criss-cross elastics.

Fig 4-454 Mounted plaster casts in centric relation showing a single contact on teeth 17 and 47.

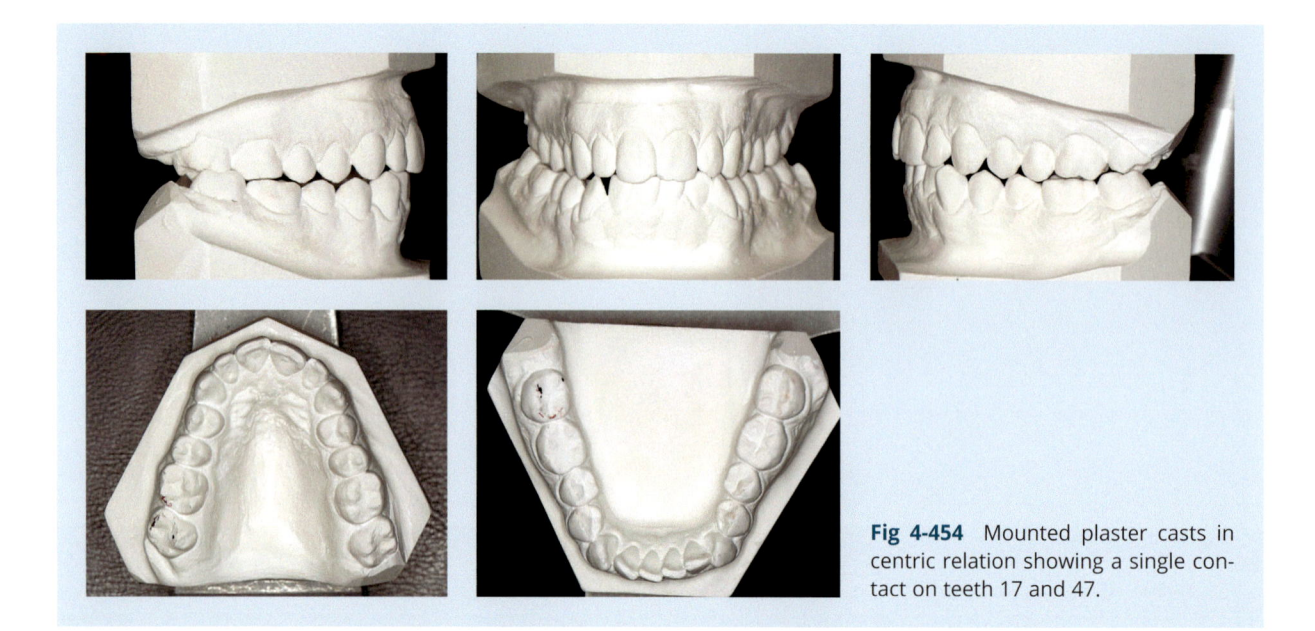

Treatment

The mounted plaster casts in centric relation show a single contact on teeth 17 and 47. During closure, the mandible slides from this occlusal contact into the habitual occlusion (Fig 4-454).

In severe crossbite situations such as this, combination of Invisalign with criss-cross elastics is recommended, as the aligner is posteriorly too weak to correct the crossbite sufficiently.

The orthodontic treatment plan (Fig 4-455) shows the planned movements, which were transferred into the ClinCheck software. An expansion of 5 mm was needed in the anterior area of the maxillary arch and 6 mm in the posterior area, with an overcorrection of 1 mm and an additional three aligners. Intrusion of 1.5 mm in the mandibular incisor area was needed to level the excessive curve of Spee. A second step would intrude the mandibular canines 1 mm and extrude the mandibular premolars 0.75 mm. Attachments would be necessary on mandibular canines and premolars to obtain anchorage for the intrusion of the incisors and extrusion of the premolars. Teeth 41 and 42 would be retracted.

The first ClinCheck analysis was asked for IPR from mesial of the mandibular molars to mesial of the canines, to obtain space for alignment and distalization of mandibular premolars, followed by canines into the spaces obtained with IPR; this would provide sufficient space anterior to solve the incisor crowding (Fig 4-456). The advantage of this procedure is that, if a later refinement was needed, additional IPR could be performed in the incisor area, as this enamel was not reduced in the first phase.

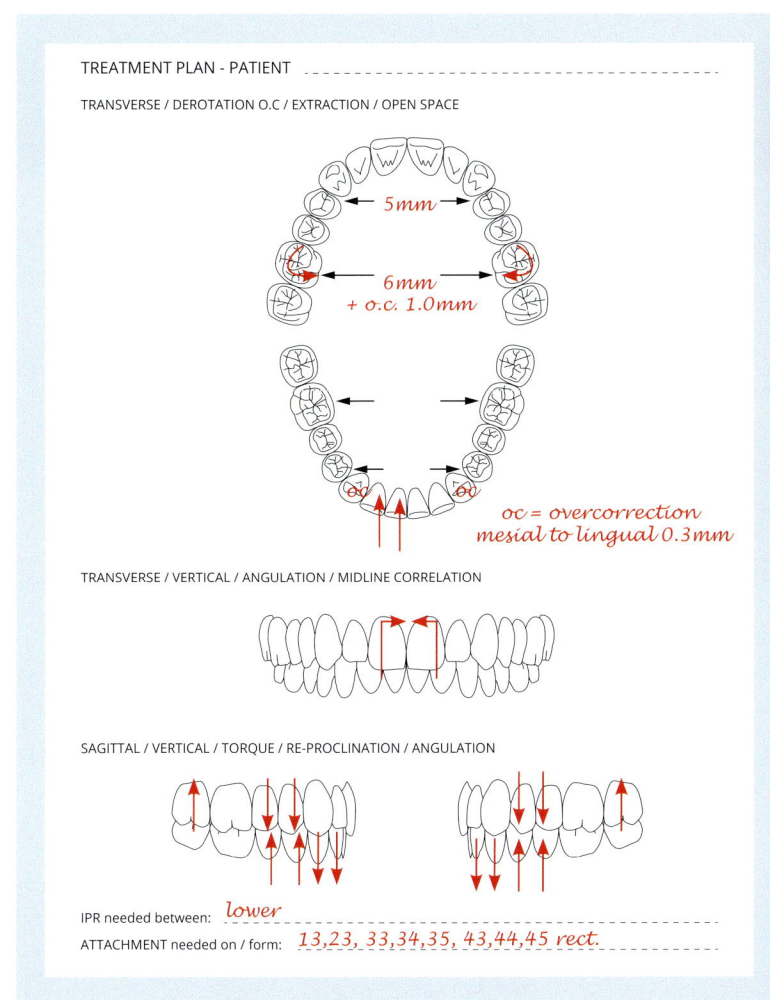

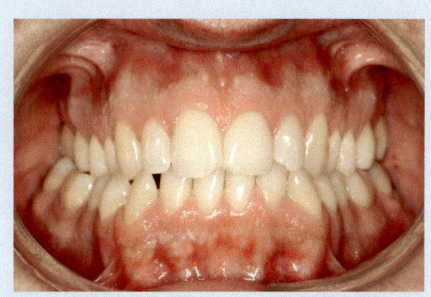

Fig 4-455 Treatment plan and intraoral view. oc., overcorrection.

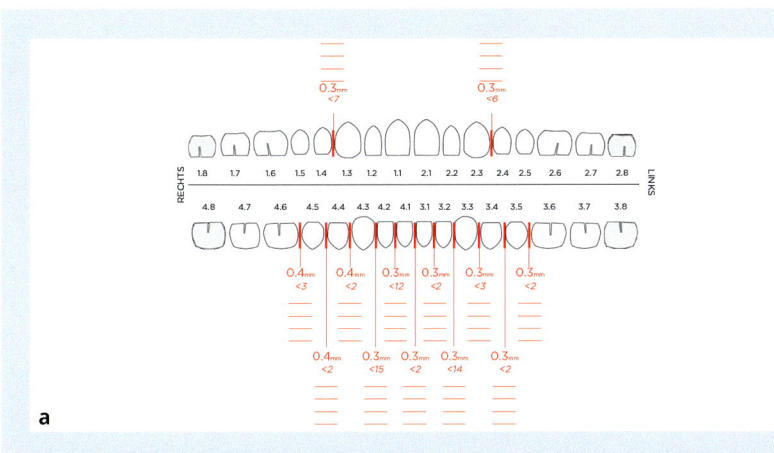

Fig 4-456 ClinCheck software results. (a) IPR chart. (b) Initial situation with crossbite on the right side. (c) Final planned situation with aligned arches and solved crossbite. (d) Superimposition to show planned movements, particularly the transversal expansion in the maxillary arch (blue, initial tooth position; white, final tooth position).

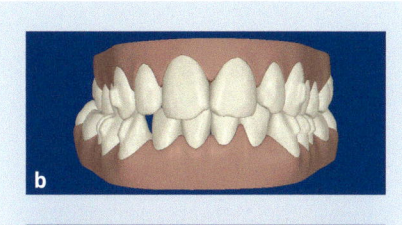

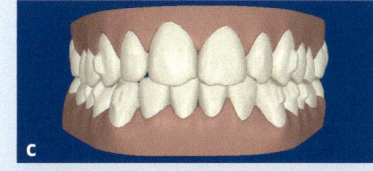

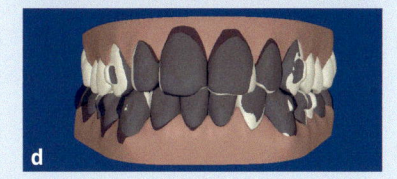

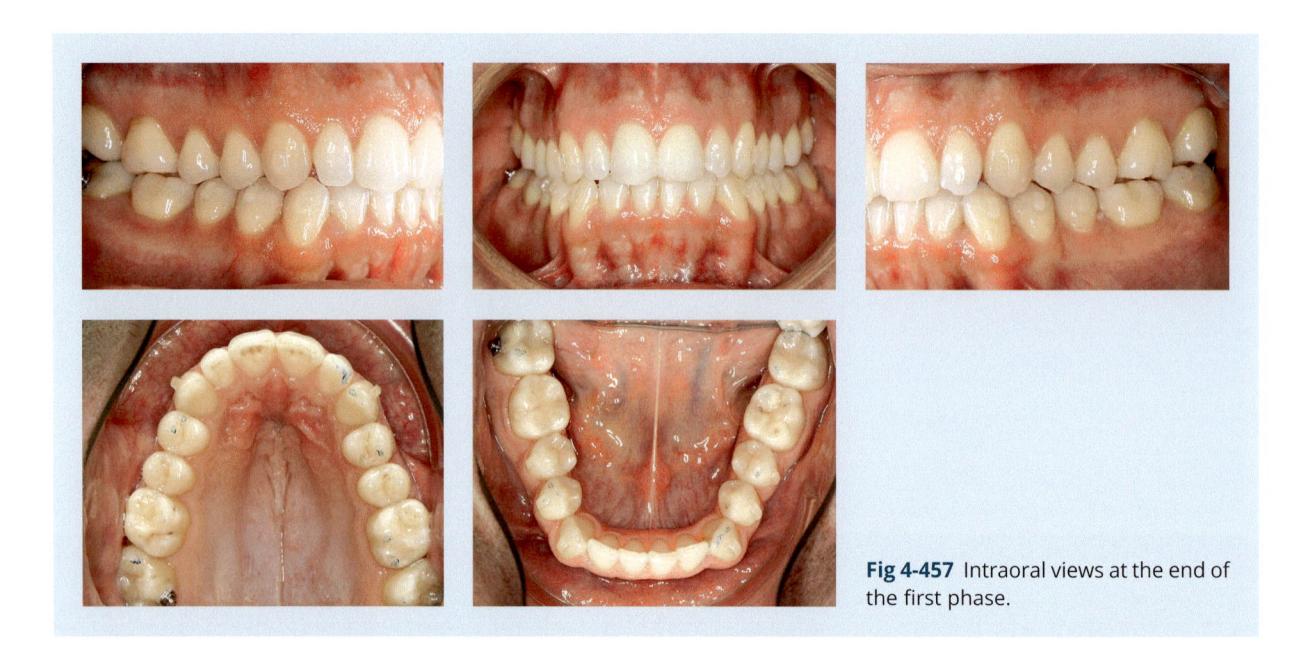

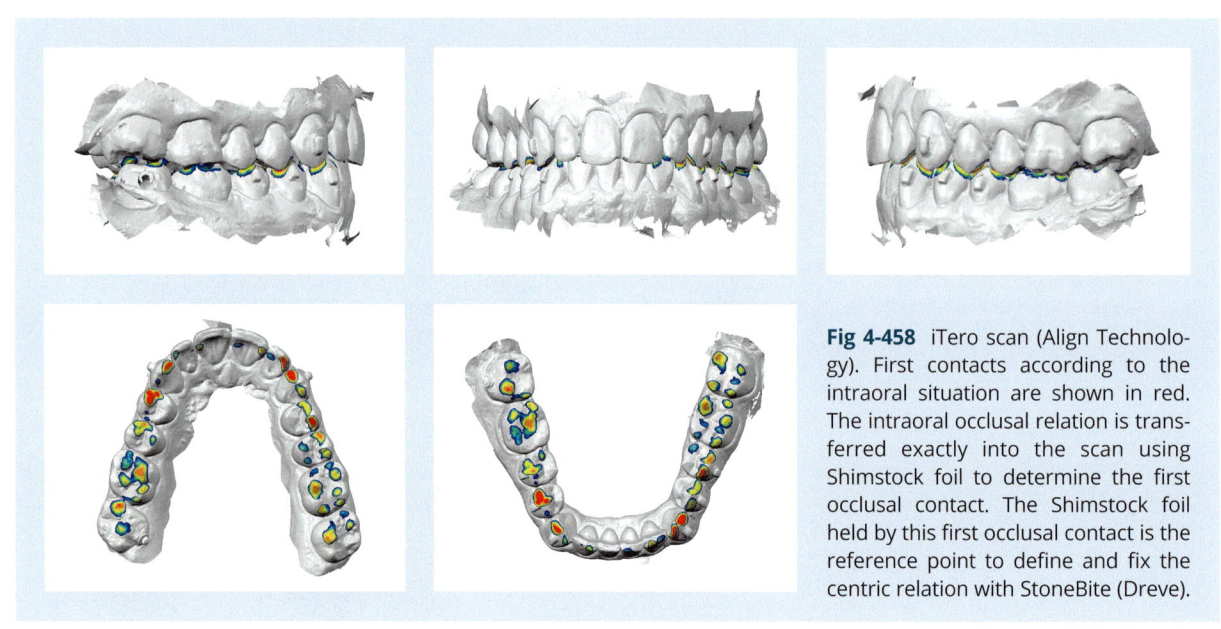

Fig 4-457 Intraoral views at the end of the first phase.

Fig 4-458 iTero scan (Align Technology). First contacts according to the intraoral situation are shown in red. The intraoral occlusal relation is transferred exactly into the scan using Shimstock foil to determine the first occlusal contact. The Shimstock foil held by this first occlusal contact is the reference point to define and fix the centric relation with StoneBite (Dreve).

The first stage used 24 maxillary and 25 mandibular aligners. After this first phase, a refinement commenced for detailing the occlusion.

At that point, the patient showed centric contact points on premolars and molars. Buttons were still in place on teeth 17 to 47 for the criss-cross elastics, which the patient wore during the night for retention in the refinement (Fig 4-457).

Teeth 33 and 43 needed more derotation, and overcorrection of both teeth with the mesial aspect to lingual and distal aspect to labial was ordered. Tooth 22 showed a heavy occlusal contact, which was eliminated in the refinement to obtain physiologic front relationship.

An iTero scan allows checking an occlusion pattern in detail (Fig 4-458). This particular procedure allows the

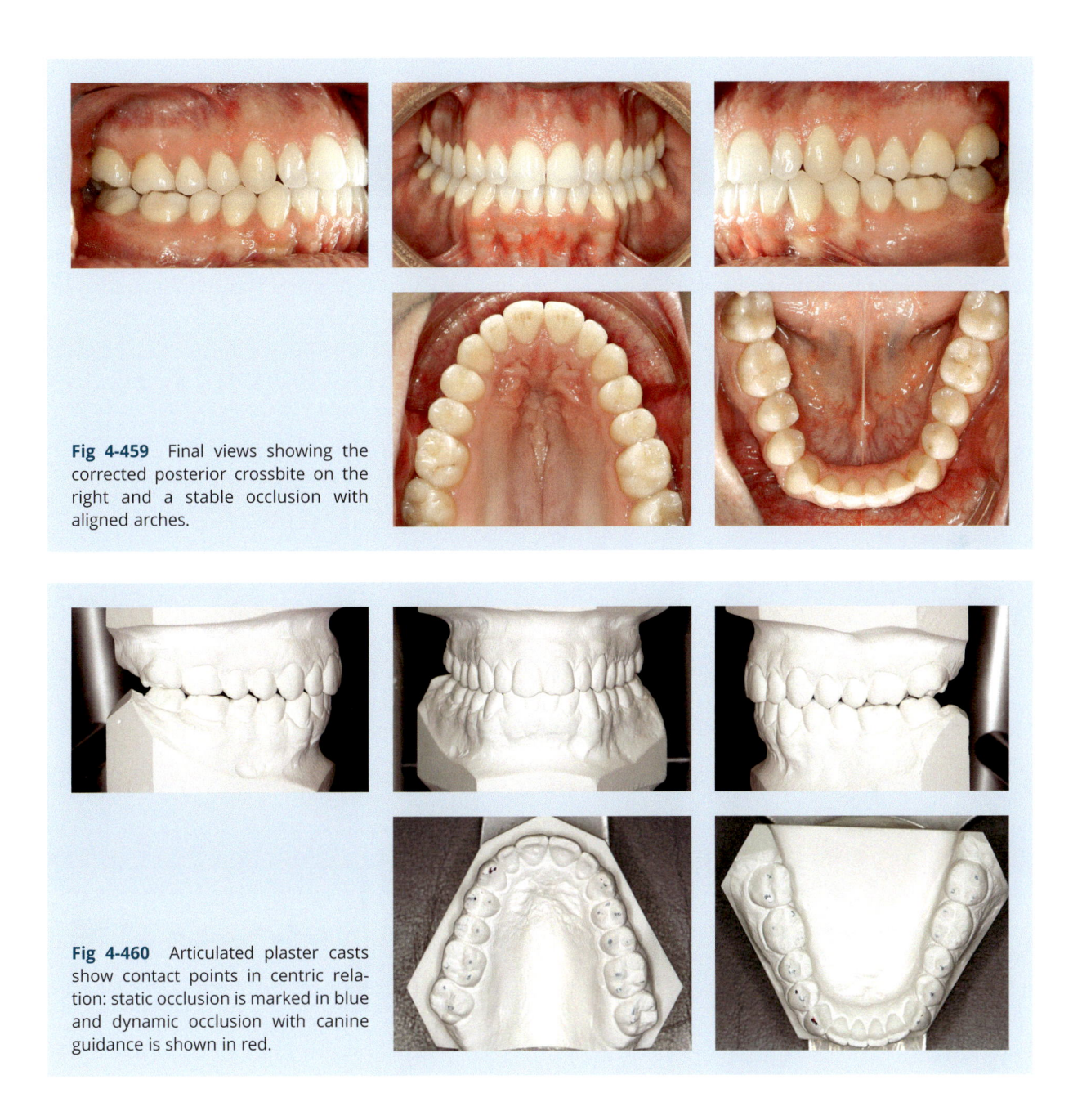

Fig 4-459 Final views showing the corrected posterior crossbite on the right and a stable occlusion with aligned arches.

Fig 4-460 Articulated plaster casts show contact points in centric relation: static occlusion is marked in blue and dynamic occlusion with canine guidance is shown in red.

centric relation to be transferred directly into the scan and, therefore, into the ClinCheck software.

At the end of treatment, the posterior crossbite on the right has been corrected and a stable occlusion has been achieved with aligned arches in slight transversally widened overcorrection (Figs 4-459 and 4-460).

Topic 55
CMD and chronic pain, partial centric contact only on two molars

Treatment:
- two phases of Invisalign treatment

Unfortunately, it is not possible to simulate a closure of the mandible on a hinge axis with the ClinCheck software, which would be particularly helpful in patients with preliminary contact points. This closure can only be seen using a virtual articulator, which is not yet available in the ClinCheck software.

In patients, in whom the elimination of a disturbing preliminary contact is part of the treatment, sometimes two or more phases of Invisalign treatment are needed. The first step is to solve the disturbing first contact and this is followed by a midcourse correction with a new centric relationship.

This patient had suffered from severe chronic pain for 2.5 years and missed school because of the pain and muscle weakness. She had orthodontic treatment elsewhere with a fixed multibracket appliance and a Bionator. A pain questionnaire filled out by the patient indicated the following symptoms:
- headache
- TMJ pain
- neck pain
- back pain
- muscle pain.

Mounted plaster casts and intraoral views showed exclusively contact points initially only on teeth 17 to 47, followed by contact on 11 to 41 (Figs 4-461 and 4-462).

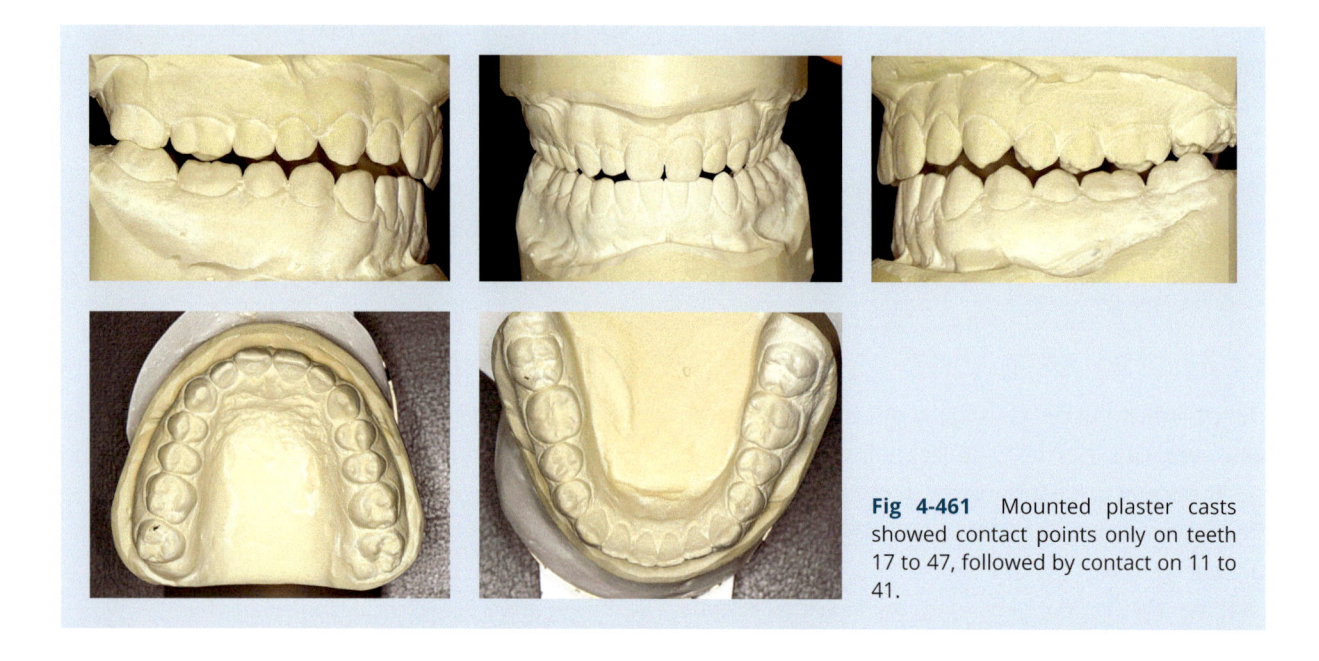

Fig 4-461 Mounted plaster casts showed contact points only on teeth 17 to 47, followed by contact on 11 to 41.

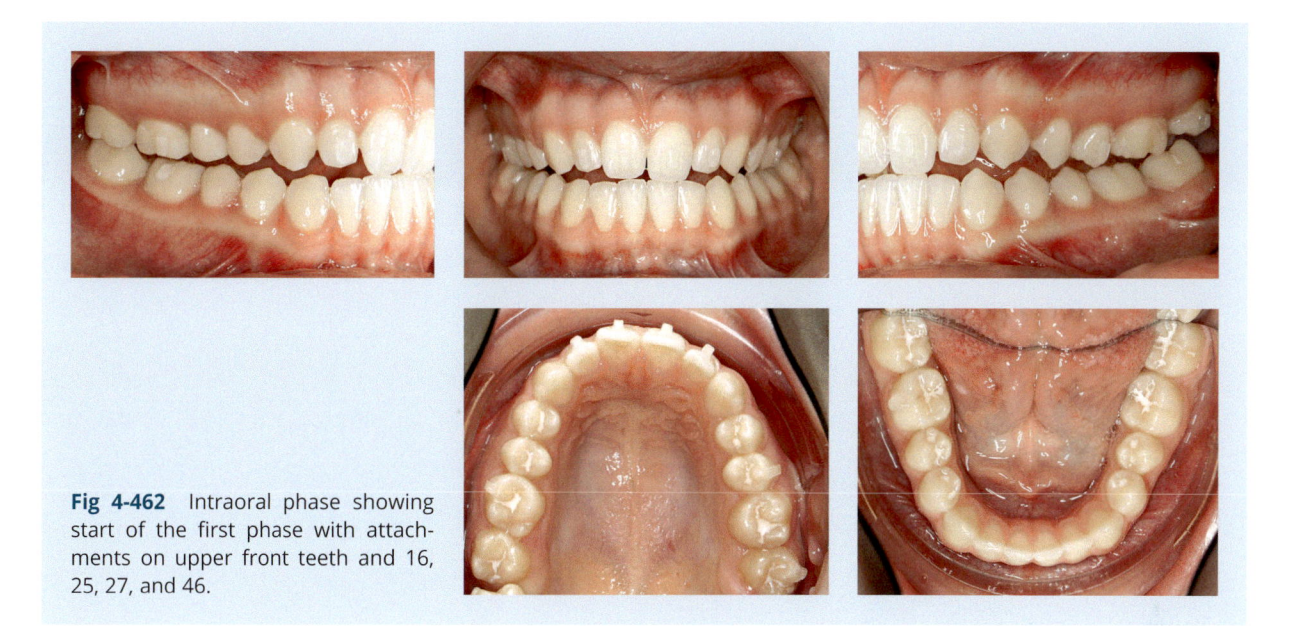

TREATMENT OF DIFFERENT MALOCCLUSIONS WITH ALIGNERS 4

Fig 4-462 Intraoral phase showing start of the first phase with attachments on upper front teeth and 16, 25, 27, and 46.

Diagnosis:
- CMD
- pain in neck and back plus headaches
- initial contact only on teeth 17 to 47.

Therapy:
- two phases of Invisalign therapy.

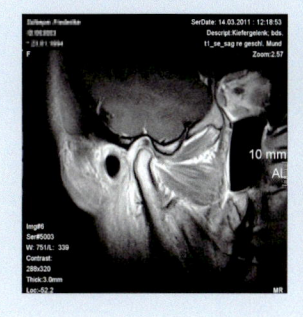

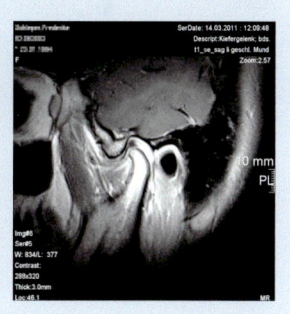

Fig 4-463 MRT of TMJs in habitual intercuspation. **(left)** Right TMJ, showing physiologic, slightly to anterior positioned discus articularis. **(right)** Left TMJ, showing a physiologic, slightly to anterior positioned discus articularis. (Dr M Andersson, Dr T Steimel, MediaPark Clinic, Cologne.)

Treatment

MRT was used to assess the TMJs (Fig 4-463).

The treatment plan asked for attachments on maxillary central and lateral incisors to obtain major anchorage for maxillary incisor movement and on molars. The patient also underwent myofunctional therapy.

The first phase of treatment used 15 aligners, leading to an increased overjet of 0.5 mm and eliminating first contact of teeth 11 to 41 (Figs 4-464 and 4-465). After elimination of this first contact, the mandible was liberated and free to rotate anteriorly into the position with the following occlusal contacts:
- 13, 14, 16 to 43, 44, 45, 46
- 23 to 33
- 25 to 35, 36.

289

Fig 4-464 Intraoral views at the end of the first phase.

Fig 4-465 Mounted plaster casts at the end of the first phase. Incisor contact has been eliminated and the mandible has rotated to anterior and shows the following occlusal contacts: 13, 14, 16 to 43, 44, 45, 46, 23 to 33, 25 to 35, 36.

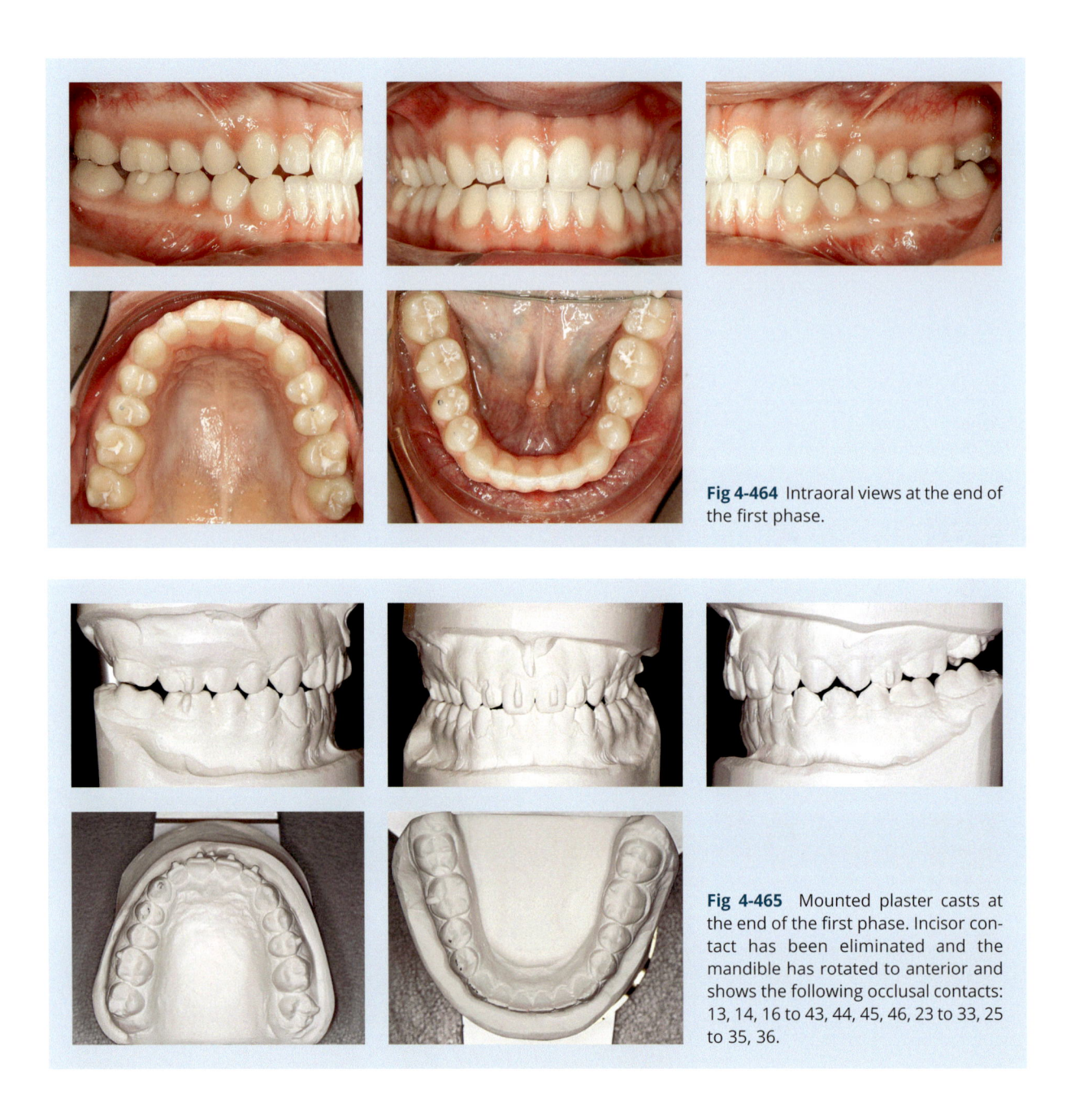

At this point, scans were taken for the second phase of treatment (Fig 4-466). With the iTero scan it is possible to diagnose in detail the static occlusion using the occlusal color pattern generated and then compare it directly with the intraoral situation or articulated plaster casts.

This second stage started with an additional 15 aligners to align the maxillary and mandibular arches and to create a posterior hard collision and physiologic anterior relationship. Vertical rectangular attachments were added on all teeth with planned extrusive movement (Fig 4-467).

The second phase created a stable occlusion with occlusal contacts on all premolars and molars. The maxillary and mandibular arches have been aligned and a physiologic anterior relation achieved (Figs 4-468 to 4-470). The patient was almost pain free and integrated normally into everyday life.

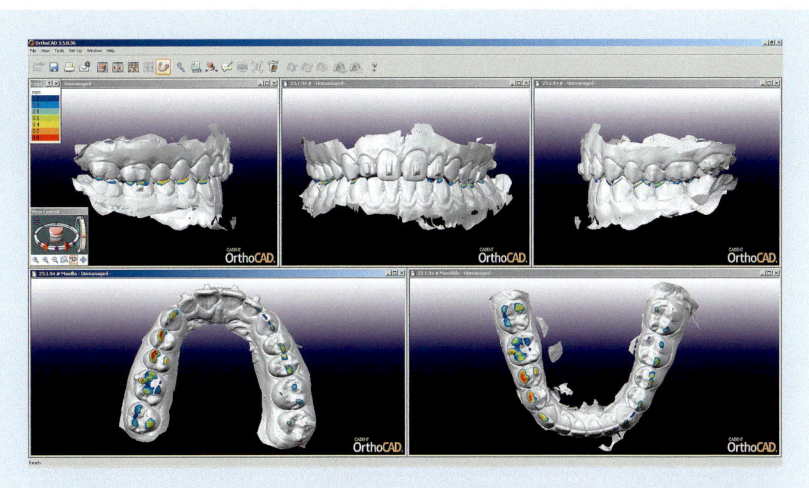

Fig 4-466 Scan for the refinement performed in centric occlusion shows the contacts in detail with the color marker: first contacts (red) are on 14, 15 to 44, 45.

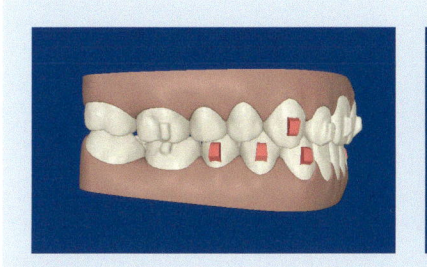

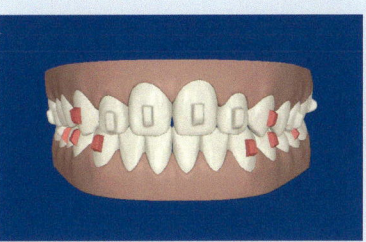

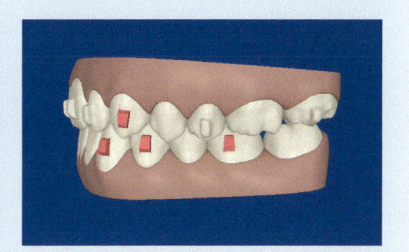

Fig 4-467 ClinCheck software for the second phase, showing the attachments.

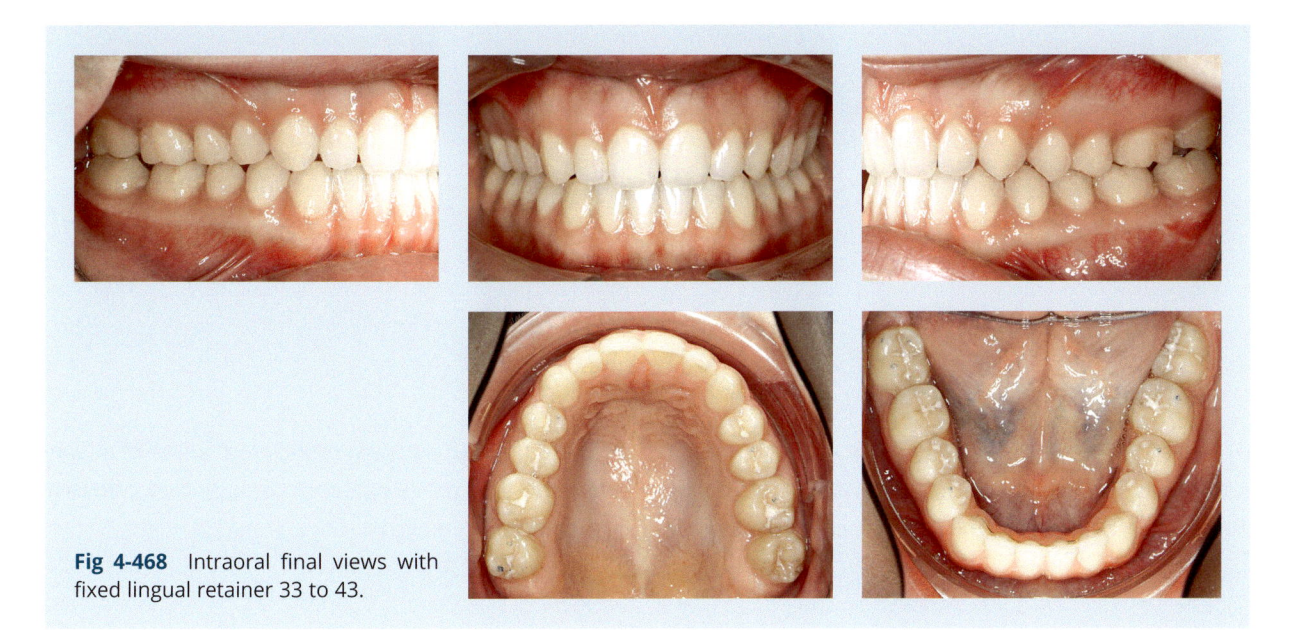

Fig 4-468 Intraoral final views with fixed lingual retainer 33 to 43.

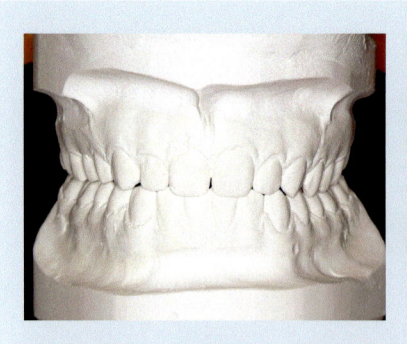

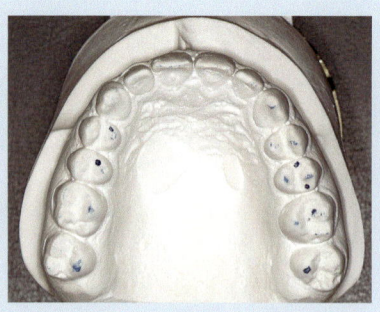

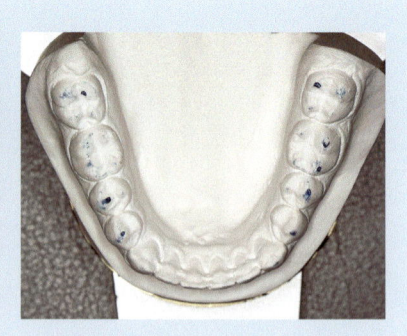

4 TREATMENT OF DIFFERENT MALOCCLUSIONS WITH ALIGNERS

Fig 4-469 Centric mounted casts show the final occlusal vertical support on all premolars and molars.

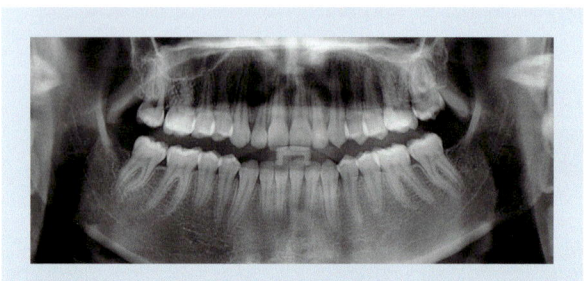

Fig 4-470 Final orthopantomogram showing no pathology.

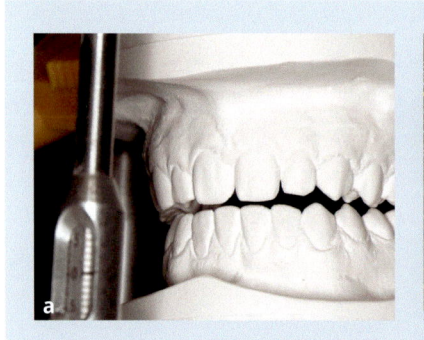

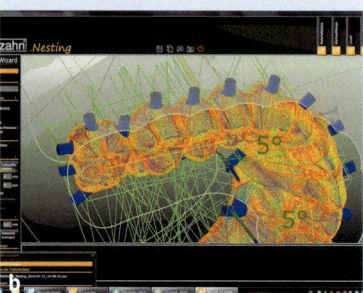

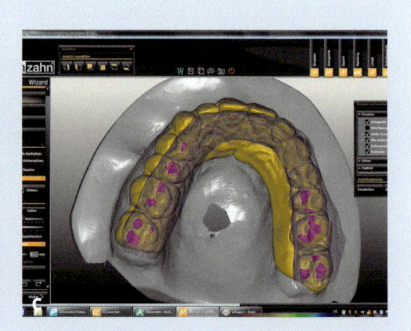

Fig 4-471 Fabrication of the maxillary splint. (a) Articulated plaster casts. (b) Computer simulation of the dimensions. (c) Occlusal contact points on the splints during the virtual set-up process (Zirkonzahn).

Retention was performed with a fixed lingual retainer in the mandibular arch from canine to canine (Fig 4-471). The stress from bruxistic activity needed to be controlled after orthodontic treatment. This was achieved with a milled splint for the maxillary arch that was worn at night (Figs 4-472 and 4-473).

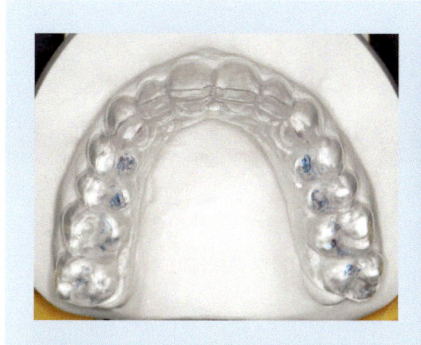

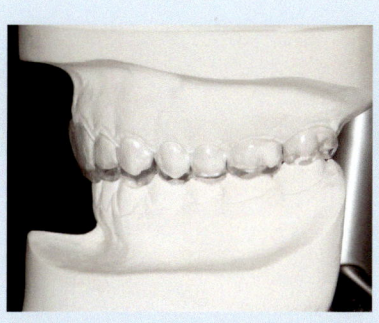

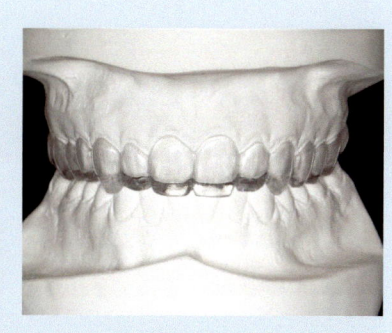

Fig 4-472 Finished milled splint (Temp Premium Flexible Transparent; Zirkonzahn) in the articulator, demonstrating an equally balanced occlusal pattern with occlusal foil and canine guidance. (Fabrication by M Läkamp).

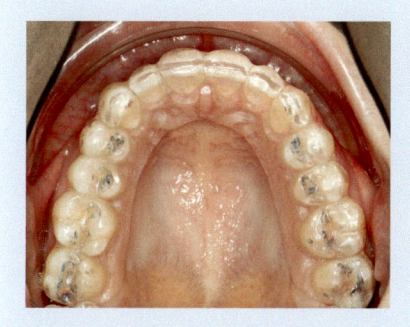

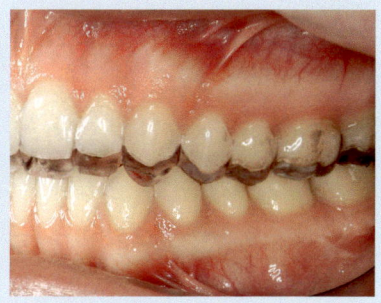

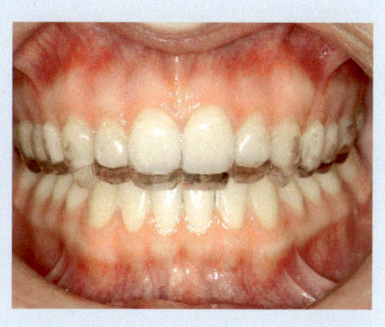

Fig 4-473 Intraoral views with the splint in place. The occlusal pattern in the mouth is identical to the occlusal pattern shown on the articulated plaster casts (Fig 4-471a).

The course of treatment is shown in Figures 4-474 and 4-475. The two phases resolved the incisor edge-to-edge bite first, followed by adjustment to get a stable occlusion with occlusal contacts on all premolars and molars.

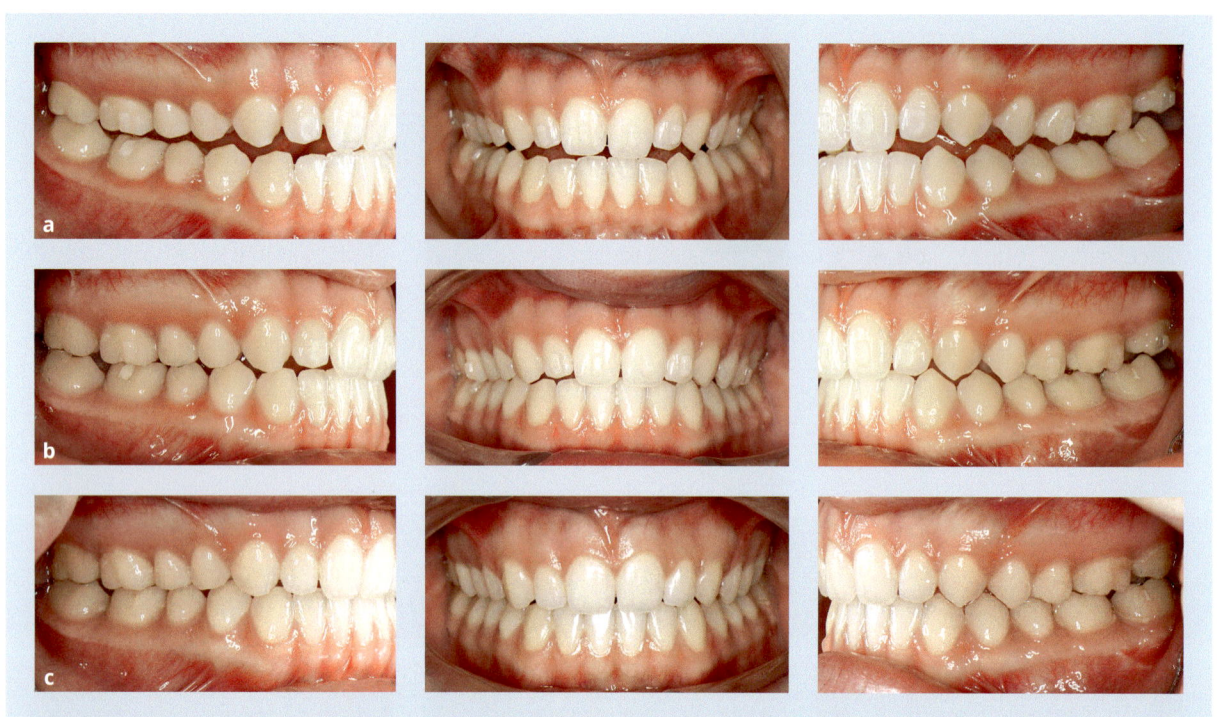

4 TREATMENT OF DIFFERENT MALOCCLUSIONS WITH ALIGNERS

Fig 4-474 Intraoral views initially **(a)**; at start of the second phase **(b)**; and, finally, with full vertical support **(c)**.

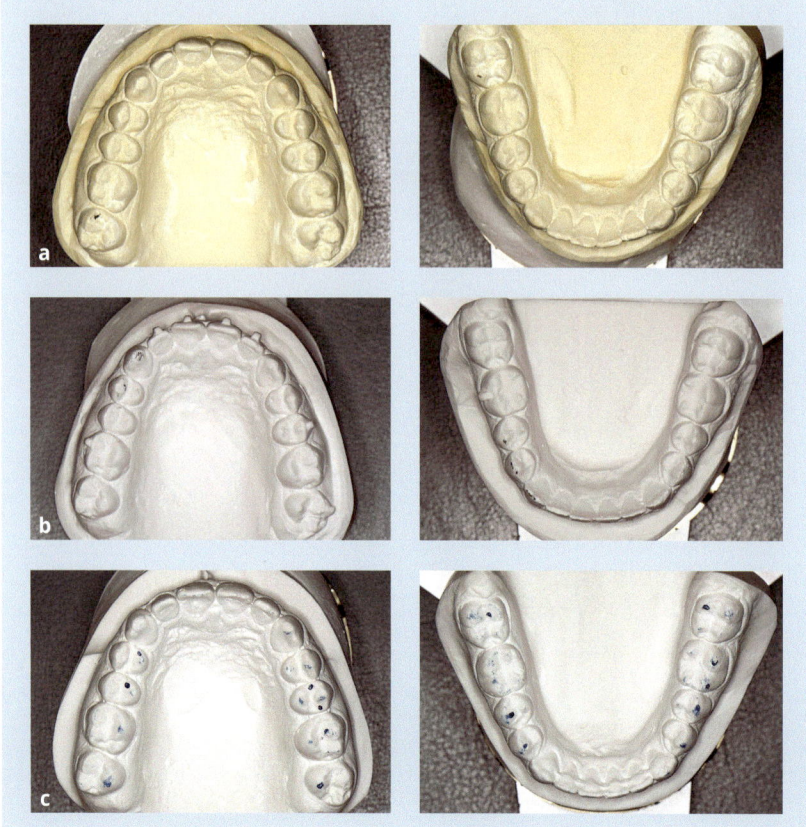

Fig 4-475 Articulated plaster casts at the start of treatment, with contact points exclusively on teeth 17 to 47 **(a)**; after the first phase of treatment, with overjet of 0.5 mm in a new centric relation **(b)**; and at the end of treatment, with full vertical support with posterior contact points **(c)**.

Topic 56
Craniomandibular disorder with partial centric contact on two incisors

Treatment:
- two phases of Invisalign treatment

As discussed in Topic 55, it is not currently possible to simulate a closure of the mandible on a hinge axis with the ClinCheck software. This would require a virtual articulator, which is not yet available.

This patient had TMJ dysfunction and reduced contacts in centric relation, these being exclusively on teeth 21 to 32 (Fig 4-476).

Fig 4-476 Initial presentation. **(a)** Frontal view. **(b)** In maximal intercuspation, the chin deviates to the left and the face shows a convexity to the right with a shortening of the left side. **(c-e)** Because of the deviation of the mandible in maximal intercuspation, the TMJ condyles move into a more retral/cranial position. CBCT of the TMJs shows this deviation, particularly of the left condyle.

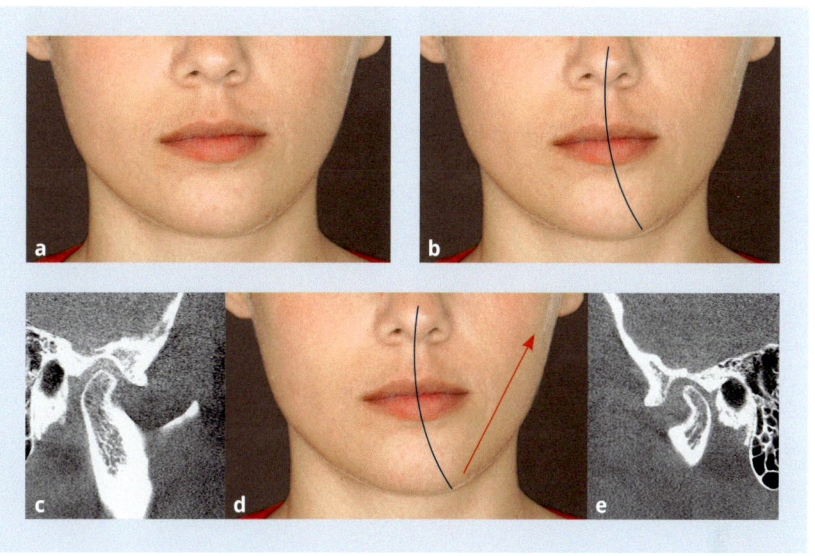

Diagnosis:
- CMD
- neck pain and pain with mouth opening
- headache
- retral/cranial dislocated condyle and anterior disc displacement, with inflammation in the bilaminar zone.

Therapy:
- occlusal splint
- Invisalign therapy in two phases.

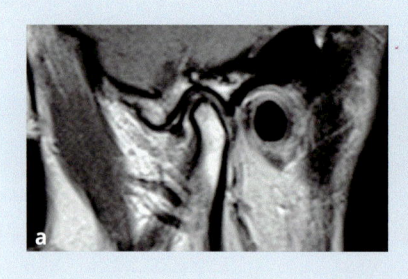

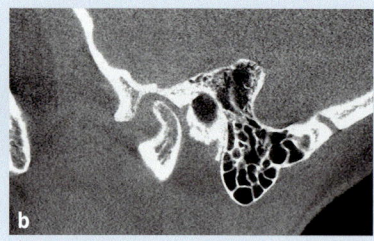

Fig 4-477 Imaging of the left TMJ. **(a)** MRT shows the anterior disc displacement in detail. **(b)** CBCT performed several months later, also shows the retral/cranial position of the condyle.

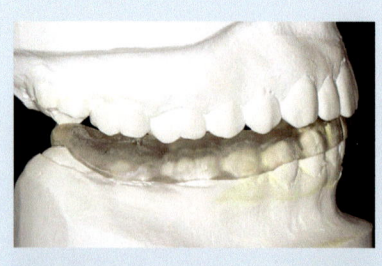

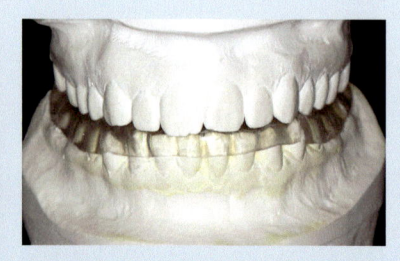

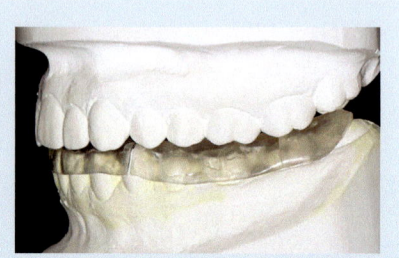

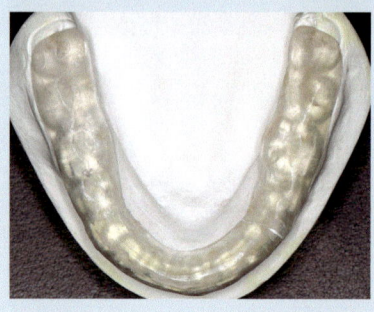

Fig 4-478 Plaster casts with the occlusal mandibular splint (Prof Dr S Kopp, Frankfurt).

Treatment

The patient was pretreated with an occlusal splint (Prof Dr S Kopp, Frankfurt) for the craniomandibular dysfunction, neck pain, headache, and pain during mouth opening. The patient was then transferred to our orthodontic office, as the patient had moved to Cologne. The centric setting achieved with the existing removable occlusal splint was included as a basis of the orthodontic treatment plan.

Because of the deviation of the mandible in maximal intercuspation, the condyles moved into a more retral/cranial position, particularly on the left (Fig 4-477).

Use of the occlusal splints gradually reduced pain until the patient was completely pain free. Plaster casts show the teeth relations with the occlusal mandibular splint in place, creating a physiologic centric mandibular position, which was the pain-free position for the patient (Fig 4-478); casts were then mounted in the articulator to plan the orthodontic treatment (Fig 4-479).

At the start of Invisalign therapy, intraoral views showed contact on maxillary central incisors and tooth 12. Contrary to the mounted casts, the intraoral views show a mandibular shift to the left in maximal intercuspation. Attachments were bonded on teeth 13, 23, 33, 34, 35, 43, 44, and 45.

TREATMENT OF DIFFERENT MALOCCLUSIONS WITH ALIGNERS 4

Fig 4-479 Mounted plaster casts according to the removable splint show the posterior open bite and the contact points exclusively on incisors. Midlines of maxillary and mandibular arches are in line.

Fig 4-480 Intraoral situation at the start of Invisalign therapy, with contact on the maxillary central incisors and tooth 12. There is a mandibular shift to the left in maximal intercuspation.

297

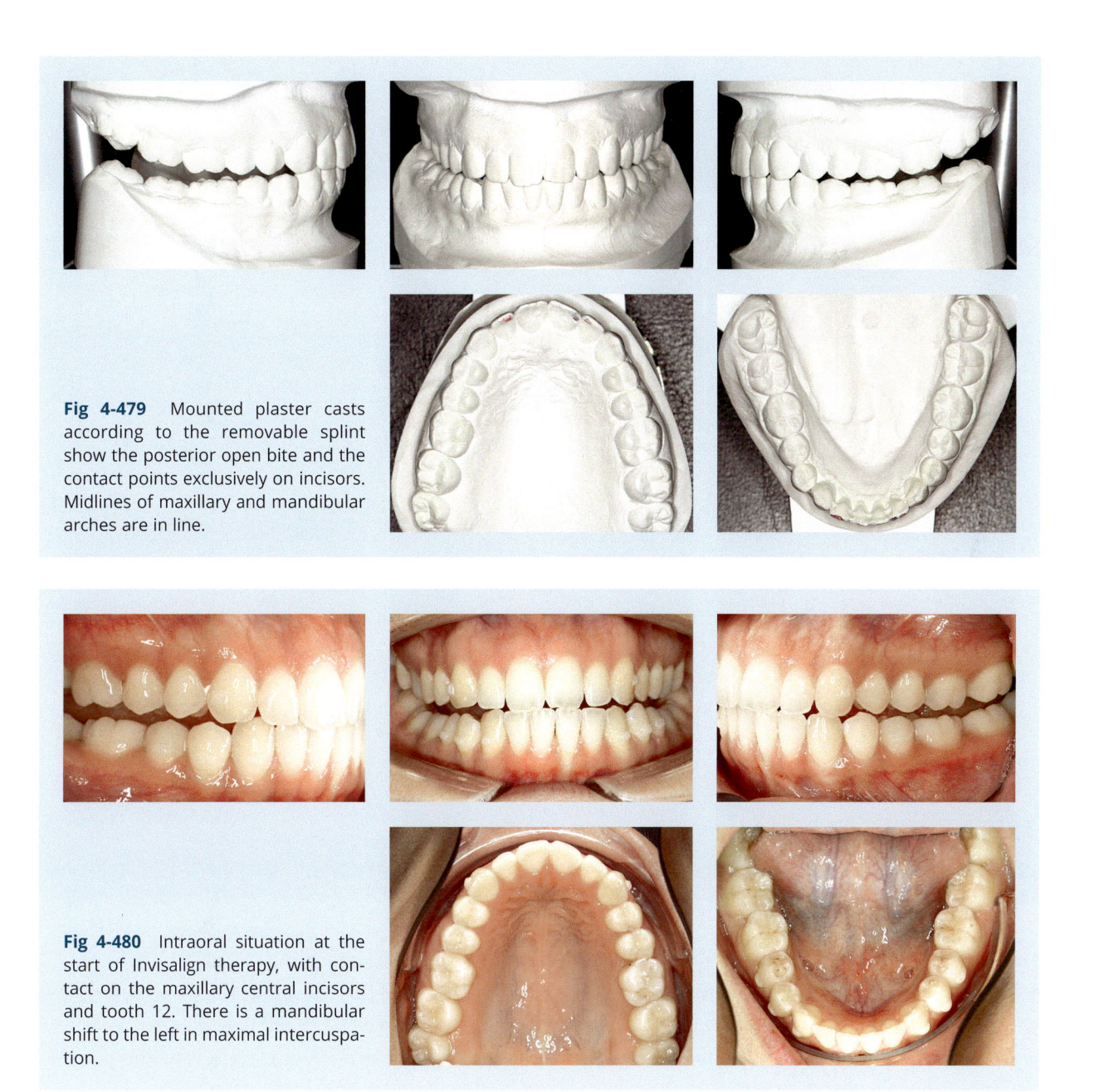

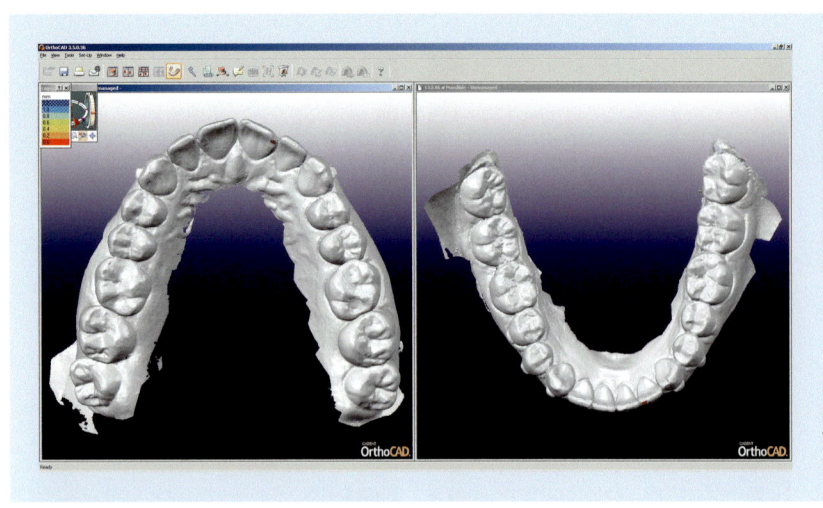

4 TREATMENT OF DIFFERENT MALOCCLUSIONS WITH ALIGNERS

Fig 4-481 Scan in centric relation demonstrates exclusive contact on tooth 21 (red) to tooth 32. Tooth 21 shows abrasion.

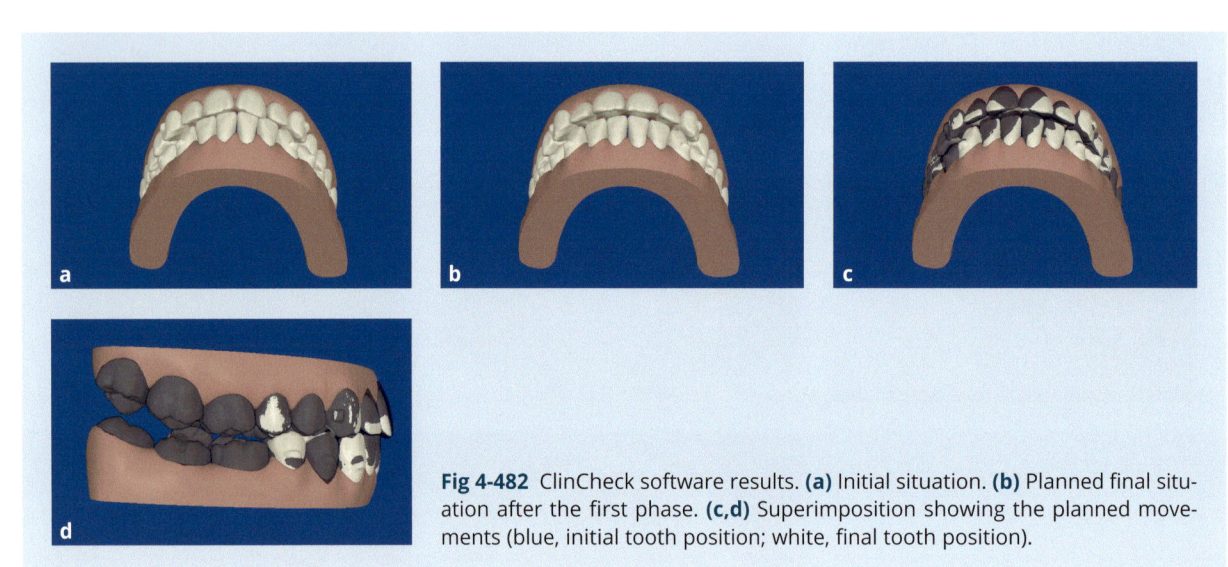

Fig 4-482 ClinCheck software results. **(a)** Initial situation. **(b)** Planned final situation after the first phase. **(c,d)** Superimposition showing the planned movements (blue, initial tooth position; white, final tooth position).

A scan in centric relation demonstrated exclusive contact on tooth 21 to tooth 32. Tooth 21 showed abrasion on the palatal enamel ridge facets, indicating that the patient was sliding from this habitual intercuspation to the left (Fig 4-481).

The first phase in the ClinCheck planning included the alignment and torque of maxillary incisors, as well as intrusion of the mandibular incisors (Fig 4-482). These movements, using 11 aligners, were intended to treat the unphysiologic and preliminary anterior contact. No posterior tooth movements were included in this first phase. A Speed Up was fabricated (Fig 4-483) to be worn in addition to the aligners for posterior support (see also Topic 16).

At the end of the first phase, torque and derotation of the maxillary incisors and intrusion of mandibular incisors had been achieved (Fig 4-484). The midlines were corrected and the mandible showed a physiologic orthopedic position. The malposition of the left condyle was successfully treated and the patient was still pain free. From this situation, scans were performed (Fig 4-485) to obtain the subsequent ClinCheck set-up (Fig 4-486) for starting the second phase of treatment.

For the second phase, vertical rectangular conventional attachments were bonded on all lower molars for anchorage during extrusion (Fig 4-487). At the end of this phase, the posterior side still showed some

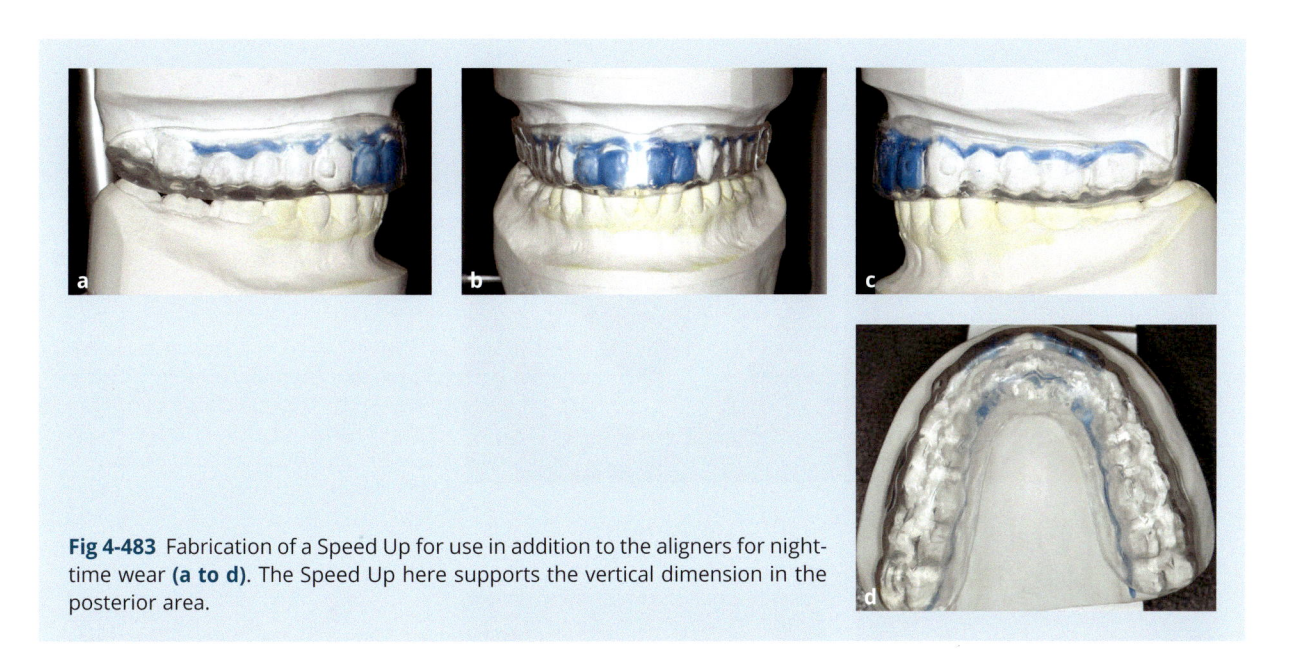

Fig 4-483 Fabrication of a Speed Up for use in addition to the aligners for nighttime wear **(a to d)**. The Speed Up here supports the vertical dimension in the posterior area.

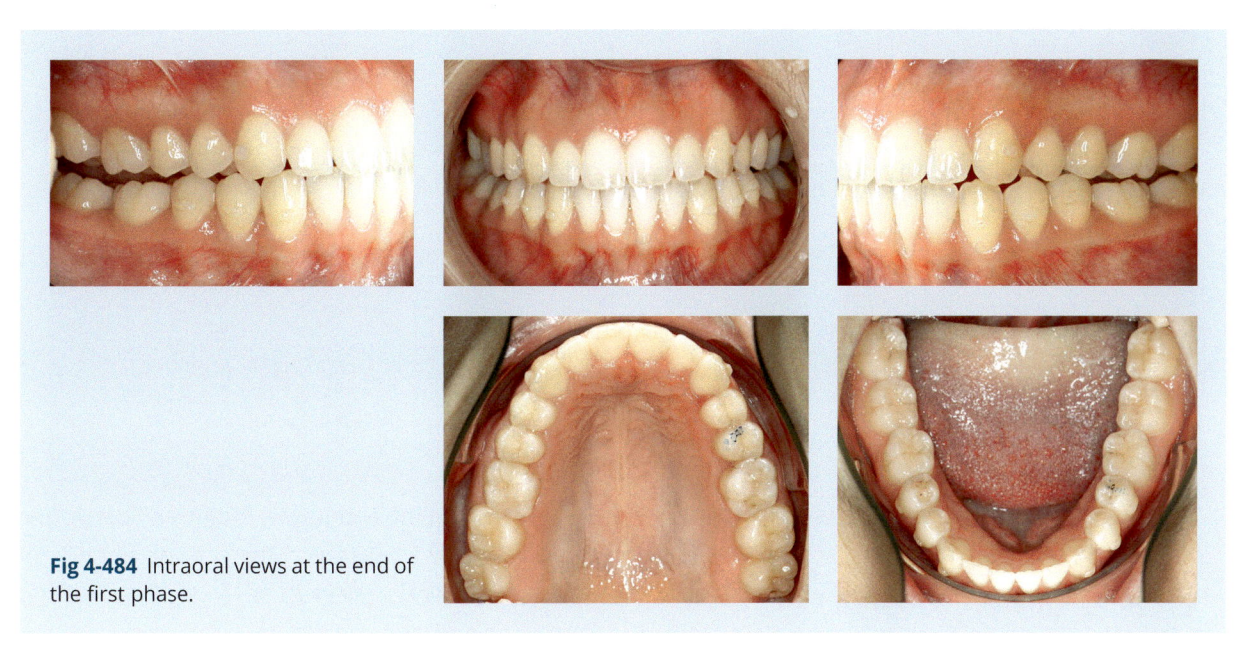

Fig 4-484 Intraoral views at the end of the first phase.

open bite and a further refinement with additional extrusion of teeth 35, 36, 37, 45, 46, 47, 48 was performed to obtain full contact. The patient was pain free but continued to wear the aligner full-time and the Speed Up during the night.

Teeth 16 and 17 were showing occlusal contacts only of the palatal cusps, the buccal aspect were still slightly missing contact after the refinement (Fig 4-488). Due to this slightly open posterior bite on the right side, buttons were bonded on teeth 16, 17, 46, 47 and the patient was advised to wear up and down elastics. The upper and lower last aligner was cut off distally of tooth 15 and 45 to allow extrusion. Retention was performed with a lingual retainer in the lower arch and a removable aligner in the upper arch.

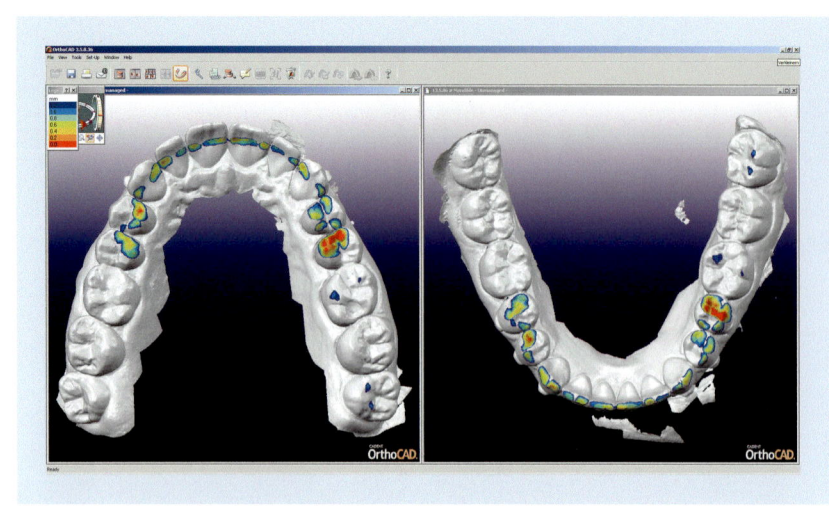

4 TREATMENT OF DIFFERENT MALOCCLUSIONS WITH ALIGNERS

Fig 4-485 Scan after the first phase showed bilateral support on maxillary and mandibular premolars, with decent equal contact points on the incisors.

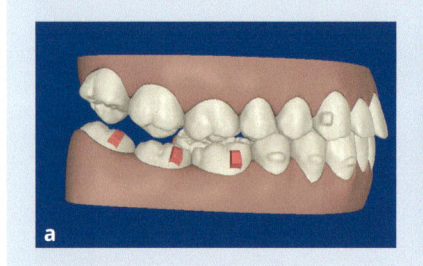

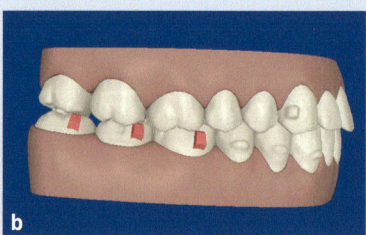

Fig 4-486 ClinCheck images for the second phase. **(a)** Right side with posterior open bite at start of second phase. **(b)** Final situation with extrusion of all molars into posterior contact and support. Attachments shown in red.

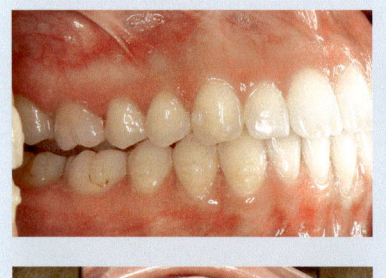

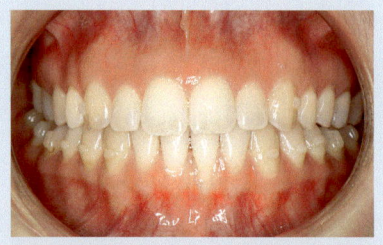

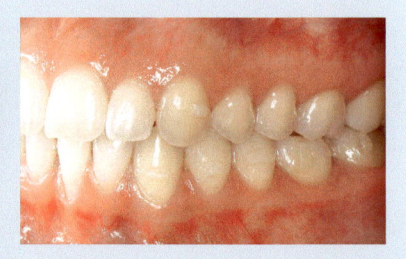

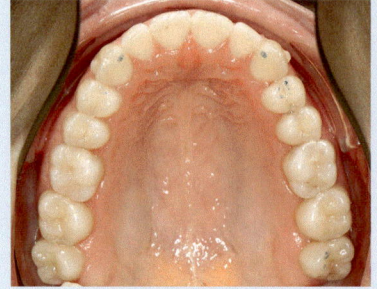

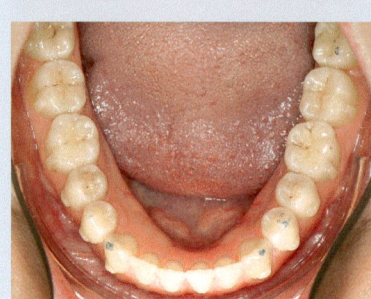

Fig 4-487 Intraoral view after the end of the second phase and before the final refinement.

300

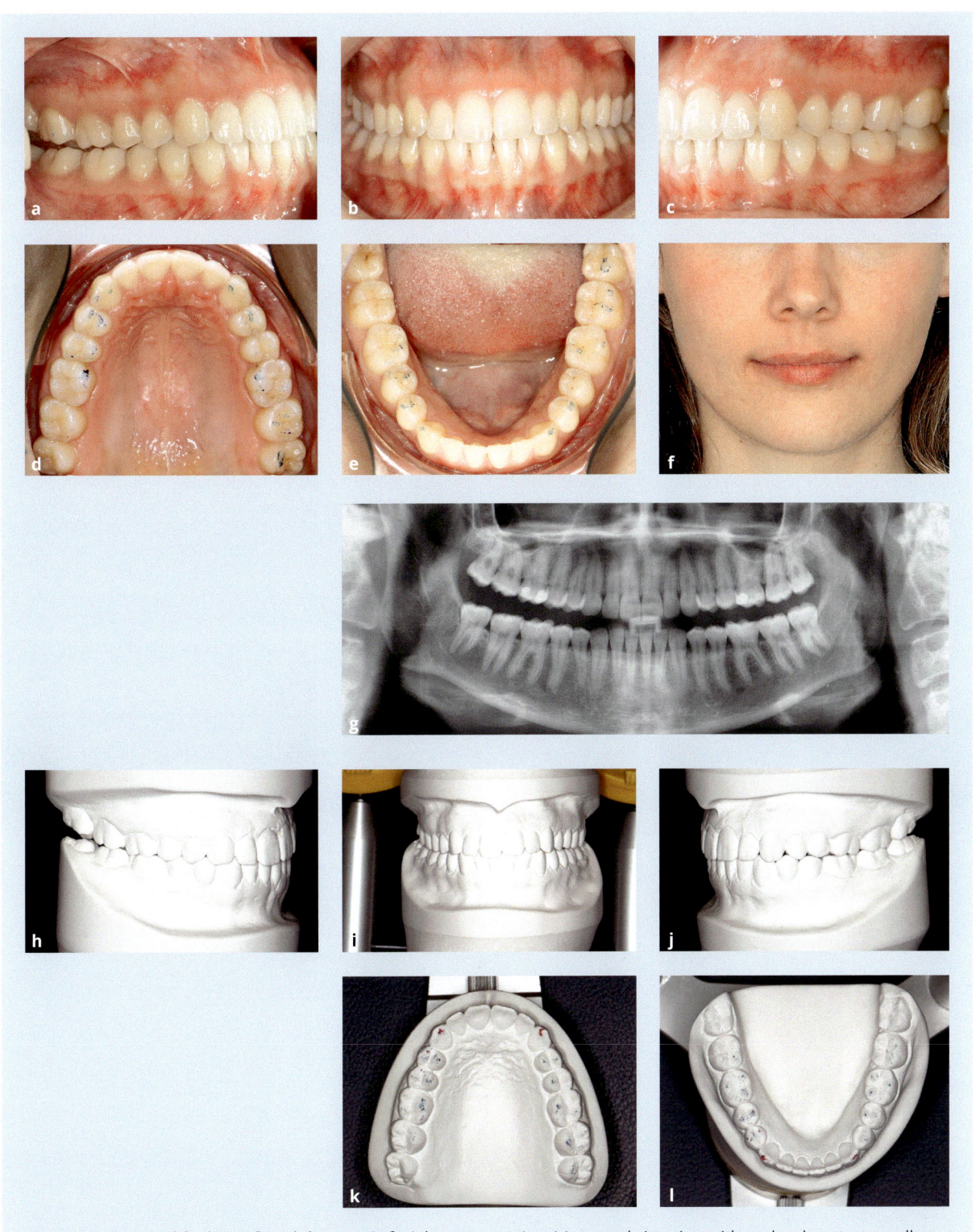

TREATMENT OF DIFFERENT MALOCCLUSIONS WITH ALIGNERS 4

Fig 4-488 Extraoral findings **(f)** with harmonic facial symmetry. **(a–e)** Intraoral situation with occlusal contact on all premolars and first molars, slightly posterior open bite of buccal aspect of teeth 16 and 17. **(g)** Final orthopantomography. **(h–l)** Plaster cast models in the articulator showing occlusal contacts in static (blue color) and dynamic occlusion (red color).

Topic 57
Craniomandibular disorder with centric contact only on first premolars

Treatment:
- orthodontic therapy with removable and fixed appliance
- Invisalign treatment

There are a number of questions that arise when incorporating aligner therapy into orthodontic practice. Is finishing and detailing possible with the Invisalign system or can it be performed better with a fixed appliance? Is it possible to plan and work out details in esthetics and in function with the Invisalign system? Fixed mechanics have side effects; does the Invisalign system also have these side effects?

This patient had a combined treatment as she was first treated elsewhere with a removable and then a fixed appliance before Invisalign treatment was started in our office.

Previous treatment

The patient started orthodontic treatment at 9 years of age with activator therapy (Fig 4-489). At this point she had:
- class II relationship
- anterior crowding with an increased overbite and overjet.

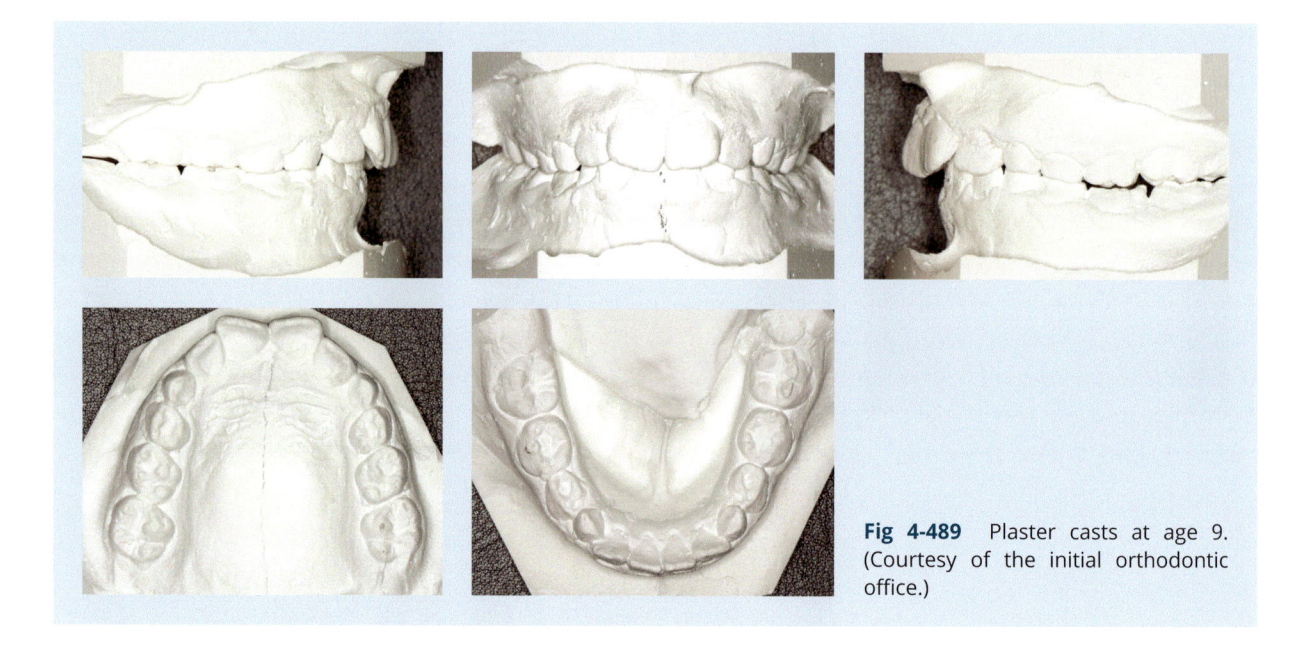

Fig 4-489 Plaster casts at age 9. (Courtesy of the initial orthodontic office.)

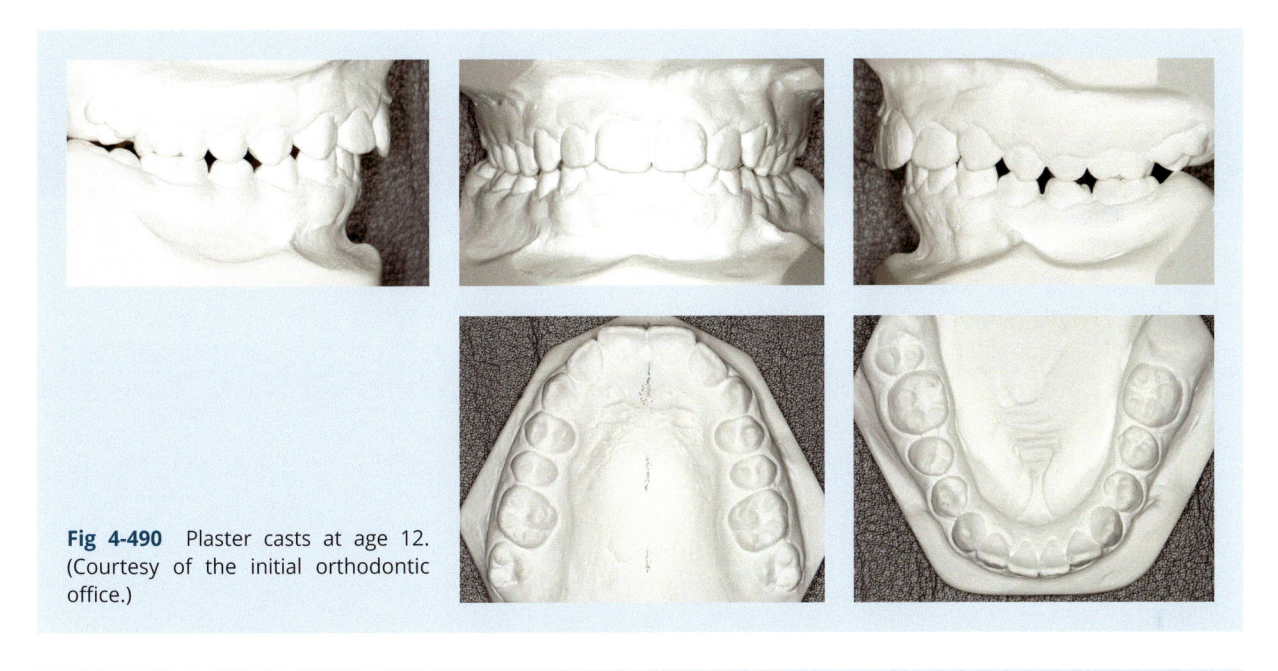

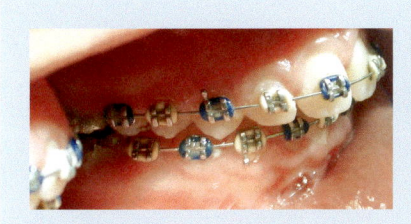

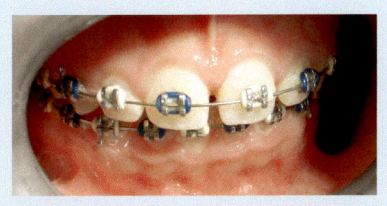

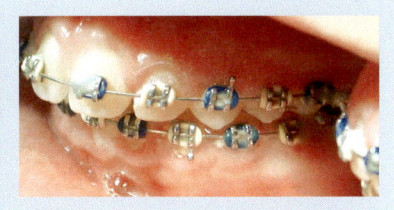

TREATMENT OF DIFFERENT MALOCCLUSIONS WITH ALIGNERS 4

Fig 4-490 Plaster casts at age 12. (Courtesy of the initial orthodontic office.)

Fig 4-491 Intraoral views a few weeks after starting treatment with the fixed appliance alio loco (photos taken by mother).

At age 12, she had a class II relationship with crowding and increased overbite and overjet (Fig 4-490). Treatment continued with fixed multibracket therapy (Fig 4-491). A gap opened between teeth 11 and 21. We prefer to avoid use of elastic ligatures (blue and yellow on the brackets in Fig 4-491) as we believe that ligating the archwire onto the bracket with an elastic ligature creates a good environment for bacterial growth, and hence increases the risk for decalcification or caries during treatment. We use only metal ligatures or self-ligating bracket systems (Damon System) in the few fixed appliance treatments.

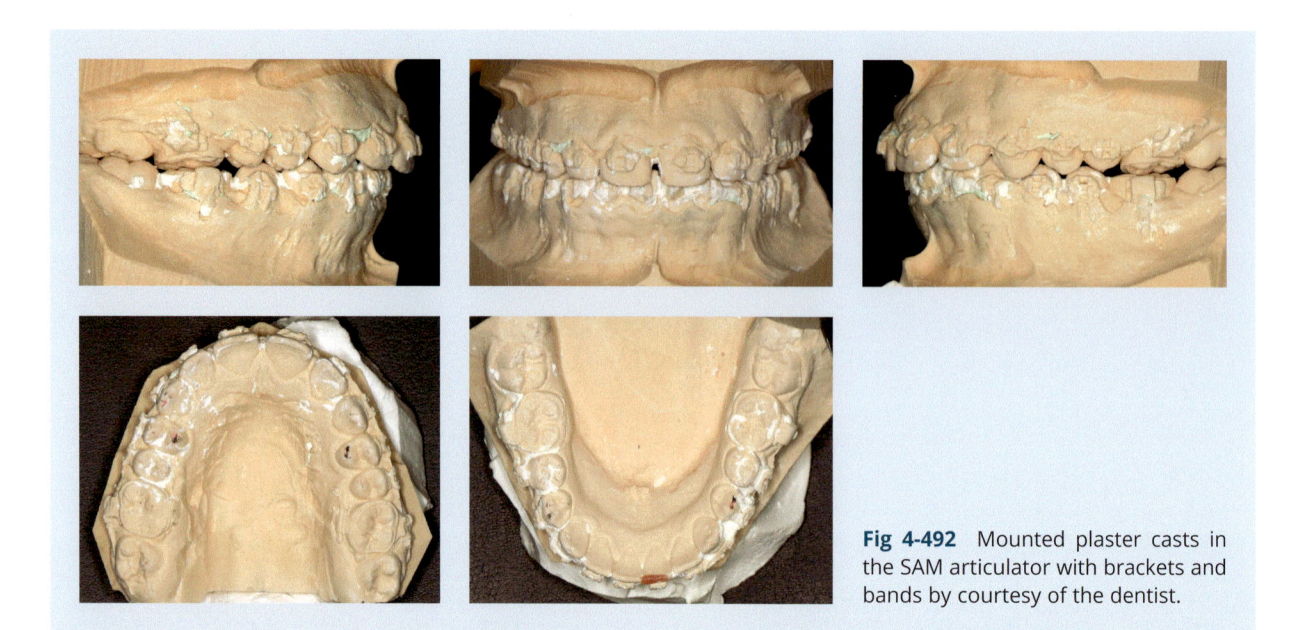

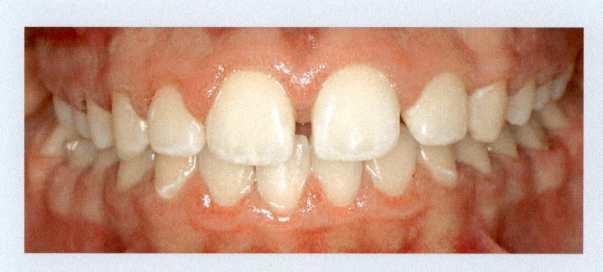

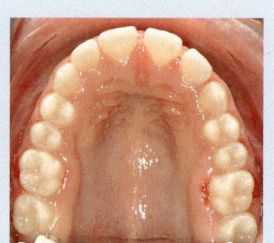

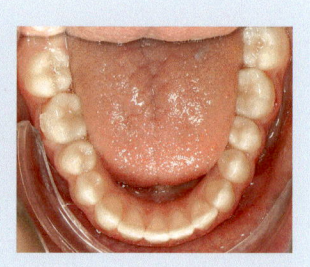

Fig 4-492 Mounted plaster casts in the SAM articulator with brackets and bands by courtesy of the dentist.

Fig 4-493 Intraoral findings after debonding at the patient's first appointment in our practice.

Invisalign treatment

After 2 years of fixed appliance treatment elsewhere, the young patient came to our office for the first time at the age of 13. After a detailed examination, it was decided to remove the fixed appliance immediately because of the large amount of decalcification and decay shown on several teeth. The examination showed

- TMJ dysfunction with a partially displaced disc and pain
- class I canine relation with increased overbite and overjet
- diastema
- severe caries lesions on the distobuccal aspect of tooth 27 after the removal of the band
- white spots and decalcification on eight teeth.

The mounted casts in centric relation demonstrate occlusal contact points on the first premolars only, with complete lack of posterior support (Fig 4-492). The intraoral views (Fig 4-493) showed:

- well-aligned mandibular arch with mild rotations
- spaces in the maxillary anterior region
- increased overjet and overbite
- lack of posterior support with reduced occlusal contacts on first premolars
- severe decay of tooth 27 distobuccal with the need for subsequent root filling
- white spots on eight teeth
- gingival hyperplasia and inflammation.

TREATMENT OF DIFFERENT MALOCCLUSIONS WITH ALIGNERS 4

Fig 4-494 The treatment plan. oc., overcorrection.

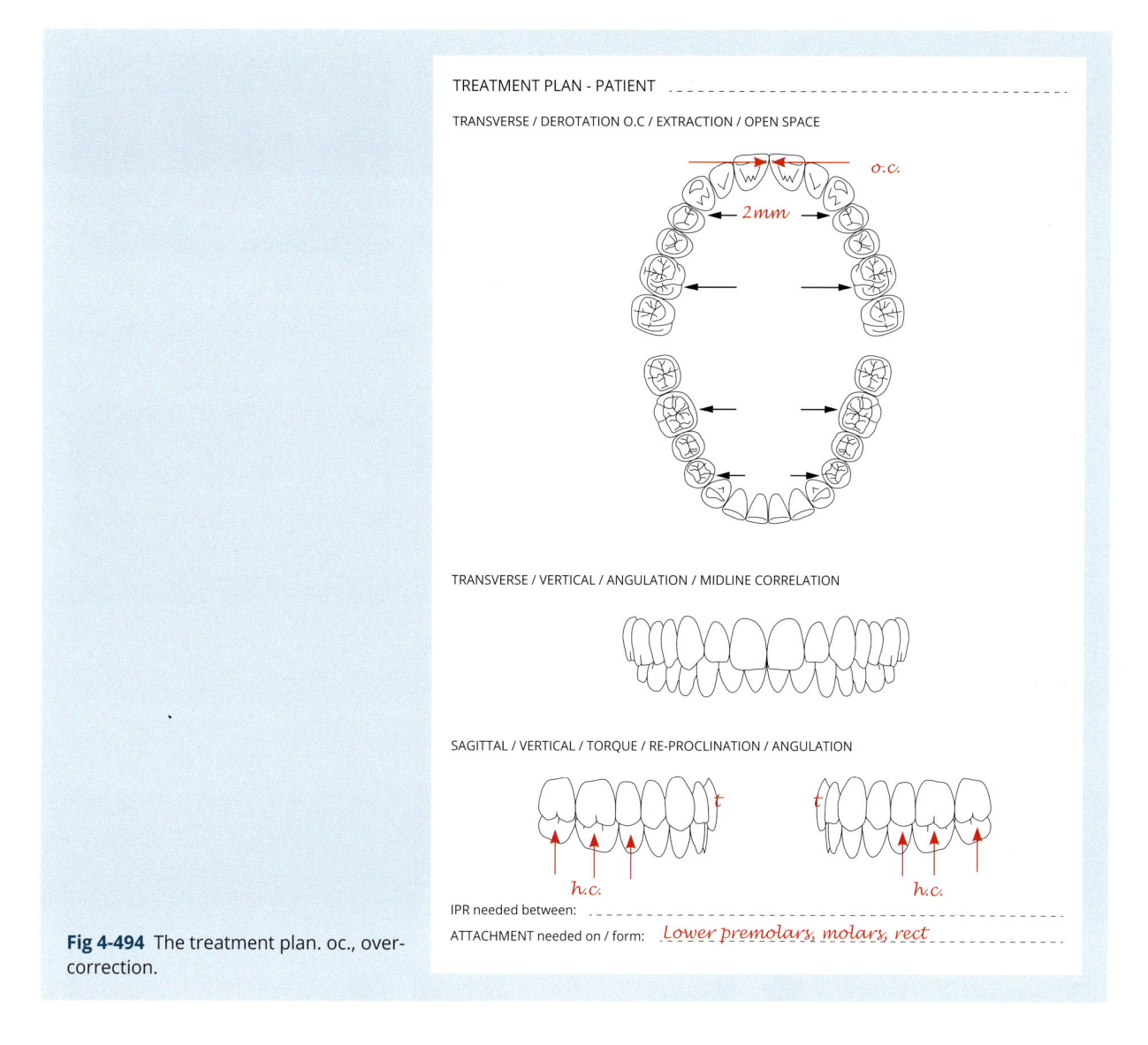

After removal of the fixed appliance and dental treatment of the caries lesions, it was planned to treat the patient with the Invisalign system.

The treatment plan (Fig 4-494) included:
- closure of diastema with power chain effect and overcorrection, keeping the roots together
- closure of the space in the maxillary incisor area with retraction and torque control (power ridge)
- leveling of the curve of Spee by extrusion of mandibular premolars and molars to close the lateral open bite with hard collision
- no extrusion in the maxillary arch
- expansion of maxillary premolar by a distance of 2 mm.

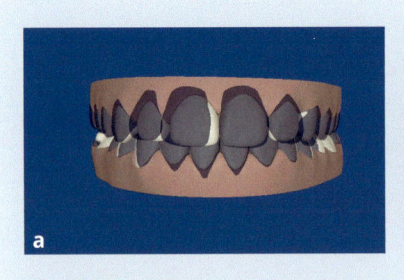

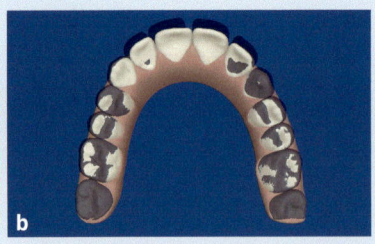

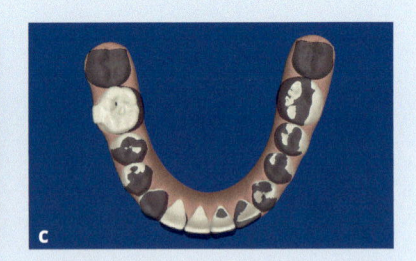

4 TREATMENT OF DIFFERENT MALOCCLUSIONS WITH ALIGNERS

Fig 4-495 ClinCheck software results. **(a)** Both arches. **(b,c)** Retraction in the maxillary and mandibular anterior region **(b)** and transversal expansion in both arches **(b,c)** (blue, initial tooth position; white, final tooth position).

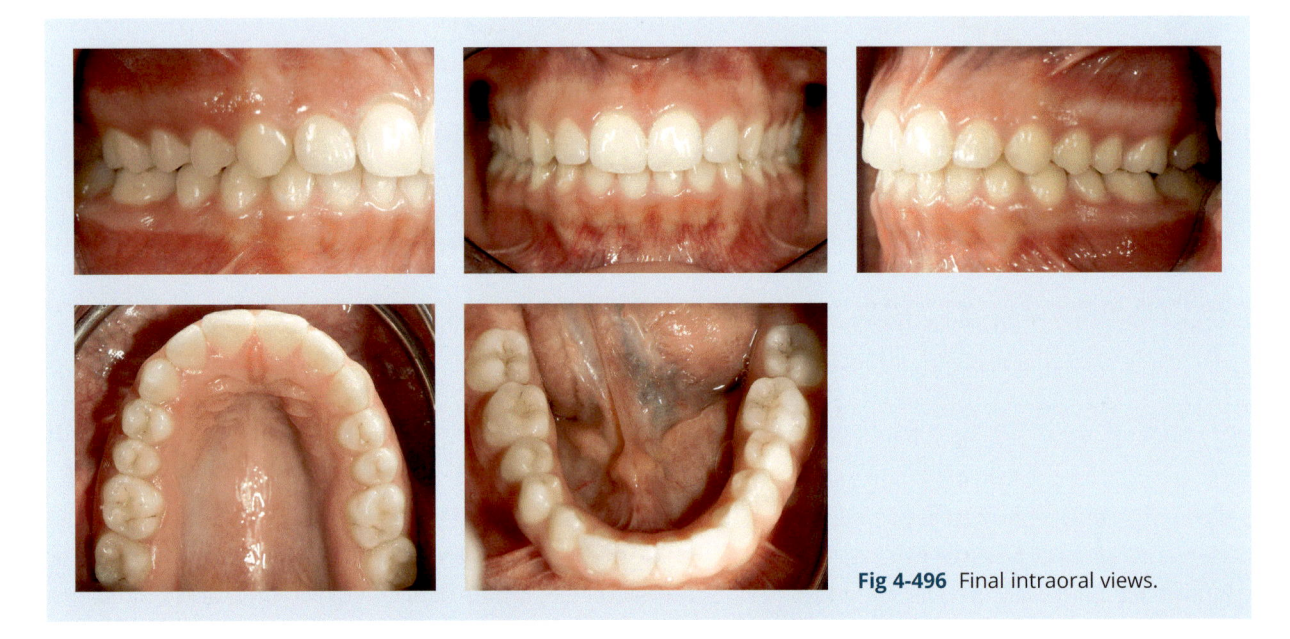

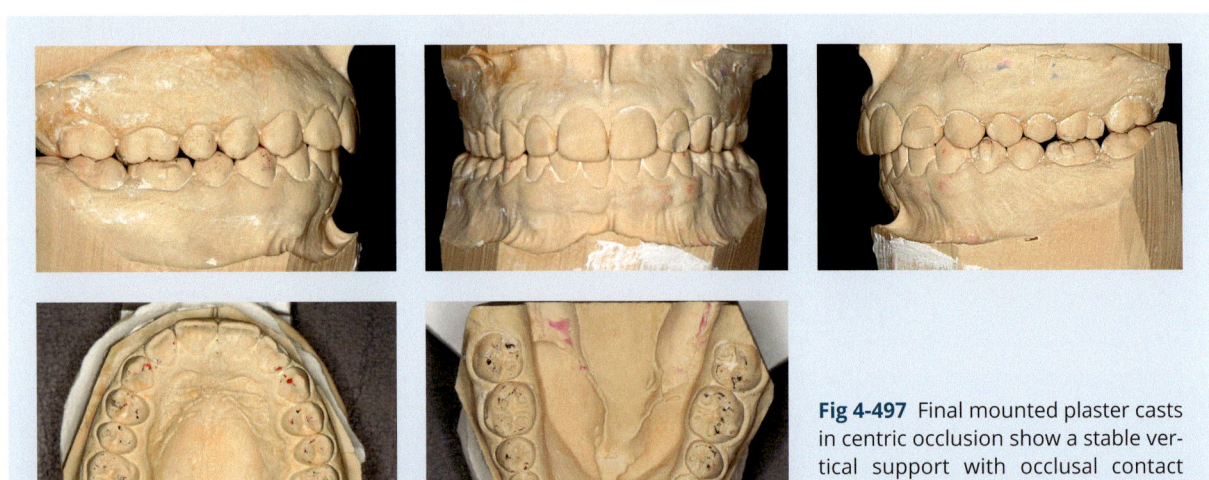

Fig 4-496 Final intraoral views.

Fig 4-497 Final mounted plaster casts in centric occlusion show a stable vertical support with occlusal contact points on all premolars and molars. The red color indicates the selective canine guidance (canines and first premolars).

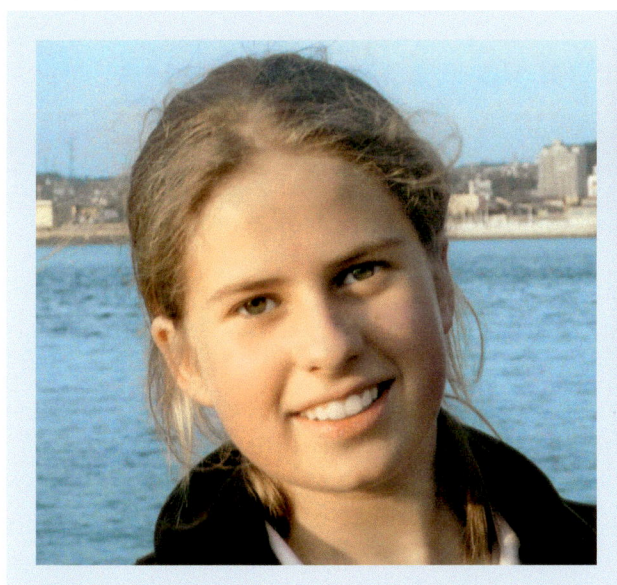

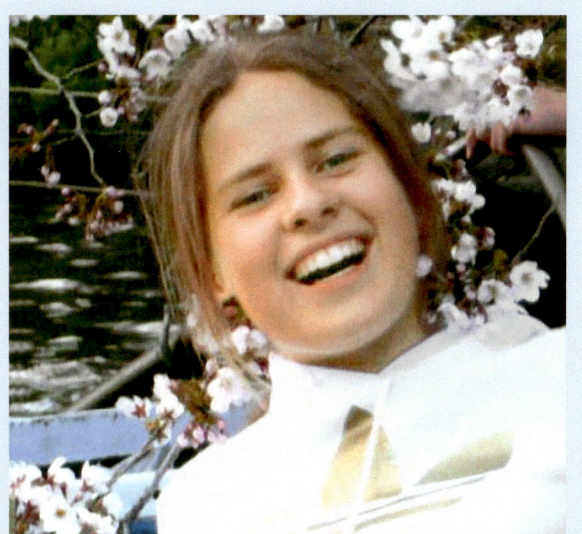

Fig 4-498 After completion of Invisalign treatment (mother's photographs).

The superimposition tool of the ClinCheck software showed the amount of planned movements in both arches with the closure of the diastema, retraction in the maxillary anterior region, and transversal expansion in both arches (Fig 4-495). Vertical rectangular attachments were added to all mandibular teeth that required extrusion.

The final intraoral views after the Invisalign treatment show stable occlusion with full occlusal contact and posterior vertical support (Figs 4-496 and 4-497). The patient was pain free and showed a physiological craniomandibular system. The incisors are just out of contact in full intercuspation (as shown with Shimstock foil) and, therefore, in a physiologic anterior relationship. The maxillary and mandibular arches are harmonically aligned with closure of all spaces. Pictures show a happy and pain-free girl with a beautiful smile (Fig 4-498).

The conclusion from the treatment pathway for this girl, which had included multibracket appliance and Invisalign treatment, is that the former had side effects of decay and decalcification but the latter appeared to be free of side effects.

Topic 58
Craniomandibular disorder with anterior disc displacement

Treatment:
- Invisalign treatment
- finishing with palatal tooth reshaping

It is taught that orthodontic treatment should finish without incisor contact in habitual intercuspation as even small disturbances in the incisor region during static occlusion can lead to neuromuscular disorders and malfunctions of the mandible.

This patient showed a class II relationship on the left side with a midline shift and a full class I on the right side (Fig 4-499). The maxillary midline was correct while the mandibular midline was deviated to the left because of missing tooth 36. Tooth 37 was in its position and so was in crossbite. The arches were well aligned, the maxillary arch showed small lateral incisors. As the class II area was in a stable one tooth to two teeth position and so did not need correction from an occlusal standpoint, was treatment required? Mounted plaster casts showed the actual problem (Fig 4-500): the incisor contact due to reclined teeth 11 and 21 and the extruded position of the mandibular incisors. Maxillary and mandibular incisors demonstrated a high amount of enamel abrasion, which suggested a mandibular centric position.

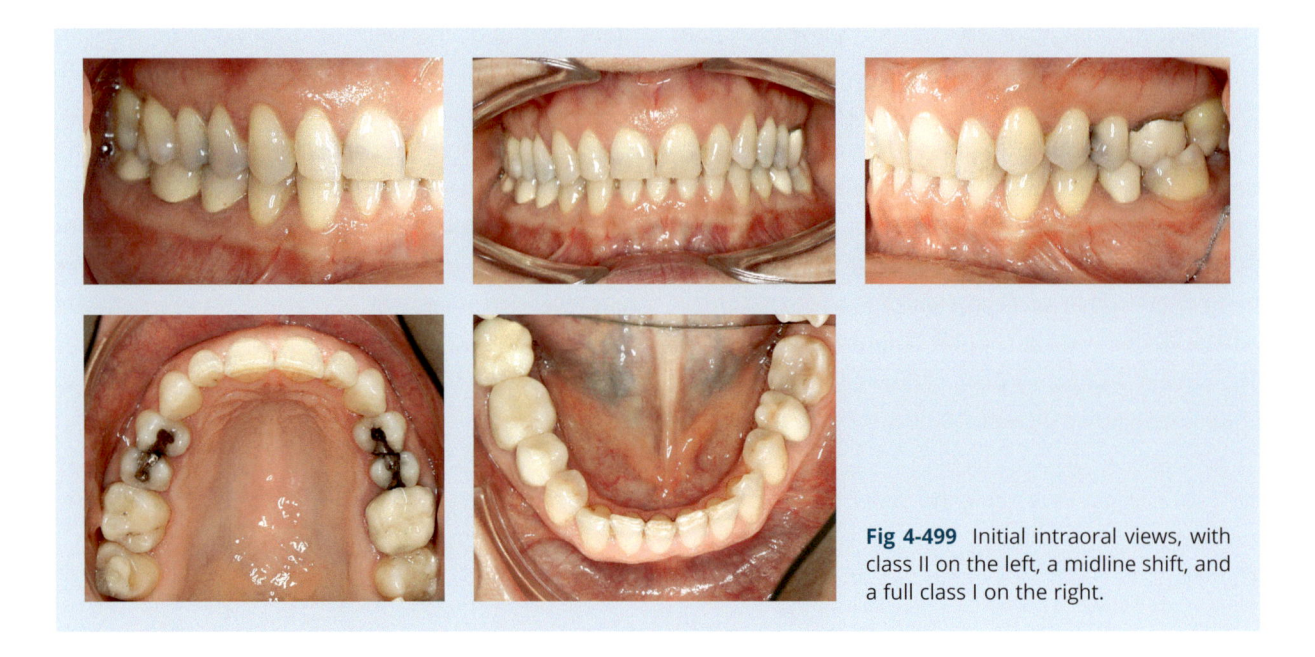

Fig 4-499 Initial intraoral views, with class II on the left, a midline shift, and a full class I on the right.

Diagnosis:
- incisor contact because of reclined teeth 11 and 21
- extruded mandibular incisors
- mandibular midline deviated to the left
- cross bite of tooth 37.

Therapy:
- Invisalign treatment
- finishing with palatal tooth reshaping.

Fig 4-500 Mounted plaster casts show incisor contact and enamel abrasion on maxillary and mandibular incisors.

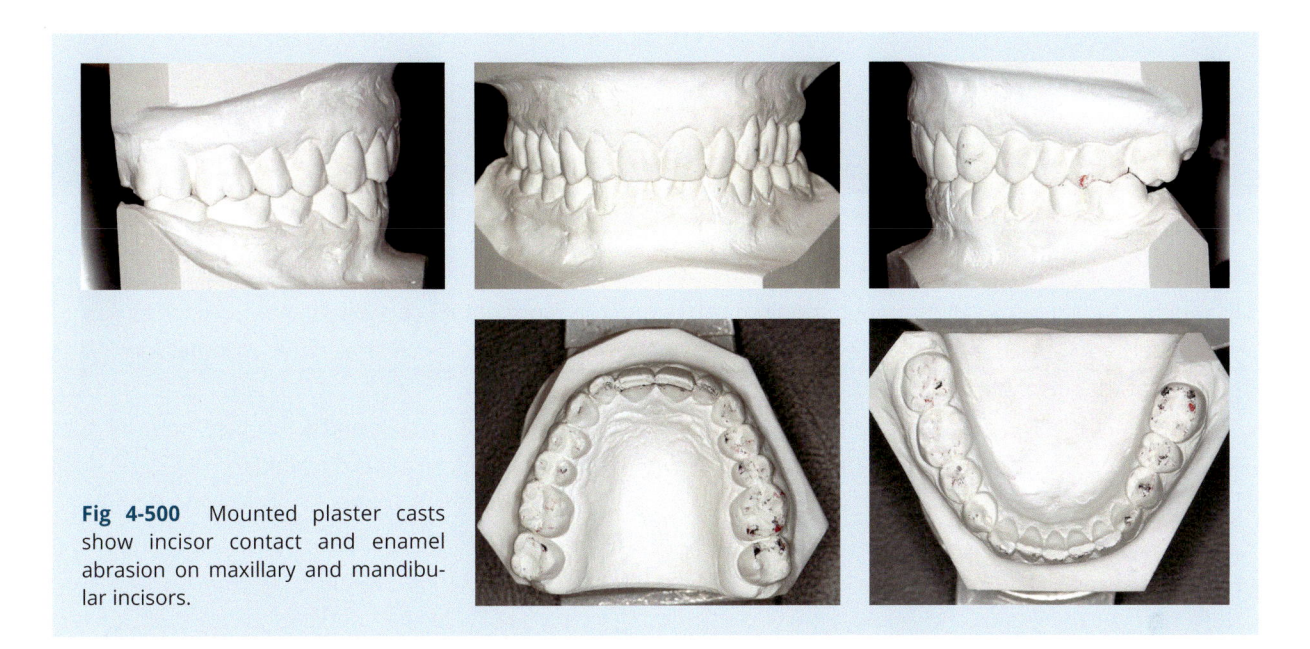

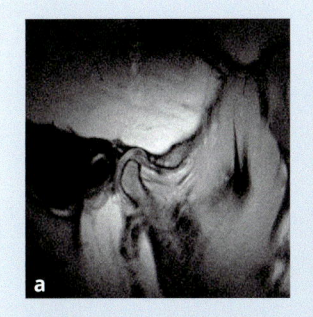

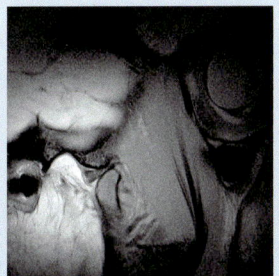

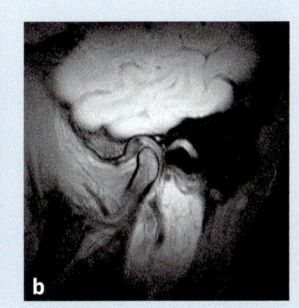

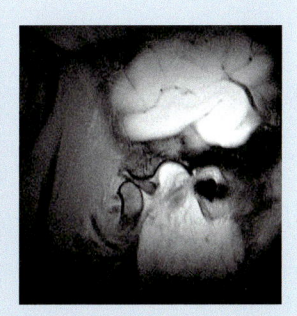

Fig 4-501 MRT. **(a)** Right TMJ showing anterior disc position in habitual intercuspation with repositioning of the disc during opening. **(b)** Left TMJ, showing anterior disc position in habitual intercuspation with repositioning of the disc. (Dr M Andersson, Dr T Steimel, MediaPark Clinic Cologne.)

Treatment

MRT was used to assess the TMJs (Fig 4-501). The movement of the discus articularis position when changing from habitual intercuspation to mouth opening has led to alterations in disc shape, which makes its recapture to its correct position difficult or impossible without surgery.

Fig 4-502 The treatment plan. t, torque.

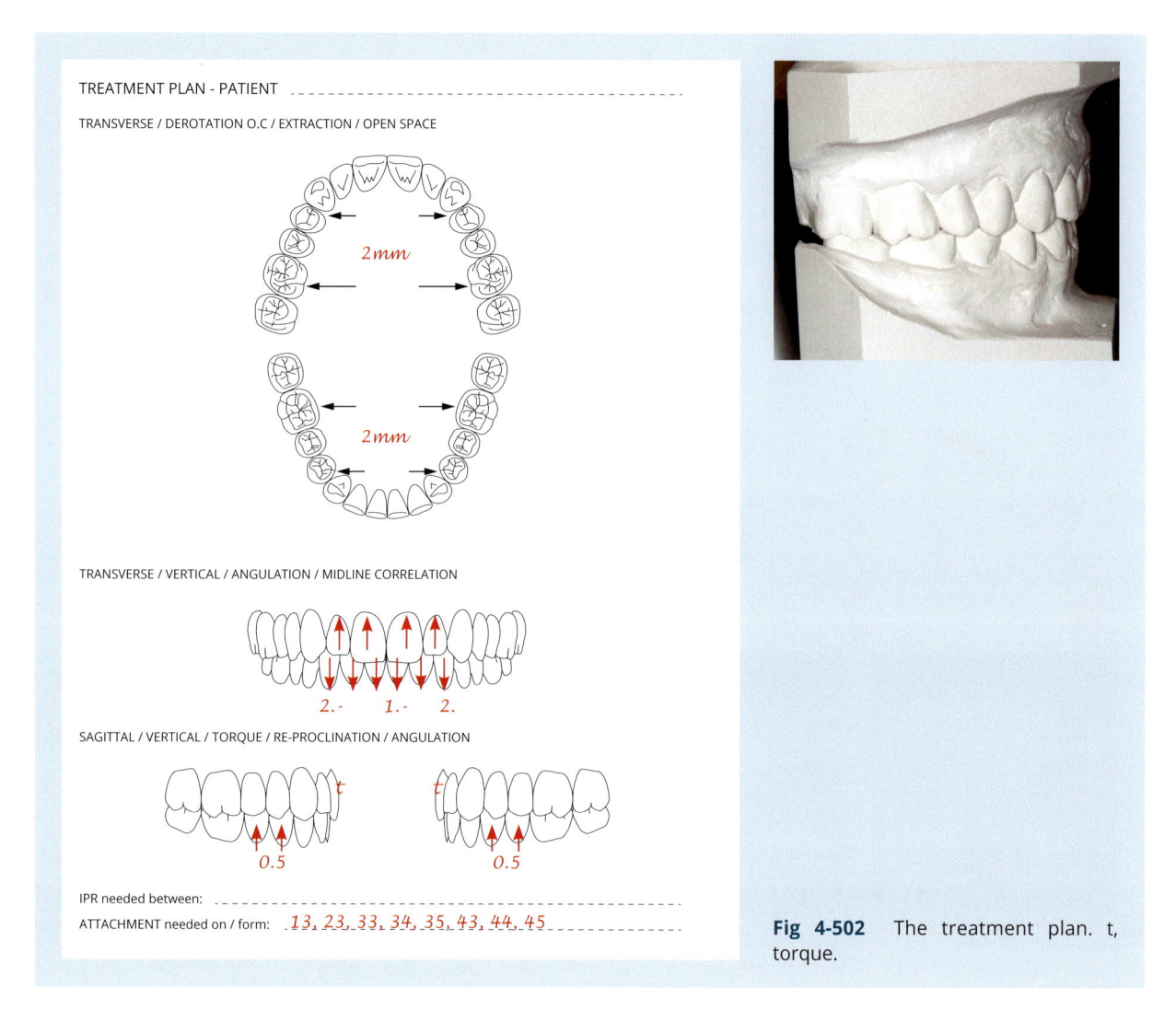

The treatment plan (Fig 4-502) included:
- expansion of the maxillary and mandibular arches of 2 mm
- torque of the maxillary central incisors with power ridges
- intrusion of maxillary incisors
- intrusion of mandibular incisors
- extrusion of mandibular premolars 0.5 mm
- end with an overbite of 1.5 mm
- end with an overjet of 0.3 mm.

Attachments would be needed on teeth 13 and 23 for anchorage during torque of the maxillary incisors as well as on teeth 33, 34, 35, 43, 44, and 45 for intrusion and extrusion. This was transferred into the ClinCheck software (Fig 4-503). This phase would require 24 aligners in the maxillary arch (Fig 4-504) and 17 in the mandibular arch.

The fitting of the power ridges on teeth 11 and 21 is excellent and the incisal edges are covered by the aligner without any gaps.

According to our experience power ridges obtain higher efficiency with attachments on the neighboring teeth, which allows increased anchorage to apply the torque movement.

The final intraoral views showed full vertical support of premolars and molars at the end of the Invisalign therapy. The incisor area is open, as indicated with Shimstock foil, except for contact on the distal aspect of tooth 21 (Fig 4-505). This occlusal pattern

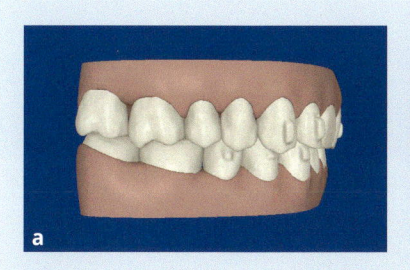

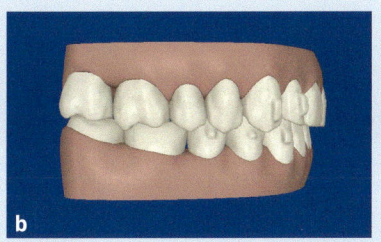

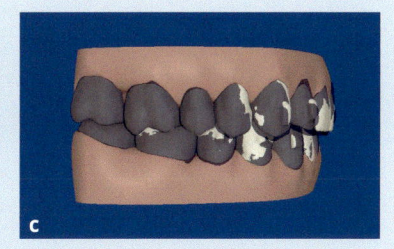

Fig 4-503 ClinCheck software results for right side. **(a)** Initial situation. **(b)** Planned final result. **(c)** Superimposition showing the planned torque of maxillary central incisors (blue, initial tooth position; white, final tooth position).

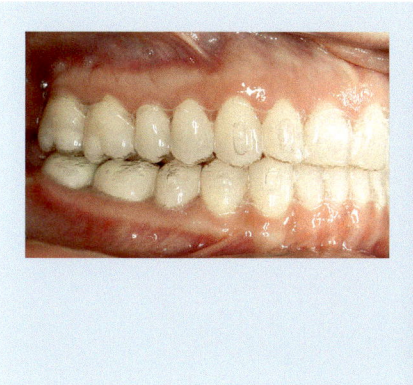

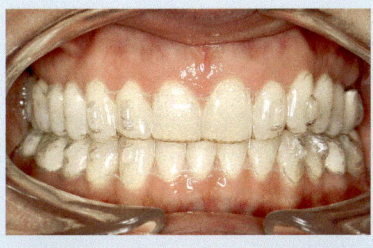

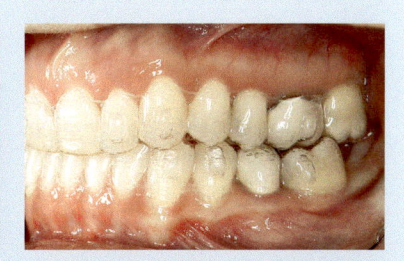

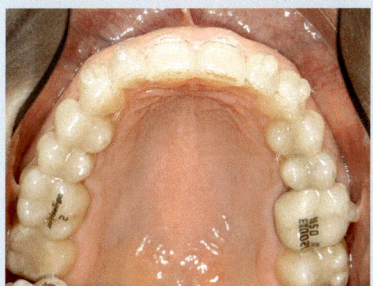

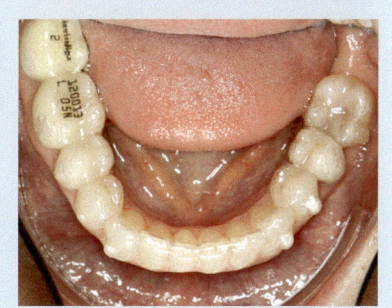

Fig 4-504 Intraoral views with aligner 24 in place.

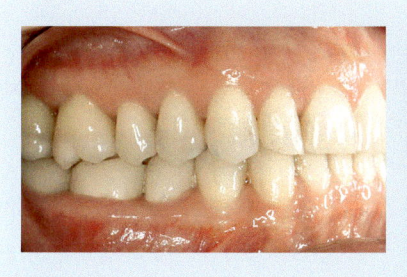

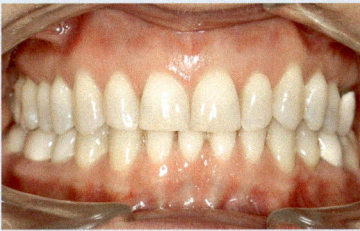

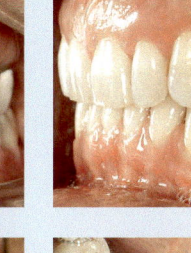

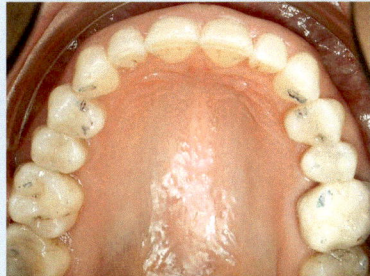

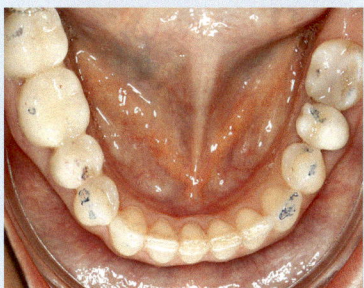

Fig 4-505 Final intraoral views with occlusal contact points shown in blue.

4 TREATMENT OF DIFFERENT MALOCCLUSIONS WITH ALIGNERS

Fig 4-506 Final mounted plaster casts showing occlusal contact points on molars and premolars (black) and canine guidance (red). Restoratives were planned on all teeth marked with "c."

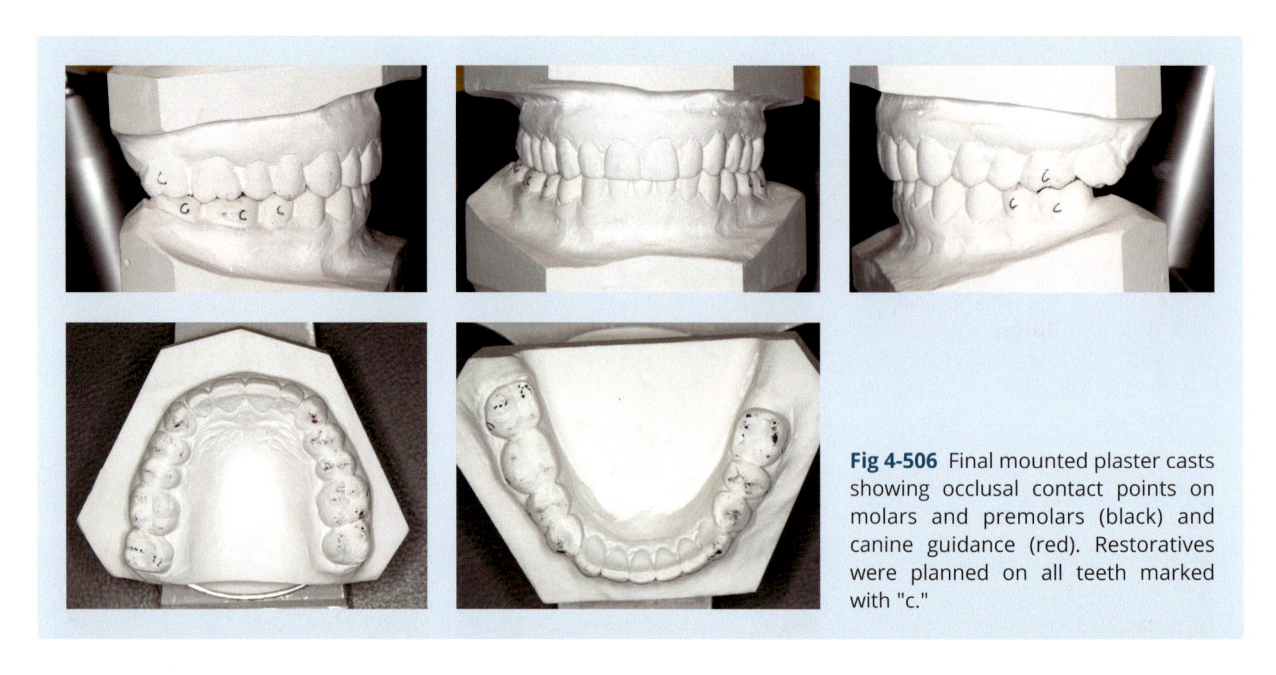

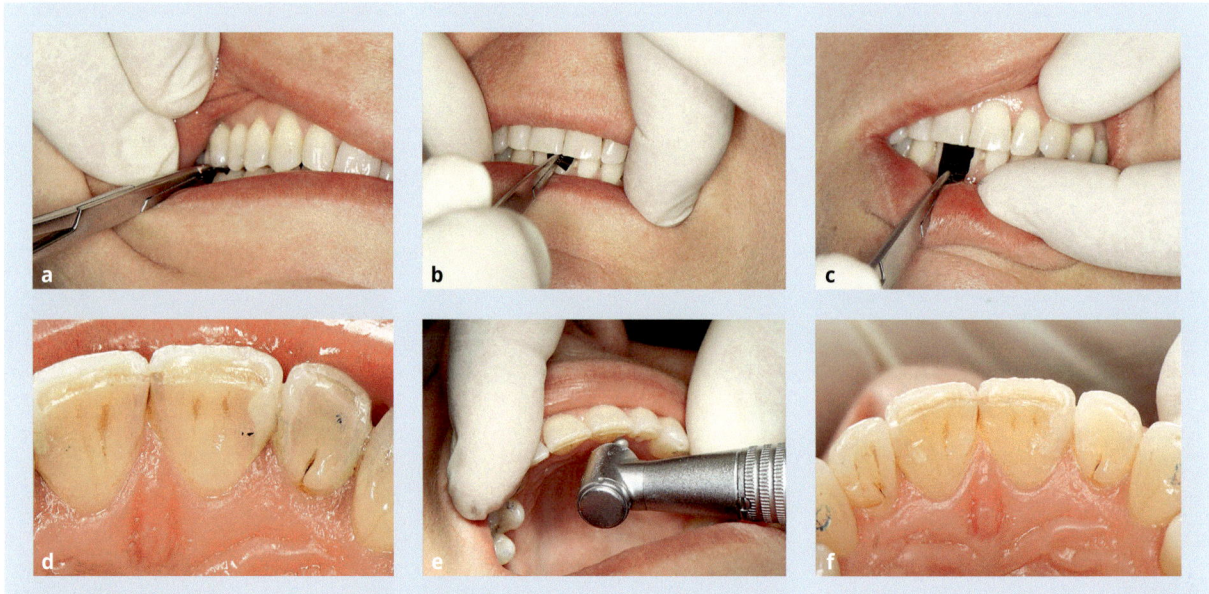

Fig 4-507 Final finishing of occlusion. **(a–c)** Occlusal testing with the Shimstock foil. The molars and premolars should hold the foil **(a)**, while the incisor area should be "Shimstock open," meaning that the foil can be pulled through the incisors in habitual occlusion in the upright sitting patient **(b,c)**. **(d)** Small occlusal contact on teeth 21 and 22. **(e)** Enamel reshaping to eliminate this contact. **(f)** Final view after reshaping.

was confirmed with mounted plaster casts (Fig 4-506).

Testing with Shimstock foil (8 µm) for occlusion enables finishing and reshaping to deal with minor issues still present (Fig 4-507).

The patient was transferred to the dental office for restoratives.

Topic 59
Digital workflow in interdisciplinary dentistry

Treatment:
- Invisalign treatment
- restorative dentistry

This topic describes in detail the digital workflow using the Invisalign system combined with the "Zirkonzahn" system, when dental restoratives are made of zirconium. As the digitial dentistry is becoming more and more important nowadays, the use of mounted plaster casts in a articulator will certainly be reduced in the future, working more with digital model findings.

From a scientific point of view, occlusal or chewing dysfunctions alone do not lead to increased sustained muscular activity over a long period. The most decisive initiating or reinforcing factor for TMJ disorders is emotional stress, which leads to an increase of oral muscle function through clenching and bruxism. While these might be ways of decreasing psychological stress, they do increase muscular activity and the load on the TMJs. According to Meyer and Asselmeyer (2005), it is not the occlusal dysfunction, but the "hyperactive, tender on palpation chewing muscles, facial and head musculature which are a significant correlate for the neuromuscular incoordination and accordingly a sign of the craniomandibular disorder."

Bruxism can lead to muscular hypertonus with painful trigger points in the muscle. These can be treated with injections of local anesthetic, manual therapy (Gautschi, 2010), or myoreflex therapy (Mosetter, 2006).

This patient has significant enamel abrasions from bruxism as well as poor smile esthetics (Figs 4-508 and 4-509). There is slight vertical bone loss in the region distal of tooth 36 because of the profound filling margin (Fig 4-510). Insufficient fillings and caries can be observed on teeth 16, 26, 25, 35, 36, and 46.

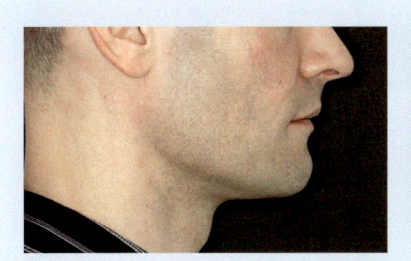

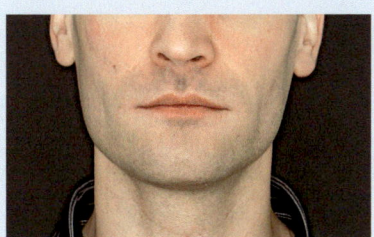

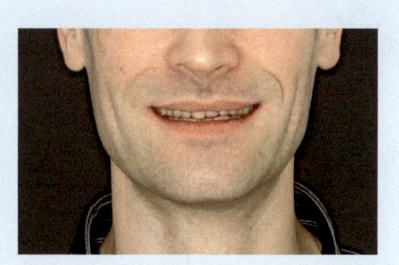

Fig 4-508 Initial presentation showing lip position and smile.

Diagnosis:
- bruxism
- trigger points, neck pain, back pain
- attrition
- buccal non-occlusion of teeth 18 to 48 and 28 to 38
- anterior edge-to-edge position.

Therapy:
- provisional fillings for decayed teeth
- criss-cross elastics 18/48 and 28/38
- Invisalign therapy
- restorative dentistry.

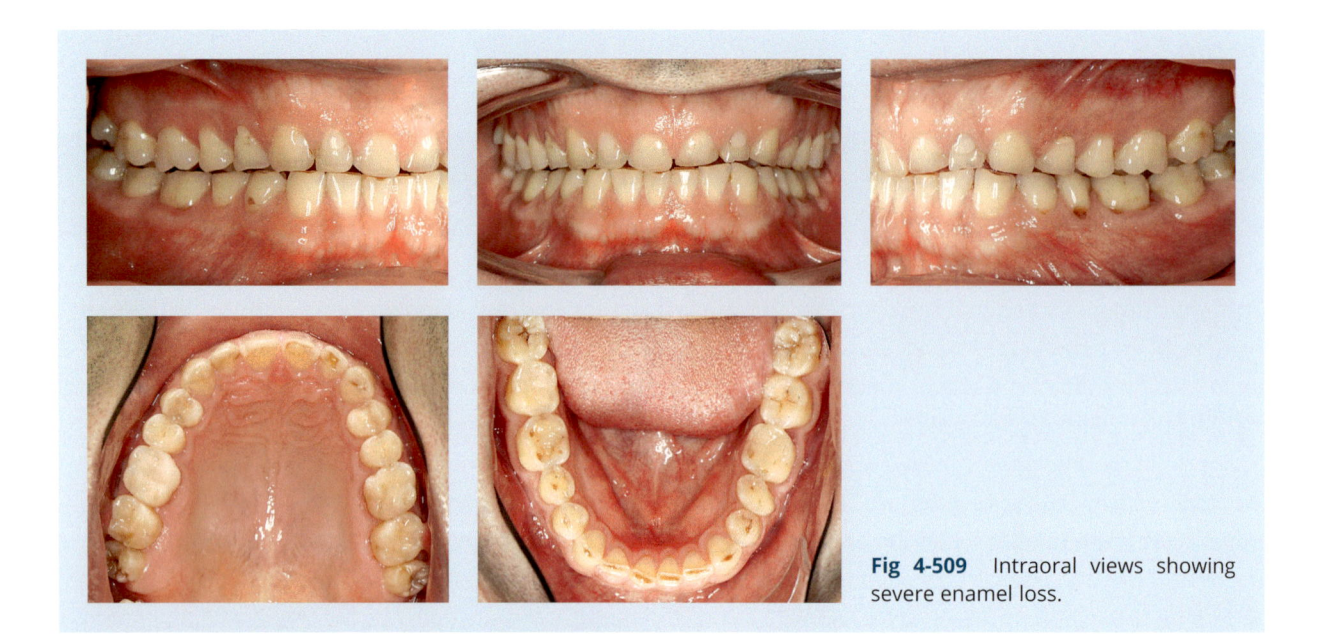

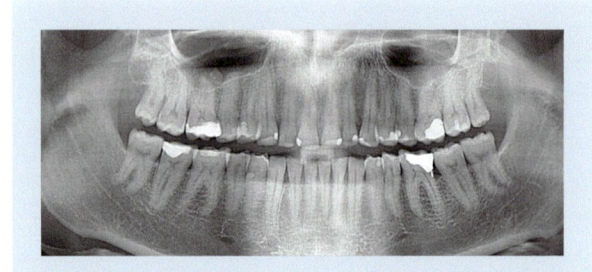

4 TREATMENT OF DIFFERENT MALOCCLUSIONS WITH ALIGNERS

Fig 4-509 Intraoral views showing severe enamel loss.

Fig 4-510 Initial orthopantomography showing slight vertical bone loss and caries lesions.

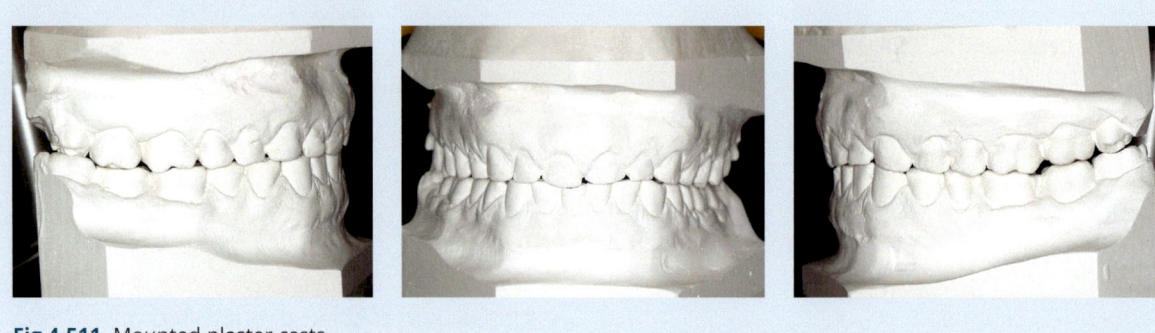

Fig 4-511 Mounted plaster casts.

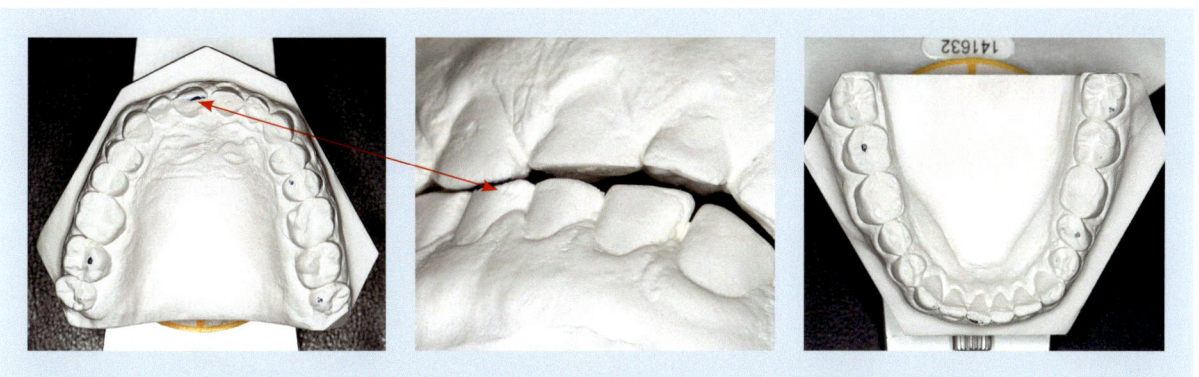

TREATMENT OF DIFFERENT MALOCCLUSIONS WITH ALIGNERS 4

Fig 4-512 Upper and lower casts showed in centric relationship with contact points on 17/47 and 11/41.

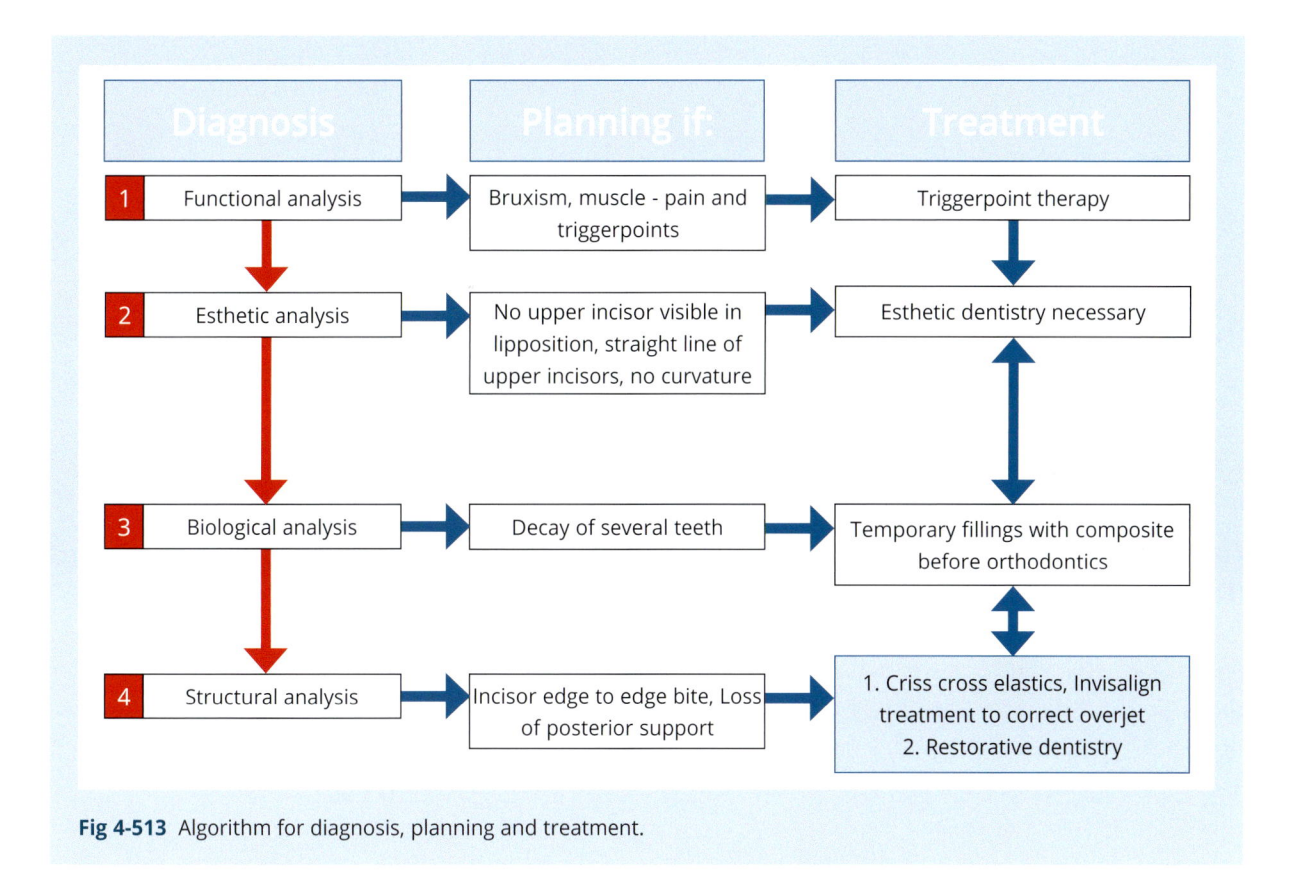

Fig 4-513 Algorithm for diagnosis, planning and treatment.

Preliminary treatment

Prior to orthodontic treatment, the osseous defect distal to tooth 36 was treated and caries lesions were treated with provisional fillings (Dr W Boisserée, Cologne). Mounted plaster models confirmed a slight class II relationship with an anterior edge-to-edge relationship. Teeth 18 and 28 showed buccal non-occlusion (Fig 4-511). The upper and lower casts showed exclusive contact points on the antagonists 17/47 and 11/41 in centric relationship. The latter led to the retrally forced guidance of the mandible (Fig 4-512).

Orthodontic treatment

Therapy was started with functional analysis (Fig 4-513).

The patient was advised to undergo manual triggerpoint therapy. The first appointment included an

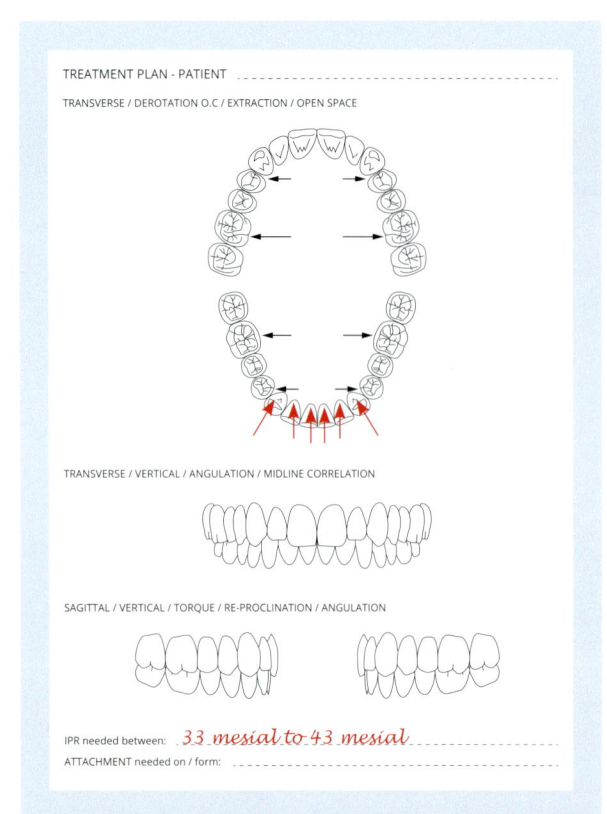

Fig 4-514 Treatment plan for phase 1 with arrows showing the retraction of the lower incisors and canines.

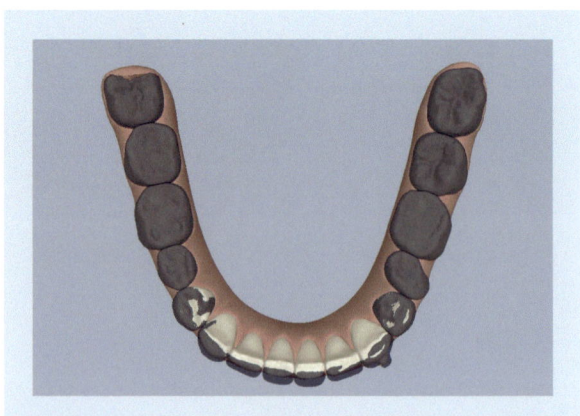

Fig 4-515 ClinCheck software for first phase movements (blue, initial tooth position; white, final tooth position).

esthetic analysis, radiographic examination, and mounting of the plaster casts. The radiographic examination showed the need for filling of the caries lesions, while the structural analysis showed the need for orthodontic therapy followed by restorative therapy.

The treatment plan (Fig 4-514) set the sequence for the first phase of treatment:
- criss-cross elastics and bonded buttons buccal on teeth 18, 28 and lingual on teeth 38, 48 to solve the buccal non-occlusion of all wisdom teeth
- Invisalign phase 1 to obtain a sufficient overjet to allow the setting of the mandible in centric relation and retraction of the lower incisors and canines.

ClinCheck software shows the first phase movements of the lower canines and incisors to create more overjet (Fig 4-515).

The treatment plan (Fig 4-516) set the sequence for the second phase of treatment after the centric position was defined:
- torque of upper incisors
- derotation of 13 and 23
- retraction of lower incisors and canines with IPR to create more overjet for the restoratives (interdisciplinary approach with Dr W Boisserée and M Läkamp).

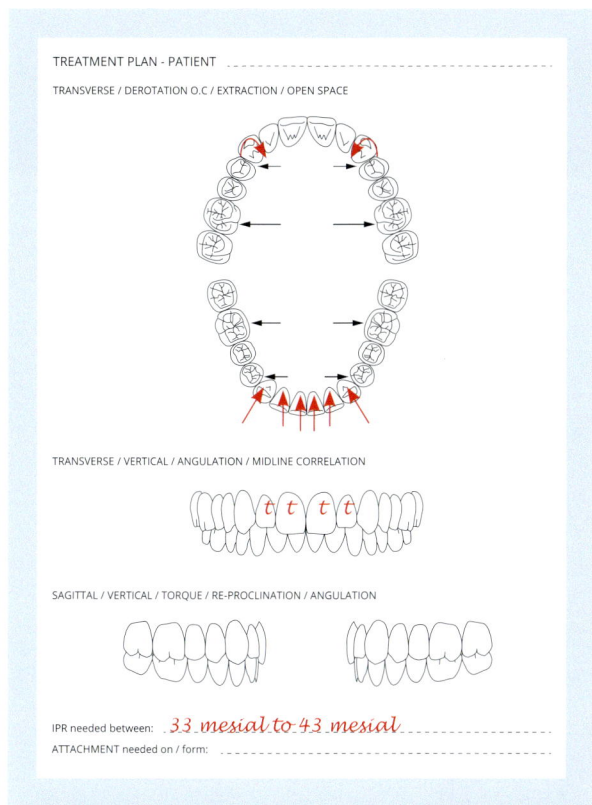

Fig 4-516 Treatment plan for phase 2 with red arrows showing the planned tooth movements. t, torque.

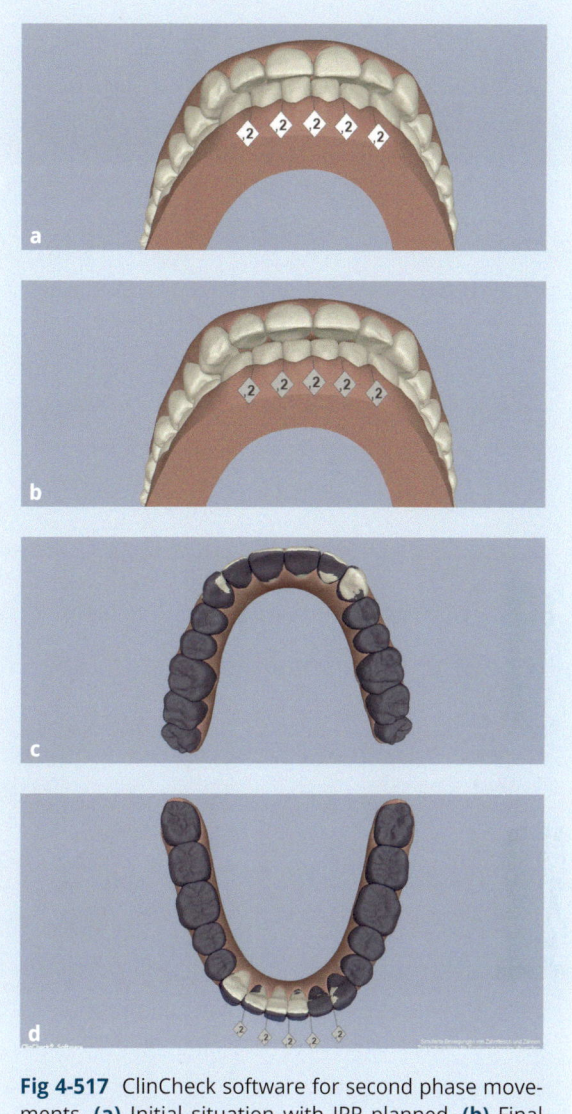

IPR needed between: 33 mesial to 43 mesial

Fig 4-517 ClinCheck software for second phase movements. **(a)** Initial situation with IPR planned. **(b)** Final planned result. **(c,d)** Superimposition compares end of phase 1 and the planned outcome after the second phase in maxilla **(c)** and mandible **(d)** (blue, initial tooth position; white, final tooth position).

After the first phase of treatment, the centric relationship was determined and the centric bite was transferred into the scan: the centric bite was fixed with StoneBite (Dreve) and the centric contact was scanned, allowing its transfer directly into the ClinCheck software (Fig 4-517). The second phase was planned to increase the overjet and further retract the lower incisors, with additional IPR from mesial 33 to mesial 43. The plan included an overjet that seems quite unphysiologically big but was intended to obtain sufficient space for the planned restorations of the upper and lower incisors after orthodontic therapy (see below).

At the end of Invisalign therapy, there was little change in esthetics as no vertical change occurred (Fig 4-518). This was planned to occur with the subsequent restorative dentistry. The final intraoral views

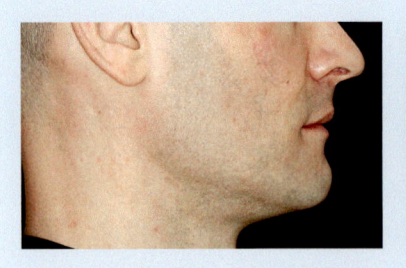

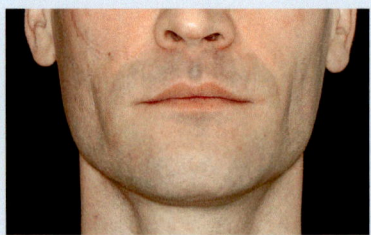

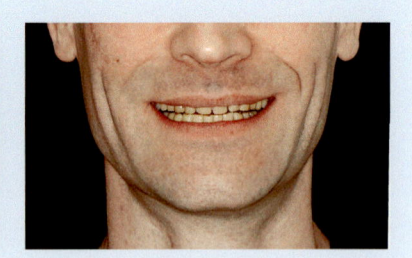

Fig 4-518 Extraoral views at the end of Invisalign therapy.

Fig 4-519 Intraoral views at the end of Invisalign therapy.

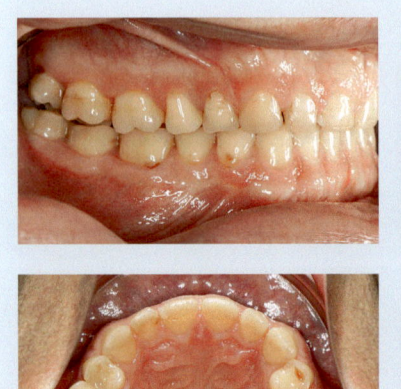

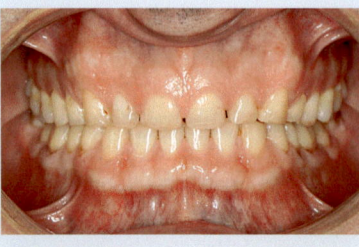

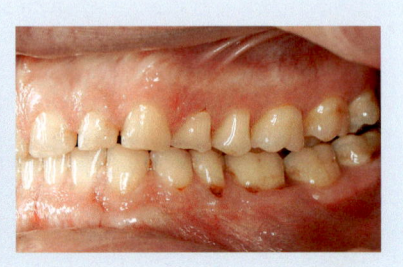

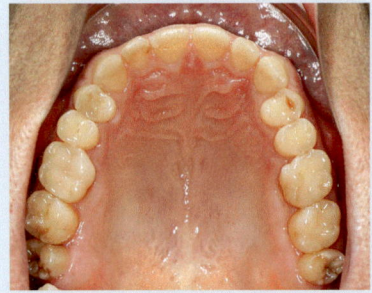

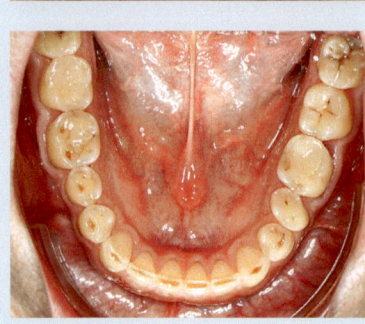

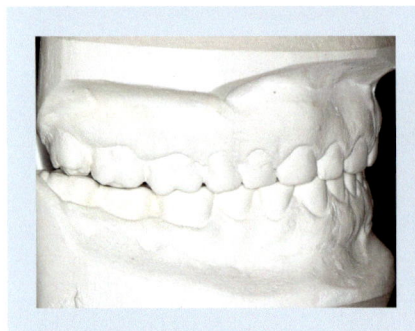

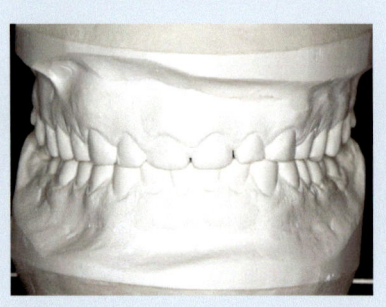

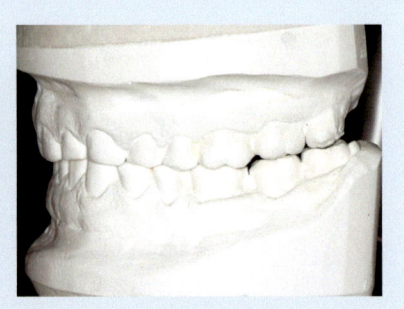

Fig 4-520 Plaster casts showing the improvement of the dental relationship from class II to class I.

after the Invisalign treatment showed aligned arch forms with equal spaces between the upper front teeth and sufficient overjet for the planned anterior restoratives. There was posterior support but reduced vertical height (Fig 4-519). The improvement in dental relationship from class II to class I was not obtained with distalization in the upper arch but with adjustment of a physiological overjet, which allowed the mandible to move forward into its physiological position (Fig 4-520). Occlusal contacts on teeth 11 to 41

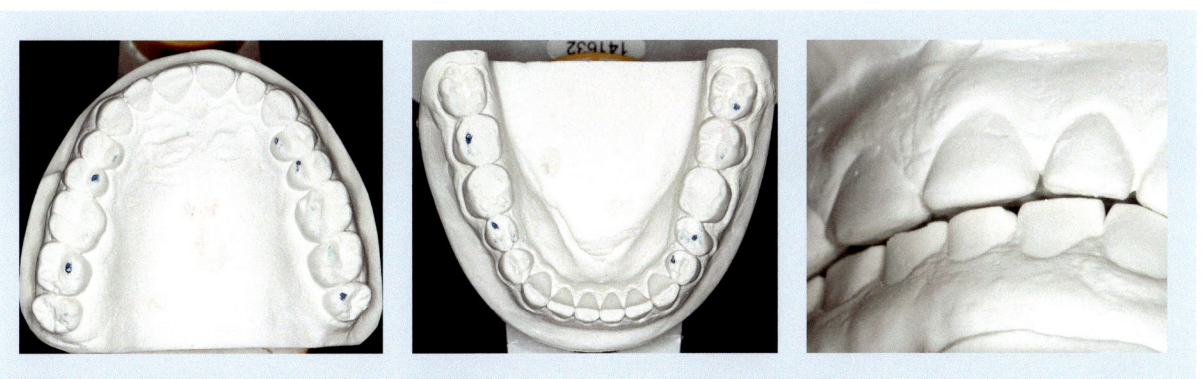

TREATMENT OF DIFFERENT MALOCCLUSIONS WITH ALIGNERS 4

Fig 4-521 Final plaster casts with contact points marked and obtained increased overjet.

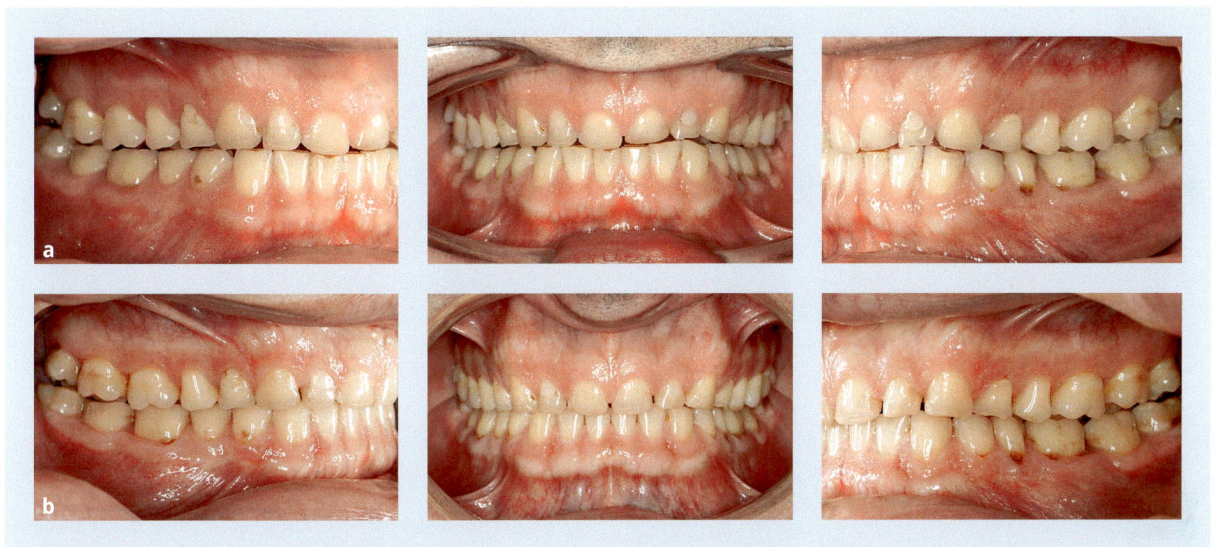

Fig 4-522 Initial (a) and final (b) intraoral views.

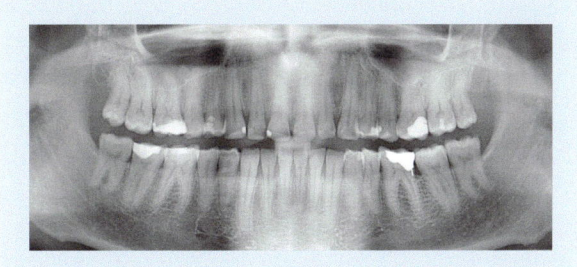

Fig 4-523 Orthopantomography at the end of Invisalign therapy.

had been eliminated and posterior support was adjusted from premolar to third molar, although the vertical posterior relationship would change further during the restorative dental treatment (Fig 4-521).

Figure 4-522 shows the course of treatment. Orthopantomography (Fig 4-523) showed a stable osseous situation with significantly improved bone situation distal of tooth 36 after periodontal treatment.

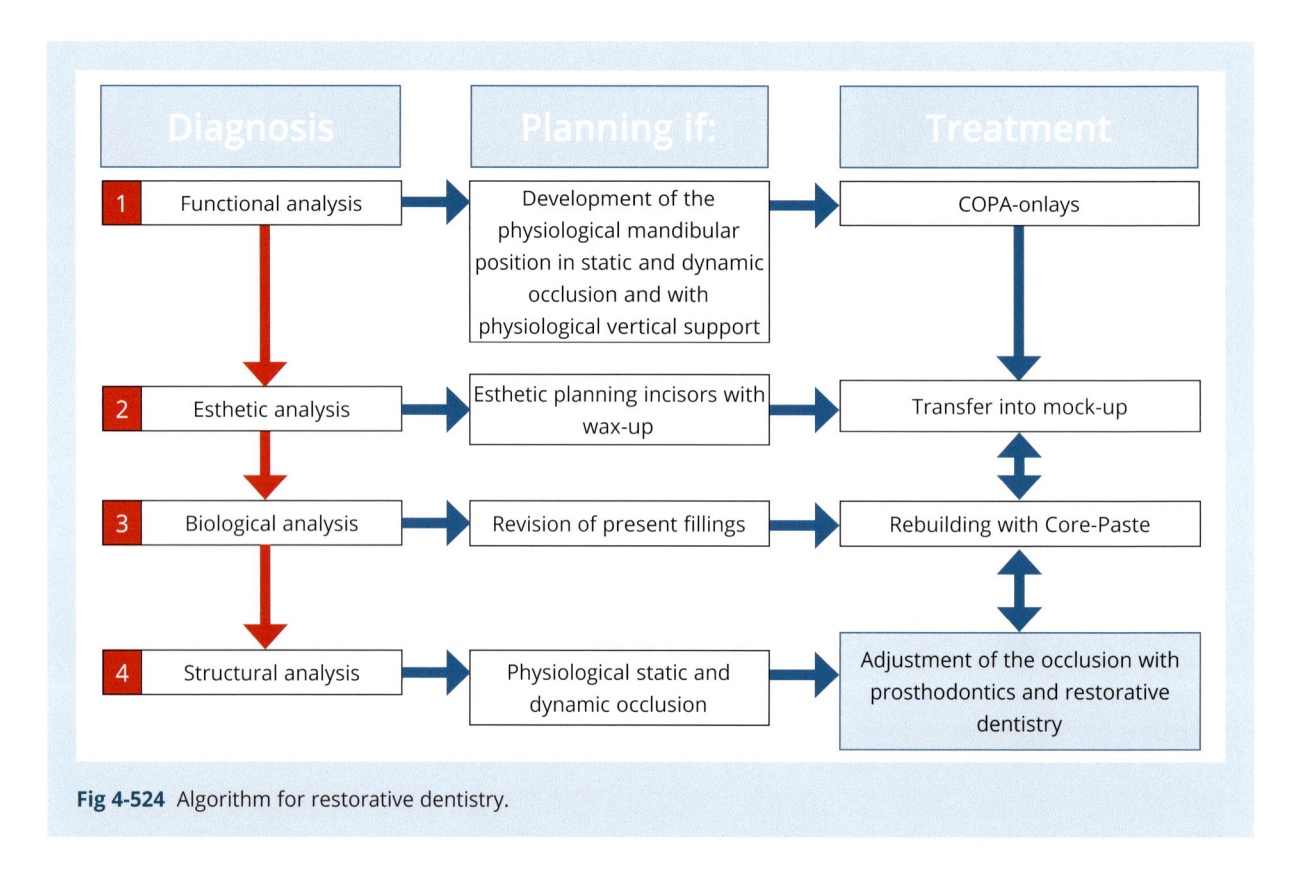

Diagnosis	Planning if:	Treatment
1 Functional analysis	Development of the physiological mandibular position in static and dynamic occlusion and with physiological vertical support	COPA-onlays
2 Esthetic analysis	Esthetic planning incisors with wax-up	Transfer into mock-up
3 Biological analysis	Revision of present fillings	Rebuilding with Core-Paste
4 Structural analysis	Physiological static and dynamic occlusion	Adjustment of the occlusion with prosthodontics and restorative dentistry

Fig 4-524 Algorithm for restorative dentistry.

Restorative treatment

Over the entire treatment time for restorations, extreme care was taken to maintain the exact therapeutic occlusion.

Because of the insufficient vertical support which we did not treat orthodontically but was planned to be restored by the dentist because of the enamel defects, a functional analysis was performed again (Fig 4-524).

This stage of treatment (Dr W Boissereé; laboratory M Läkamp) took place over a number of steps dealing with:
- maintenance of therapeutic occlusion over the whole treatment process using fixed splints (COPA onlays)
- esthetic analysis using a wax-up, and mock-up to produce provisional crowns
- the definitive prosthetic restoration, using CAD/CAM processes.

Pathway for restorative treatment

The general process that is followed, through wax-up to mock-up to provisional crowns, and the final restorations is described here.

In order to construct the physiologic vertical dimension in a reversible manner, fixed splints (COPA onlays) are bonded. This allows planning and treatment of the esthetic, biologic, and structural parameters.

For the functional analysis of the musculoskeletal system, new accurate plaster casts are mounted in centric jaw relation (Fig 4-525). The vertical dimension can then be adjusted with bondable COPA onlays in relation to the intended prosthetic rehabilitation. The COPA onlays are inserted by bonding the splint elements to the mandibular teeth quadrant by quadrant, with a thin flowing orthodontic bonding sealant (Fig 4-526). In order to avoid changes from attrition, the wearing time for the onlays should be limited to 4–8 weeks. Figure 4-527 shows the onlays in the mouth.

Subsequently, the therapeutic occlusion can be tested before further prosthetic changes occur. This set-up forms the basis for the later one-to-one transfer of the therapeutic jaw relation into the final prosthetic rehabilitation.

TREATMENT OF DIFFERENT MALOCCLUSIONS WITH ALIGNERS 4

Fig 4-525 Plaster casts mounted in centric jaw relation **(a)** and then adjusted with bondable COPA onlays **(b)**.

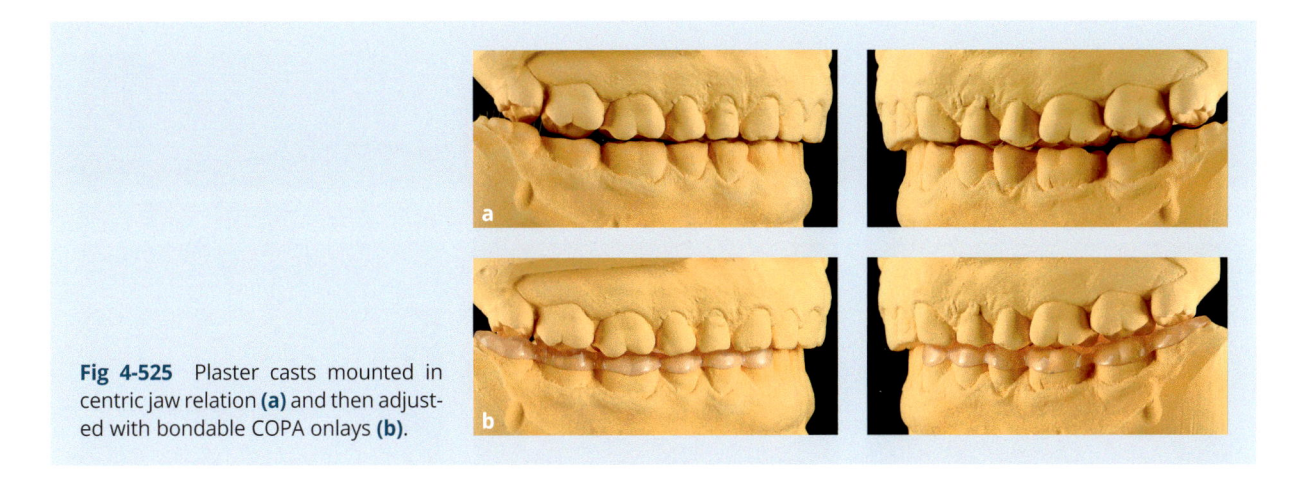

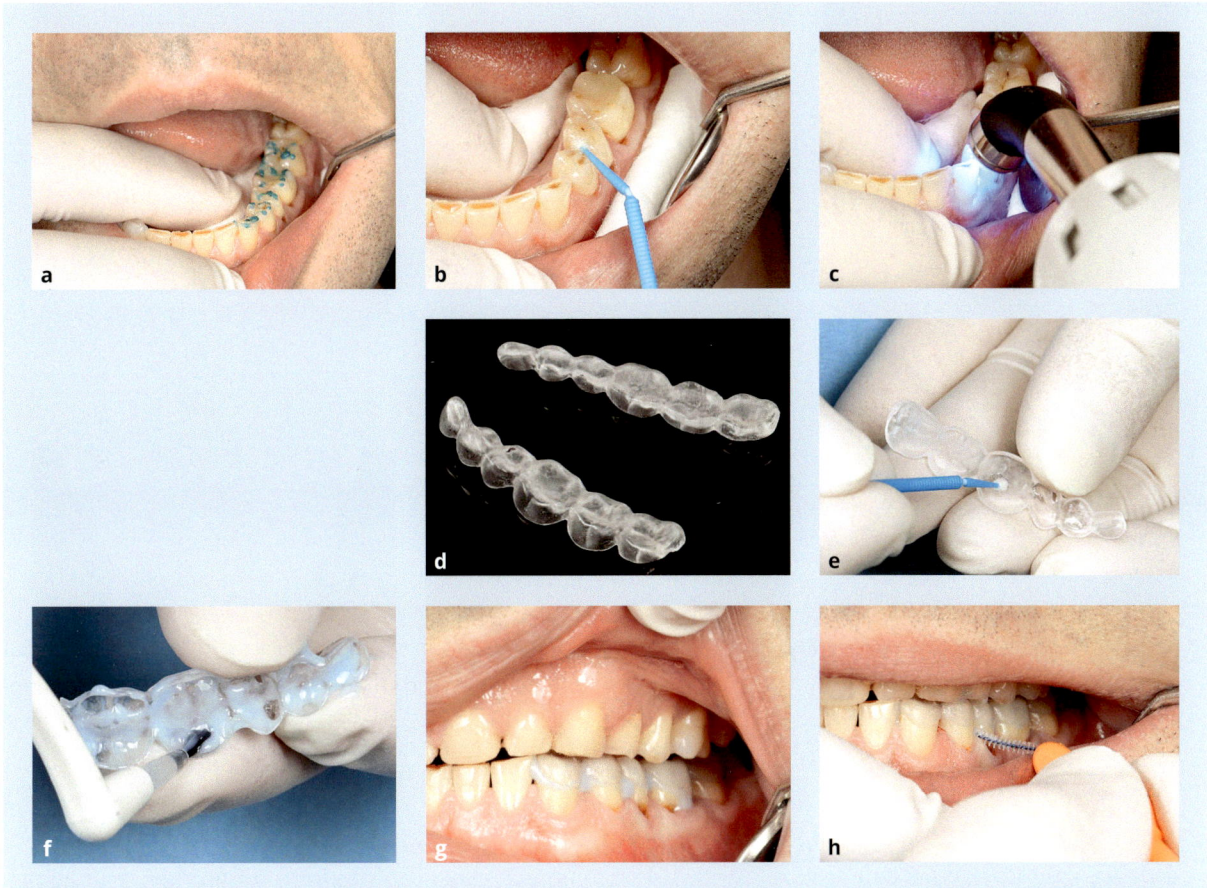

Fig 4-526 Insertion of COPA onlays. **(a–c)** After the teeth have been cleaned, the occlusal surfaces are sandblasted with 50 μm aluminum oxide powder and the occlusal surfaces of the prepared teeth are etched for 5 seconds (phosphoric acid 35%), rinsed and dried, before the surface is prepared for bonding (Reliance Bonding Resin). **(d,e)** The lower surface of the onlays is also sandblasted with aluminum oxide powder, treated with saline for 60 seconds and bonded (Monobond S, Ivoclar Vivadent), then dried. **(f–h)** The onlays are bonded according to the manufacturer's instructions (e.g. with Excel Regular Blue, Reliance Ortho). Excessive adhesive can be removed with foam pellets and interdental brushes.

4 TREATMENT OF DIFFERENT MALOCCLUSIONS WITH ALIGNERS

Fig 4-527 COPA onlays in the mouth. **(a)** In static occlusion. **(b)** In dynamic occlusion (laterotrusion to the right, protrusion–laterotrusion to the left). **(c)** Onlays showing equal contacts in static (black) and dynamic occlusion (laterotrusion red; protrusion blue).

Fig 4-528 Frontal views for esthetic analysis.

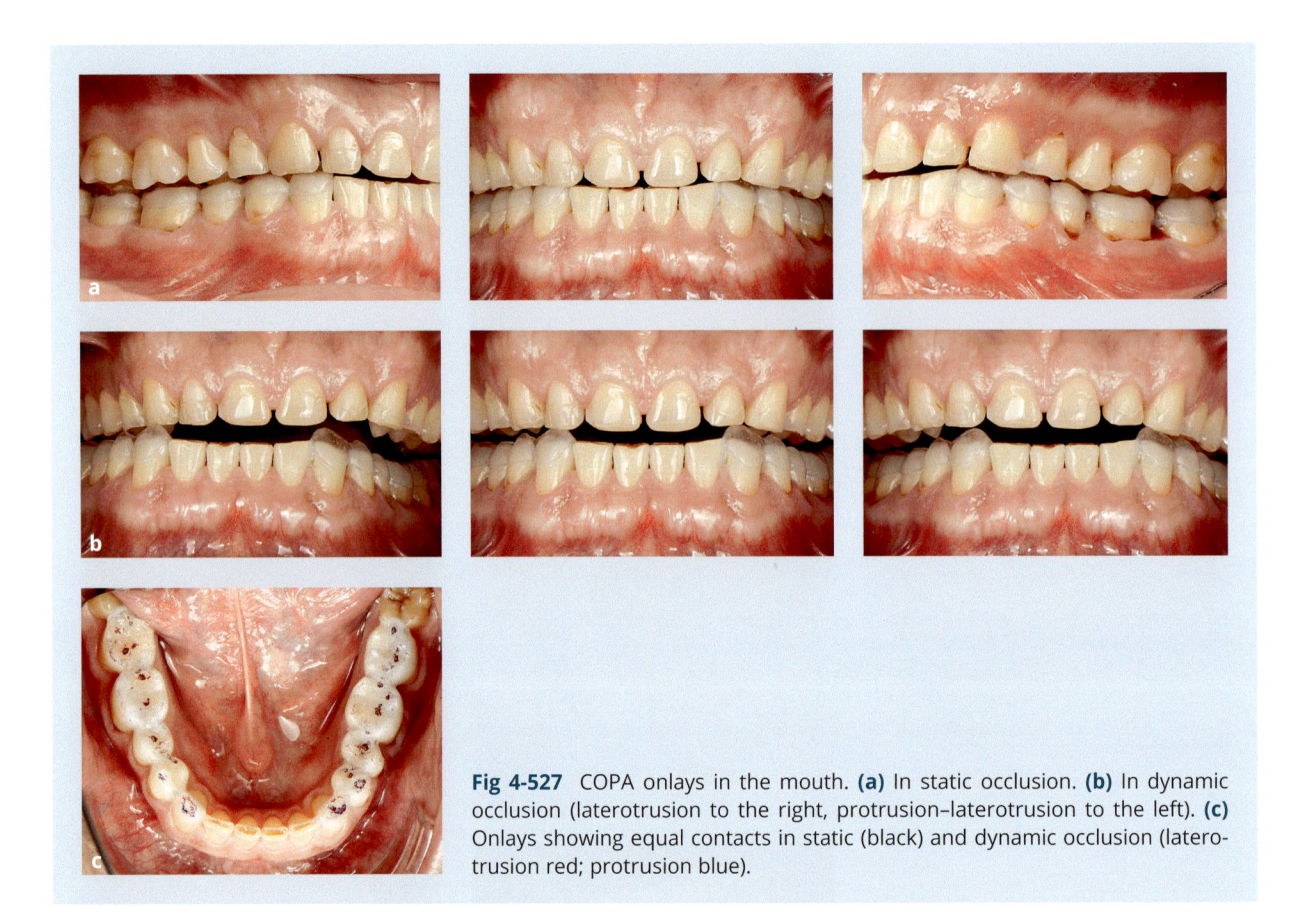

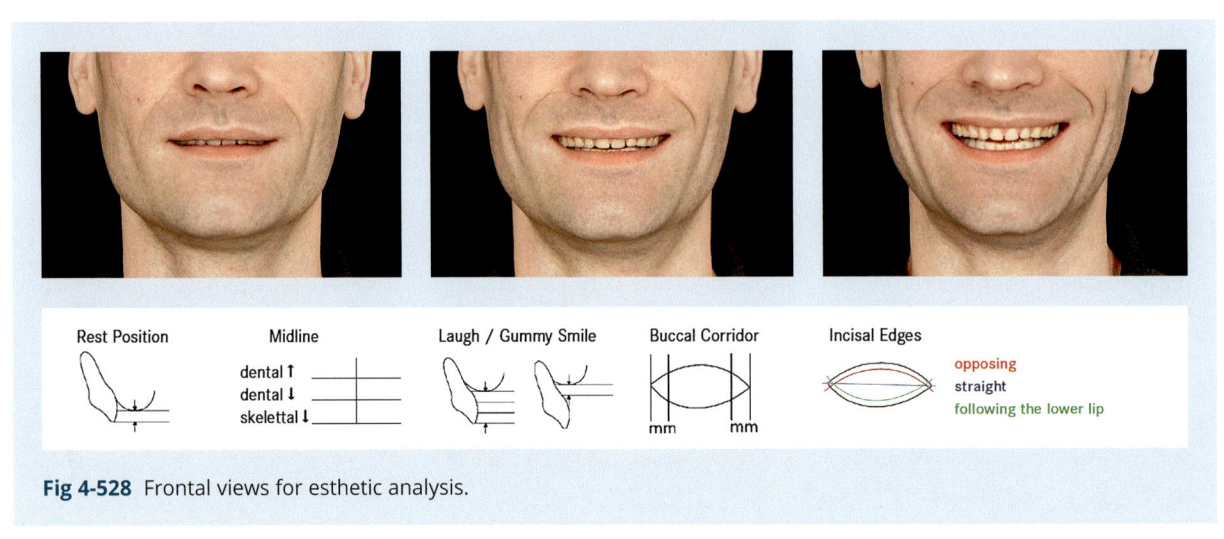

For precise prosthetic rehabilitation, it is necessary to use a backward planning for the prosthetic construction. Apart from the therapeutic jaw relationship, patient esthetics must be considered as the final rehabilitation, and should be not only functional but also pleasing and fitting for the individual. Photographic documentation uses frontal views of the patient with the mouth slightly open with the upper lip in a rest position (the so-called "Emma view" according to B Zacchrisson), smiling, and laughing, as well as lateral views (Fig 4-528).

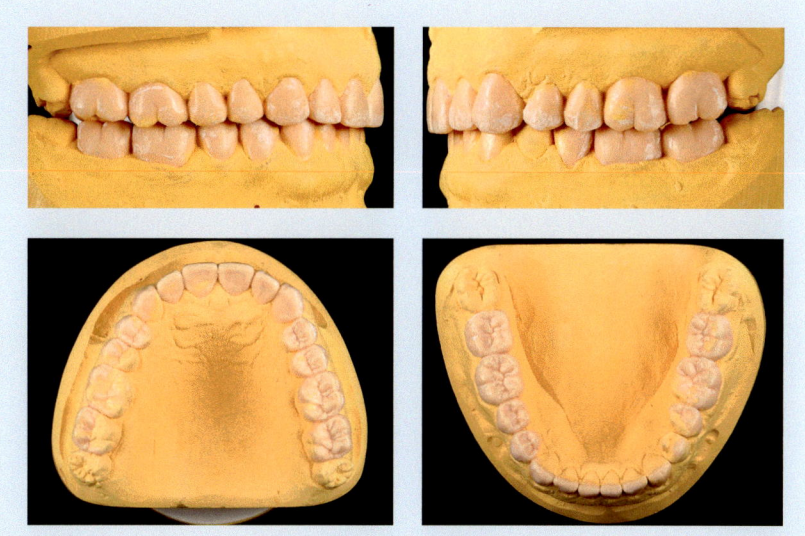

TREATMENT OF DIFFERENT MALOCCLUSIONS WITH ALIGNERS 4

Fig 4-529 The wax-up with perfect match of the upper and lower teeth in both arches.

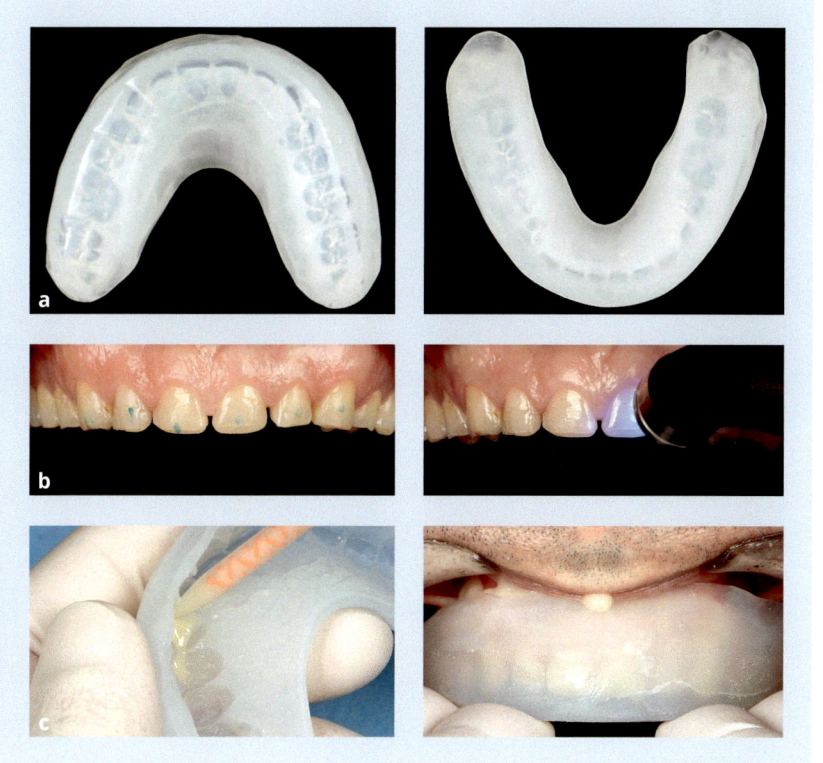

Fig 4-530 Formation of the mock-up. **(a)** For precise transfer of the wax-up into a mock-up, special molding forms were made of clear silicone (Regofix, Dreve), which guarantee a reliable and accurate fit on the arches. **(b)** To obtain permanent anchorage of the mock-up, the maxillary anterior teeth were etched punctually and then bonded. **(c)** The transfer of the wax-up into a mock-up is performed using the silicone components and with Luxatemp (DMG), which is inserted into the silicone molding form with a cartridge. The prepared silicone form can be precisely positioned onto the teeth.

For the esthetic analysis, an exact three-dimensional wax-up is made that is used to anticipate diagnostics.

The wax-up is made in the laboratory on a new pair of casts that are assembled in the current therapeutic occlusion in the articulator (Fig 4-529).

In this particular patient, rehabilitation of the posterior teeth was required for conservative and functional reasons. The significant amount of abrasion and loss of substance in the upper and lower anterior teeth have been included, therefore, in the prosthetic

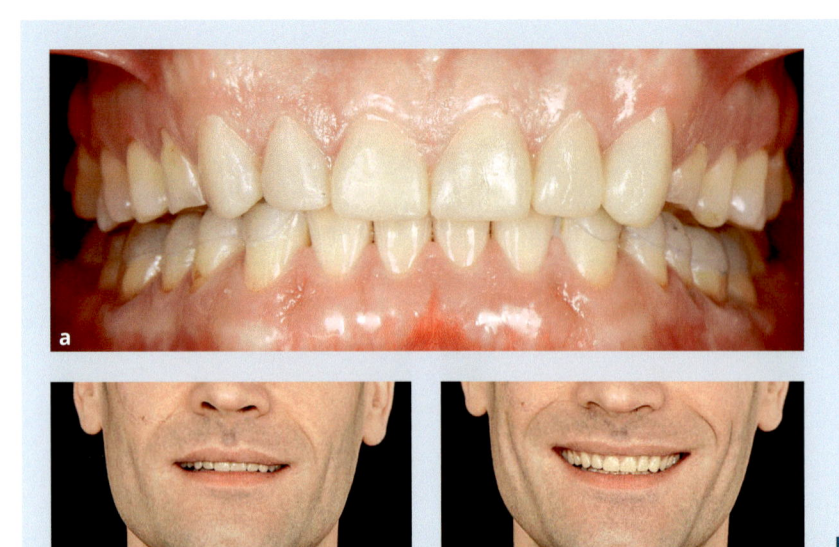

Fig 4-531 The upper incisors transferred into the mock-up in intraoral **(a)** and extraoral **(b)** views.

plan. A reconstruction of the anterior teeth only with composite was not possible because of the extent needed, and dental crowns on all teeth was favored as it would improve protection from decay. In fact, teeth 17 and 27 could not be supplied with a partial crown for occlusal rehabilitation, and the wisdom teeth were excluded from the prosthetic rehabilitation. In order to avoid contact points of the restorations during mediotrusion (balances), care was taken in the wax-up to keep the curve of Spee as flat as possible.

The wax-up was transferred into a mock-up (Fig 4-530).

Figure 4-531 shows the upper incisors transferred into the mock-up to verify the esthetic appearance of the planning. Since the course of treatment included preparation of the posterior teeth, the anterior mock-up should initially be used to contribute to ensuring therapeutic occlusion, while the posterior region has bonded COPA onlays, formed and fitted.

Since the bonded splints need to be removed for the preparation of the posterior teeth, there is risk of iatrogenic loss of the therapeutic jaw relation. Even the smallest occlusal inaccuracies can lead to renewed peripheral disorders and can challenge the entire treatment outcome. This is why the following rules should be followed to enable a safe transfer into the definitive prosthetics:

- the front is initially untreated and secured with a frontal reference bite in the therapeutic starting position
- treatment of the posterior teeth takes place quadrant by quadrant, with a subsequent quadrant only started once the prepared quadrant is supplied with a stable and exact fitting temporary onlay.

Right at the beginning of prosthetic treatment, a removable frontal reference bite is directly made in the patient's mouth to match exactly the therapeutic occlusion (Fig 4-532). If the reference bite is made precisely, the patient occludes when closing in therapeutic jaw relationship (which is determined by the onlays) quite naturally and accurately with the maxillary incisors in the impressions of the bite. The reference bite can be used for orientation during the preparation process, to avoid needing support zones, and for the fabrication of provisional restorations and registrations. To that extent, the frontal reference bite is an essential and simple instrument for securing the therapeutic jaw relation in the course of treatment.

Fig 4-532 (a) The frontal reference bite (Pattern Resin, GC Germany) that has been set on the mandibular incisors with impressions of the incisal edges of teeth 12–22. (b) The reference bite in the mouth.

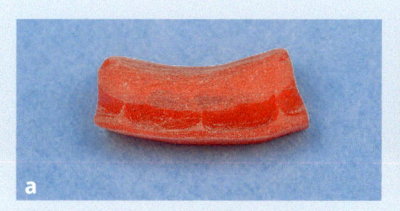

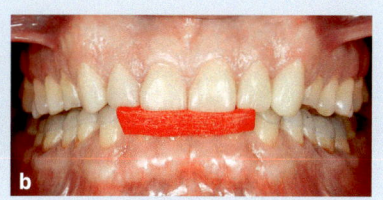

Fig 4-533 Making the mock-up in the maxilla on the right posterior side. (a) The teeth can be selectively etched to improve adhesion (5 seconds). (b) Bonding. (c,d) Luxatemp (DMG) is inserted into the silicone molding and the mold is placed on the teeth.

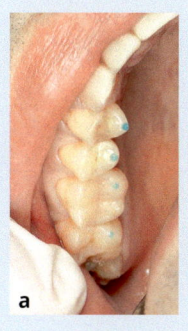

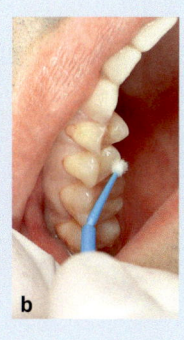

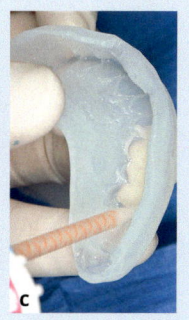

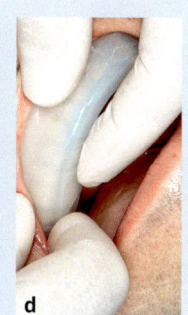

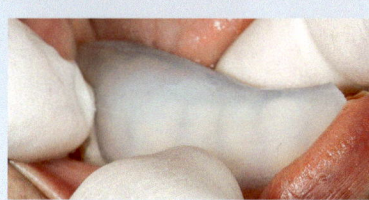

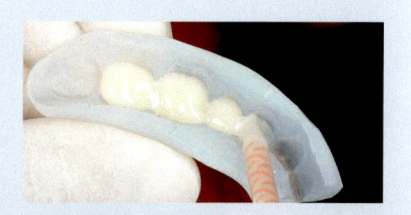

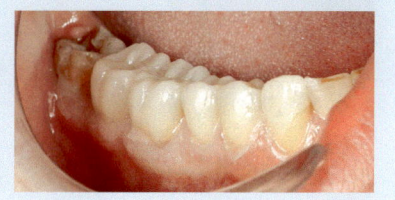

Fig 4-534 Making of the mock-up in the mandible.

The mock-up is transferred to one side of the mouth on the maxillary posterior teeth with the help of a silicone molding (Fig 4-533). The occlusion is checked in coordination with the front reference bite. Once the therapeutic starting position is confirmed, the silicone bite can be used for making the provisional crowns.

The mock-up for the mandible is also done with the frontal reference bite to obtain precise transfer of the predetermined mandibular position into the planned, future tooth shapes (Fig 4-534). The COPA onlays must be removed beforehand.

Figure 4-535 shows the mock-up on the right mandible for this patient. The frontal reference bite and the contralateral remaining COPA onlays maintain the exact therapeutic initial situation while the mock-up is precisely ground to fit. Once the reference bite is removed, an impression tray can be inserted in the patient's mouth with silicone material to transfer the shape. After hardening, the silicone tray shows the exact shape of the mock-up (Fig 4-536).

Once the prosthetics have been determined, the mouth is prepared quadrant by quadrant under the rubber dam technique (Fig 4-537). The preparation is

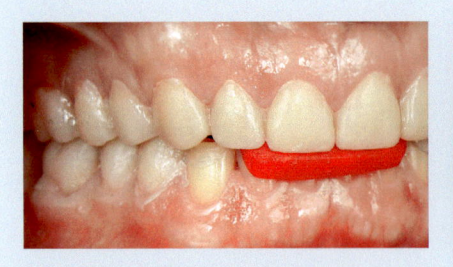

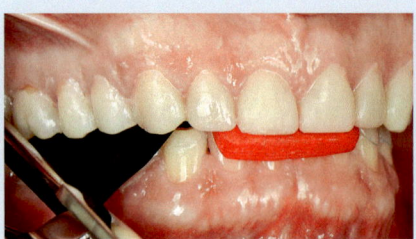

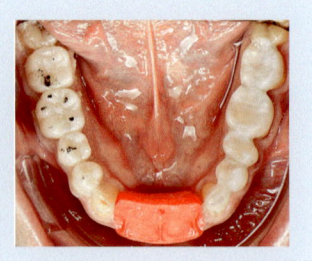

Fig 4-535 Intraoral views showing the inserted mock-up on the mandibular right with the frontal reference bite and the contralateral COPA onlays in place.

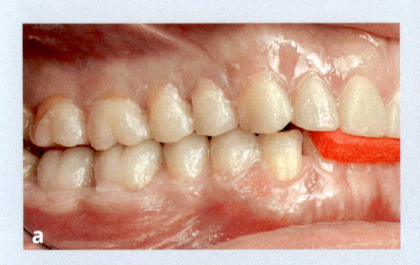

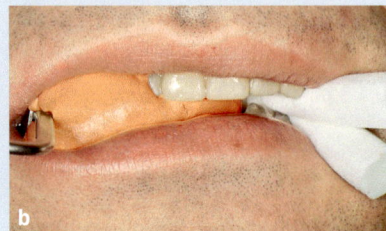

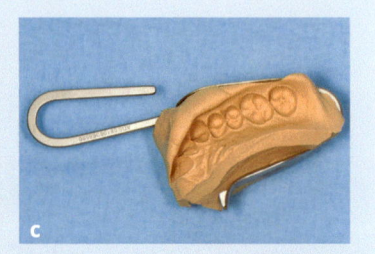

Fig 4-536 Transfer of information from the mock-up. **(a)** The mock-up on the mandibular right and the reference bite. **(b)** An impression tray (Scheufele Löffel (George Dental), Silicone (Affinis, Coltène)) is inserted with silicone material. **(c)** After hardening of the silicone, the tray shows the exact shape of the mock-up.

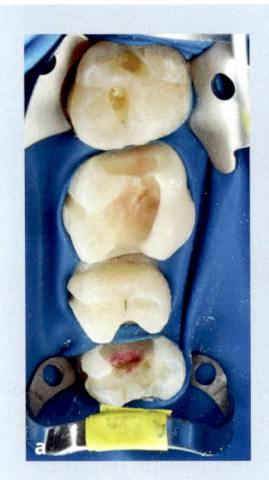

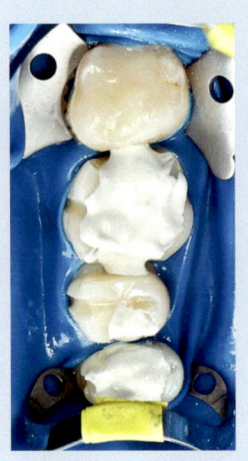

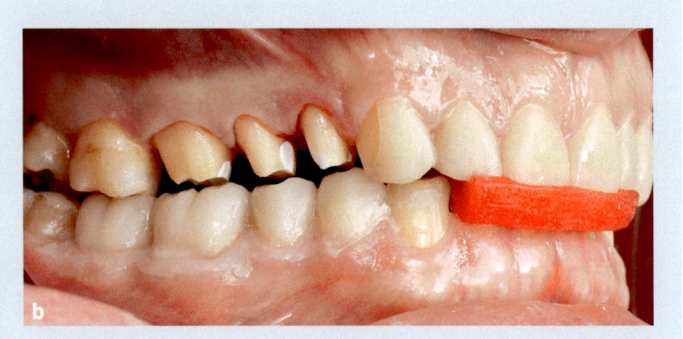

Fig 4-537 Preparation for insertion of prosthetics. **(a)** Teeth for restoration and the prepared teeth. **(b)** The frontal reference bite and the contralateral splint provides further information for occlusal orientation.

performed in orientation to the mock-up and the opposite side of the jaw to ensure that the treatment goal of the final prosthetic reconstruction is maintained.

After the completed preparation of one quadrant, provisional crowns are made with the silicone key in coordination with the frontal reference bite to transfer the correct support exactly. PMMA resin (Tempron, GC) is favorable for making provisional crowns (Fig 4-538). The material is very hard and resistant and it bonds well with other methacrylates (e.g. Super-T, George Dental). It can, therefore, be combined or readjusted easily. The provisional crown can be occlusally corrected if needed with the frontal reference

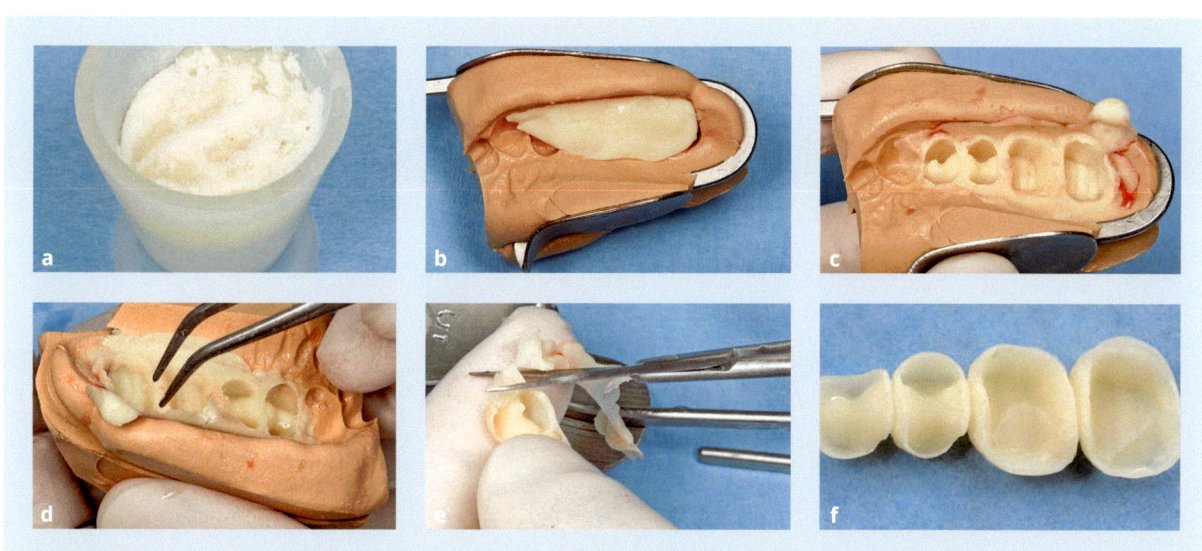

Fig 4-538 Preparation of PMMA resin. **(a)** The liquid and resin powder are mixed in an elastic container (Resimix cup, George Dental) and covered with water until a viscoplastic state is reached. **(b)** The material can then be filled into the silicone mold and put onto the prepared arch region. **(c)** The patient is asked to occlude. After about 20 seconds the mold can be removed. **(d)** The resin is still viscoplastic. To avoid damage, the silicone mold can be removed from the impression tray and bent so that plastic provisional crown can be removed safely. **(e)** After removal, it can be reduced and cut with scissors and reinserted into the patient's mouth, while still soft. It remains in the patient's mouth until it has hardened with occlusion controlled, and with the frontal reference bite in place. **(f)** Finally, it can be removed, elaborated, and polished in detail in the laboratory.

Fig 4-539 Intraoral views of the arches showing the right side supplied with provisional crowns. The left side still shows the bonded COPA onlay.

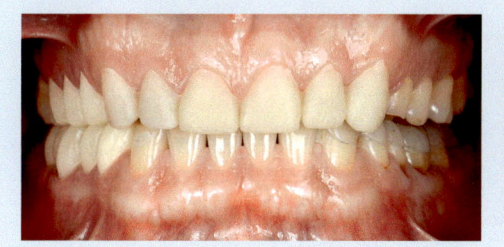

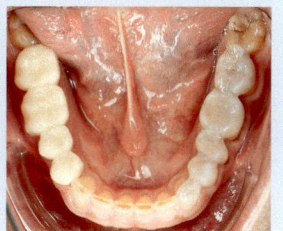

bite and the onlay on the contralateral side giving the correct occlusion. Once finished, the provisional crowns can be fitted (Fig 4-539).

With a careful quadrant by quadrant approach, all posterior teeth can be precisely prepared and supplied with provisional crowns without losing the therapeutic starting position. The provisional crowns correspond exactly to the treatment planned in the wax-up and mock-up. The orientation for the therapeutic starting position is still guaranteed by the upper front teeth, as supplied by the mock-up in relation to the frontal reference bite.

In this treatment phase, the wax-up treatment goal has almost entirely been transferred into the shape of the posterior provisional restorations and the mock-up of the maxillary anterior teeth.

At this point, structural analysis and control can take place. The structural analysis deals with the question of whether the planned prosthetic restoration is able to reconstruct the patient's situation satisfactory in function and esthetics. Corrections to the shape of the provisional crowns can be made and these need to be considered in the making of the final restoration. The future static and dynamic occlusion should be reviewed (Fig 4-540).

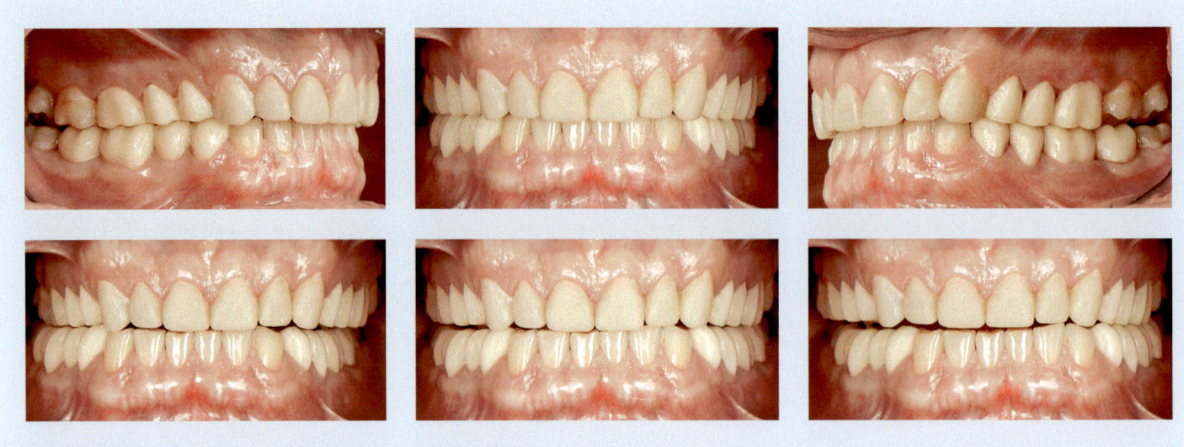

Fig 4-540 Intraoral views with provisional restorations.

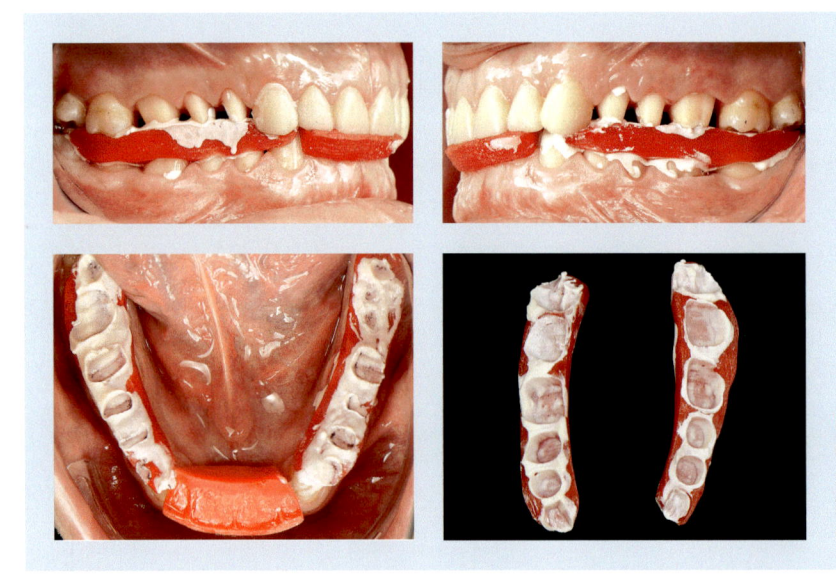

Fig 4-541 Preparation of the posterior bite registrations. These are made side by side, with constant coordination and adjustment to the frontal reference bite.

If the design of the provisory supply and the mock-up is satisfactory, the next step is treatment of the anterior teeth. To maintain the therapeutic intermaxillary relationship, which has been fixed until now with the frontal reference bite, posterior bite registration of the posterior regions needs to be performed before the frontal reference orientation is lost by the treatment of the anterior teeth. The bite registration is carried out, preferably without anesthesia, in a separate visit. The bite registration elements are made side by side, with constant coordination and adjustment to the frontal reference bite (Fig 4-541). For stability reasons, PMMA is particularly well suited as material for these reference bites. The PMMA is coated with a cement or a thin liquid plastic layer (Super-T, American Dental Systems) to display the impressions of the prepared teeth in detail.

After securing therapeutic occlusion with stable, perfectly fitting provisonal crowns and registrations, anterior treatment can begin. If the mock-up still needs to be corrected for esthetic reasons, it is convenient to build a new, directly built silicone molding form for fabricating the provisional crowns. The preparation of the maxillary front teeth takes place with the mock-up in situ. To secure a dimensionally accurate final preparation, it is helpful to use depth mark-

Fig 4-542 Preparation of provisional structures for the anterior teeth.

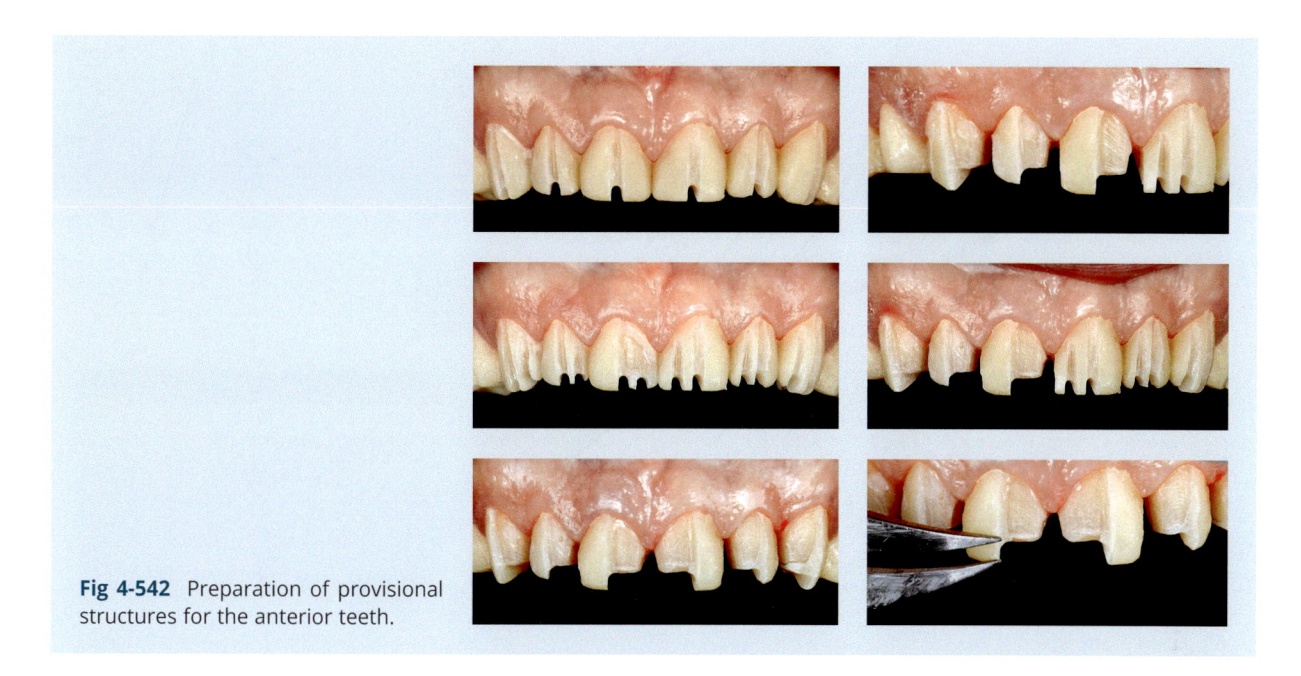

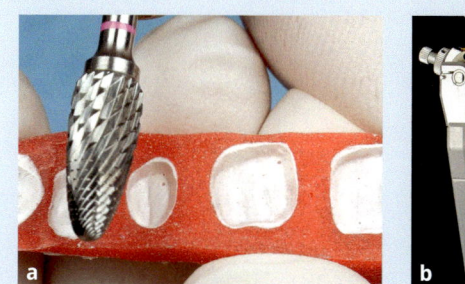

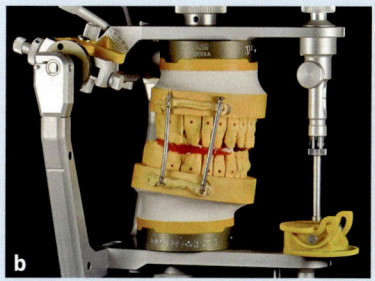

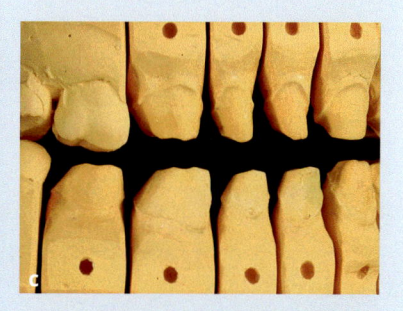

Fig 4-543 Mounting of casts for restoration fabrication. **(a)** Centric registration for assembly of casts. **(b)** Casts secured with wire pins set with a hot glue gun. **(c)** The saw casts mounted in the therapeutic horizontal and vertical jaw relationship and ready for scanning.

ings within the preparation of the teeth. Each tooth is prepared initially on one half only, which facilitates the preparation and helps to reduce the tooth structure dimensionally for accuracy of the proposed restoration (Fig 4-542). The preparation can be completed under dimensional control through the transparent silicone molding. Once the preparation has also been carried out for the mandibular incisors, impressions of both arches can be taken.

The prosthetic restorations were planned to be fabricated in a CAD/CAM process (Zirkonzahn). Because of the treatment extent and technical uncertainties in digital workflow, it is still necessary to make conventional saw casts, which are arbitrarily mounted in the articulator (Fig 4-543). The mandibular cast is mounted using the registration and oriented to the maxillary cast. Since the vertical dimension of the therapeutic initial situation has been accurately maintained in the course of treatment, no change is made to the support pin height of the articulator, which had been set at "zero" at the beginning of treatment. After the mounting process, magnetic split-control is essential. If even small differences occur, the casts should be reassembled so that the therapeutic starting position is not changed.

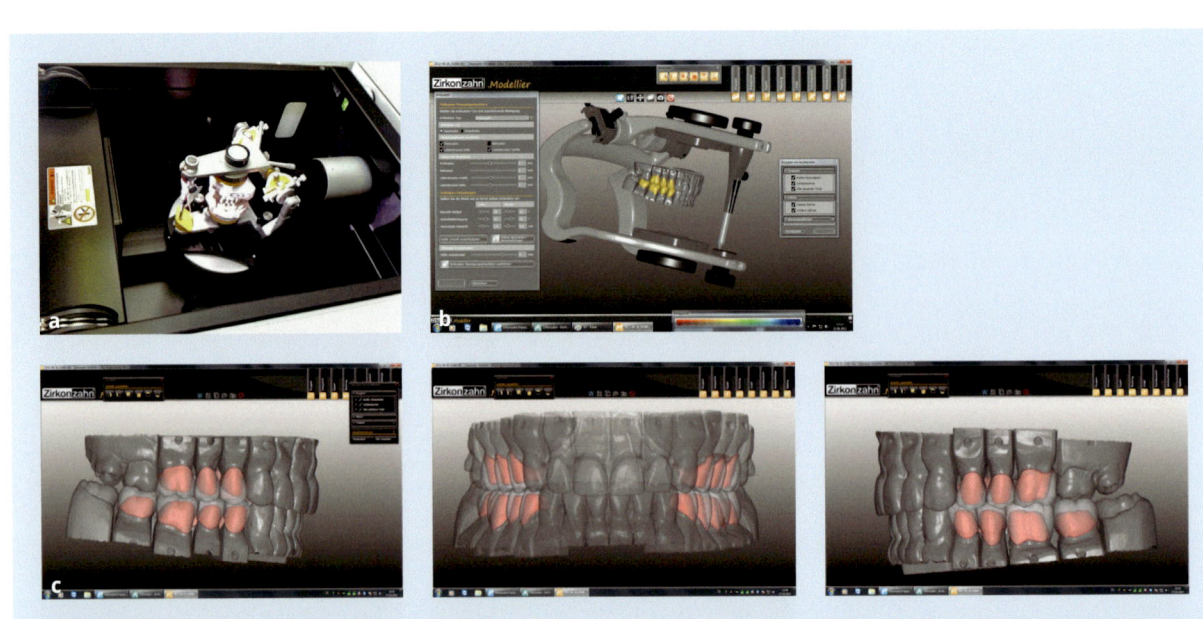

Fig 4-544 Scanning for CAD. **(a)** Digital articulator scan to allow exact spatial assignment of the maxillary and mandibular casts. **(b)** An arbitrary facebow was used to scan the reference positioning for the SAM system. Based on the facebow transfer, the scanned casts are positioned virtually in the center of the articulator and transferred onto the screen. Mean or individual values can be regulated and changed with the use of controllers that allow individual measurements of the simulated movements. **(c)** Wax-up casts were additionally scanned, digitized and virtually laid over the already existing virtual work models, a procedure called "matching."

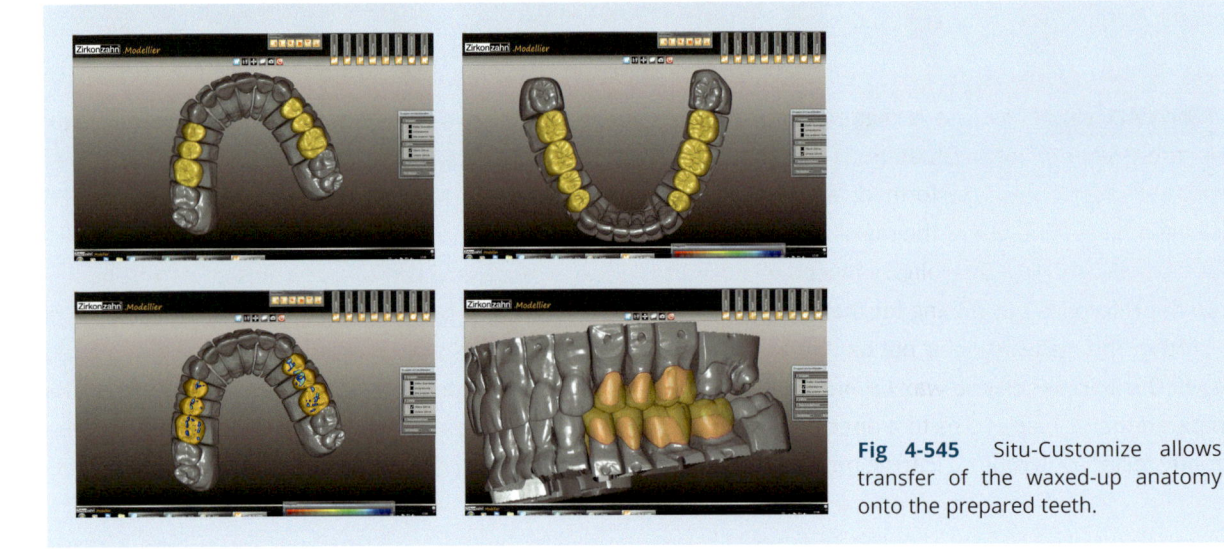

Fig 4-545 Situ-Customize allows transfer of the waxed-up anatomy onto the prepared teeth.

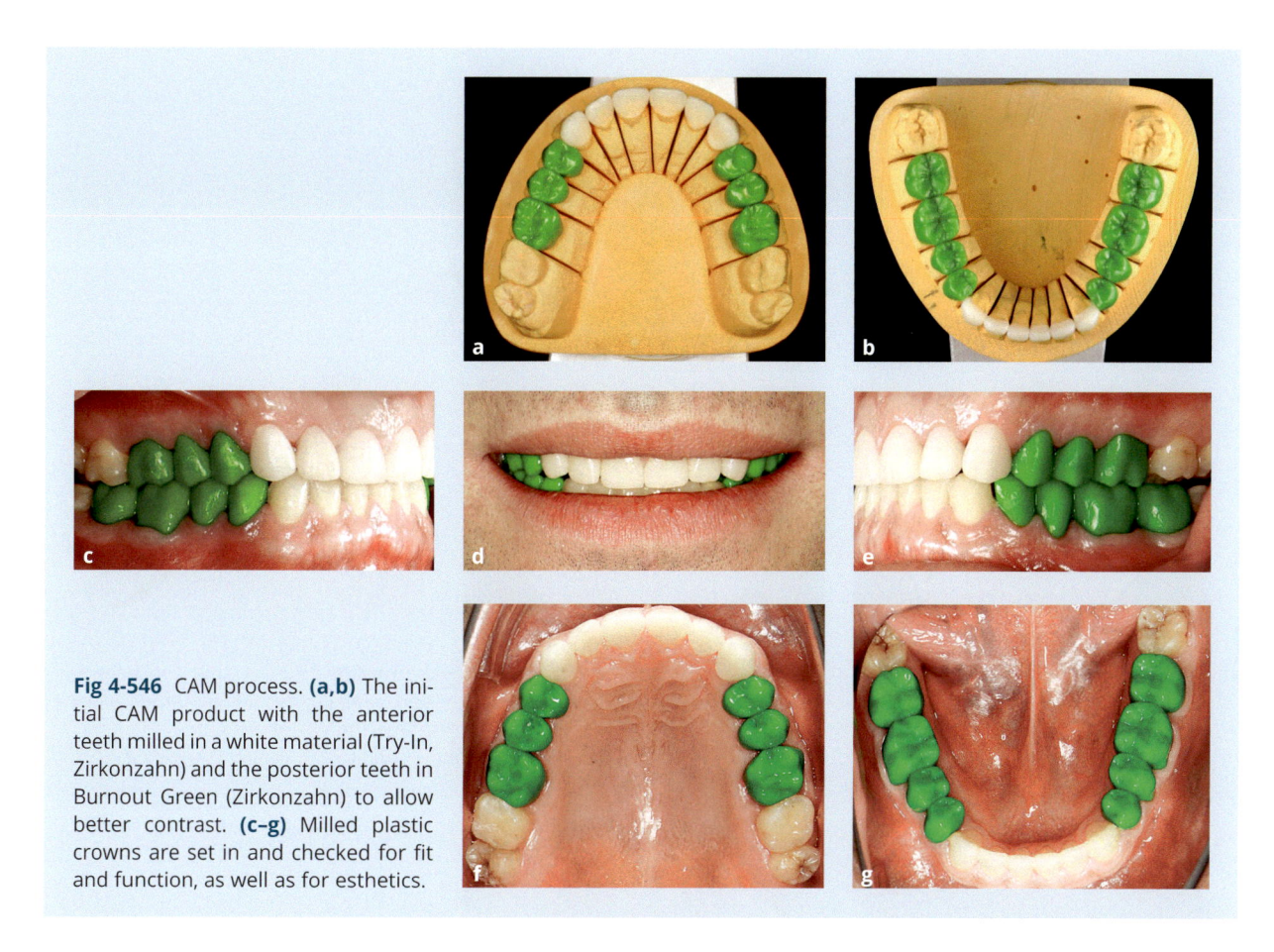

Fig 4-546 CAM process. **(a,b)** The initial CAM product with the anterior teeth milled in a white material (Try-In, Zirkonzahn) and the posterior teeth in Burnout Green (Zirkonzahn) to allow better contrast. **(c–g)** Milled plastic crowns are set in and checked for fit and function, as well as for esthetics.

For CAD, each saw cast is digitized and scanned with the prepared teeth situation. A so-called digital articulator scan is also performed, which allows the exact spatial assignment of the maxillary and mandibular casts (Fig 4-544). An arbitrary facebow is used to scan the reference positioning for the SAM system.

Within the software, the option "Situ-Customize" allows the transfer of the wax-up anatomy onto the prepared teeth, which leads to a direct transfer of the already tested provisional restorations into the future reconstruction (Fig 4-545). Intricacies of the design can be adjusted manually in the program to optimize the occlusal contact and guide relations. The preparation margins are automatically recognized by the program and, if necessary, can also be adjusted manually.

The CAM process is initially in plastic, which can be tried in before the completion of the restoration to ensure fitting, function, and esthetics are checked in detail (Fig 4-546).

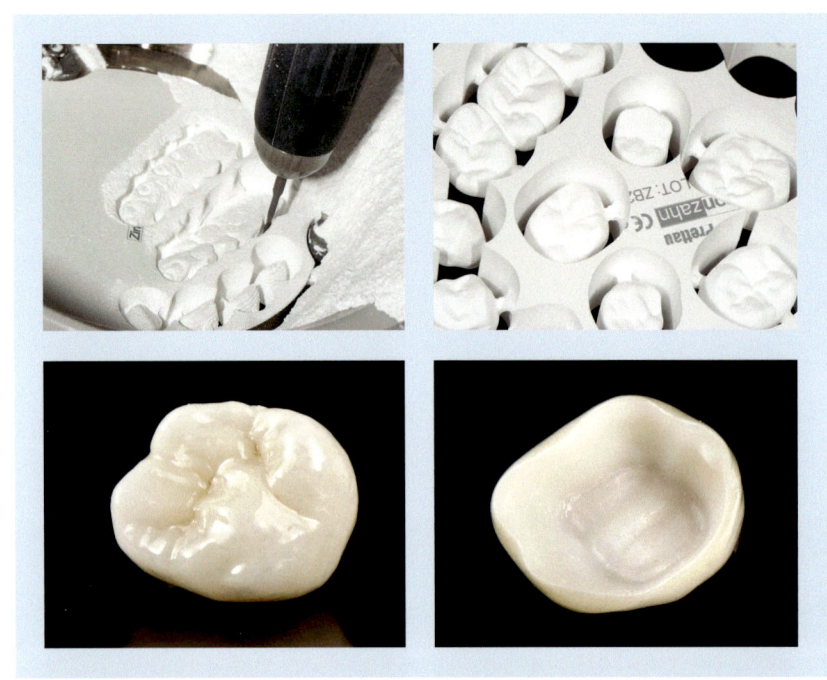

4 TREATMENT OF DIFFERENT MALOCCLUSIONS WITH ALIGNERS

Fig 4-547 Posterior crowns were milled in a monolithic procedure into translucent zirconium (Prettau Zirkon), painted, and afterwards sintered for 12 hours at 1600°C.

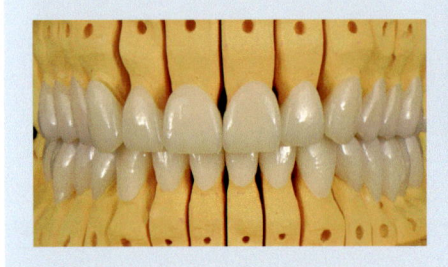

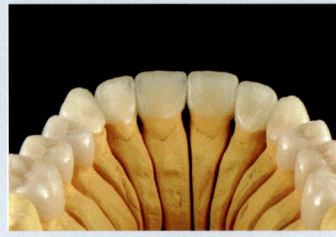

Fig 4-548 Press ceramic has a burn-out capacity to 100% and so the crowns can be produced, embedded, burned out, and pressed with e.max (Ivoclar). They can then be ground back in the cut-back method and individually layered to overcome the monolithic character.

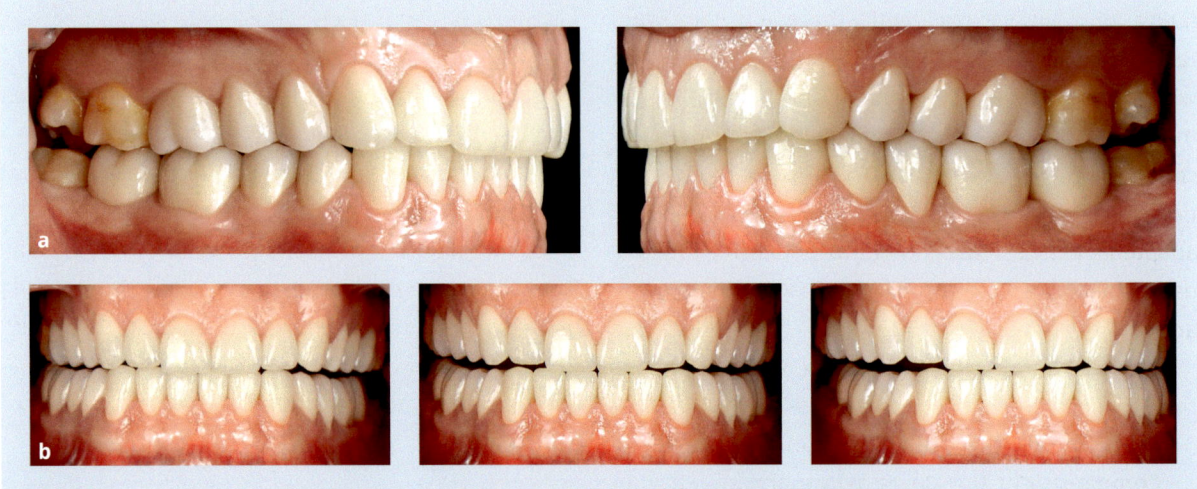

Fig 4-549 Final views showing optimal function in static **(a)** and dynamic **(b)** occlusion.

332

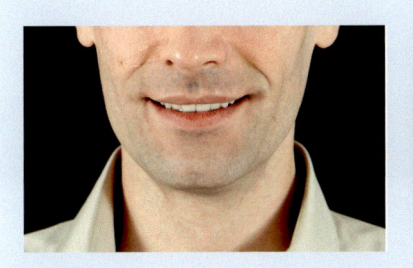

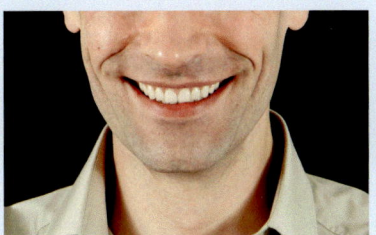

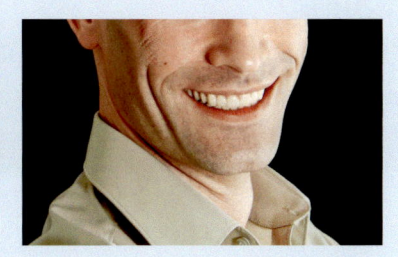

Fig 4-550 Final esthetic result with the upper lip in a resting position and an ideal upper arch form showing harmonic dentofacial relations during smile.

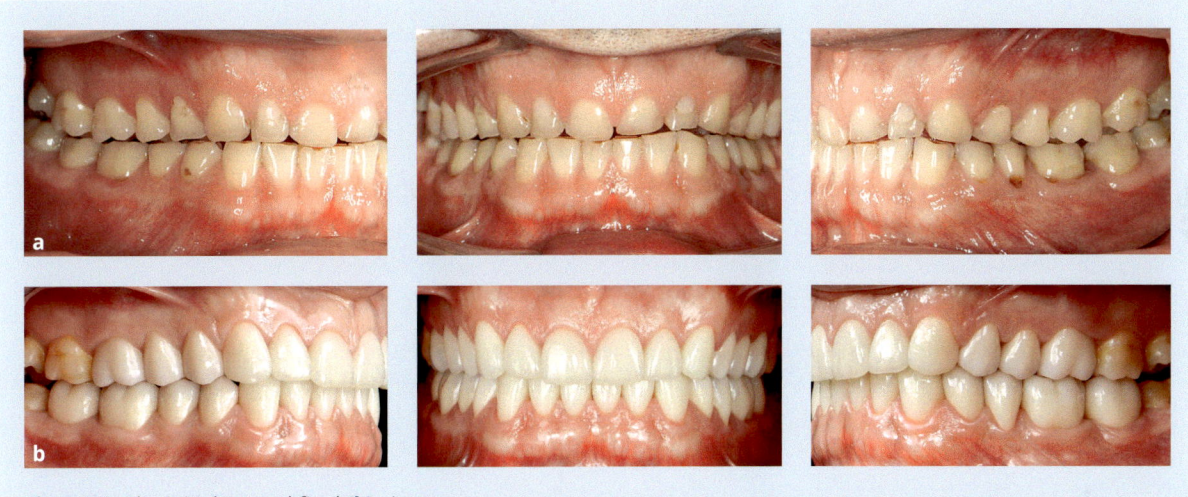

Fig 4-551 The initial (a) and final (b) views.

If there are any changes to the restorations during fitting, it is necessary to identify these and to incorporate them into the definitive reconstruction. This is why all the parts are re-scanned and transmitted by matching into the existing digital planning before final crown production (Fig 4-547). The finished crowns can be fitted onto the plaster casts and readjusted and adapted by other stain firings to obtain the optimal desired color. A final glaze layer guarantees the longevity of the crown (Fig 4-548).

After a 4-week period of testing, the restorations can be inserted definitely with a glass-ionomer cement (Fuji banner, GC, Japan) (Figs 4-549 and 4-550).

Comparison of the views before and after orthodontic treatment and restorative dentistry (Fig 4-551) show that the large mount of enamel loss in both arches has been treated with inserted ceramic crowns on all teeth apart from teeth 17, 27, 18, 28, 38, and 48.

In order to ensure retention of teeth position after orthodontic therapy, patients are advised to wear removable aligners that have been occlusally adjusted in both arches. The patient can alternate which arch uses the aligner from night to night. The removable retainer can be deep drawn with Biolon (Dreve) and if necessary build up with plastic directly in the mouth. Polishing can be performed in the laboratory or chair side as for any occlusal appliance.

Topic 60
Posterior open bite at the end of Invisalign treatment

Treatment:
- refinement or retainers

At the end of Invisalign treatment, posterior teeth should show a stable occlusion with full vertical support. A lateral posterior open bite is not acceptable as a final result. Patients with loss of posterior support due to missing teeth or the absence of occlusal contact in maximum intercuspation had a higher incidence of TMJ sounds and tenderness (see Wiegelmann et al, 2015). However, some patients will in fact have a bilaterally open posterior bite at the end of treatment. There are several factors that can lead lead to this problem (Fig 4-552):
- final outcome was planned without sufficient overjet (use IPR in the lower arch or leave spaces distal of upper lateral incisors)
- final outcome was planned with too much overbite
- final outcome was planned with insufficient upper incisor torque
- final outcome was planned with insufficient upper canine torque (use positive canine torque according to Ricketts or buccal crown tipping as final position)
- final outcome was planned with too much crown tipping, e.g. after crossbite correction
- final outcome with mesially tipped molars due to insufficient anchorage during mesialisation
- final outcome was planned without posterior hard collision (check occlusal points in the cc Pro Software)
- aligner thickness might lead some patients to intrude their posterior teeth if they have severe bruxism (the use of a Speed Up as descibed in Topic 16 might help to avoid this).

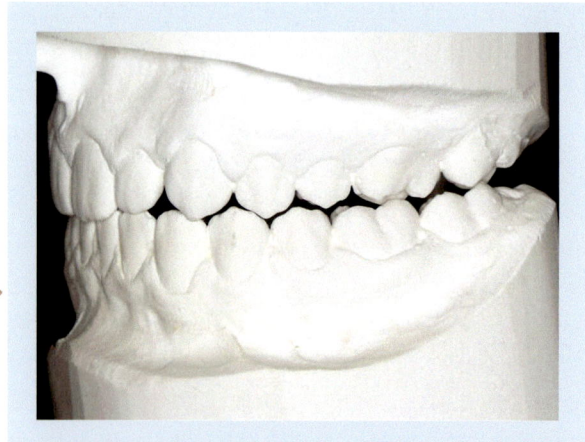

Fig 4-552 Plaster casts showing open posterior bite and insufficient overjet.

Treatment
Already in the first phase of the treatment, it should be clear if a movement of molars is useful and necessary. Certainly in some treatments molar movements are indispensable. In some cases though, treatment might be necessary only in the front and canine region, or eventually in the premolar region. Even in these treatments, the ClinCheck software moves the molars, though minimally, changing former stable posterior occlusions visible intraorally and in the mounted plaster casts. This is why due to stability reasons and anchorage, the molar relationship should rather be maintained. In the online treatment plan for patients undergoing this treatment, we plan to not change the posterior relationship at all.

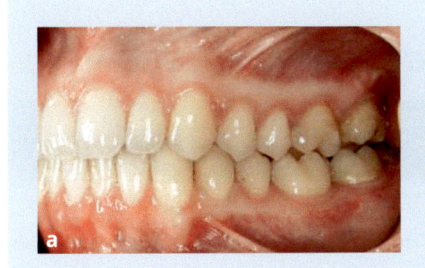

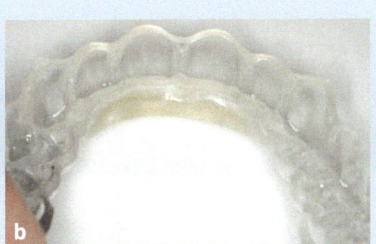

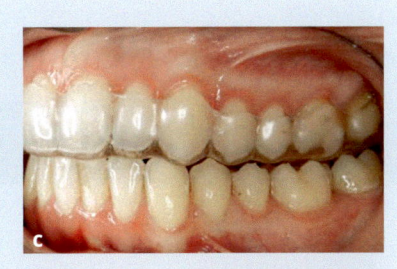

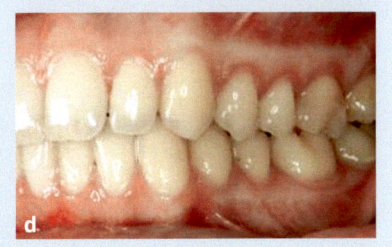

Fig 4-553 Treatment of a posterior missing contact after Invisalign treatment. **(a)** Intraoral view. **(b,c)** Mandibular lingual retainer from 33 to 43 and a maxillary splint with anterior build up **(d)**. Final posterior occlusion with full occlusal contact.

Treatment options for posterior open bite after the first phase of the Invisalign therapy

There are several options to deal with this problem of a posterior open bite after Invisalign treatment:
- perform a refinement to solve potential preliminary contacts on incisors and canines. Extrusion of premolars and molars into hard collision is needed
- reduce/grind tooth substance in the anterior region (depends on the amount of posterior open bite)
- cut out the last aligner posterior of canines to allow settling of premolars and molars (with additional up and down elastics on bonded buttons if necessary)
- provide a mandibular lingual retainer from 33 to 43 and a maxillary splint with anterior build up to allow extrusion of the mandibular posterior teeth over the following weeks (Fig 4-553).

The treatment used depends on the severity of the problem. The situation shown in Figure 4-552 is sufficiently severe that a refinement would be needed. By comparison, the missing posterior contact in Figure 4-553 might easily be treated with retainers, as shown.

Topic 61
Selective tooth grinding in centric and/or excentric supraocclusions

Treatment:
- selective grinding

Selective grinding of teeth may be indicated in patients with centric and/or excentric supraocclusions. As grinding of natural teeth reduces not only restorative and filling material but potentially also healthy tooth substance, it should be performed with great care. However, grinding can reduce the vertical dimension in static occlusion.

The goal of selective grinding is a physiologic cusp-to-fossa relationship (Fig 4-554). Dynamic occlusion should be guided bilaterally from anterior teeth and canines.

This patient was treated with the Invisalign system but at the end of treatment showed missing bilateral equal posterior contacts (Figs 4-555 to 4-557).

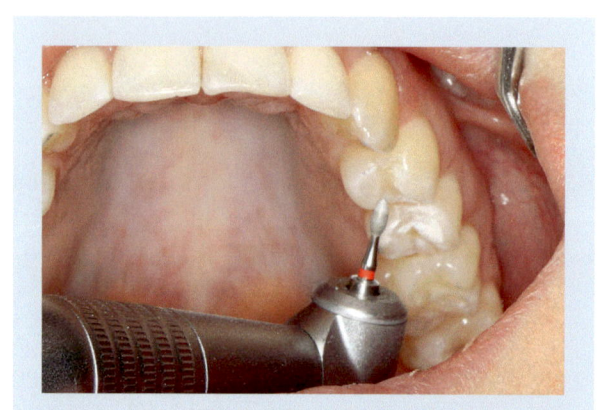

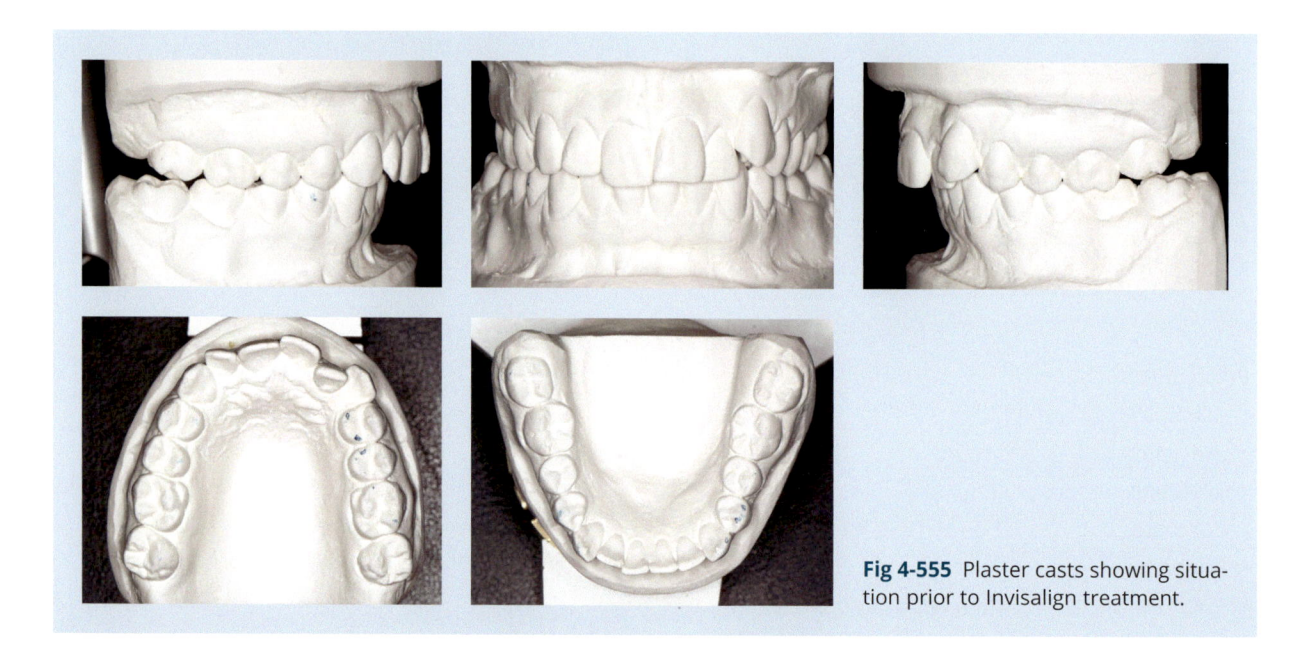

Fig 4-554 Occlusal grinding of tooth 24 with a diamond bur.

Fig 4-555 Plaster casts showing situation prior to Invisalign treatment.

Fig 4-556 Plaster casts after Invisalign treatment showing a class I relationship but missing bilateral equal posterior contacts.

Fig 4-557 Intraoral views at the end of Invisalign treatment.

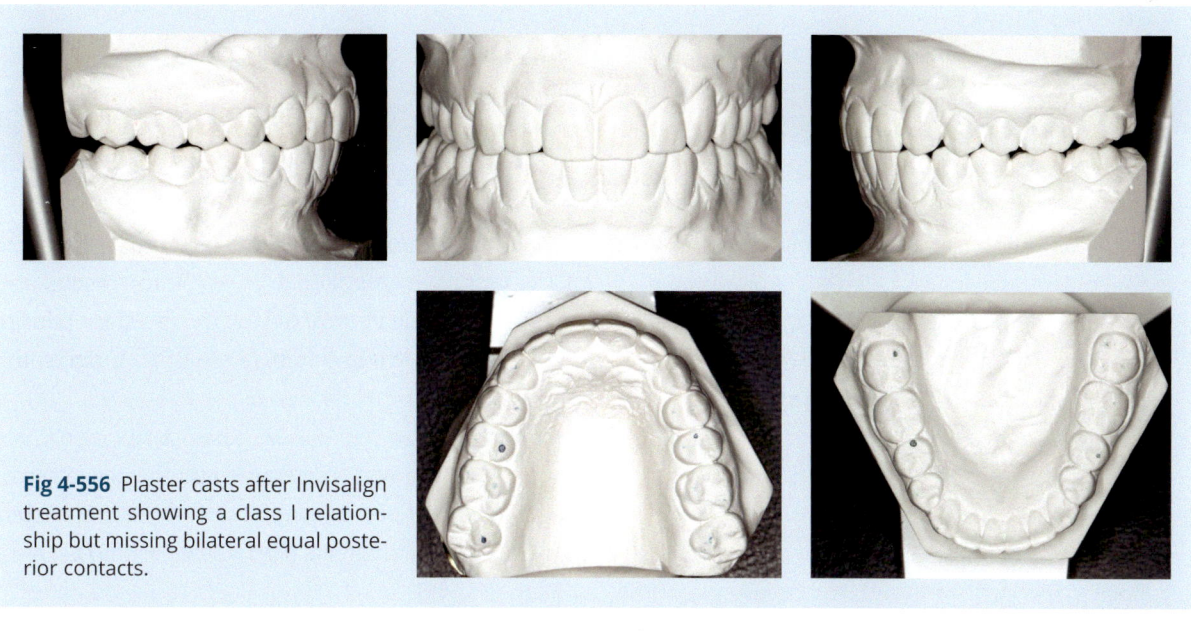

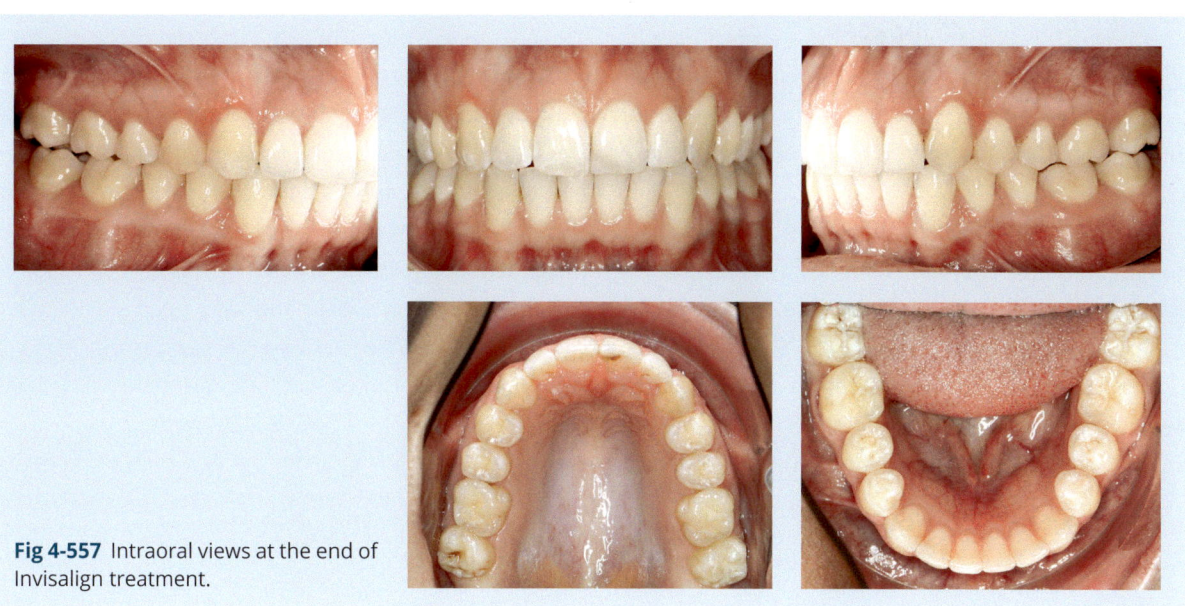

Initial diagnosis:
- class II relationship
- reclined maxillary incisors
- rotations and crowding
- excessive curve of Spee
- deep bite
- occlusal contacts on the left side, unilateral missing support.

Therapy:
- Invisalign treatment with class II elastics.

Treatment

Although Invisalign treatment achieved a class I relationship on both sides, there were missing bilateral equal posterior contacts. This was treated with selective grinding, which was tested first on the plaster casts.

Casts of Super Stone class IV were fabricated and mounted in relation to the cranium in an articulator (e.g. SAM). The first phase of selective grinding was performed on the plaster casts in three stages (Freesmeyer, 2009):

1. Analysis of cusps and fossa relationship to assess if grinding is appropriate
2. Grinding of teeth in static occlusion
3. Grinding of teeth in dynamic occlusion.

Grinding on the cast starts with the correction of the static occlusion. If incisor contacts start to develop with posterior grinding, it must be decided whether additional grinding of the anterior teeth is necessary to further reduce the vertical height of the occlusion. Alternatively, a refinement might be indicated to optimize the occlusion.

The goal of grinding in dynamic occlusion is to obtain an incisor–canine guidance with equal and simultaneous disocclusion of posterior teeth. The static occlusal contacts need to be maintained. The priority objective are the "routes of escape" on the non-supporting cusps. If there is interference on the mediotrusion side, grinding should be performed on the inner versants of the supporting cusps, always maintaining the static contacts. Interferences in protrusive movements can be eliminated in the direction of movement of the protrusion facets from posterior to anterior, until an incisor–canine guidance with equal and simultaneous disocclusion of posterior teeth is established. The ground contacts on the plaster casts can be marked with color to transfer the occlusal protocol more easily to the patient (Fig 4-558a,b). Grinding is continued to optimize the occlusion on the plaster casts.

If grinding on the plaster casts shows significant improvement in occlusal pattern and the possibility of obtaining static and dynamic occlusion without interference, grinding can be performed in the patient's mouth (Fig 4-559a,b). Occlusal contacts are marked with colored occlusal foil on the upright sitting patient. If contacts are identical with the ones on the mounted plaster casts, the grinding pattern is transferred onto the teeth. The final result of the grinding should be an equal occlusal pattern with contact points that hold Shimstock foil and a contact-free anterior relation (Figs 4-558 and 4-559). If the contact points seem to be slightly uneven in the two sides, this can be assessed again a few weeks later and may need slightly more grinding. Generally, settling of the molars leads to improved posterior contact points and this may simply resolve.

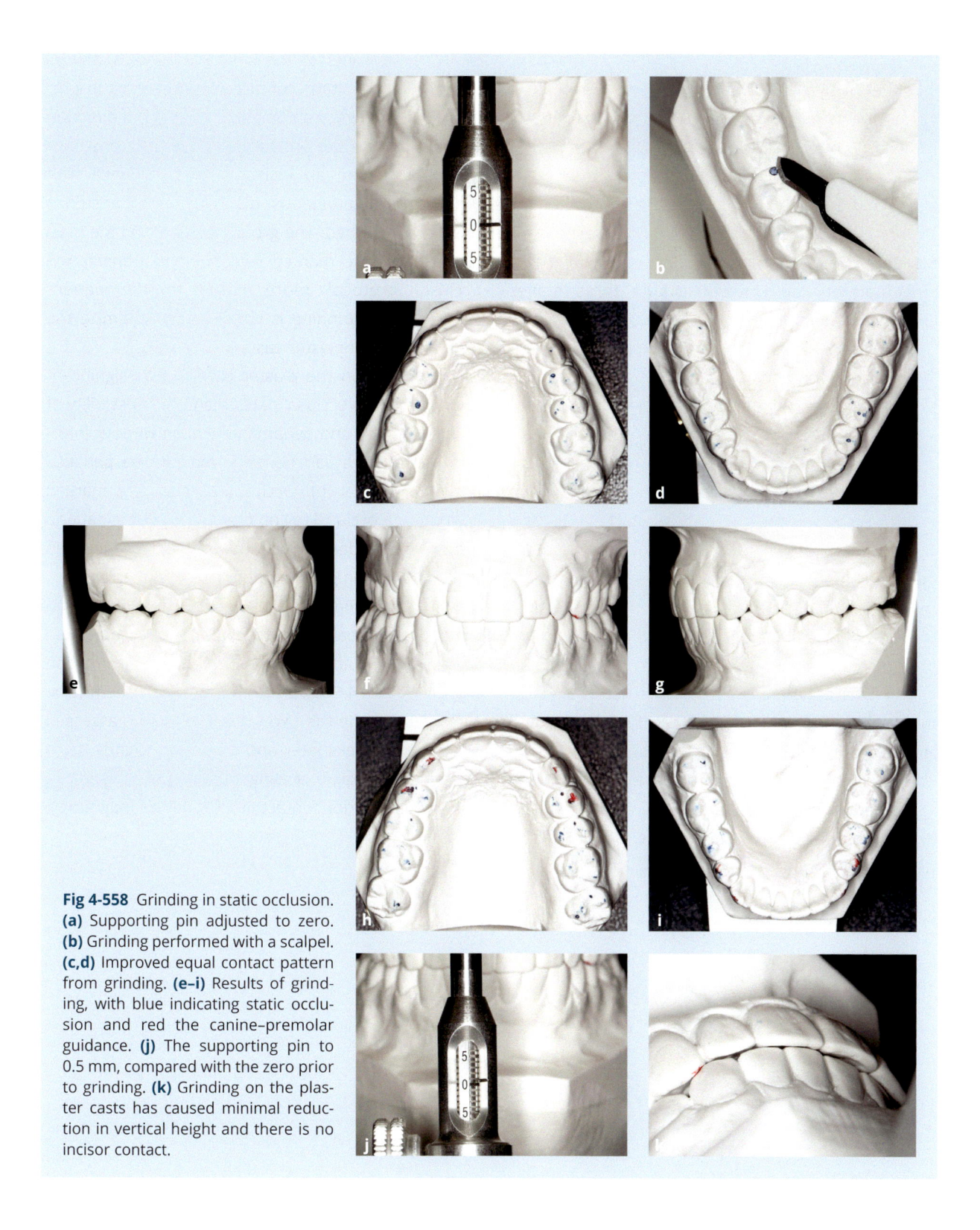

Fig 4-558 Grinding in static occlusion. **(a)** Supporting pin adjusted to zero. **(b)** Grinding performed with a scalpel. **(c,d)** Improved equal contact pattern from grinding. **(e–i)** Results of grinding, with blue indicating static occlusion and red the canine–premolar guidance. **(j)** The supporting pin to 0.5 mm, compared with the zero prior to grinding. **(k)** Grinding on the plaster casts has caused minimal reduction in vertical height and there is no incisor contact.

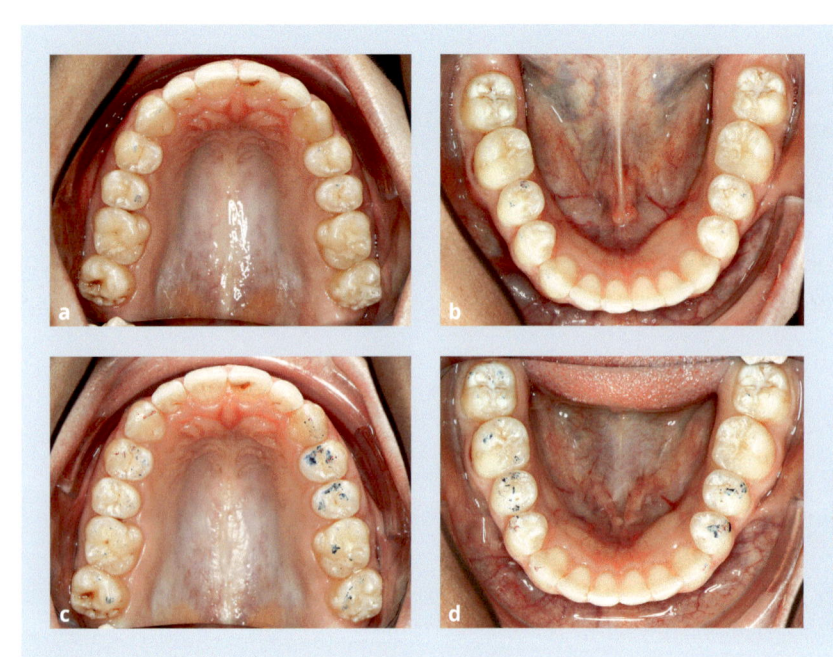

Fig 4-559 Grinding of teeth in the mouth. **(a,b)** Maxillary and mandibular contact points (blue) marked for grinding. **(c,d)** Bilateral supported occlusal pattern after grinding but contact points seem to be slightly heavier on the left and so will be assessed again after several weeks.

Topic 62
Retention after the Invisalign technique

Treatment:
- retainers after orthodontic therapy

Every orthodontic treatment needs subsequent retention, sometimes even lifelong retention. Retention after the Invisalign therapy does not differ from retention after fixed appliances. As Maurits Persson (2006) said, "cells remember force, not appliance."

Fig 4-560 Lingual retainer. **(a)** Golden twist wire (Goldenbraces) and transfer fixture (Orthocryl, Vertex). **(b)** The lingual retainer in the mouth bonded and built up with composite resin (Enamel Plus, Vanini) on teeth 34 to 44.

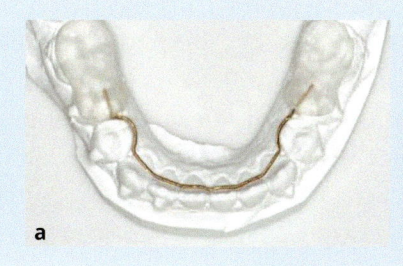

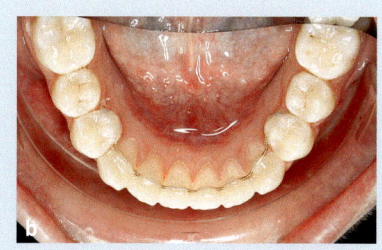

Treatment

When retaining the arch form with a lingual retainer, easy inset of the wire into the optimal position during the bonding process is achieved using a fabricated transfer fixture (Fig 4-560).

The bonding procedure requires sandblasting and etching of the tooth before application of bonding material (e.g. Optibond, Kerr 4). The lingual retainer is inserted with a floating composite resin (e.g. Tetric Evo-Flow, Ivoclar) on every tooth surface. The transfer caps are removed with a diamond burr and then the adhesive surfaces on each single tooth are built up with composite resin.

A well established concept of retention, particularly in adults who have had problems with their TMJs and/or ceramic crowns is the lingual retainer from canine to canine in the mandibular arch and a maxillary retention splint or milled splint (Fig 4-561, see also Topic 55).

The patient is advised to wear the last aligner or a Vivera retainer for 12 weeks, for a couple of hours in the day and the retention splints at night. Afterwards, the wearing time can be reduced step by step, most of the time ending with wearing of one of the two splints on alternate nights. In general, retention after Invisalign therapy does not differ from the retention after fixed appliances.

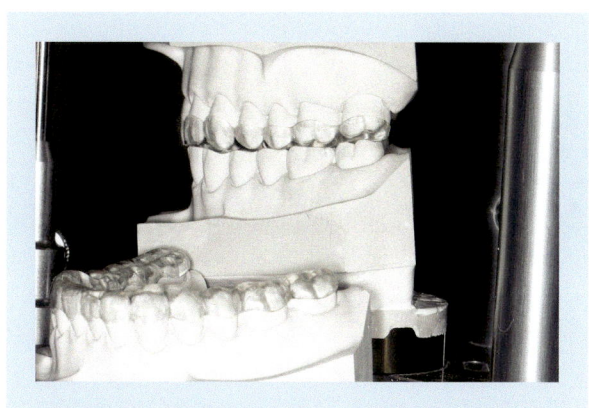

Fig 4-561 Maxillary and mandibular retention splints on plaster casts in the SAM articulator.

Topic 63
Scanning procedure with the iTero scanner

Treatment:
- scanning of the centric occlusion

The iTero system employs a parallel confocal imaging technique. An array of incident red laser light beams, passing through a focusing optics and a probing face, is shone on the teeth. The focusing optics defines one or more focal planes on the probing face in a position that can be changed by a motor. The beams generate illuminated spots on the structure and the intensity of returning light rays is measured at various positions of the focal plane, determining spot-specific positions (SSP) yielding maximum intensity of the reflected light beams. Data are generated that represent the three-dimensional structure of the teeth. This captures all structures and materials found in the mouth without the need to apply any reflective coating to the teeth. The SSP is always a relative position as the absolute position depends on the position of the sensing face. However, the generation of surface topology does not require knowledge of the absolute position, as all dimensions in the cubic field of view are absolute. By determining surface topologies of adjacent portions from two or more different angular locations and then combining such surface topologies, a complete three-dimensional representation of the entire structure may be obtained.

While the ability of the iTero camera to scan without the need for coating the teeth may be advantageous, it does require the inclusion of a color wheel into the acquisition unit; consequently, the camera has a larger scanner head than other systems (Fig 4-562). In fact, a two-dimensional color image of the three-dimensional structure of teeth is also taken at the same angle and orientation with respect to the structure. As a consequence, each x–y point on the two-dimensional image corresponds to a similar point on the three-dimensional scan having the same relative x–y values. The imaging process is based on illuminating the target surface with three differently colored illumination beams that in combinable provide white light; this captures a monochromatic image of the target portion of teeth, corresponding to each illuminating radiation, and combines the monochromatic images to create a full color image. The three differently colored illumination beams are provided by a white light source optically coupled with color filters. The filters are arranged on sectors of a rotatable disc coupled to a motor.

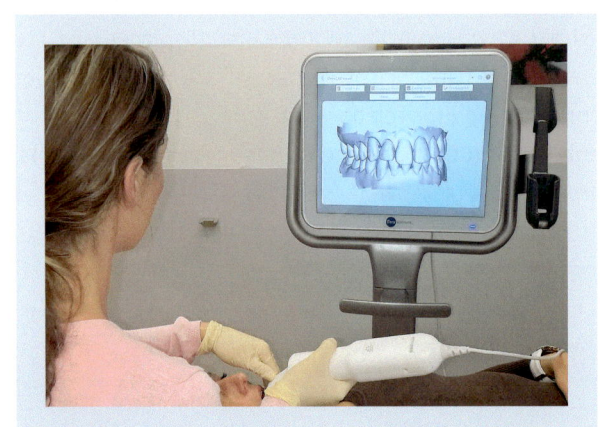

Fig 4-562a iTero element scanner during scanning procedure.

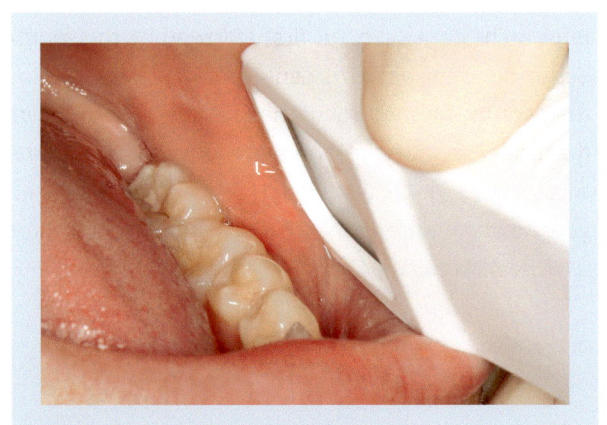

Fig 4-562b Detail of iTero element scanner head during intraoral scanning procedure.

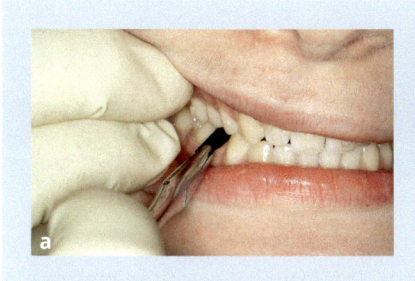

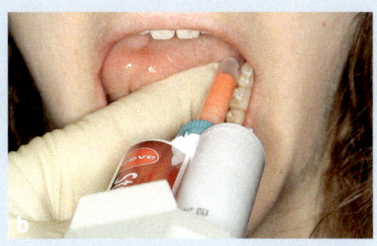

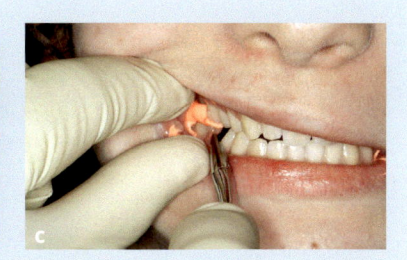

Fig 4-563 Scanning centric occlusion. **(a)** The first centric occlusal contact is determined with Shimstock foil in the upright sitting patient. **(b)** Silicone (StoneBite) is applied to the two teeth that do not have the first centric contact. **(c)** The patient occludes into the StoneBite, which fixes the first centric occlusal contact with Shimstock foil.

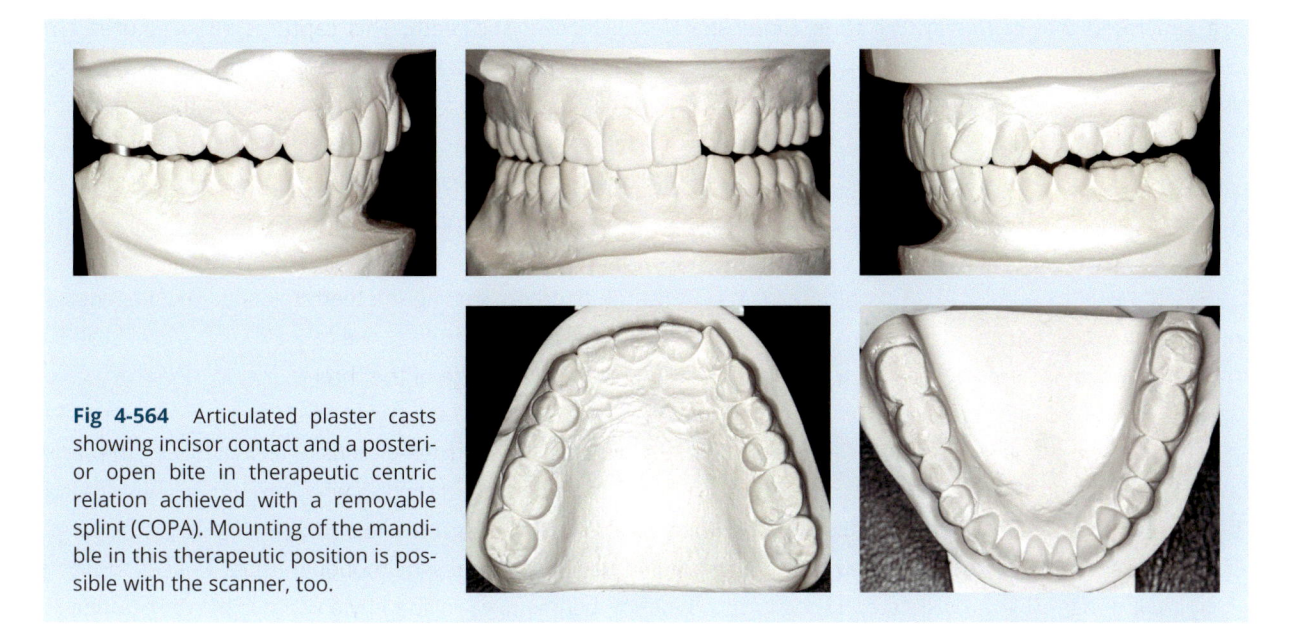

Fig 4-564 Articulated plaster casts showing incisor contact and a posterior open bite in therapeutic centric relation achieved with a removable splint (COPA). Mounting of the mandible in this therapeutic position is possible with the scanner, too.

Scanning procedure

Both arches are scanned first followed by the centric occlusion (Fig 4-563). The centric occlusion is fixed and then scanned anteriorly of the fixed bite position with the StoneBite material. The scanner mounts the lower to the upper arch accordingly in this position, thus guaranteeing direct transfer of the bite into the ClinCheck software.

In the example here, the articulated plaster casts show a patient with anterior disc displacement and neck pain with incisor contact and a posterior open bite; therapeutic relation was achieved with a removable splint (COPA), as shown in the articulated plaster models in Figures 4-564 and 4-565.

Fig 4-565 Articulated plaster casts showing occlusal points (black) on teeth 12, 11, 21, and 24, and on 31, 41, 42, and 34 in centric relationship after the treatment with the removable splint (COPA).

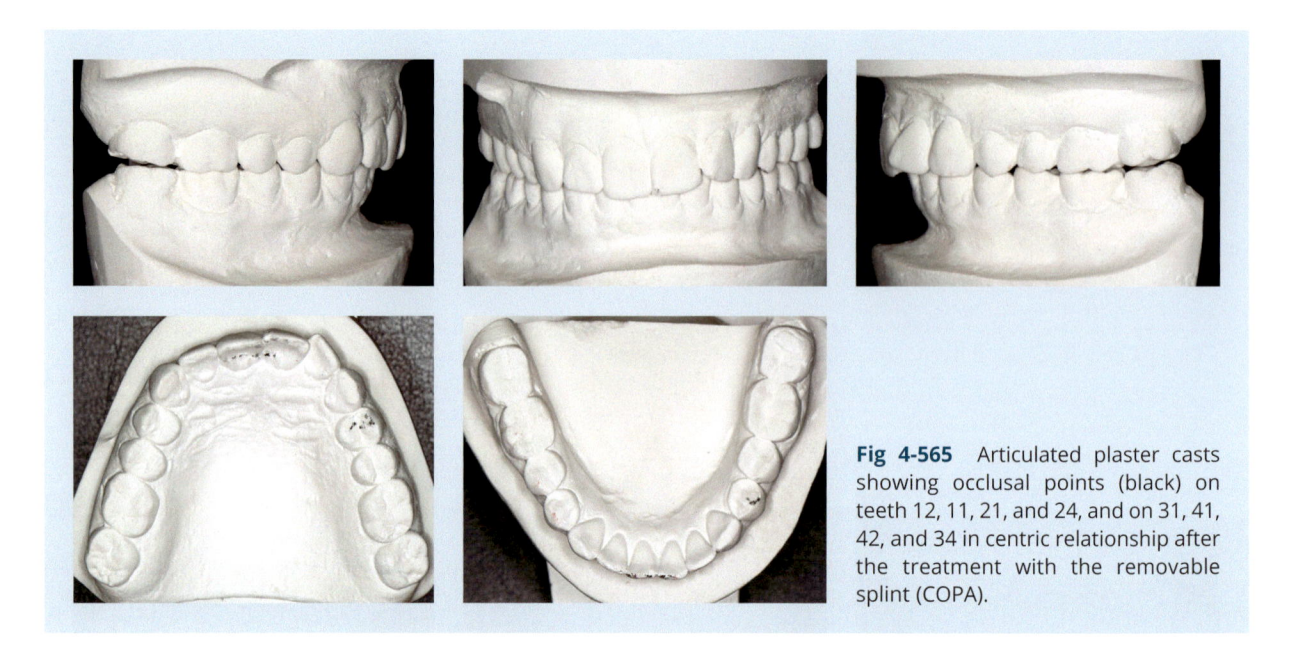

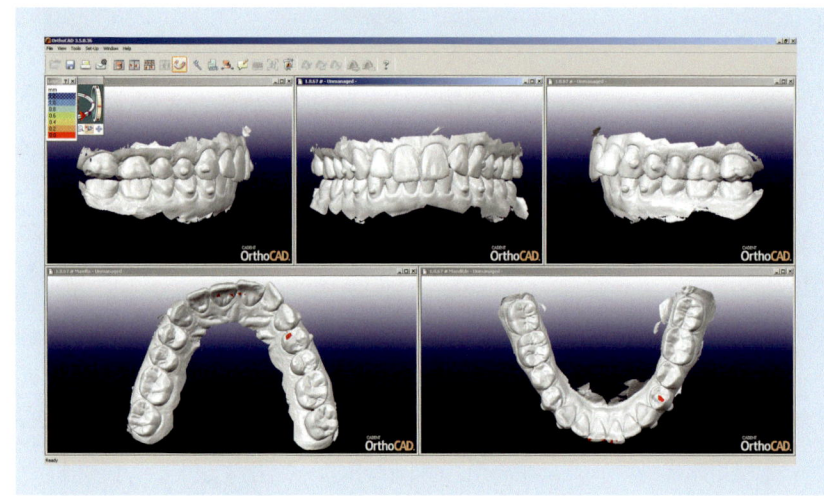

Fig 4-566 Scan taken in centric relation. Contact points (red) are seen on teeth 12, 11, 21, and 24, and 31, 41, and 42, which matches exactly those on the casts.

The intraoral situation can then be scanned with iTero (Fig 4-566). The scans including the contact points and therefore the exact occlusal relationship can be transferred into the ClinCheck software (Fig 4-567), allowing planning of the Invisalign treatment.

Based on the mantra that "centric needs time to develop," now the Invisalign treatment can be planned in the exact centric position. The use of the removable splint to adjust the mouth into therapeutic centric relation will also help to achieve a pain-free state.

This scanning approach helps in ensuring maximum precision when transferring information on the exact occlusion into the ClinCheck software, and thence into the Invisalign treatment. Once the ClinCheck software has a virtual articulator tool, this precision might even improve. The future of dentistry is digital (Figs 4-568 to 4-581).

TREATMENT OF DIFFERENT MALOCCLUSIONS WITH ALIGNERS 4

Fig 4-567 Scanned situation transferred into the ClinCheck software.

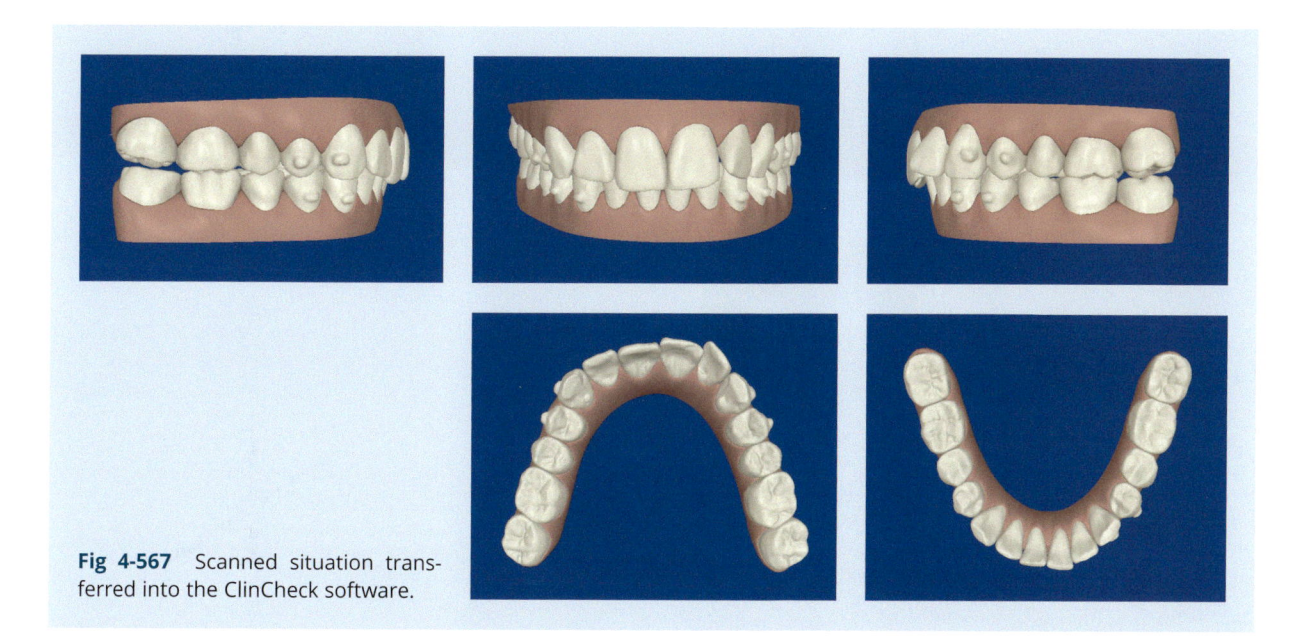

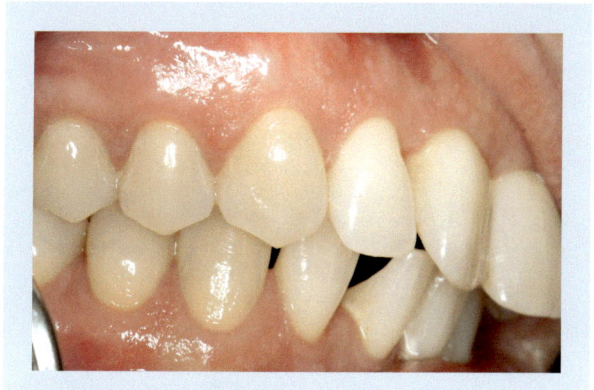

Fig 4-568 Initial situation with planned extraction of tooth 14.

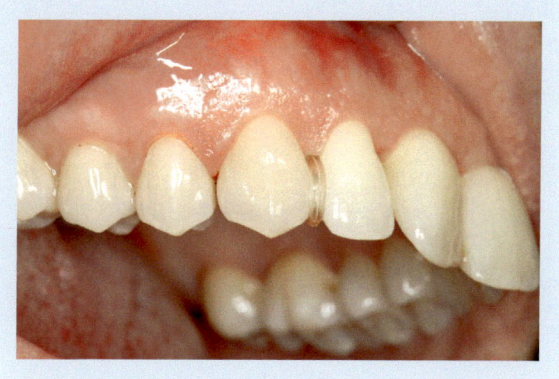

Fig 4-569 The preparation prior to the scanning procedure included IPR mesial of tooth 14 of 1,5mm followed by insertion of an alastic mesial of tooth 13.

A precise impression, but especially the intraoral scan allows an exact representation of interproximal spaces. Our course of the extraction treatment is based on this fact. The following example will show this procedure within the planning of the extraction of tooth 14 (Fig 4-568).

The tooth movement with aligners is performed in the most precise manner in cases when the aligner can cover and grip the tooth completely. This is why we start this treatment by "exposing" the canine mesially and distally prior to the scan procedure or alternatively the impressions (Figs 4-569 to 4-571). The course of treatment shows the good axial position of tooth 13 during the posterior movement into the extraction space with perfect aligner fitting. The patient is currently wearing aligner 32, total treatment will be finished with planned 53 aligners (Figs 4-572 to 4-579).

345

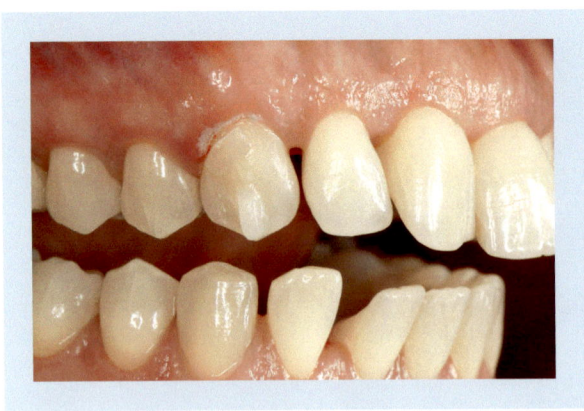

4 TREATMENT OF DIFFERENT MALOCCLUSIONS WITH ALIGNERS

Fig 4-570 The alastic was removed after 3 days, leading to a posterior movement of tooth 13 with opening of space mesially, allowing the future aligner to capture tooth 13 perfectly.

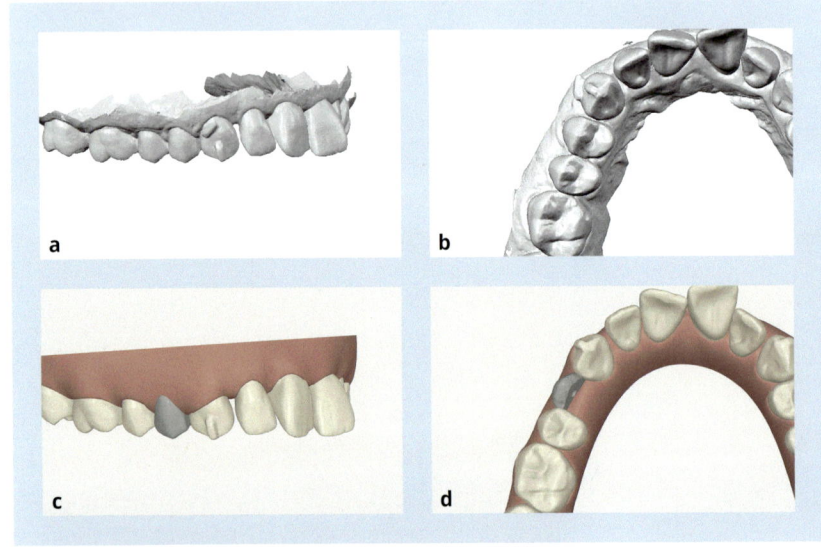

Fig 4-571 Scan **(a, b)** and Clincheck Software **(c, d)** demonstrating space mesial of tooth 13 due to elastic force and distal due to IPR according to intraoral situation

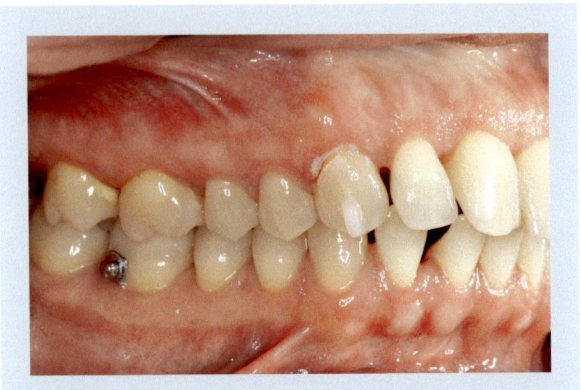

Fig 4-572 With aligner 3 the space distal of tooth 13 was closed and tooth 14 was advised for extraction to the dentist. The patient was using class II elastics for anchorage.

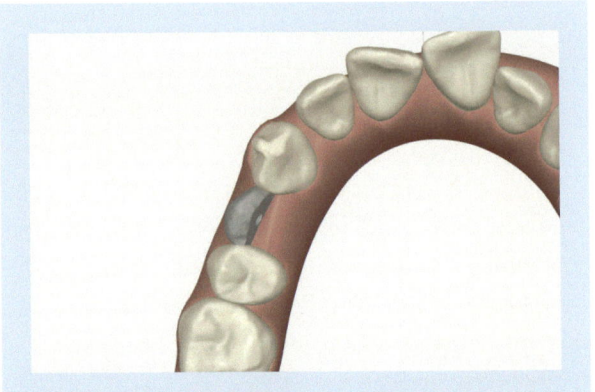

Fig 4-573 ClinCheck Situation with aligner 3: extraction of tooth 14 was virtually performed and a pontic added in the aligner. Tooth 13 had moved to contact of tooth 14 with the first three aligners.

TREATMENT OF DIFFERENT MALOCCLUSIONS WITH ALIGNERS 4

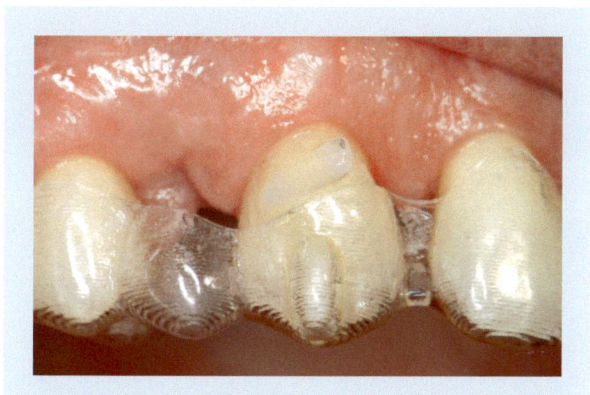

Fig 4-574 Situation with aligner 11 in situ: tooth 13 is distalized slightly more with increased space to tooth 12, the aligner captures the tooth precisely.

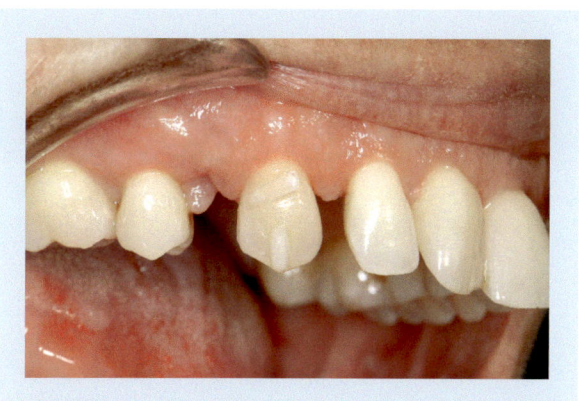

Fig 4-575 Intraoral situation with aligner 11, showing good axial root position of tooth 13

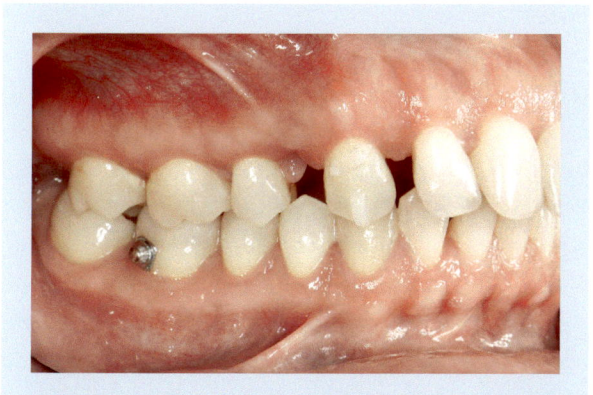

Fig 4-576 Intraoral situation with aligner 11, showing the occlusal relationship

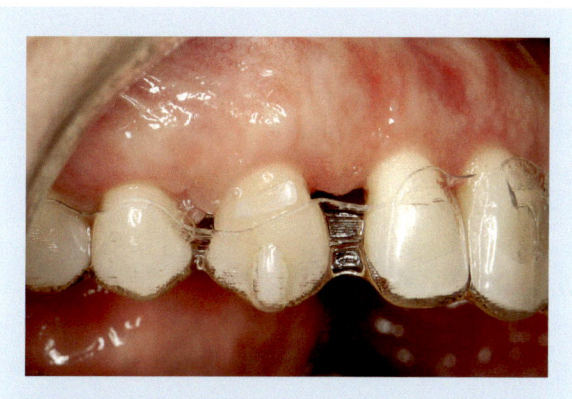

Fig 4-577 Intraoral situation with aligner 22 in situ, again the aligner shows perfect fitting of tooth 13

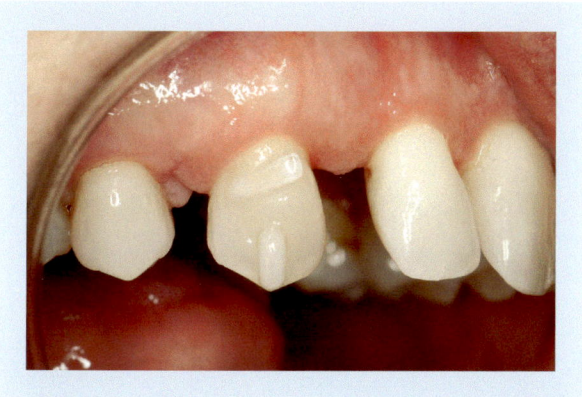

Fig 4-578 Intraoral situation without aligner 22, showing the bodily movement of tooth 13 into the extraction space.

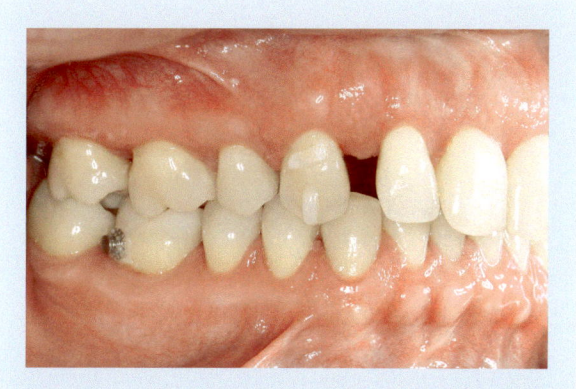

Fig 4-579 Intraoral situation at the stage of aligner 32, showing the occlusal relationship. The change of the aligner was performed every 10 days.

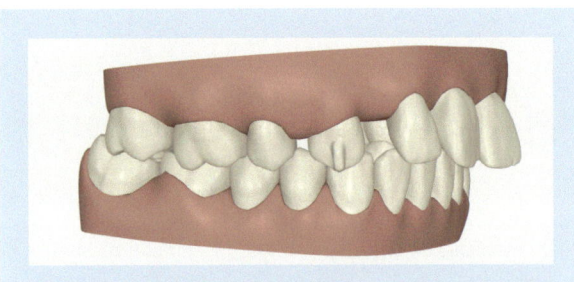

Fig 4-580 ClinCheck Situation with aligner 22, showing spaces mesial and distal of tooth 13 according to the shown intraoral situation.

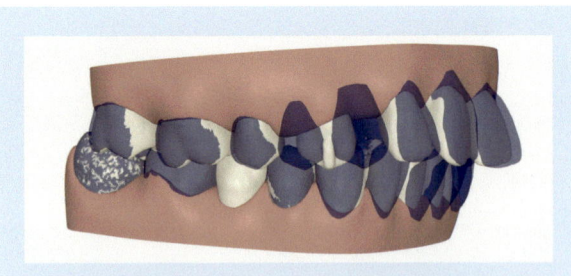

Fig 4-581 ClinCheck superimposition with aligner 22, showing the amount of already performed tooth movement (blue color = initial situation, white color = planned tooth position).

The nature of malocclusion that requires first premolar tooth extraction is an orthodontic problem that affects more than 50% of patients in Asia, 20% in Europe, and 12% in North America (Soh J et al). Invisalign G6 for first premolar extraction is the culmination of continuous clinical innovation at Align offering comprehensive features and functionality, engineered to improve clinical outcomes for orthodontic treatment of severe crowding and bimaxillary protrusion. Align's first premolar extraction solution provides vertical control and root parallelism using new SmartStage technology and SmartForce features that optimize the progression of tooth movements for first premolar extraction treatment planned for maximum anchorage. The SmartStage technology is programmed to optimize the progression of tooth movements and provide aligner activation, engineered to eliminate unwanted tipping and unwanted anterior extrusion during retraction, while the new SmartForce features are designed to deliver the force systems necessary to achieve predictable tooth movements. These new features include Optimized Retraction Attachments, designed to work with SmartStage technology for effective bodily movement during canine retraction, with or without elastics, and new Optimized Anchorage Attachments, designed to work with SmartStage technology to maximize posterior anchorage (announced by Align Technology in November 2014). Results with the new features have been developed and demonstrated lately by Dr H Samoto and Dr V Vlaskalic.

References

Aquilio C. Presentation at the 2013 Invisalign European Summit, Rome, 23–26 May 2013.

Barrer HG. Protecting the integrity of mandibular incisor position through keystoning procedure and spring retainer appliance. J Clin Orthod. 1975;9:486–494.

Castroflorio T, Garino F, Lazzaro A, Debernardi C. Upper-incisor root control with Invisalign appliances. J Clin Orthod 2013;47:346–351.

Dizidienda G. Vermessung und vergleichende Untersuchung der Gelenkspaltbreite von physiologischen und pathologischen Kiefergelenken mittels digitaler Volumentomographie. Dip Med, University Clinic of Innsbruck, 2011.

Fillion D. Zur approximalen Schmelzreduktion in der Erwachsenenkieferorthopädie. Teil 2: Vor- und Nachteile der approximalenSchmelzreduktion. Inf Orthod Kieferorthop 1995;27:64–90.

Freesmeyer W. Quintessenz Focus Zahnmedizin. Funktionsdiagnostik und –therapie. Berlin: Quintessenz, 2009.

Gautschi R. Manuelle Triggerpunkt-Therapie. Stuttgart: Thieme, 2010.

Gelb H (ed). New Concepts in Craniomandibular and Chronic Pain Management. St Louis, MO: Mosby-Wolfe, 1994.

Ioi H, Nakata A. Counts AL. Comparison of the influences of buccal corridors on smile esthetics between Koreans and Japanese. Ortho Waves 2009;68:166–170.

Jarjoura K, Gagnon G, Nieberg L. Caries risk after interproximal enamel reduction. Am J Orthod Dentofac Orthoped 2006;130:26–30.

Jing Y, Han X, Guo Y, et al. Nonsurgical correction of a class III malocclusion in an adult by miniscrew-assisted mandibular dentition distalization. Am J Orthod Dentofacial Orthop 2013;143:877–887.

Knak S. Praxisleitfaden Kieferothopädie. Munich: Urban & Fischer, 2004.

Lin JCY, Liou JWJ, Bowman SJ. Simultaneous reduction in vertical dimension and gummy smile using miniscrew anchorage. J Clin Orthod 2010;44:157–170.

Lin JC, Tsai SJ, Liou EJ, Bowman SJ. Treatment of challenging malocclusions with Invisalign and miniscrew anchorage. J Clin Orthod 2014;48:23–36.

Masella RS, Meister M. Current concepts in the biology of orthodontic tooth movement. Am J Orthod Dentofacial Orthop 2006;129:458–468.

Melsen B, Verna C, Luzi C. Mini-implants and their Clinical Applications: The Aarhus Experience. Bologne: Edizioni Martina, 2014.

Meyer G, Asselmeyer T (eds). ABC der Schienenterhapie. Cologne: Deutscher Zahnärzteverlag, 2005.

Meyer, HP. Myofascial pain syndrome and its suggested role in the pathogenesis and treatment of fibromyalgia syndrome. Curr Pain Headache Rep 2002;6(4):274–283.

Mosetter K, Mosetter R. Myoreflextherapie: Muskelfunktion und Schmerz. Konstanz: Vesalius, 2006.

Nakao K, Goto T, Gunjigake KK, Konoo T, Kobayashi S, Yamaguchi K. Intermittent force induces high RANKL expression in human periodontal ligament cells. J Dent Res 2007;86:623–628.

Persson M. Presentation at the Warsaw Congress, Polish Orthodontic Society, 28.09-01.10.2006.

Ricketts RM. Bioprogressive therapy as an answer to orthodontic needs. Part II. Am J Orthod 1976;70:359–397.

Samoto H, Vlaskalic V. A customized staging procedure to improve the predictability of space closure with sequential aligners. J Clin Orthod 2014 Jun;48(6):359-367.

Soh J et al. Occlusal Status in Asian Male. Angle Orthod 2005;75(5):814-820.

Wiegelmann S, Bernhardt O, Meyer G. The associations between occlusal parameters in static and dynamic occlusion and the signs and symptoms of craniomandibular disorders. Zeitschr Kraniomand Funkt 2015;7(1):27–38.

Yamaguchi, M, Inami T, Ito K, Kasai K, Tanimoto Y. Mini-implants in the anchorage armamentarium: new paradigms in the orthodontics. Int J Biomater 2012; 2012:394121

Yang, C. et al New arthroscopic disc repositioning and suturing technique for treating an anteriorly displaced disc of the temporomandibular joint: part 1 - technique introduction. Int J Oral Maxillofac Surg 2012:41:1058–1063

Yasuda H. Bone and bone related biochemical examinations. Bone and collagen related metabolites. Receptor activator of NF-kappaB ligand (RANKL). Clin Calcium 2006;16:964–1970.

Zachrisson BU. Tooth movements in the periodontally compromised patient. In: Lindhe J, Lang NP, Karring T (eds) Clinical Periodontology and Implant Dentistry. Oxford: Wiley-Blackwell, 2008:1241–1279.

Zachrisson BU, Minster L, Ogaard B, Birkhed D. Dental health assessed after interproximal enamel reduction: caries risk in posterior teeth. Am J Orthod Dentofacial Orthop 2011;139:90–8.

Zheng X. Use of interproximal enamel reduction in adult malocclusion patients with periodontitis. Shanghai Kou Qiang Yi Xue 2010;19:485–489.

ADVANTAGES OF THE INVISALIGN SYSTEM   5

Treatment with aligners requires patient compliance and it is important to make this clear to the patient and parents at the very start of discussing orthodontic treatment. However, aligner therapy does have a number of advantages compared with fixed multibracket appliances. These are listed here and then discussed in more detail.

- Virtual treatment planning
    - interdisciplinary coordination
    - more predictable end result
- Easier to maintain oral and periodontal health during treatment
    - aligner can be removed for eating and teeth cleaning
    - no brackets, bands, or wires to interfere with continuing periodontal treatment
- Reduced risk of decalcification and decay
    - aligner can be removed for teeth cleaning
    - no brackets, bands, or wires, which can create an enviroment for decalcification and decay
- Few or no complications during aligner therapy
    - few or no emergencies
    - minimal or no mucosa defects
    - minimal or no inflammation
    - no enamel abrasion
    - no allergic reactions
- Force can be adjusted
    - light and intermitted force possible (less risk of root resorptions)
    - decrease in staging can minimize forces
    - interproximal enamel reduction (IPR) can be calculated before treatment starts
- Less pain with treatment
    - less pain with changing an aligner than with changing a wire
    - less discomfort with debonding of attachments
- Reduced blocking of the maxilla
    - no osteopathic side effects
- Compliance is assisted because daily activities can continue
    - no metal components to be a risk in sporting activities
    - playing musical instruments can continue

ADVANTAGES OF THE INVISALIGN SYSTEM 5

Virtual treatment planning

- interdisciplinary coordination
- more predictable end result

Backward planning, beginning with the end in mind, is a core feature of the Invisalign technique. The virtually planned treatment outcome in the ClinCheck software can be discussed by all who will be involved in treatment. This is particularly important in patients who need restorative dentistry or implants after orthodontics. The interdisciplinary team can discuss the Invisalign treatment outcome and, therefore, the basis that will be available for subsequent prothetics (Fig 5-1).

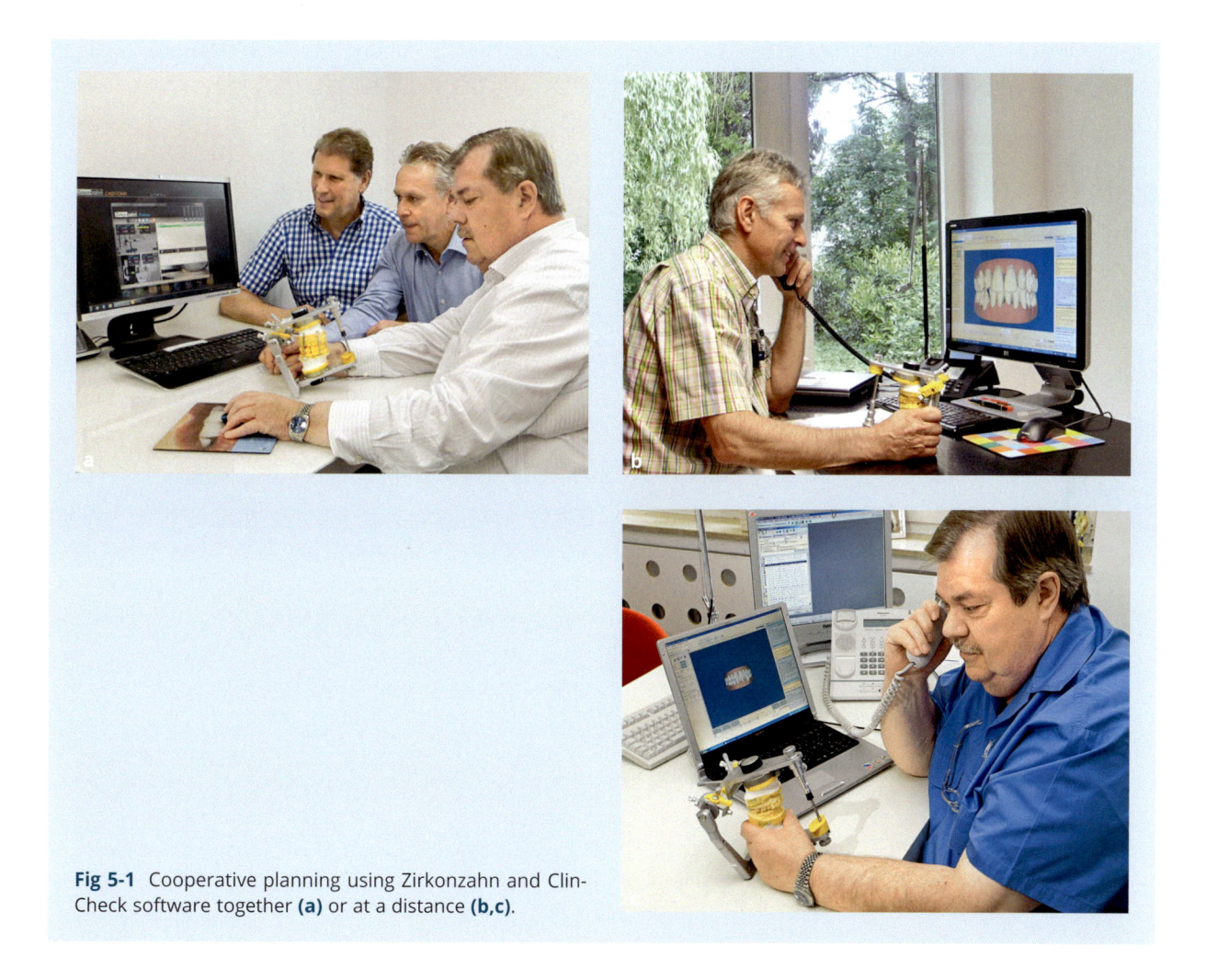

Fig 5-1 Cooperative planning using Zirkonzahn and ClinCheck software together **(a)** or at a distance **(b,c)**.

5 ADVANTAGES OF THE INVISALIGN SYSTEM

Easier to maintain oral and periodontal health during treatment

Advantages:
- aligner can be removed for eating and teeth cleaning
- no brackets, bands, or wires to interfere with continuing periodontal treatment

As aligners can be removed for tooth cleaning, it is easier for the patient to maintain oral health during treatment with the Invisalign system than with fixed orthodontic appliances (Miethke and Vogt, 2005) (Fig 5-2).

Conclusion

Periodontal health is not jeopardized during Invisalign therapy even though aligners cover all the teeth and part of the keratinized gingiva. This may be because aligners are removable and so allow unimpeded oral hygiene.

Reduced risk of decalcification and decay

Advantages:
- aligner can be removed for teeth cleaning
- no brackets, bands, or wires, which can create an enviroment for decalcification and decay

One of the potential side effects with fixed orthodontic appliances is the occurrent of decalcifications and periodontal lesions under brackets (Mattousch et al, 2007) (Fig 5-3; see also Topic 57). White spot lesions developed during orthodontic treatment have very limited ability to improve after appliance removal. On average, 40% of surfaces in males and 22% in females showed white spots after treatment with fixed appliances ($P < 0.01$) (Boersma et al, 2005; Lovrov et al, 2007).

Conclusions

Despite improvements in materials and preventive efforts, fixed orthodontic treatment continues to carry considerable risk of enamel demineralization. Each patient's prophylactic efforts, including fluoride use, are of paramount importance in preventing white spot lesions. Use of a technique that makes this prophylaxis easier reduces unwanted effects.

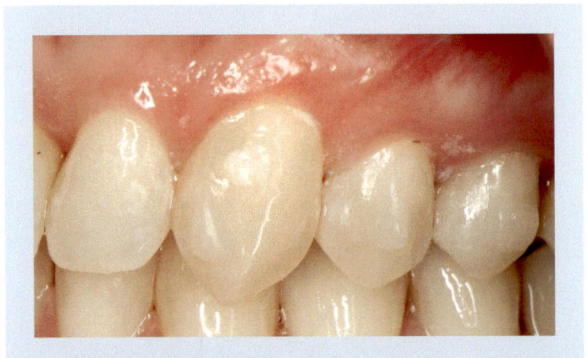

Fig 5-2 A patient during aligner treatment with G4 attachments on teeth 23, 24, and 25.

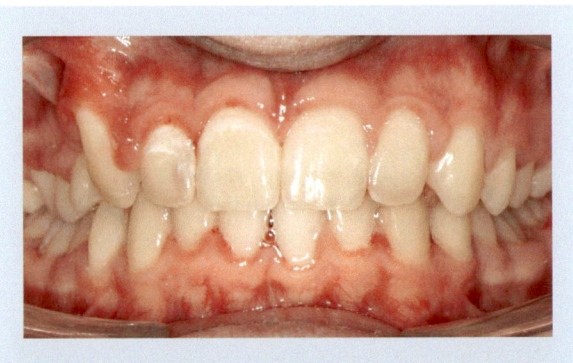

Fig 5-3 Decalcification and periodontal lesions (situation immediately after debonding of brackets).

Few or no complications during aligner therapy

Advantages:
- few or no emergencies
- minimal or no mucosa defects
- minimal or no inflammation
- no enamel abrasion
- no allergic reactions

As Invisalign therapy does not use metal components, it avoids the problems that can arise from abrasion and metal content (Fig 5-4). As there is no bracket contact, there is no need for bite ramps. One study, although with limitations, suggested that gingival overgrowth induced by orthodontic treatment could be linked to a low dose of nickel released to the epithelium from metal appliances (Sokucu et al, 2007). A study of eluents from aligner material showed no evidence of cytotoxicity or estrogenicity in vitro (Eliades et al, 2009).

Conclusions

The use of Invisalign appliances did not seem to have adverse effects from the physical position or from the materials of the aligners.

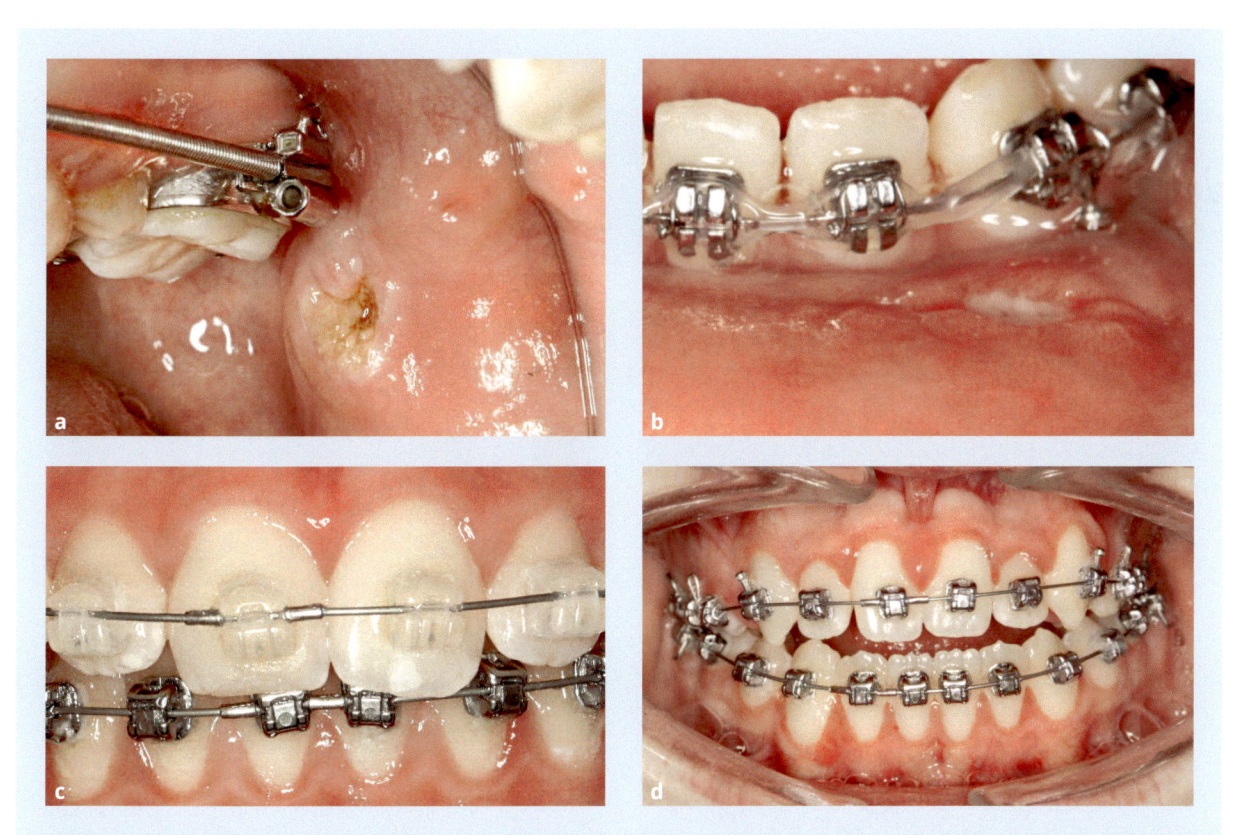

Fig 5-4 Complications with fixed appliances. **(a,b)** Mucosa defects; **(c)** enamel abrasion; **(d)** gingival inflammation.

Force can be adjusted

Advantages:
- light and intermitted force possible leading to less risk of root resorptions
- decrease in staging can minimize forces
- IPR can be calculated before the treatment starts

The ClinCheck software enables proposed IPR and force systems to be assessed before implementation (Fig 5-5). If needed, aligner staging can be slowed and more aligners can be used. Initial tooth movement benefit from light forces. Heavier forces tend to increase the rate and the amount of canine retraction but lose their advantage because of unwanted clinical side effects (Yee et al, 2009). Similarly, there appear to be advantages from using intermittent orthodontic forces in terms of reducing root resorption. A study of the use of intermittent or continuous orthodontic forces showed that osteoclast numbers in the intermittent force group were 100.5% of the continuous force group at mesial sites, and osteoclast surfaces in the intermittent force group were 68.2% of those in the continuous force group. At the mesial sites, root resorption in the intermittent force group was approximately 30.0% of that in the continuous force group ($P < 0.01$) (Kumasako-Haga et al, 2009; see also Chapter 3 and Topic 8 in Chapter 4).

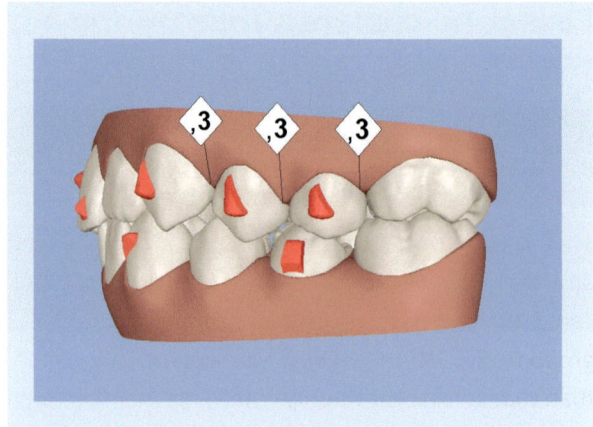

Fig 5-5 ClinCheck image showing IPR and attachments.

Conclusions

The potential for adjustment of force magnitude, duration, and consistency with the Invisalign system may help in avoiding unwanted tooth movements.

Reduced blocking of the maxilla

Advantages:
- no osteopathic side effects

Paired cranial bones such as the maxilla show a symmetrical movement in terms of internal and external rotation around their suture (Fig 5-6). All the bones of the cranium are linked by sutures that allow some transmission of movements. Motion patterns between cranium and sacrum can be thought of as a "closed kinematic chain," where movement of one bone affects another. If movement is blocked at one place over a long period, this can affect other bones and the effect of the blockage can continue even when the stimulus is removed. Although such dysfunction can be treated osteopathically, it is better to avoid its emergence in the first place. Consequently, any orthodontic blocking of the maxilla should be avoided.

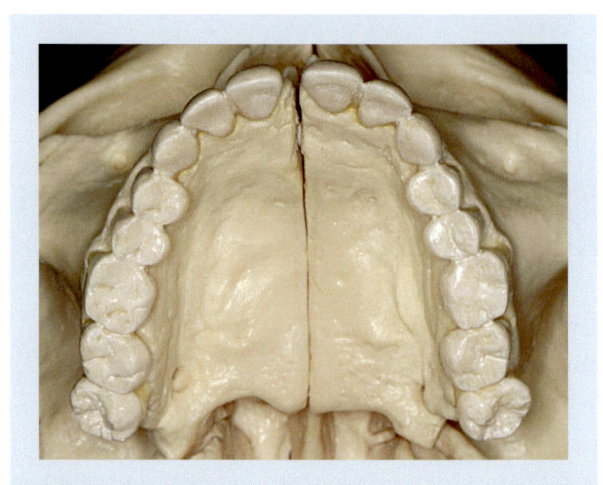

Fig 5-6 The maxilla with its suture.

Conclusion

Use of aligners avoids a rigid structure across the whole of the palate with the potential knock-on effects.

Less pain with treatment

Advantages:
- less pain with changing an aligner than with changing a wire
- less discomfort with debonding of attachments

A study of pain intensity in the first week following the application of light and heavy continuous forces indicated that biting pain in the heavy-force (200 cN) group from 6 hours to 4 days was significantly greater than that at force initiation ($P < 0.05$). It was also rated using a visual analog scale as greater than that assessed by patients in a light-force group (20 cN) ($P < 0.05$) (Ogura et al, 2009).

Conclusion
The Invisalign system, by offering the option of reducing heavy forces, can be advantageous in reducing pain in treatment.

Compliance is assisted because daily activities can continue

Advantages:
- no metal components to be a risk in sporting activities
- playing musical instruments can continue

Compliance is a major factor in the success of orthodontic treatment, and this has been a significant factor in the use of fixed appliances. The aligners of the Invisalign system, by allowing daily activities such as sport and playing wind instruments to continue are ideal, particularly for teenagers.

Easier to treat patients with enamel hypoplasia

Advantages:
- easier to treat patients with enamel hypoplasia

In patients with existing hypoplasia, particularly of posterior teeth, insertion of brackets can lead to problems with changes of the tooth surface and tooth material (Fig 5-7).

Conclusion
The Invisalign system offers the possibility to treat even patients with enamel hypoplasia without the difficulty of bonding brackets or bands.

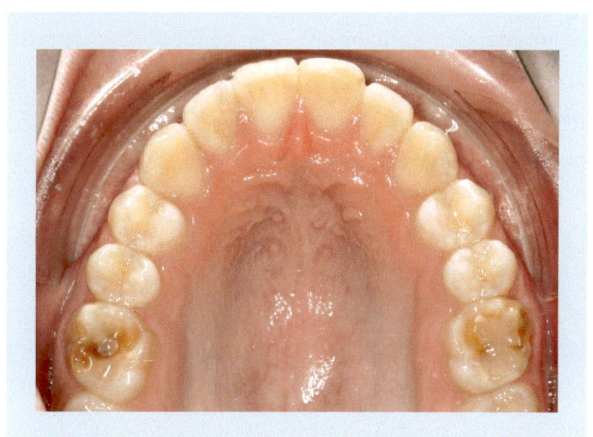

Fig 5-7 Hypoplasia of upper first molars.

References

Boersma JG, van der Veen MH, Lagerweij MD, Bokhout B, Prahl-Andersen B. Caries prevalence measured with QLF after treatment with fixed orthodontic appliances: influencing factors. Caries Res 2005;39:41–47.

Eliades T, Pratsinis H, Athanasiou AE, Eliades G, Kletsas D. Cytotoxicity and estrogenicity of Invisalign appliances. Am J Orthod Dentofacial Orthop 2009;36:100–103.

Gursoy UK, Sokucu O, Uitto VJ, et al. The role of nickel accumulation and epithelial cell proliferation in orthodontic treatment-induced gingival overgrowth. Eur J Orthod 2007;29:555–558.

Kumasako-Haga T, Konoo T, Yamaguchi K, Hayashi H. Effect of 8-hour intermittent orthodontic force on osteoclasts and root resorption. Am J Orthod Dentofacial Orthop 2009;135:278; discussion 278–279.

Lovrov, K, Hertrich K, Hirschfelder U. Enamel demineralization during fixed orthodontic treatment: incidence and correlation to various oral-hygiene parameters. J Orofac Orthop 2007;68:353–563.

Mattousch TJ, van der Veen MH, Zentner A. Caries lesions after orthodontic treatment followed by quantitative light-induced fluorescence: a 2-year follow-up. Eur J Orthod 2007;29(3):294–298.

Miethke RR, Vogt S. A comparison of the periodontal health of patients during treatment with the Invisalign system and with fixed orthodontic appliances. J Orofac Orthop 2005;66:219–229.

Ogura M, Kamimura H, Al-Kalaly A, et al. Pain intensity during the first 7 days following the application of light and heavy continuous forces. Eur J Orthod 2009;31:314–319.

Yee JA, Türk T, Elekdağ-Türk S, Cheng LL, Darendeliler MA. Rate of tooth movement under heavy and light continuous orthodontic forces. Am J Orthod Dentofacial Orthop 2009;136:150; discussion 150–151.

Further reading

Experience with the Invisalign system has increased rapidly in recent years, leading to increasing numbers of publications. It was not the aim of this book to give a full overview of these references. However, some references have been specifically cited in the chapters and listed at the end of each. Here a few further references of interest given for Invisalign and related orthodontic therapies.

Ali SA, Miethke HR. Invisalign, an innovative invisible orthodontic appliance to correct malocclusions: advantages and limitations. Dent Update 2012;39:254–256, 258–260.

Boisserée W, Schupp W. Two-stage approach to mandibular splint therapy with craniomandibular orthopedic positioning appliances. Zeitschr Kraniomand Funkt 2012;4(1):79-94.

Boyd RL. Esthetic orthodontic treatment using the invisalign appliance for moderate to complex malocclusions. J Dent Educ 2008;72:948–967.

Garino F, Garino GB, Castroflorio T. The iTero intraoral scanner in Invisalign treatment: a two-year report. J Clin Orthod 2014;48:98–106.

Giancotti A, Farina A. Treatment of collapsed arches using the Invisalign System. JCO 2010;44,7:416-25

Guarneri MP, Gracco A, Siciliani G. Trattamento estetico di due casi clinici con metodica Invisalign. Mondo Ortodontico 2010:35(2);95-105

Gracco A, Mazzoli A, Favoni O, et al. Short-term chemical and physical changes in invisalign appliances. Aust Orthod J 2009;25:34–40.

Haubrich, J. Die Invisalign-Behandlung als Bestandteil interdisziplinärer Therapie – Möglichkeiten und Grenzen des Systems. ZWR- Das Deutsche Zahnärzteblatt 2013;122: 372–376.

Haubrich J, Schupp W. Optimierung dentofazialer Ästhetik. KN 2015;4:1-8.

Haubrich J, Schupp, W. Die unsichtbare Zahnspange. Teamwork 2005;5:59–69.

Hönn M, Göz GA. premolar extraction case using the Invisalign system. J Orofac Orthop 2006;67:385–394.

Krieger E, Seiferth J, Marinello I, Jung BA, Wriedt S, Jacobs C, Wehrbein H. Invisalign treatment in the anterior region. J Orofac Orthoped 2012;73:1-12

Li S, Zhou J, Ren C. Adult orthodontic technique development and challenge. Hua Xi Kou Qiang Yi Xue Za Zhi 2013;31:449–451.

Mampieri G, Giancotti A. Invisalign technique in the treatment of adults with pre-restorative concerns. Prog Orthod 2013;20:40.

Mehta J. An interview with Dr. Harold Gelb, part II. Funct Orthod 1987;4:18–24.

Neumann I, Schupp W, Heine G. Distalbewegung oberer 1. Molaren mit dem Invisalign-System – Ein Patientenbericht. Kieferorthopädie 2004;2:133–137.

Miller KB, McGorray SP, Womack R, Quintero JC, Perelmuter M, Gibson J, Dolan TA, Wheeler TT. A comparison of treatment impacts between Invisalign aligner and fixed appliance therapy during the first week of treatment. Am J Orthod Dentofacial Orthop 2007;131(3):302.e1-9.

Ojima K, Dan C, Nishiyama R, Ohtsuka S, Schupp W. Accelerated extraction treatment with Invisalign. J Clin Orthod 2014;48:487–499.

Premaraj T, Simet S, Beatty M, Premaraj S. Oral epithelial cell reaction after exposure to Invisalign plastic material. Am J Orthod Dentofac Orthop 2014;145:64–71.

Schaefer I, Braumann B. Halitosis, oral health and quality of life during treatment with Invisalign and the effect of a low-dose chlorhexidine solution. J Orofac Orthop 2010;71:430–441.

Schott T, Gernot Goz. Korrektur eines Deckbisses mit einseitiger Prämolarenextraktion mittels Invisalign und Langzeitstabilität des Ergebnisses. Kieferorthopadie 2010; 24(4): 249-256

Schupp W, Haubrich J. Möglichkeiten und Grenzen der Invisalign-Behandlung. Quintessenz 2010; 61:951–962.

Schupp W, Haubrich J, Neumann I. Treatment of anterior open bite with the Invisalign system. J Clin Orthod 2010;44:501–507.

Schupp W, Haubrich J, Neumann I. Invisalign treatment of patients with craniomandibular disorders. Int Orthod 2010;8:253–267.

Schupp W, Haubrich J, Neumann I. Class II correction with the Invisalign system. J Clin Orthod 2010;44:28–35.

Schupp W, Haubrich J, Hermens E, Boisserée W. Diagnose und Therapie des kraniomandibulären und muskuloskelettalen Systems in der kieferorthopädischen Praxis unter besonderer Berücksichtigung des Invisalign-Systems. Inf Orthod Kieferorthop 2013;45:93–103.

Schupp W, Haubrich J, Hermens E. Möglichkeiten und Grenzen der Schienentherapie in der Kieferorthopädie. Zahnmed Up2date 2013;2:171–184.

Simon M, Keilig L, Schwarze J, Jung BA, Bourauel C. Forces and moments generated by removable thermoplastic aligners: incisor torque, premolar derotation, and molar distalization. Am J Orthod Dentofac Orthop 2014;145:728–736.

Tunkay O, Bowman, J, Amy B, Nicozisis J. Aligner Treatment in the Teenage Patient. JCO 2013;47:115-119

Wu D. Oral epithelial cell reaction and Invisalign treatment. Am J Orthod Dentofac Orthop 2014;145(5)551.

Yee JA, Kimmel DB, Jee WS. Periodontal ligament cell kinetics following orthodontic tooth movement. Cell Tissue Kinet 1976;9:293–302.

Quintessence Publishing Co. Ltd,
Grafton Road, New Malden, Surrey KT3 3AB,
United Kingdom
www.quintpub.co.uk

QUINTESSENCE PUBLISHING

Copyright © 2016, Quintessence Publishing Co. Ltd
All rights reserved. This book or any part thereof may not be reproduced, stored in a retrieval system, or transmitted in any form or by any means, electronic, mechanical, photocopying, or otherwise, without prior written permission of the publisher.

Editing: Quintessence Publishing Co. Ltd, London, UK
Layout and Production: Quintessenz Verlags-GmbH, Berlin, Germany
Printed and bound in Germany

ISBN: 978-1-85097-284-6